Introduction to Neuropsychopharmacology

D0882165

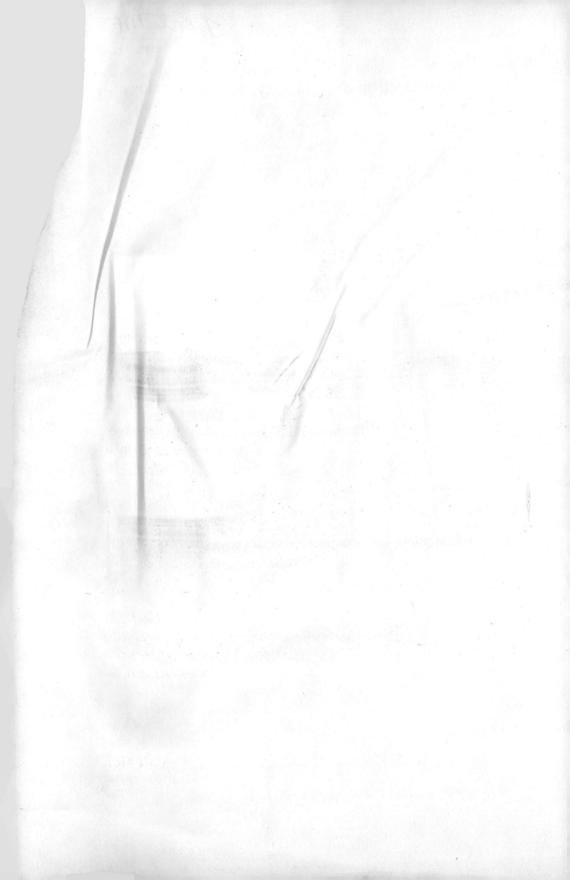

Introduction to Neuropsychopharmacology

Leslie L. Iversen, PhD, FRS
Professor of Pharmacology
University of Oxford
Oxford, UK

Susan D. Iversen, PhD
Professor of Experimental Psychology
University of Oxford
Oxford, UK

Floyd E. Bloom, MD
Emeritus Professor
Molecular and Integrative Neuroscience Department
The Scripps Research Institute
La Jolla, CA

Robert H. Roth, PhD
Professor of Pharmacology and Psychiatry
Yale University School of Medicine
New Haven, CT

OXFORD
UNIVERSITY PRESS
2009

OXFORD
UNIVERSITY PRESS

Oxford University Press, Inc., publishes works that further
Oxford University's objective of excellence
in research, scholarship, and education.

Oxford   New York
Auckland   Cape Town   Dar es Salaam   Hong Kong   Karachi
Kuala Lumpur   Madrid   Melbourne   Mexico City   Nairobi
New Delhi   Shanghai   Taipei   Toronto

With offices in
Argentina   Austria   Brazil   Chile   Czech Republic   France   Greece
Guatemala   Hungary   Italy   Japan Poland   Portugal   Singapore
South Korea   Switzerland   Thailand   Turkey   Ukraine   Vietnam

Copyright © 2009 by Oxford University Press, Inc.

Published by Oxford University Press, Inc.
198 Madison Avenue, New York, New York 10016
www.oup.com

Oxford is a registered trademark of Oxford University Press

Library of Congress Cataloging-in-Publication Data

Introduction to neuropsychopharmacology / Leslie L. Iversen . . . [et al.].
p. ; cm.
Includes bibliographical references and index.
ISBN: 978-0-19-538053-8
1. Neuropsychopharmacology. I. Iversen, Leslie L.
[DNLM: 1. Central Nervous System Agents—therapeutic use. 2. Drug
Design. 3. Mental Disorders—drug therapy. 4. Nervous System
Diseases—drug therapy. 5. Psychopharmacology. QV 76.5 I617 2009]
RM315.I589 2009
615'.78—dc22

                                        2008035833

The science of medicine is a rapidly changing field. As new research and clinical experience broaden our knowledge, changes in treatment and drug therapy occur. The author and publisher of this work have checked with sources believed to be reliable in their efforts to provide information that is accurate and complete, and in accordance with the standards accepted at the time of publication. However, in light of the possibility of human error or changes in the practice of medicine, neither the author, nor the publisher, nor any other party who has been involved in the preparation or publication of this work warrants that the information contained herein is in every respect accurate or complete. The opinion and suggestions herein are solely that of the author and not necessarily shared by the publisher. Readers are encouraged to confirm the information contained herein with other reliable sources, and are strongly advised to check the product information sheet provided by the pharmaceutical company for each drug they plan to administer.

9 8 7 6 5 4 3 2 1
Printed in the United States of America
on acid-free paper

To Our Families

Preface

When we put the Eighth Edition of the *Biochemical Basis of Neuropharmacology* down for a long winter's nap five years ago, we were definitely conflicted. The pressures of meeting deadlines, deciding what new information to include, and what of the old to exclude were definite downsides to a ninth edition. However, every time we heard from our student readers that the book had been their lure into the neurosciences, and into neuropharmacology in general, moments of regret flashed by. Furthermore, the look of astonishment when we told them that the eighth edition would be the last made us wonder whether we had reached the right decision.

After serious soul-searching, we think we have found a way to serve our loyal readers and not overly strain the authors by developing this new book – admittedly based heavily on the old "Cooper Bloom and Roth" – but relinquishing a lot of the academic minutiae we so enjoyed. Along with two co-conspirators expert in the new content, we agreed to take a new path. With so many new drugs based on so much new evidence, we focus now on the principles by which the effects of drugs on behaviors, as well as cells and circuits, are determined. By way of describing their theory and mechanisms, it is our intent to now make clear which of the drugs are actually being prescribed by clinicians for the benefit of their patients.

We aim this new book squarely at medical students, graduate students in the neurosciences and behavioral sciences, at House Officers and Fellows, and those in search of an introduction to one of the most exciting and heavily applied fields, the study of drugs that affect the cells and circuits of the brain, and the brain's behavioral, emotional, and cognitive operations. We offer you an *Introduction to Neuropsychopharmacology*.

We thank our Editor Craig Panner, who convinced us we could do this and meet his deadlines, Jamie Simon of The Salk Institute for the new artwork, Dr Jim Johnson of the University of Oxford for the new chemical structures, and Dan Hays for the excellent copy-editing.

Floyd Bloom, La Jolla, CA
Bob Roth, New Haven, CT
Les Iversen, Oxford, UK
Sue Iversen, Oxford, UK

Contents

Introduction to Neuropsychopharmacology

Introduction to Neuropsychopharmacology

Neuropsychopharmacology is the branch of neurosciences devoted to the study of drugs that affect nervous tissue and alter behaviors. Specifically, the study of the effects of drugs on neurons, their synapses, and circuits is *neuropharmacology* (see Chapter 2), while the study of the effects of drugs on behaviors, including emotional and cognitive mental activities, is *psychopharmacology* (see Chapter 3); thus, these comprise neuropsychopharmacology *in toto*. This text purposely constrains the coverage of such drugs to those that are currently employed by practicing physicians to treat diseases of the brain and nervous system, ranging from psychotropic drugs that affect mood and behavior to anesthetics, sedatives, hypnotics, narcotics, anticonvulsants, and analgesics, as well as a variety of drugs that affect the autonomic nervous system. Although the precise mechanisms of action of many such drugs remain to be determined, this coverage views their actions from the perspective of the chemical messengers that serve to communicate signals between neurons, namely the neurotransmitters. With those anchor points, we seek to explain the ways in which systems of interconnected neurons may be regulated by the drugs to change behaviors such as cognitive performance, emotions, and appetite and combat the addictive properties of abused drugs.

No single logical pathway exists to illustrate the process of modern drug development. Rather, the relationship between insights into the molecular operations of the nervous system and drugs that can alleviate the symptoms of neurological and psychiatric diseases often appears to be more a random exploitation of actions initially considered to be side effects, such as sedation. In part, this illogical developmental process arose because many of the pioneering medications that now appear to be transmitter specific were discovered long before the selective actions of the neurotransmitters on which the drugs work were known. Similarly, in attempts to compete commercially, many similarly targeted drugs with unique chemical structures often exposed novel therapeutic properties that could later be further exploited. In this context, we survey the pipeline of drugs currently in development and with the potential to be added to the clinical armamentarium in the realizable future.

The very existence of drugs having specific chemical structures that can control a given pathological condition of the brain and behavior is itself an exciting experimental finding since such a drug can also be a tool to clarify normal as well as abnormal brain chemistry and previously unknown neuronal physiology, such as the uptake, storage, and release of the specific neurotransmitters. Furthermore, recognition of the analogy between curare poisoning in animals and myasthenia gravis in humans led to the understanding of the cholinergic neuromuscular transmission problem in myasthenia gravis and to subsequent treatment with anticholinesterases. What is not understood in such simple terms is why in some cases, such as the treatments for depression or schizophrenia, the therapeutic actions require days to weeks of treatment even though the molecular action on the target process may well occur with maximal effectiveness in seconds. One inference made but not established has been that the drug and its intended biochemical reaction do not produce the therapeutic effect but require an adaptation by the brain to the presence of the drug effect to become beneficial. Thus, building better drugs could require understanding the nature of this unknown adaptation.

Lastly, a goal of this book is to guide students of neuropsychopharmacology in the appraisal of new data that will certainly emerge during their careers: Learn not to accept data without a critical appraisal of the procedures that were employed to obtain the results and the reinterpretations these new data would compel of the data previously available. Currently, discovery in the neurosciences pertinent to neuropsychopharmacology is occurring at a very rapid pace, revealing novel forms of signaling between neurons, novel forms of ion channels, and novel adaptive mechanisms beginning with genes whose expression is activated or suppressed by the emergence of disease or exposure to drugs. In this book, it is presumed that the reader has some prior understanding of neuroanatomy, neurochemistry, and neurophysiology. This book is therefore purposely titled *Introduction to Neuropsychopharmacology*. Let us begin.

SELECTED REFERENCES

Cooper, J. R., F. E. Bloom, and R. H. Roth (2003). *The Biochemical Basis of Neuropharmacology*, 8th ed. Oxford University Press, New York.

Nestler, E. J., S. E. Hyman, and R. C. Malenka (2001). *Molecular Neuropharmacology*. McGraw-Hill, New York.

Siegel, G. J., B. W. Agranoff, R. W. Albers, S. K. Fisher, and M. D. Uhler (1999). *Basic Neurochemistry*, 6th ed. Lippincott-Raven, Philadelphia.

Squire, L. R., D. Berg, F. E. Bloom, S. du Lac, A. Ghosh, and N. Spitzer, Eds. (2008). *Fundamental Neuroscience*, 3rd ed. Academic Press, New York.

Cellular and Molecular Foundations of Neuropsychopharmacology

As we begin to consider the particular problems that underlie the analysis of drug actions in the central nervous system, the curious student will ask "Just what is so special about nervous tissue?" Nerve cells have three special properties that distinguish them from all other cells in an individual. First, they are morphologically highly heterogeneous in size and shape. Second, neurons can conduct bioelectric signals for long distances in the body without any loss of signal strength. Third, they possess specific intercellular connections with other nerve cells and with innervated tissues such as muscles and glands. These connections determine the types of information a neuron can receive and the range of responses it can yield in return.

CYTOLOGY OF THE NERVE CELL

Neuroscientists have recognized the heterogeneous size and shape of neurons since the classic studies of the Spanish Nobel Prize-winning cytologist Santiago Ramón y Cajal. The shape of the nerve cell body (also called the *soma* and the *perikaryon*—literally, "the part that surrounds the nucleus") provides a simple classification of different kinds of neurons. Neurons, such as the sensory neurons of the dorsal root ganglion, have only one process—an axon that conducts signals from peripheral sensory receptors in skin to neurons in the dorsal part of the spinal cord. The sensory receptor nerve cells of the retina, the olfactory mucosa, and the auditory nerve are all bipolar neurons with an axon and a single dendrite that receives inputs from other local neurons, as are a class of small nerve cells of the brain known as granule cells.

All other nerve cells tend to fall into the class known as multipolar nerve cells. Their main differences relate to the size and complexity of the neuron's *dendritic tree*, whose branches may be long and smooth, short and complex, or bear short spines like a cactus. It is on these dendritic branches as well as on the cell body where the termination of axons from other neurons makes the specialized interneuronal communication point known as the synapse.

Regardless of their shape and size, neurons have very characteristic cytoplasmic organelles. Neuronal cytoplasm in the perikaryon and dendrites, but not in the axons, is rich in rough and smooth endoplasmic reticula, connoting an emphasis on their secretory activity. In all structural compartments, neurons are rich in mitochondria, connoting their dependence on high rates of adenosine triphosphate (ATP) generation. The axons and dendrites exhibit prominent microtubules to maintain their polarized shapes.

The Synapse

The characteristic specialized contact zone that has been presumptively identified as the site of functional interneuronal communication is the *synapse*. It contains special organelles. As the axon approaches the site of its termination, it exhibits structural features not found more proximally. Most striking is the occurrence of dilated regions of the axon (*varicosities*), within which are clustered large numbers of microvesicles (*synaptic vesicles*). Synaptic vesicles tend to be spherical in shape, with diameters varying between 400 and 1200 Å. Depending on the type of fixation used, the shape and staining properties of the vesicles can be related to their neurotransmitter content. One or more varicosities may form a specialized contact with one or more dendritic branches before the axon's ultimate termination. Such endings are known as *en passant* terminals. In this sense, the term *nerve terminal*, or *nerve ending*, connotes a functional transmitting site rather than the end of the axon, although some varicosities may not transmit (i.e., release their neurotransmitter) with every impulse.

Electron micrographs of synaptic regions in the central nervous system reveal a specialized contact zone between the axonal nerve ending and the postsynaptic structure (Fig. 2–1). One of the areas in which molecular biology has advanced the neurosciences has been the identification of many of the specific proteins that have precise functional properties in and on the surface of the synaptic vesicles and at sites along the inside of the presynaptic membrane

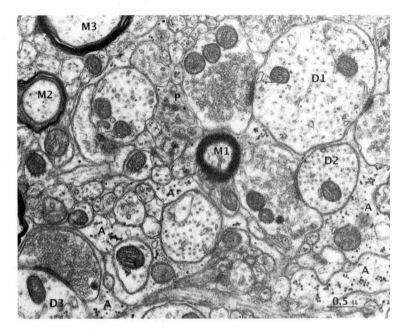

FIGURE 2–1. This electron micrograph illustrates the neuropil of the rat cerebral cortex containing the essential elements of axo-dendritic synapses, astrocytes, and myelinated axons. At the upper right, a dendritic shaft (D1) receives two synapses, one on the right side with modest post-synaptic membrane thickening (asymmetric) , and one on the left with no apparent membrane thickening (symmetric). Below it, another dendrite (D1) receives a symmetric synapse. All three axon terminals have mainly small, lucent synaptic vesicles, but that on D2 and D3, also show 1 large granular vesicle. Three myelinated axons are seen in cross section (M1, M2, and M3) with some oligodendrocyte cytoplasm seen beneath the myelin in M2. Astrocyte processes (A) containing very electron-dense glycogen granules surround the axons and dendrites. The scale bar at lower right equals 0.5 micra. (Bloom and Battenberg, unpublished).

associated with vesicle docking and release. Similarly, the direct chemical identification at discrete sites within the postsynaptic surface of the special-ized contacts of receptor proteins and other proteins capable of modifying the response to neurotransmitters has given near consensus to the functional infer-ence of a synaptic active zone. In some neurons, especially the single-process and small granule cell types, the dendrite may also be structurally specialized to store and release transmitter.

Glia

A second element in the maintenance of the neuron's integrity depends on a type of cell known as *neuroglia*. There are two main types of neuroglia, together termed *macroglia*.

The *fibrous astrocyte* is named for its starlike shape and abundant microtubules. Astrocytes are found mainly in gray matter—regions of axons and dendrites. They tend to surround and closely contact the outer surface of blood vessels, and they may serve to surround and separate functional units of nerve endings and dendrites. Astrocytes can accumulate glucose, synthesize glycogen, and provide two-carbon energy substrates to neurons, a functional linkage that is also activity dependent and regulated by extracellular cations as well as by at least some neurotransmitters. These findings have led to the suggestion that the regional localization of glucose uptake, as demonstrated in the human brain by positron emission tomography and in the brain of other species by 2-deoxyglucose autoradiography, reflects primarily the uptake of glucose by astrocytes and not by neurons.

Oligodendroglia are the second major type of neuroglia (also termed a *satellite cell* when it occurs close to nerve cell bodies and the *Schwann cell* when it occurs in the peripheral nervous system). Its most prominent characteristic is the formation of *myelin*—an enclosure of concentric layers of oligodendroglia surface membrane around the axon that come together so closely that the original internal surfaces of the membrane become fused, presenting the ringlike appearance of the myelin sheath in cross section. Along the course of an axon, which may be many centimeters, many oligodendrocytes are required to constitute its myelin sheath. At the boundary between adjacent portions of the axon covered by separate oligodendrocytes there is an uncovered axonal portion known as the node of Ranvier.

Many central axons and certain elements of the peripheral autonomic nervous system do not possess myelin sheaths. Even these axons, however, are not bare or exposed directly to the extracellular fluid; rather, they are enclosed within single invaginations of the astrocyte surface membrane. Because of this close relationship between the conducting portions of the nerve cell, its axon, and the astrocyte, it is easy to see the origin of the proposition that the astrocyte may contribute to the nurture of the nerve cell.

A third nonneuronal cell class in the brain, termed *microglia*, is of mesodermal origin and related to macrophages and monocytes. Some microglia reside within the brain, often around blood vessels. However, during events that cause tissue necrosis, such as stroke, trauma, or infection, macrophages enter the brain and secrete chemical signals to recruit lymphocytes and leukocytes to seal off and repair the tissue damage.

Brain Permeability Barriers

Chemical substances pass from the bloodstream into the brain at rates that are far slower than those for entry from the blood into all other organs in the body. These permeability barriers appear to be the result of numerous contributing diffusional obstacles based on their molecular size, charge, solubility, and specific carrier systems. The difficulty has not been in establishing the existence of these barriers but, rather, in determining their mechanisms. The endothelial cells of brain capillaries differ from those of other tissues in that the intercellular zones of membrane apposition are much more highly developed in the brain and virtually continuous along all surfaces of these cells. Furthermore, cerebral vascular endothelial cells lack pinocytotic vesicles, which are considered to be the transvascular carrier systems of both large and small molecules in other tissues. Possibly, these features of cerebral endothelial cells constitute the blood–brain barrier. The functional barrier also underlies the restricted access into the brain for highly charged lipophobic small molecules such as the neurotransmitters norepinephrine and serotonin, their amino acid precursors, or drugs that affect the metabolism of these and other neurotransmitters. However, charged molecules can diffuse widely through the extracellular spaces of the brain when permitted entry via the cerebrospinal fluid.

Substances that have difficulty entering the brain, in general, also have difficulty leaving it. Thus, when monoamines are increased in concentration by blocking their catabolism (see Chapter 7), high levels of amine persist until the inhibiting agents are metabolized or excreted. One such excretory route is the acid-transport system, by which the *choroid plexus* cells actively secrete acid catabolites into the cerebrospinal fluid, as well as drugs such as penicillin or zidovudine, which one might like to keep in. This excretory step can be blocked by the drug probenecid, resulting in increased brain and cerebrospinal fluid amine catabolite and drug levels. Specialized sets of neurons known as the *circumventricular organs* exist within discrete sites along the linings of the cerebroventricles that are functionally on the blood side of the blood–brain barrier. Considered to be "windows" through which the normally excluded central milieu can monitor the components of the bloodstream, these neurons can communicate directly with neurons well within the enclosure of the blood–brain barrier.

BIOELECTRIC PROPERTIES OF THE NERVE CELL

Given these structural details, we can now turn to the second striking feature of nerve cells, namely their bioelectric properties. The basic concepts of the physical phenomena of bioelectricity hold that a difference in electrical potential exists within a charged field when ions and other charged particles are separated by lipid membranes and prevented from randomly redistributing themselves because the membranes provide a resistance to current flow. If the resistance tends to 0, no net current will flow since no potential difference can exist in the absence of a measurable resistance. If the resistance is extremely high, only a minimal current will flow; this will be proportional to the electromotive force or potential difference (or voltage) between the two sites. The relationship between voltage, current, and resistance is Ohm's law: $V = I \times R$.

When we measure the electrical properties of living cells, these basic physical laws apply with one exception. The pioneer electrobiologists, who did their work before the discovery and definition of the electron, developed a convention for the flow of charges based not on the electrons but on the flow of positive charges. Therefore, since in biological systems the flow of charges is not carried by electrons but by ions, the direction of flow is expressed in terms of the movement of positive charges. To analyze the electrical potentials of a living system, we use small electrodes (a microprobe for detecting current flow or potential), electronic amplifiers for increasing the size of the current or potential, and oscilloscopes or polygraphs for displaying the potentials observed against a time base.

Membrane Potentials

If we take two electrodes and place them on the outside of a living cell or tissue, we will find little, if any, difference in potential. However, if we puncture a neuron with an ultrafine electrode across the otherwise intact membrane, we will measure a potential difference with the inside of the neuron 50 mV or more negative with respect to the extracellular electrode (Fig. 2–2). This transmembrane potential difference is found in almost all living cells and indicates that cells are *electrically polarized*. If positive current is applied to the inside of the cell, the transmembrane potential difference is decreased and the neuron becomes *depolarized*. Conversely, passing negative ions into the cell through the microelectrode makes the neuron more negative (*hyperpolarized*). The potential difference across the membrane of most living cells can be accounted for by the relative distribution of the intracellular and extracellular ions: Extracellular fluid is particularly rich in sodium (Na) and relatively low in potassium (K), whereas intracellular cytoplasm is relatively high in K content and very low in Na. While the membrane of the neuron permits K ions (K^+) to flow back and forth with relative freedom, it resists the movement of Na ions (Na^+) from the extracellular fluid to the inside of the cell. Since K^+ can cross the membrane, they tend to flow along the concentration gradient, which is highest inside the cell. K^+ diffusion out of the cell leaves a relative negative charge behind due to the negative charges of the macromolecular proteins. As the negative charge inside the cell begins to build, the further diffusion of K^+ from inside to outside is retarded. Eventually, an equilibrium point will be reached that is proportional to certain physical constants and to the relative concentrations of intracellular and extracellular K^+ and chloride (Cl^-) ions.

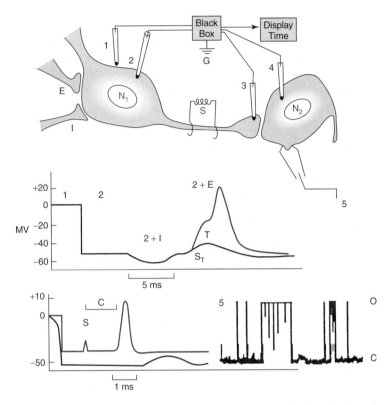

FIGURE 2–2. At the top is shown a hypothetical neuron (N_1) receiving a single excitatory pathway (E) and a single inhibitory pathway (I). A stimulating electrode (S) has been placed on the nerve cell's axon; microelectrode 1 is extracellular to nerve cell 1, whereas microelectrode 2 is in the cell body and microelectrode 3 is in its nerve terminal. Microelectrode 4 records from within postsynaptic cell 2. The potentials and current, recorded by each of these electrodes, are compared through a "black box" of electronics with a distant extracellular grounded electrode and displayed on an oscilloscope screen. When the cell is resting and the electrode is on the outside of the cell, no potential difference is observed (1). In the resting state, electrode 2 records a steady potential difference between inside and outside of approximately −50 mV (2). While recording from electrode 2 and stimulating the inhibitory pathway, the membrane potential is hyperpolarized during the inhibitory postsynaptic potential (2 + I). When recording from electrode 2 and stimulating the excitatory pathway, a subthreshold stimulus (S_T) produces an excitatory postsynaptic potential indicated by a brief depolarization of the resting membrane potential (2 + E). When the excitatory effects are sufficient to reach threshold (T), an action potential is generated that reverses the inside negativity to inside positivity (2 + E). On the lower scale, potentials recorded by electrodes 3 (blue line) and 4 (black line) are compared on the same time base following axonal stimulation of nerve cell 1, which is assumed to be excitatory. The point of stimulus is seen as an electrical artifact at point S. The action potential generated at the nerve terminal occurs after a finite lag period due to the conduction time (C) of the axon between the stimulating electrode and the nerve terminal. The action potential in the nerve ending does not directly influence postsynaptic cell 2 until after the transmitter has been liberated and can react with nerve cell 2's membrane, causing the excitatory postsynaptic

These concepts of ionic diffusion potentials across semipermeable membranes apply generally not only to nerve and muscle but also to blood, glandular, and other cells large enough to have their transmembrane potential measured.

Membrane Ion Pumps

Membrane potential bears a linear relationship to the external K^+ concentration at normal to high K^+ concentrations but deviates from this linear relationship when the external K^+ concentration is less than normal. Although the plasma membranes of nerve and muscle cells and other types of polarized cells are relatively impermeable to the flow of Na ions along the high concentration gradient from extracellular to intracellular, they are not completely impermeable. Enough Na enters to double the intracellular Na concentration in approximately 1 hour if there is not an opposing process to maintain the relatively low intracellular Na concentration. The process that continuously maintains the low intracellular Na concentration is known as *active Na transport* or, colloquially, the *sodium pump*. This pump mechanism ejects Na from the inside of the cell against the high extracellular concentration and electrical gradients forcing it in. However, the pump does not handle Na exclusively but requires the presence of extracellular K^+. Thus, when an Na ion is ejected from the cell, a K ion is incorporated into the cell, giving the mechanism yet another apt name, the Na–K ATPase exchanger. Thus, two factors operate to drive K^+ into the cell in the presence of relatively low external K^+ concentration: (1) the electrical gradient across the membrane and (2) the Na–K pump mechanism. The pump is immediately dependent on metabolic energy and can be blocked by several metabolic poisons, such as dinitrophenol and the rapid-acting cardiac glycoside ouabain. Astrocytes also have such pumps.

The Uniqueness of Nerves

All that we have said regarding the transmembrane ionic distributions applies equally to the red blood cell or glia as it does to the neuron. Thus, possession of a transmembrane potential difference is not sufficient to account for the neuron's

---

potential. The time between the beginning of the action potential recorded by microelectrode 3 and the excitatory postsynaptic potential recorded by electrode 4 is the time required for excitation secretion coupling in the nerve terminal and the liberation of sufficient transmitter to produce effects on nerve cell 2. Electrode 5 is a patch clamp electrode attached to neuron 2; it indicates the effects of transmitters acting through receptors located elsewhere on the neuron's surface, mediating channel opening (O) and closing (C) events through intracellular second messengers.

bioelectric properties. However, applying depolarizing currents across the membrane reveals the essential difference between neurons and other cells. When a nerve cell membrane is depolarized from a resting value of approximately −70 mV to approximately −10 to −15 mV, an explosive self-limiting process occurs, namely the action potential. In the *action potential*, the transmembrane potential is reduced (depolarized) not merely to 0 but beyond 0 so that the inside of the membrane now becomes transiently positive with respect to the outside, up to 10 to 30 mV in the positive direction. Because of this explosive response to an electrical depolarization, the nerve membrane is said to be "electrically excitable," and the resultant voltage polarity shift is the action potential. Although astrocytes can also show variable membrane potentials, they do not exhibit this degree of excitability.

Once the axon has been sufficiently depolarized to reach threshold for an action potential, the wave of activity travels at a rate proportional to the diameter of the axons (through which the bioelectric currents will flow). In large axons, the rate is further accelerated by the insulation provided by myelin sheaths, restricting the flow of transmembrane currents to the opening at the nodes of Ranvier. This *saltatory* conduction is consequently much more rapid. The threshold level for an all-or-none action potential is also inversely proportional to the diameter of the axon: Large myelinated axons respond to low values of imposed stimulating current, whereas fine and unmyelinated axons require much greater depolarizing currents. Local anesthetics block activation of Na⁺ conductance, preventing depolarization.

Once the threshold has been reached, a complete action potential will not develop if it occurs too soon after the preceding action potential, an interval termed the *refractory phase* attributable to the finite activation cycle of the process that increases Na⁺ conductance. K⁺ conductance increases with the action potential and lasts slightly longer than the activation of Na⁺ conductance, resulting in a prolonged phase of after-hyperpolarization.

Ion Channels

The discovery that drugs can selectively block cation movement and that Na⁺ permeability (blocked by tetrodotoxin) can be separated from K⁺ permeability (blocked by tetraethylammonium [TEA]) made more detailed analysis of ion movement mechanisms feasible. Membrane physiologists now agree that there are several ion-specific pathways that form separate and independent "channels" for passive movement of Na⁺, K⁺, Ca²⁺, and Cl⁻. Due to several spectacular advances in the molecular biology of ion channels, it is becoming clear that these conductance mechanisms are actually quite complex arrays of interacting proteins. In some cases, the channel proteins open and close in an all-or-nothing fashion on timescales of 0.1 to 10 milliseconds to provide

aqueous channels through the plasma membrane that ions car
precisely, channel macromolecules can exist in several inter
formations, only one of which permits ion movement. Th
shifts from one form to another are sensitive to the bioelectrı ˍ
on the membrane; by facilitating or retarding the conformational shıˍ.
ion channels are "gated." In this concept, Ca^{2+} acts at the membrane surface to
alter permeability only by virtue of the effect its charge has on the electric
fields of otherwise fixed (mainly negative) organic charges. The altered fields
in turn can gate the channels because a part of the channel protein is able to
sense the field and, thus, modulate the conformational shifts that open or close
the gate. When ions flow across the membrane, the ionic current changes the
membrane potential and other membrane properties.

Four types of ion channel are recognized: (1) nongated, passive ion channels, previously referred to as "leakage channels," which are continuously
open; (2) voltage-gated (i.e., voltage-sensitive) channels, in which channel
opening and closing is affected by the membrane potential inside of the cell;
(3) chemically gated channels, the opening and closing of which is affected by
receptors on the external plasma membrane, such as those affected by drugs
and other transmitters; and (4) ion-gated channels, whose opening and closing
is affected by shifts in intracellular ion concentrations. Ion-gated channels are
often also sensitive to membrane potential and to external regulatory receptors, and chemically gated channels are often also voltage sensitive. These
various modes of interaction provide an extremely rich spectrum of responses,
thus greatly complicating what were once simple rules of excitability and ion
conductance regulation. Additional forms of more complex ion flow regulation provide the means by which neurons communicate to their target cells
through junctional transmission.

Junctional Transmission

At the nerve ending, the membrane of the axon is separated from the membrane of the postjunctional nerve cell (dendrite or soma), muscle, or gland by
an intercellular space of 50 to 200 Å (Fig. 2–1). With the advent of microelectrode techniques for recording the transmembrane potential of nerve cells
in vivo, it became possible to determine the effects of stimulation of nerve pathways that had previously been shown to cause either excitation or inhibition of
synaptic transmission. From such studies, Eccles (1964) observed that subthreshold excitatory stimuli would produce postsynaptic potentials with time
durations of 2 to 20 milliseconds. The excitatory postsynaptic potentials alge-
braically accumulate with other contemporaneous excitatory and inhibitory
postsynaptic potentials. Most important, the duration of these postsynaptic
potentials is longer than can be accounted for on the basis of electrical activity

in the preterminal axon or on the electronic conductive properties of the post-synaptic membrane (Fig. 2–2). This latter observation, combined with the fact that synaptic sites are not directly electrically excitable, provides conclusive evidence that central synaptic transmission must be chemical: The prolonged time course is only compatible with a rapidly released chemical transmitter whose time course of action is terminated by local enzymes, diffusion, and reuptake by the nerve ending.

When an ideal excitatory pathway is stimulated, the presynaptic element releases an excitatory transmitter, which activates ionic conductances of the postsynaptic membrane, depolarizing the membrane toward the Na^+ equilibrium potential. If the depolarization reaches the threshold for activating adjacent voltage-dependent conductances, an all-or-none action potential (spike) will be triggered. The postsynaptic potential resulting from the stimulation of an ideal inhibitory pathway selectively activates channels for Cl^- or K^+, resulting in diffusion of ions and hyperpolarization of the membrane. This counterbalances the excitatory postsynaptic potentials. Experimentally, it is possible to poise the neuronal membrane potential at or near the so-called equilibrium potentials for each of the ionic species and to determine the ionic species whose equilibrium potential corresponds to the conductance change caused by the synaptic transmitter. This is the most molecular test for the identification of synaptic transmitter substance actions.

Whereas classically acting neurotransmitters produce their effects on receptor-coupled ion conductances that are voltage independent, many other transmitters operate on receptors coupled to voltage-sensitive mechanisms. Transmitters whose receptors are associated with intracellular second messenger systems (e.g., activation of cyclic nucleotide synthesis) frequently produce these more complex forms of interaction (see Chapter 4). Similarly, many neuropeptides appear to affect certain of their target cells by modifying responses to other transmitters while not showing any direct shifts in membrane potential or conductance when tested for actions on their own (see Chapter 10). For example, the β-adrenergic actions of locus ceruleus neurons on their central targets produce excitability changes that depend on which other afferent systems are activated synchronously (see Conditional Actions of Transmitters).

This simplified ideal version of ionic mechanisms may be only one of many regulatory mechanisms between connected cells. The most numerous central nervous system neurons, the small bipolar-process type of granule-like cell, may conduct its neuronal business within its restricted small spatial domain with no need to ever fire an action potential. Those neurons that do fire action potentials may sometimes do so unconventionally, using an influx of Ca^{2+} ions (voltage-sensitive Ca conductance) rather than Na^+. This Ca^{2+} spike may represent a mechanism to transmit activity from the cell body out to the dendritic system. The student is advised to maintain an appreciative awareness of these potentially complex interaction systems. Given the onslaught of molecular biological characterizations for ion channels, it is important for the student to recognize that within a specific functional category of ion conductance (i.e., Na^+, K^+, Ca^{2+}), there are subtypes of functional responses that are ligand specific and that may be carried out by more than one ion channel protein (ionophore) complex. These precisely defined channel proteins can now be examined in intimate molecular detail to dissect how drugs, toxins, and imposed voltages can alter the excitability of a neuron.

Calcium Channels

Among the multiple voltage-sensitive Ca^{2+} conductances described in neurons, three are most consistent. The first is a transient, low-threshold Ca^{2+} conductance (termed *T*). This Ca^{2+} conductance is inactive at resting membrane potentials but is "deinactivated" by modest hyperpolarizations, providing an oscillatory behavior. It is most frequently inhibited by Cd^{2+} or Co^{2+} and, in some cases, by Ni, Mg, or Mn as well; it can be activated by Ba^{2+}. The second Ca^{2+} conductance channel is a slowly inactivating, high-threshold Ca^{2+} conductance (termed *L*) and is seen mainly in nerve terminals. The third Ca^{2+} conductance channel is a transient, high-threshold Ca conductance (termed *N*) observed in the soma and dendrites of large neurons in the neocortex, olfactory cortex, and hippocampal formation. The latter are blocked by Mn^{2+}, Co^{2+}, and Cd^{2+} and activated by Ba^{2+} and TEA; these responses may be inhibited functionally by endogenous purinergic receptors (see Chapter 11). The N-type Ca^{2+} channels have also been well studied in sympathetic neurons, where they are regulated through three separate transductive pathways, each of which may be engaged by different neurotransmitters and their specific intracellular mechanisms (see Chapter 4).

Potassium Channels

At least three types of K channel have been described in central neurons: (1) the "A" or "A-like" fast, transient K conductances inhibited by 4-aminopyridine, Ba^{2+}, or Co^{2+}; (2) the so-called anomalous rectifying K conductances, of which the M current (closed by cholinergic muscarinic receptors) is one example; (3) the Ca-activated K conductances, blocked by Co, Mn, Cd, and some neurotransmitters (see Aston-Jones and Siggins, 1994, and Hille, 1992). Although most data on these K^+ channel effects are pharmacological, the properties can clearly regulate cell firing and response patterns in distinct manners. By closing the M current, muscarinic receptors transduce cholinergic signals into more effective depolarization, once partial depolarization brings this channel into play. Somatostatin can oppose this effect, forcing the M channel to open. The latter effect may be mediated intracellularly by second messengers derived from arachidonic acid metabolism (see Chapter 4).

By blocking the Ca-activated K channel of central neurons, the transmitter receptors for β-adrenergic agonists, 5-hydroxytryptamine, histamine, and corticotropin-releasing hormone enhance the ability of responsive neurons to follow long depolarizing pulses, thereby generating longer trains of action potentials per afferent impulse.

Depending on the specific cells in which they were recognized (even Ca-activated K channels exist in many glands and completely nonneural cell types) and the conditions and possible inhibitors that may have been evaluated, as many as 12 different K conductances have been proposed. For example, many K channels are linked to second messenger mediation (e.g., the channels activated by GABA$_B$ receptors [see Chapter 5] and by D$_2$ dopamine receptors on rat substantia nigra neurons [see Chapter 7]).

Slow Postsynaptic Potentials

Most of the postsynaptic potentials described by Eccles (1964) were relatively short, usually 20 milliseconds or less, and appeared to result from passive changes in ionic conductance. Postsynaptic potentials of slow onset and several seconds' duration have been described (Fig. 2–2), both of a hyperpolarizing nature and of a depolarizing nature. Many of these slow synaptic potentials are not accompanied by the expected increase in transmembrane ionic conductances but, rather, by increased transmembrane impedance. Although multiple hypothetical explanations have been offered for such responses, the actual molecular mechanisms remain obscure. The phosphorylation of a membrane-mounted ion channel protein after neuotransmitter signals are transduced into an intracellular second messenger would be expected to alter its ionic permeability, and perhaps such changes lie at the root of the membrane effects of several types of neurotransmitter.

Conditional Actions of Transmitters

Not all neurotransmitter actions comply with the classically conceived transmitter profile and may benefit from broader conceptualizations of transmitter actions. For example, when the β-adrenergic effects of locus ceruleus stimulation are examined, target cell responses no longer adhere to standard concepts of inhibition. Rather, they appear to fit better the designation of "biasing" or "enabling." The latter indicates that the enabling transmitter (in this example, norepinephrine) can enhance or amplify the effectiveness of other transmitter actions converging on the common target neurons during the time period of the enabling circuit's activity (see Chapter 7). These β-adrenergic actions can enhance either excitatory or inhibitory afferents, a general effect referred to as *enabling* or, more ambiguously, *modulatory*. Some pharmacological actions of neuropeptides have been described as having the opposite effect, or *disen-abling* (e.g., the effects of opioid peptides on the excitatory actions of sensory transmitters within the spinal cord) (see Chapter 10). This story is more complex (surprised?) because neuropeptides coexist with amino acid and amine transmitters.

Considering the issue of neurotransmitter time course suggests some principal physiological characteristics of conditional and unconditional actions. *Unconditional actions* are those that a given transmitter evokes by itself (i.e., in the absence of other transmitters acting on the common target cell). *Conditional actions*, occurring either pre- or postsynaptically, include, but are not limited to, the type of enhancement that is subsumed by enabling. In such a conditional interaction, each transmitter would act at its own pre- or postsynaptic transmitter receptor and interact on that target cell when both transmitters occupy their receptors simultaneously. Clearly, neurons have a broad but finite and as yet incompletely characterized repertoire of molecular responses that messenger molecules (transmitters, hormones, and drugs) can elicit. The power of the chemical vocabulary of such components is their combinatorial capacity to act conditionally and coordinately and to integrate the temporal and spatial domains within the nervous system.

Transmitter Release

Secretion of synaptic transmitters is the activity-locked expression of neuronal activity induced by depolarization of the nerve terminal. Evidence strongly favors the view that a voltage-sensitive Ca^{2+} conductance is required for transmitter secretion. Biochemical, ultrastructural, and physiological experiments have led to the concept that transmitter molecules are stored within vesicles in the nerve terminal and that the Ca-dependent excitation–secretion coupling within the depolarized nerve terminal requires the transient exchange of vesicular contents into the synaptic cleft. It is unclear whether the vesicle simply undergoes rapid fusion with the presynaptic specialized membrane to allow the transmitter stored in the vesicle to diffuse out or whether the process of exocytotic release simultaneously requires insertion of the vesicle membrane into the synaptic plasma membrane, reappearing later by the reverse process, namely endocytosis. Information on the lipid and protein components of the two types of membrane once suggested that long-term fusion–endocytosis cycles were unlikely, but recent data are compatible with either fusion release or contact release. Unfortunately, neurochemically homogeneous vesicles from central synapses have never been completely purified; therefore, all such analyses remain somewhat open to interpretation.

In some cases, release of the transmitter can be modulated "presynaptically" by the neuron's own transmitter (autoreceptors). Autoreceptors are conceived to be receptors that are generally distributed over the surface of a neuron and are sensitive to the transmitter secreted by that neuron. In the case of the central dopamine-secreting neurons, such receptors have been related to the release of the transmitter and to its synthesis. Such effects seem to be achieved through receptor mechanisms different from those by which the same transmitter molecule acts postsynaptically. Presynaptic release may also be modified (by receptors other than autoreceptors) by coreleased neuropeptides or by the effects of transmitters released by other neurons in the vicinity of the terminal or the cell body.

APPROACHES TO DRUG ACTION ANALYSIS

If, as modern-day neuropsychopharmacologists, we are chiefly concerned with uncovering the mechanisms of action of drugs in the brain, there are several avenues along which we can organize our attack. We could choose to examine the way in which drugs influence the perception of sensory signals by higher integrative centers of the brain. This is compatible with a single-neuron and ionic conductance types of analysis, directed, for example, at how drugs affect inhibitory postsynaptic potentials. Drugs that cause convulsions, such as strychnine, have been analyzed in this respect; but all types of inhibitory postsynaptic potential are not affected by strychnine.

A second basic approach would be to use both macroelectrodes and microelectrodes to compare the drug responses of single units and populations of units in the same brain region. This approach is clearly limited, however, unless we understand the intimate functional relations between the multiple types of cells found even within one region of the brain.

A third approach is also possible. We could choose to separate the effects of drugs between those affecting the generation of action potential and its propagation and those acting on junctional transmission. For this type of analysis, we must identify the chemical synaptic transmitter for the junctions to be studied. Many of the interpretative problems already alluded to can be attacked through this approach. Thus, as might be expected, there is likely to be more than one type of excitatory and inhibitory transmitter substance, and a convulsant drug may affect the response to one type of inhibitory transmitter without affecting another. Moreover, a drug may have specific regional effects in the brain if it affects a unique synaptic transmitter there. In fact, using this approach, it may be possible to find drug effects not directly reflected in electrical activity but related more to the catabolic or anabolic systems maintaining the required functional levels of transmitter. We conclude this chapter by considering the techniques for identifying the synaptic transmitter for particular synaptic connections. The chapters that follow are organized to present in detail our current understanding of putative central neurotransmitter substances and the therapeutic application of agonists, antagonists, or modifiers of transmitter in neurological and psychiatric diseases.

IDENTIFICATION OF SYNAPTIC TRANSMITTERS

How then do we identify the substance released by nerve endings? The entire concept of chemical junctional transmission arose from the classic experiments of Otto Loewi, who demonstrated chemical transmission by transferring the ventricular fluid of a stimulated frog heart onto a nonstimulated frog heart, thereby showing that the effects of the nerve stimulus on the first heart were reproduced by the chemical activity of the solution flowing onto the second heart. Since the phenomenon of chemical transmission originated from studies of peripheral autonomic organs, these peripheral junctions have become convenient model systems for central neuropharmacological analysis.

Certain interdependent criteria have been developed to identify junctional transmitters. In the central nervous system, however, satisfaction of these criteria presumes (1) that the proper nerve trunk or set of nerve axons can be selectively stimulated and (2) that release of the transmitter can be detected in the amounts released by single nerve endings after one action potential. This last subcriterion would be necessary if we wish to restrict our analysis to the first set of activated nerve endings and not to examine the substances released by the secondary and tertiary interneurons in the chain, some of which might reside quite close to the primary endings. For many years, satisfaction of the local release criterion was almost impossible because collection devices were so large as to injure the brain and detection methods were insufficiently sensitive. However, newer technologies, such as *in vivo* microdialysis, tissue voltammetry, and antibody-coated carbon filaments, have been applied to detect release effectively.

Localization

Because it is difficult, if not impossible, to identify the substance released from single nerve endings by selective stimulation, the next best evidence would be to prove that a suspected synaptic transmitter resides in the presynaptic terminal of our selected nerve pathway. Normally, we would expect the enzymes for synthesizing and catabolizing this substance to also be in the vicinity of this nerve ending, if not actually part of the nerve ending's cellular machinery. To document the presence of neurotransmitter, several types of specific cytochemical methods for microscopy have been developed. More commonly employed is the biochemical population approach, which analyzes the regional concentrations of suspected synaptic transmitter substances. However, presence per se indicates neither releasability nor neuroeffectiveness. Although it has generally been considered that a neuron makes only one transmitter and secretes that same substance everywhere that synaptic release occurs, neuropeptide exceptions to this rule have become common (see Chapter 10).

Synaptic Mimicry: Drug Injections

A third criterion arising from peripheral autonomic nervous system analysis is that the suspected exogenous substance mimics the action of the transmitter released by nerve stimulation. The student will now realize how important it is to have methods of drug administration equal in sophistication to those with which the electrical phenomena are detected. The most practical micromethod of drug administration yet devised is based on the principle of electrophoresis. Micropipettes are constructed in which one or several barrels contain an ionized solution of the chemical substance under investigation. The substance is applied by appropriately directing the current flow. The microelectrophoretic technique, when applied with controls to rule out the effects of pH, electrical current, and diffusion of the drug to neighboring neurons, has overcome the major limitations of classic neuropharmacological techniques. An alternative especially effective for testing poorly ionized molecules, such as neuropeptides, is to fill the delivery capillary with lower concentrations and then to "puff" very small volumes onto the test neuron by air pressure. When tested on single neurons in brain slice preparations, the methods of patch clamp electrodes can be employed to test tiny areas of responsive neuronal surfaces. This is only one of the reasons why *ex vivo* brain slice methods and short-term tissue culture preparations, analyzed with voltage clamping and patch clamping, have gained in popularity.

Pharmacology of Synaptic Effects

The fourth criterion for identifying a synaptic transmitter requires identical pharmacological effects of drugs potentiating or blocking postsynaptic responses to both the neurally released and the administered samples. Because the pharmacological effects are often not identical (most "classic" blocking agents are extrapolated to the brain from effects on peripheral autonomic organs), this fourth criterion is often satisfied indirectly with a series of circumstantial pieces of data. With the advent of drugs that block the synthesis of specific transmitter agents, or genetic methods to inactivate the genes encoding transmitter receptors, the pharmacology for certain families of transmitters has been improved.

MOLECULAR FOUNDATIONS OF NEUROPSYCHOPHARMACOLOGY

Complete understanding of the basis for a drug's actions on the brain requires knowledge of all the molecules involved. However, until approximately the past decade, most of the molecules involved in drug actions on the nervous system were recognized by their actions rather than their precise molecular structures or cellular compartmentalization. Due to advances in molecular biology, a growing number of these critical molecules can be specified in highly accurate terms to the level of their atomic structure. Nevertheless, as neuropharmacologists, the terms of reference remain very much the same. A drug is said to act *selectively* when it elicits responses from discrete populations of cells that possess "drug-recognizing" macromolecules, or receptors. Most drug receptors involve sites where neurotransmitters act. Some resemble, at the molecular level, specific molecular features of a neurotransmitter. However, drugs may also act by regulating intracellular enzymes critical for normal transmitter synthesis or breakdown or removal from the extracellular spaces of the brain. Receptors recognize drugs for a variety of reasons, which will be explored in subsequent chapters. Once having made that recognition, the activated receptor usually interacts with other molecules to alter membrane properties or intracellular metabolism. These cellular changes in turn regulate the interactions between cells in circuits. These circuit changes regulate the performance of functional systems (e.g., the sensory, motor, or vegetative control systems) and eventually the behavior of the whole organism.

Thus, understanding the actions of drugs on the function of the brain, whether it be in terms of single cells or behavior, is a multilevel, multifaceted process that begins with and builds on the concept of molecular interactions. Even beginning students of drug action on the nervous system will probably accept this statement as a reasonable hypothetical principle. In practice, however, this principle is severely compromised because most of the molecules in a very complex organ such as the brain remain unknown.

When Watson and Crick deduced the three-dimensional, double-helical structure of DNA in 1953, the implications for the coding and replication of genetic information were recognized but could not be experimentally tested. Almost 25 years of effort were required before the new biological technology was launched. During this interval, it became clear how to combine genes and gene fragments from multicellular organisms with those of viruses, fungi, and bacteria to produce new genetic instructions and novel gene products. At last, the concept of a *gene* and its cellular *product* attained concrete form. Almost immediately, neuroscientists, who are always ready to exploit new technologies, began to apply these methods to the brain.

The power of molecular biological methods is realized from several related but independent developments: (1) the ability to clone genetic information (i.e., to isolate a selected segment and accurately reproduce it in large amounts), (2) the ability to determine the nucleic acid sequence of the selected gene segment (i.e., to read the complete molecular structure of a gene), and (3) the ability to practice genetic engineering (i.e., to perturb and control gene expression and to alter the structure of gene products by chemically modifying precise sites in the molecular structure of the genes). Within a decade, the possibilities for applying this basic triad of powerful tools were dramatically revealed by two additional innovative technologies: the *polymerase chain reaction* (PCR; by which large amounts of specific nucleic acid sequences can be produced without prior purification, cloning, or even a complete knowledge of their sequences) and the ability to create *transgenic animals* (i.e., to transfer synthetic genes into embryonic cells to make new mice, pigs, and cows to the experimentalist's specifications). Second-generation refinements of the latter two technologies have allowed PCR to serve as a means to find novel gene products within a family of genes in which some segments have been conserved (e.g., the transmembrane domains of certain receptors and transporters). The transgenic strategy can now reproducibly provide mice that are good disease models, either by creating mice lacking a specific gene (*knockout mutations*) presumed to be essential for one or another transductive pathway or by extending the original application of transgenic mice to overexpress selected genes, such as the mutated forms identified in human monogenic diseases such as Huntington's disease (see Chapter 14). All of these developments have contributed to a very rapid advance toward a truly molecular basis for the understanding of the nervous system and the way it can be altered by drug actions.

MOLECULAR STRATEGIES IN NEUROPHARMACOLOGY

The immediate applications of molecular biological strategies within neuropharmacology are shortcuts in molecular isolation and sequence determination—for instance, to uncover new peptides or proteins or to provide more complete understanding of enzymes, receptors, channels, or other integral proteins of the cell. A likely premise holds that the phenotype of a cell within the nervous system depends on the structural, metabolic, and regulatory proteins by which it establishes its recognizable structural and functional properties. If this is valid, then complex, multifaceted neurons will probably rely on hundreds, if not thousands, of special-purpose proteins, many of which may exist in limited amounts. Purifying such rare proteins by the methods that existed before molecular cloning, especially in the absence of a functional assay to guide the purification process, is an overwhelming task requiring exceptional patience, resources, and a very large supply of the proper starting tissue material. For some of the very rare hypothalamic hypophysiotropic releasing factors (see Chapter 10), hundreds of thousands of hypothalami were required as well as the development of unique purification schemes for each subsequent factor to be pursued.

Converting the quest for the structure of specific proteins into a molecular biological quest for the mRNA or gene segment that encodes this protein greatly facilitates the experimental analysis simply because of the powers of cloning, complementarity, and rapid sequencing. Several methods have been developed that increase the chances of finding whatever the researcher is seeking. These methods depend in part on the nature of the cDNA being pursued and how the investigator probes either for the insert or for the translation of the fusion gene product in a cell system capable of processing the primary translation product into a structural form that will resemble its natural configuration and sometimes even its natural function. Given the possibility of protein–protein interactions, synthetic genes can be translated into tools to detect unknown proteins with affinity for the newly discovered gene product, a strategy exploited shamelessly in the isolation of the vesicle proteins needed for transmitter secretion.

In addition to their capacity to accelerate the discovery of new molecules participating in the nervous system's response to disease or to self-administered drugs, molecular biological strategies can be used to determine how critical a particular gene product may be in mediating a cellular event with behavioral importance—for example, the role of a specific transmitter's receptor subtype in a cellular event (e.g., long-term potentiation), which may in turn underlie behavioral phenomena such as memory formation or recall (see Chapter 3). These functional probes can be achieved through advanced methods for transgenic animal construction in which specific mutations are engineered into any targeted gene of an experimental animal's genome, leading eventually to the production of homozygous animals lacking either that gene completely or the capacity to turn it on and off as experimentally desired.

Less demanding and less vulnerable to potential confounding roles of the targeted gene in the developing nervous system are more short-term manipulations, such as the intracerebral or intraventricular injection of special nucleotide constructs to deliver *ribozymes* (RNA constructions that can target and degrade specific mRNAs) or *antisense oligonucleotides* (which can bind to mRNAs, delay their translation, and enhance their degradation) and, more recently, small inhibitory RNAs that can selectively suppress translation of a specific mRNA. Experimentally, virally transmitted vectors allowing uptake and then localized expression of growth factors or transmitters lost with degenerating neurons may deliver a means for more chronic therapies. Exploration of neuronal

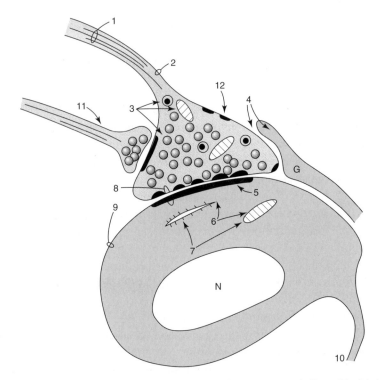

FIGURE 2–3. Twelve steps in the synaptic transmission process are indicated in this idealized synaptic connection. Step 1 is transport down the axon. Step 2 is the electrically excitable membrane of the axon. Step 3 involves the organelles and enzymes present in the nerve terminal for synthesizing, storing, and releasing the transmitter, as well as for the process of active reuptake. Step 4 includes the enzymes present in the extracellular space and within the glia for catabolizing excess transmitter released from nerve terminals. Step 5 is the postsynaptic receptor that triggers the response of the postsynaptic cell to the transmitter. Step 6 shows the organelles within the postsynaptic cells that respond to the receptor trigger. Step 7 is the interaction between genetic expression of the postsynaptic nerve cell and its influences on the cytoplasmic organelles that respond to transmitter action. Step 8 includes the possible "plastic" steps modifiable by events at the specialized synaptic contact zone. Step 9 includes the electrical portion of the nerve cell membrane that, in response to the various transmitters, is able to integrate the postsynaptic potentials and produces an action potential. Step 10 is the continuation of the information transmission by which the postsynaptic cell sends an action potential down its axon. Step 11, release of transmitter, is subjected to modification by a presynaptic (axoaxonic) synapse; in some cases, an analogous control can be achieved between dendritic elements. Step 12, release of the transmitter from a nerve terminal or secreting dendritic site, may be further subjected to modulation through autoreceptors that respond to the transmitter that the same secreting structure has released. Glia (G) can accumulate (4) released transmitters.

progenitor cell properties may ultimately allow for a replaceme
cally vulnerable neurons to disease. An alternative strategy cre
whole transgenic animals with novel mutations of the proteins in c
closely resemble but can outcompete the protein at its natural bin
sites (a so-called dominant negative mutation).

In addition to preparing novel mutant animals by transgenic technologies, it is possible to insert the special constructs into *null cells* (cells that normally do not express the transduction system under investigation) and, when they express a new receptor in their membrane, to probe these receptors for more conventional pharmacological characterization of natural or synthetic agonists and antagonists. In this way, one might not only develop novel drugs unique to such receptors but also detect previously unknown natural ligands for functionally uncharacterized "orphan" receptors (see Chapter 4).

THE STEPS OF SYNAPTIC TRANSMISSION

We conclude this chapter by briefly examining the mechanisms of presumed synaptic transmission for the mammalian central nervous system. Each step in such transmission constitutes one of the potential sites of central drug action (Fig. 2–3). A stimulus activates an all-or-none action potential in a spiking axon by depolarizing its transmembrane potential above the threshold level. The action potential propagates unattenuated to the nerve terminal, where ion fluxes activate a mobilization process leading to transmitter secretion and transmission to the postsynaptic cell. When the transmitter is released from its storage site by the presynaptic action potential, the effects on the postsynaptic cells cause either excitatory or inhibitory postsynaptic potentials, depending on the nature of the postsynaptic cell receptor for the particular transmitter agent. If sufficient excitatory postsynaptic potentials summate temporally from various inputs onto the cell, the postsynaptic cell will integrate these potentials and give off its own all-or-nothing action potential, which is then transmitted to each of its own axon terminals, and the process continues.

SELECTED REFERENCES

Aston-Jones, G. and G. R. Siggins (1994). Electrophysiology. In *Psychopharmacology: The Fourth Generation of Progress* (F. E. Bloom and D. J. Kupfer, Eds.). Raven Press, New York, pp. 41–64.

Bloom, F. E. (2006). Neurotransmission and the central nervous system. In *The Pharmacological Basis of Therapeutics* (L. L. Brunton, J. S. Lazo, and K. L. Parker, Eds.), 11th ed. McGraw-Hill, New York, pp. 317–340.

Bloom, F. E. (2008). Fundamentals of neuroscience. In *Fundamental Neuroscience* (L. Squire, D. Berg, F. E. Bloom, S. du Lac, A. Ghosh, and N. C. Spitzer, Eds.), 3rd ed. Academic Press, New York, pp. 3-14.

Eccles, J. C. (1964). *The Physiology of Synapses.* Academic Press, New York.

Hille, B. (1992). *Ionic Channels of Excitable Membranes*, 2nd ed. Sinauer, Sunderland, MA.

Llinas, R. R. (1988). The intrinsic electrophysiological properties of mammalian neurons: Insights into central nervous system function. *Science* 242, 1654–1660.

Loewi, O. (1921). Uber humorale Übertragbarkeit der Herznervenwirkung. *Pflugers Arch.* 189, 239.

Magistretti, P. (2008). Brain energy metabolism. In *Fundamental Neuroscience* (L. Squire, D. Berg, F. E. Bloom, S. du Lac, A. Ghosh, and N. C. Spitzer, Eds.), 3rd ed. Academic Press, New York, pp. 271–296.

Swanson, L. (2008). Basic plan of the nervous system. In *Fundamental Neuroscience* (L. Squire, D. Berg, F. E. Bloom, S. du Lac, A. Ghosh, and N. C. Spitzer, Eds.), 3rd ed. Academic Press, New York, pp. 15–40.

3

Principles and Methods of Behavioral Pharmacology

As we have seen, chemical communication at central nervous system synapses plays a critical role throughout the brain. Behavior is the product of integrated brain function, and we now understand the role of specific neurotransmitters in the control of many aspects of behavior. Drugs have powerful effects on neurotransmitter function and thereby change behavior. The field known as behavioral pharmacology or psychopharmacology focuses on the analysis of the behavioral effects of drugs in animals and humans. In parallel, knowledge that disorders of neurotransmitter function in the brain were likely to underlie a wide range of psychiatric and neurological disorders accrued. The merging of these two lines of research led to the development of a range of behavioral models for understanding the neural and pharmacological correlates of normal and abnormal behavior and their importance for evaluating drug treatments.

Before discussing models of particular relevance to specific mental illnesses, it is important to understand the key role that behavioral models have played in the development of psychopharmacology during the past 50 years. During this period, a number of different schools of behavioral science have been influential, and at times they may have appeared to be in conflict. There are many ways of measuring behavior, and opinions differ as to which provides the most useful assays for assessing drug effects. All have a role to play.

29

The study of behavior has a long and distinguished record in the history of psychological science, but until recently there was little dialogue between traditional learning theorists and psychopharmacologists. This is changing, and it represents one of the most exciting developments in the field.

There are three sections in this chapter. In the first, we describe different aspects of behavior, the principles of their control, and the determinants of their expression. In the second, the behavioral tasks of most importance to contemporary psychopharmacology are described in more detail. In the third, models of particular significance in relation to abnormal as opposed to normal behavior are highlighted. In later chapters, their use in the evaluation of novel drugs for treating neuropsychiatric disorders is described.

THE ANALYSIS OF BEHAVIOR

Under natural conditions, animals make two kinds of behavioral responses—elicited and emitted. *Elicited responses* are those that can be induced reliably by a specific stimulus and under normal conditions only by that stimulus or one very similar to it. Such responses are reflexive, such as contraction of the pupil in response to light or salivation in response to food. The autonomic nervous system controls a variety of such reflexes. By contrast, *emitted responses* are not induced by any clearly identifiable stimulus. A rat placed in an activity box runs around to varying degrees depending on many factors, including time of day, hunger, estrous state, ambient temperature, and previous experience with the box. Ethologists traditionally study such naturalistic behaviors with observational methods, recording the elements of behavior and their duration and sequence. The behavioral patterns critical for physiological homeostasis and survival fall into this category, such as feeding and drinking, food hoarding, mating and maternal behavior, and exploratory locomotion. Responses controlled by the skeletal nervous system play a major role in these behavioral patterns. However, there are elements of such behavioral sequences that involve elicited autonomic responses. In courtship and mating, for example, emitted behavior is predominant initially, but the sequence culminates in copulation, a reflexive action.

Although under natural conditions emitted and elicited responses merge seamlessly, they can be identified individually under experimental conditions and changed by the learning experience. There are two forms of learning or conditioning—classical (Pavlovian or respondent) and operant (instrumental).

Classical Conditioning

This category of behavioral analysis was originally described by Pavlov, and many believe it to be a process of stimulus substitution. A given response, the *unconditioned response* (UR), is elicited by a specific stimulus, the *unconditioned stimulus* (US). A *neutral stimulus* (CS) that normally would not elicit the UR is presented at the same time as the natural elicitors (US). After experience responding to the paired stimuli (US + CS), the previously neutral CS now elicits the CR (appears identical to the UR). Thus, the dog is conditioned to salivate to a bell in the absence of food. The parameters of the CS and the temporal relationship between the US and CS are major variables determining the speed and strength of classical conditioning.

Taste aversion, which is of biological importance for survival, is an example of classical conditioning that does not conform to these rules. In this paradigm, thirsty rats are given access to water flavored with a highly preferred taste. Once drinking is established, sickness is induced in the rats with X-rays or drugs such as lithium chloride. After recovery from the sickness, rats given a choice of flavored or unadulterated water avoid the former. Strikingly, taste aversion can occur after a single US/UR pairing; the UR (sickness) can be induced hours after the US (taste) is experienced, and this form of learning is specific to the taste and odor of the water or food and not to its appearance (e.g., "flashing" water).

Operant Conditioning

Operant conditioning, by contrast, is controlled by the consequences of emitted behavior. If a response is followed by a pleasant or unpleasant consequence, the probability of that response changes. Operant conditioning was first studied with rats in mazes or cats in puzzle boxes, where the animal experiences trial by trial the outcome of its behavior (i.e., it finds food or escapes from the box). A pleasant outcome or *reinforcement* increases responding. Reinforcers are easily recognized as outcomes we like, such as food, but it is important to realize that escaping from or avoiding an unpleasant outcome is also reinforcing (termed *negative reinforcement*). Shock escape or avoidance is readily studied with either discrete trial tasks, in which a stimulus periodically signals an impeding shock and a response during the signal avoids the shock, or free operant schedules (nondiscriminated, often termed *Sidman avoidance*). Under these conditions, shocks are arranged to occur repeatedly but without warning, and an animal must respond steadily in order to prevent or postpone them. In these tasks, avoidance is active, but in other tasks it may be passive; that is, the subject (or animal) must learn not to respond in order to avoid the shock. Mild electric shock to the body surface is the most commonly used aversive stimulus, but loud noise, bright light, air puffs to the face, and novelty can have aversive properties.

Consider the classic discrete-trial signaled avoidance procedure. The rat is placed on one side of a two-chambered box. A tone is presented and if, while the tone is on, the rat jumps the barrier to the safe side the shock is avoided.

Initially, the rat is slow to move and jump the barrier to escape the shock. However, after approximately 40–50 trials reliable shock avoidance is seen.

Both classically and operantly conditioned responses show *extinction* when the conditioning paradigm is terminated and reinforcement no longer occurs. One theory of extinction proposes loss of association (reversal of conditioning), and the other theory, more commonly held today, proposes loss of performance (suppression of responding that can readily be reinstated). In the latter case, it is proposed that a new learning process occurs during extinction that has the effect of suppressing the CS–US association, although the memory of the association is preserved. Extinction is usually rapid, but avoidance learning shows exceptionally slow extinction, and this phenomenon may account for the development and persistence of phobic behaviors. Drugs able to enhance this extinction process could be very useful in treating such disorders by accelerating the replacement of maladaptive associations. However, no such drugs are currently available, although promising results have been obtained with the glutamate NMDA receptor partial agonist D-cycloserine, which has been shown to facilitate extinction of conditioned fear in rats and to improve fear reduction of social phobia and fear of heights in human studies.

It is generally accepted that elicited (autonomic) responses are most easily conditioned classically and emitted responses are most easily conditioned operantly. However, this is not an absolute distinction, and under special conditions operant conditioning of autonomic responses can be achieved (e.g., voluntary control of heart rate) and skeletal responses may be part of reflexive behavior (e.g., leg withdrawal as part of the response to painful stimuli). Equally, classical conditioning of operant responses can occur. *Autoshaping* is the most intensively studied paradigm. Pigeons are exposed to a simple Pavlovian conditioning procedure in a key pecking apparatus. A light is projected periodically onto a response key and the delivery of food follows regardless of the behavior of the bird. The lit key is the CS and the food is the US. After approximately 50 pairing, the birds begin to peck the lit key; that is, apparently instrumental responses emerge without the bird experiencing an operant conditioning procedure. Autoshaping provides a very important paradigm for studying the complex interplay of respondent and operant conditioning in the control of behavior.

Schedules of Reinforcement

In the 1950s, B. F. Skinner refined operant conditioning equipment (Skinner box) and made it easy to automatically record responses (cumulative recorder). He also introduced schedules of reinforcement to replace the earlier poorly controlled discrete trial procedures. Initially, working with pigeons with key pecking as the emitted response, Skinner demonstrated different and highly reproducible patterns of responding depending on the relationship between pecking the key and its outcome. One peck, one reward is termed *continuous reinforcement*; a set number of pecks for one reward is termed a *fixed ratio* schedule; and availability of reward at the end of a specific delay is termed a *fixed interval* (FI) schedule. A range of commonly used schedules is illustrated in Figure 3–1, with their parameters and characteristic patterns of

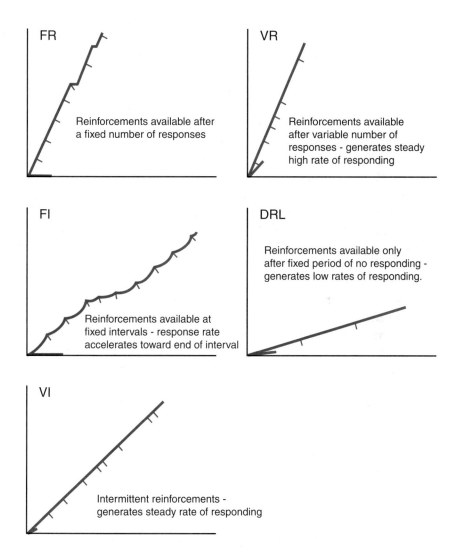

FR
Reinforcements available after a fixed number of responses

VR
Reinforcements available after variable number of responses - generates steady high rate of responding

FI
Reinforcements available at fixed intervals - response rate accelerates toward end of interval

DRL
Reinforcements available only after fixed period of no responding - generates low rates of responding.

VI
Intermittent reinforcements - generates steady rate of responding

FIGURE 3–1. Sample cumulative records of responding on different schedules of reinforcement. The slope of record indicates rate of responding. Reinforcements are indicated by short diagonal lines on the record. DRL, differential reinforcement low rates of responding; FI, fixed interval; FR, fixed ratio; VI, variable interval; VR, variable ratio. (Modified from Carlton, 1983.)

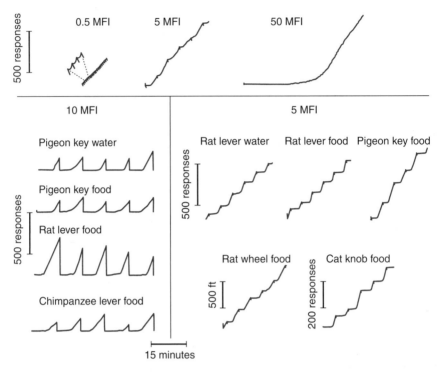

FIGURE 3–2. Generality of fixed-interval performance. A fixed-interval (FI) schedule of presentation of food or water was in operation in all examples.(*Top*) Records from a pigeon pecking a plastic key for food reward. Three different durations of FI (in minutes) are shown, with food rewards indicated by downward key strokes; the general pattern of accelerated responding as the time for food reward approaches persists, despite a 100-fold change in the FI parameter. (*Bottom left*) Performances under a 10-minute FI schedule. Food or water presentation is marked by resetting of the marker pen to baseline. Across different species, responding for water or food reward under this schedule is remarkably similar. (*Bottom right*) Responses under a 5-minute FI schedule for food or water. Responses are again similar across species and for different types of switch recording the response. (Iversen & Iversen, with permission from Kelleher, R. and Morse W. [1966] Fig 1, *Ergebn der Physiol*, 60 1–56.)

responding. A given schedule, such as the FI, generates the same pattern of responding in all species tested regardless of the operant response reinforced (Fig. 3–2).

Even more striking is the demonstration that food reinforcement and removal of electric shock (negative reinforcement) sustain indistinguishable patterns of FI responding in squirrel monkeys (Fig. 3–3). Such observations undermine motivational explanations of the behavior and suggest that the similarity of behavior lies not in the nature of the reinforcer but in the way it is programmed. By the 1960s Skinnerian schedules of reinforcement provided the first powerful methodology for characterizing and distinguishing the various classes of

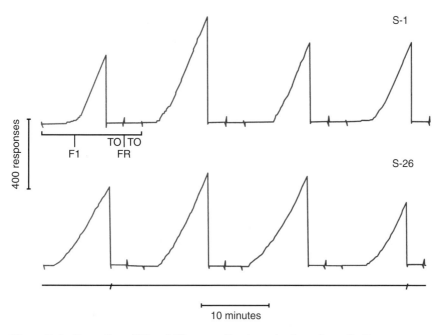

Figure 3–3. Generality of FI and FR responding in squirrel monkeys. Performance was maintained by food presentation (top, monkey S-1) or by stimulus shock termination (bottom, monkey S-26). The sequence of visual stimuli and corresponding schedules was the same in the top and bottom records. At the beginning of the records, an FI 10-minute schedule was in effect, signaled by a white light. At the termination of the FI component, the pen reset to baseline and a 2.5-minute time-out period followed, during which responding had no consequences. This was followed by an FR 30 component, signaled by a red light, indicated by a short diagonal stroke on the record. The cycle was then repeated. At the bottom of the record for monkey S-26, short diagonal strokes indicate electric shock presentations. Note the similarity in responding patterns under these multiple FI/FR food or shock schedules. (Modified from Kelleher and Morse, 1964.)

psychotropic drugs known at that time. For example, Kelleher and Morse compared the effects of amphetamine and chlorpromazine in squirrel monkeys working on multiple FI/FR schedules for either food reinforcement or shock removal. Amphetamine increased rates of responding under both conditions, with low rates of responding early in the FI being increased more than the higher rates of FR responding (Fig. 3–4). By contrast, chlorpromazine decreased responding for positive and negative reinforcement on both schedules. The schedule of reinforcement, rather than its nature, is the more important determinant of drug action. If the generated pattern of responding is identical, so is the drug response. The methodology has become extremely important in studies of addiction in which animals work on different schedules to obtain intravenous infusions of reinforcing drugs (see Chapter 20).

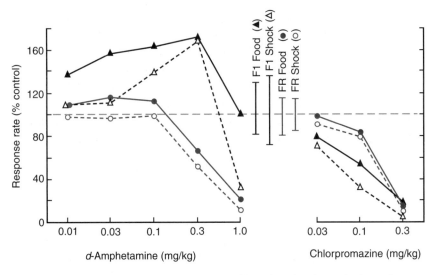

FIGURE 3–4. Effects of d-amphetamine and chlorpromazine in squirrel monkeys on responding under multiple FI/FR food and FI/FR shock schedules. Each drug was given intramuscularly 2.5 hours before the beginning of the test session. Three monkeys were studied on each schedule, with duplicate measurements at each dose level. Summary dose–response curves were calculated as mean percentage changes from responding in non-drug control sessions. Dashed horizontal lines indicate baseline control values (i.e., 100%); vertical lines indicate range of control values for each schedule. Note the general similarity of pairs of dose–effect curves for FI and FR components. (Modified from Kelleher and Morse, 1964.)

The Value of Multiple Schedules in Studying Drug Effects on Behavior

With multiple schedules it is possible to assess in a single animal, over a short period of time, a drug effect on behavior maintained by different reinforcers or different schedules of reinforcement, as we have seen, or by reinforcement as opposed to punishment, in signaled or unsignaled conditions. For example, a three-component multiple schedule was used to investigate minor tranquilizers. Hungry rats were exposed to a sequence of three signaled conditions: food on a variable interval (VI) of 30 seconds for 10 minutes, followed by 4 minutes of time-out conditions (apparatus inactive), followed by 3 minutes on a Geller–Seifter conflict schedule (VI food plus shock). The sequence was repeated twice within a testing session. Response rates were high on the reinforced VI and low during time-out and punishment components. Minor tranquilizers, including chlordiazepoxide, increased punished responding, with little effect on food-reinforced behavior. Further examples of the effects of anxiolytics on suppressed responding are discussed in Chapter 14. However, the response-releasing effects are specific insofar as equally low rates of responding controlled by time-out conditions were not increased to the same extent as punished responding. The use of multiple schedules avoids the need for independent groups of animals in order to assess drug effects on different aspects of behavioral control. The disadvantage is that the multiple schedule may introduce contrast effects between the various components; for example, switching from high to low rates of responding in order to obtain reinforcement or switching between reinforced and punished responding—effects that may be affected by the drug.

Discriminative Stimuli

If responses are emitted and reinforced in the presence of a stimulus, that stimulus is called a *discriminative stimulus*, or S^D, which subsequently has information value indicating to the animal that a particular reinforcement contingency is in operation. A stimulus indicating that reinforcement is not operating is termed an S^Δ. The use of S^D and S^Δ enables one to ask a number of questions about an animal's discriminative capacity. For example, in an operant task responding may be rewarded in the presence of a green light (S^D) and not in the presence of a red light (S^Δ). Rates of responding soon vary dramatically in the presence of green or red light, indicating that the animals can discriminate the two visual cues. Stimulus control can also be demonstrated with discrete trial procedures with the animal responding to one stimulus and not to another when given a choice between the stimuli—so-called *simultaneous discrimination tasks*. If a drug impairs discriminative performance, it may do so by impeding sensory processing or by altering the tendency of the animal to respond to the S^D. Performance on discrete trial procedures is amenable to analysis by signal detection theory. Using rates of hit and false alarm responses on the discrimination task makes it possible to distinguish changes in sensory discrimination (d') from changes in the tendency to respond (response bias; β). It may be important to know how precise the animal's idea of the S^D is, and in these circumstances a stimulus generalization gradient experiment provides the answer. For example, an animal may be trained to respond in the presence of an S^D, such as a vertical line, and then be subsequently exposed to a range of lines tilted from vertical to horizontal. The rate of responding to the generalization stimuli indicates the strength of the original discriminative control. If the animal noticed the training stimulus, a large number of responses are emitted when this stimulus subsequently appears and fewer to different but related stimuli. There is no response to unfamiliar stimuli. If for some reason the initial discrimination training is unsuccessful or if the animal has lost its discriminative capacity after training, stimuli presented during the generalization testing are responded to equally, and the gradient is said to be "flat."

The generalization gradients produced in such experiments are "sharpened" if, during training, the animal is not reinforced for responding to a stimulus at one end of the range (the S^{Δ}) while being reinforced in the presence of the S^D and if a reinforcement schedule that generates a high rate of responding is used during training.

Discriminative stimuli are usually exteroceptive sensory signals (visual, auditory, tactile, olfactory, and gustatory), but interoceptive stimuli transmitted via the sensory autonomic nervous system can also act as S^D's or S^{Δ}'s. Certain drugs provide powerful interoceptive discriminative cues. In *drug discrimination learning*, an animal is trained to make one response (e.g., press one of two levers to obtain reinforcement) when experiencing one drug state and to make a different response (e.g., press the other lever) in a nondrugged or different drug state. Just as physical stimuli demonstrate stimulus generalization, so too do interoceptive cues. This procedure is important for evaluating the "subjective" properties of drugs that may be rewarding or aversive, the properties of their antagonists, and the neuropharmacological basis of their reinforcing or aversive effects. As discussed in Chapter 20, it is also useful in demonstrating whether or not new medications with unknown behavioral actions are perceived to be the same or different from drugs known to have addictive or aversive properties.

Rate Dependency

Different schedules of reinforcement produce different patterns and, importantly, different rates of responding. It is clear that when studying the effects of drugs on behavior, it is important to recognize the nondrug baseline levels of responding. This principle was initially demonstrated for barbiturate drugs, but the effects of the stimulant drug amphetamine on behavior sustained by an FI schedule have been studied in more detail and provide the best illustration of rate dependency. Rates of responding are increased overall, but the increase is related to the baseline rate of responding. Low rates during the initial segments of the FI are increased to a greater degree than the higher rates at the end of the interval. If the analysis is extended to a range of behavioral procedures that generate variable low-to-high baseline activity (motor activity, other schedules of reinforcement, and avoidance procedures), the empirical generalization of rate dependency holds; amphetamine increases low rates of behavior in a dose-related manner while decreasing high rates of behavior over the same dose range. It is clear, therefore, that amphetamine cannot be characterized as a drug simply with stimulant or depressant properties (see Chapters 16 and 21). In addition, when drugs are compared further, interesting dissociations emerge. The benzodiazepine drug chlordiazepoxide, like amphetamine, shows rate dependency effects on nonpunished sectors of a multiple schedule, albeit weaker than the effect seen with amphetamine. However, unlike amphetamine, chlordiazepoxide releases low rates of punished responding—an effect that shows a strong rate dependency.

Conditioned Reinforcement

So far stimuli have been described that have innate reinforcing properties: food, water, accesses to sexual contact, or exploration of the environment. However, neutral stimuli devoid of this property can become conditioned or secondary reinforcers. Once acquired, conditioned reinforcers can sustain behavior and delay extinction in the absence of a primary reinforcer; for example, lever pressing for the click of the food hopper in the Skinner box in the absence of food delivery or lever pressing for a visual cue that has been paired previously with a local infusion of a drug of addiction into dopamine-rich areas of the brain (see Chapter 20). Conditioned reinforcers acquire their properties by the process of classical conditioning—that is, stimulus substitution in which the CS (click or visual cue) comes to represent the UCS in its ability to sustain operant behavior in the absence of primary reinforcement. In humans and nonhuman primates, conditioned reinforcers are powerful controllers of behavior; for example, money rewards for humans and food tokens for chimpanzees. In parallel, we should consider innate aversive stimuli such as shock. Neutral stimuli paired with shock acquire conditioned aversive properties, which are proposed to be critical for shock-avoidance behavior. The tone becomes a conditioned aversive stimulus in the way that a tone (food hopper click) becomes a conditioned positive reinforcer.

Aversive Stimuli and Punishment

Just as reinforcement powerfully influences behavior, so too does punishment. If operant responding leads to the presentation of an aversive stimulus, the probability of that response decreases. This is termed *punishment* and is best demonstrated by superimposing an aversive stimulus (commonly electric shock) on existing baselines of ongoing spontaneous or reinforced behavior. For example, if a thirsty rat, having learned to drink from a spout, subsequently receives a mild electric shock to the mouth when attempting to lick, drinking decreases. Another widely used punishment procedure was originally described by Geller and Seifter (Fig. 3–5). A rat is trained to press a lever for food on a VI schedule. After high rates of responding are achieved, shock is introduced. The rat receives a mild shock to the feet each time a response is made to the lever, and although lever presses are still reinforced, the overall rate of responding is severely depressed. This is termed *immediate punishment*, denoting the fact that it follows a lever response with a regular time

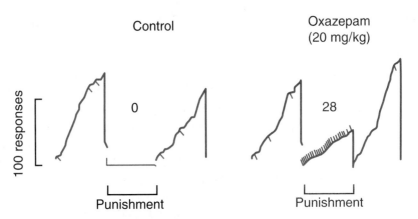

FIGURE 3–5. Geller–Seifter conflict test. Performance records from Geller–Seifter conflict test in rats. Lever presses are cumulative, so the slope of the tracing at any point indicates the response rate. When there is no lever pressing, the trace is horizontal. Punishment periods 3 minutes in duration, signaled by a tone, are flanked by equivalent periods of nonpunished responding for a milk reward (indicated by a downward pen stroke); responses during punishment periods are indicated by upward pen strokes (numbered). The anxiolytic drug oxazepam resulted in a marked disinhibition of the effect of punishment on responding but had no effect on responding during nonpunished periods. (Modified from Stein, Wise, and Berger, 1973.)

relationship and to distinguish it from *adventitious punishment*, which can be programmed to occur irrespective of the animal's responses. As discussed in Chapter 14, this paradigm involving immediate punishment is deemed to create conflict and the consequent suppression of responding can be reversed with a range of anxiolytic drugs.

The effects of aversive stimuli on behavior have long been recognized as a challenge to learning theory. On the one hand, animals may escape from or avoid shock; on the other hand, their behavior may be suppressed by shock. If we could convince ourselves that reinforcement was operating in all the procedures, we might be able to accommodate all the effects of aversive stimuli into reinforcement theory. This was Skinner's attitude regarding punishment. He viewed it as a special case of reinforcement in which avoidance of shock was mediated not by the observed reduction in responding but by an increase in the probability of an internal and unobservable response in the animal. Thus, with punishment as with reinforcement, a response probability (in this case, the response being not to respond) increases. This explanation is attractively parsimonious, but recourse to unobservable events for explanatory purposes does not produce an easily testable hypothesis. Although it would be convenient to encompass all the effects of aversive stimuli within reinforcement theory, there is a strong view that maintains that a decrease in response probability to aversive stimuli is a different process that can be procedurally distinguished from the other varied effects of shock and, more important, involves different neural systems.

Behavioral paradigms involving aversive stimuli have played a key role in the history of behavioral pharmacology. Initially, schedules of escape/avoidance versus punishment were used to differentiate the major classes of drug being investigated in the 1960s (Kelleher and Morse, 1964). As the field of neuroscience emerged and the role of the limbic structures in the responses to aversive stimuli became more clear, and its relationship to the control of emotion emerged, behavioral paradigms involving aversive stimuli were soon adopted as animal models of emotional disorders in humans.

Properties of Punishment

It is generally accepted that the most satisfactory way to measure abnormal behavior is to identify a response within the animal's normal repertoire that can be quantified readily, hence the focus on parametric studies of how aversive stimuli change elements of unconditioned or conditioned behavior in conflict situations.

Adventitious Punishment

Several procedures involving adventitious punishment have been of continuing interest with respect to abnormal behavior. Intense, unavoidable shock causes profound changes in behavior. In studies by Seligman, dogs were strapped into a hammock and given 64 inescapable electric shocks (5 s, 6.0 mA). The next day, the dogs were placed in an escape/avoidance testing chamber, where upon the presentation of a signal they could jump a barrier to avoid the shock. The dogs were found to be inactive and unable to learn this task. The term *learned helplessness* was given to this behavior, and at first it was compared to reactive depression in humans and was considered a model with considerable potential in biological psychiatry. Further work on the rat suggested that after repeated unavoidable shock, a form of conditioned immobility exists that is incompatible with the gross body movements required to successfully avoid shock by leaping a barrier. However, in an avoidance task that requires minimal movement (e.g., protrusion of the nose through a hole), animals that have received shock are able to learn to avoid further shocks and indeed learn at a faster rate than controls. This result places the term learned helplessness in an ambiguous position and demonstrates how easy it is to jump to the wrong conclusions about grossly disturbed behavior patterns.

More robust procedures superimpose shocks on behavior maintained by reinforcement. One valuable procedure was originally devised by Estes and Skinner in 1941. Rats are trained to press for food on a VI schedule that sustains high levels of responding. At this stage, Pavlovian conditioning trials are introduced. A sound (CS) is periodically sounded for approximately 30 seconds, after which a brief electric shock (US) is delivered to the rat's feet. These Pavlovian conditioning trials are completely independent of lever pressing for food; lever pressing continues to produce food but has no effect on the occurrence of either the tone or the shock. As training continues, the presentation of the CS results in suppression of lever pressing, so-called "conditioned suppression" (Fig. 3–6).The most widely accepted explanation for this phenomenon is that the tone, through its pairing with shock, induces fear and its presentation comes to disrupt responding. The sound acquires conditioned punishment status, and akin to conditioned reinforcement, it comes to sustain suppression in the absence of shock. This a form of *conditioned emotional response*.

Immediate Punishment

Azrin and Holtz (1966) provided a systematic description of *immediate punishment*. To be effective, immediate punishment must reliably follow responses. Foot shock is often unreliable because the resistance of the animal varies, particularly the skin of the feet, thus reducing the effectiveness of the shock. The speed of leg withdrawal reflexes also determines the severity of shock actually received. To overcome these problems, Azrin introduced implanted electrodes so that shock could be delivered directly to the body surface. In the pigeon, predictable relationships between ongoing food-reinforced behavior and immediate punishment can be demonstrated. The degree of suppression depends on (1) the severity of deprivation, (2) the strength of the punishing stimulus, (3) the schedule of reinforcement operating, and (4) the schedule of punishment. It is most effective when the following conditions are met: (1) The punishment should be as intense as possible, (2) the delay between behavior and punishment should be kept to a minimum, (3) the punishment should be introduced at maximum intensity, and (4) the punishment should reliably follow the behavioral response.

There appear to be two factors involved in the suppression of behavior by punishment. One factor involves a specific suppression of the punished response by the association of punishment with the emission of behavior. Since associative learning depends on the temporal relationship between the events to be associated, increasing the delay of punishment would result in poorer learning with a consequent reduction of the suppressive effects of punishment. The second factor involves a nonspecific suppression of behavior in the experimental situation, and this is relatively independent of the interval between the response and punishment. If the response–punishment interval is short, response suppression should occur because of the joint operation of these two factors. If punishment is delayed beyond the limits within which

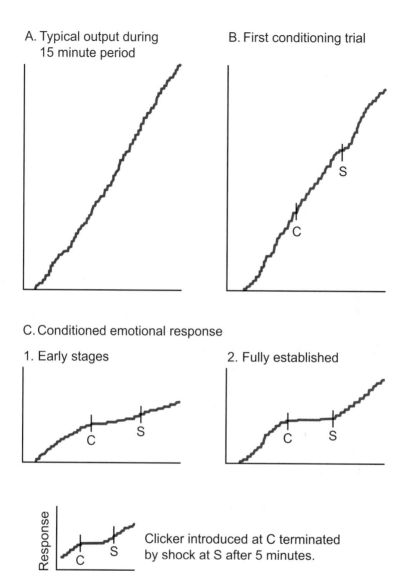

A. Typical output during 15 minute period

B. First conditioning trial

C. Conditioned emotional response

1. Early stages

2. Fully established

Response

Time

Clicker introduced at C terminated by shock at S after 5 minutes.

FIGURE 3–6. Conditioned suppression of behavior (often termed conditioned emotional response). (A) Typical VI responding for food in rats. (B) The effect of brief shock (S) was reliably preceded by an auditory signal (clicker [C]) on this VI responding. (C1 and C2) Progressive suppression of responding as this cycle is repeated, with progressively fewer responses emitted during the clicks. (Iversen & Iversen, with permission from Hunt, H.F. and Brady, J.V. [1951] Figure 1, *J Comp Physiol Psychol*, 44, 88–98.)

associative learning can occur, any suppression induced by punishment must be due solely to the nonspecific effect of shock in the situation, and further increases in delay of punishment will have no additional effect.

Aversive Stimuli Other Than Electric Shock

The preoccupation with shock as an aversive stimulus has had unfortunate theoretical implications. Some theorists have proposed that aversive stimuli induce fear, which is motivating, and that fear is always a conditioned response based on the association of some previously nonaversive stimulus with pain. However, there are good grounds for questioning the assumption that all fears are conditioned responses of this kind. Many stimuli that are not painful or do not lead to painful consequences can nevertheless be used as negative reinforcers or punishers, and they are highly aversive if their behavioral effects are observed. The termination of noise, for example, has been shown to reinforce escape behavior in humans, monkeys, cats, rats, and mice. Response-contingent noise suppresses responding in a similar range of species. Intense light will motivate escape learning and can serve as an unconditioned stimulus for avoidance learning. Forced swimming in cold water is highly aversive to rats. Being touched by a hot or cold metal plate or blasted with air evokes active escape. Complex patterns of visual and auditory stimuli are apparently aversive in that they induce typical patterns of defensive behavior in various species; for example, ducklings freeze at the sight of a hawk. It has been suggested that these responses be termed "distress reactions," and they can be observed at a very early stage of development. Encoding the familiar is a prerequisite for the fear of novelty. For example, human infants must be capable of visual memory before a fear of visual novelty can develop.

Manipulation of Reinforcement Contingencies May Also Act as Aversive Stimuli

Sudden increases or decreases in the expected magnitude of the reward disrupt behavior. Crespi reported that if rats were trained in a runway to run to a goal box for a reinforcement of a certain size, they ran faster or slower if the size of the reward was unexpectedly increased or decreased. These sudden increases and decreases in ongoing behavior have been described as "behavioral contrast." Unexpected changes in schedules of reinforcement also induce behavioral disruption. For example, when pigeons have been conditioned to receive reinforcers at a certain time and of a certain magnitude for a particular response effort, they become very disturbed and aggressive if they are not rewarded in the expected manner. Azrin and colleagues described a procedure in which a pigeon was alternately rewarded 10 times on a continuous reinforcement schedule for pecking a key and then was given a period of extinction. At the back of a cage, a suitably restrained "target" pigeon was positioned and the attack response to it recorded. The attacks occurred during extinction and were most frequent at the start of the extinction period. Similar behavior was observed in the squirrel monkey when aggression was measured by the number of bites on a piece of hose pipe placed in the animal's cage. In natural situations, random adventitious shock can result in increases in unconditioned behaviors such as aggression to conspecifics or inanimate objects, sexual behavior, or feeding.

Falk proposed that schedule-induced aggression is similar to an abnormal drinking behavior termed "schedule-induced polydipsia." If water is freely available when rats lever press for 45-mg dry food pellets on a 1-minute FI schedule, large quantities of water are consumed. During a 3.5-hour session, this can be three or four times the normal total daily intake. This does not occur with continuous reinforcement schedules but seems to occur when inter-reinforcement times exceed 30 seconds. Falk suggested that these be called "adjunctive behaviors," which resemble the "displacement activity" classically described in the ethological literature. Displacement behaviors are described as occurring when certain environmental events result in the interruption of some consummatory activity in an organism under high "drive" conditioning. These are exactly the conditions that produce adjunctive aggressive behavior as defined by Falk. Therefore, aggression should not be viewed as a behavior generated by a hypothetical internal state in the absence of eliciting stimuli but, rather, as a behavior occurring in a specific situation—a situation in which another class of reinforcers is intermittently scheduled.

BEHAVIORAL TASKS IN CONTEMPORARY PSYCHOPHARMACOLOGY

Unconditioned Behavior

Measures of Motor Behaviors in Different Environments

In rodents, spontaneous locomotor activity in a small confined area, devoid of specific stimuli, is measured by (1) jiggle cages (box balanced on a central pivot), (2) breaks in infrared light beamed across the cage, or (3) video tracking with computerized analysis capable of quantifying sequences and patterns of movement. Direct observation of animals is also important for understanding changes in behavior. For example, increasing doses of amphetamine initially increase and then decrease photocell beam breaks. Observation reveals that the reduced activity score is not due to the cessation of behavior; rather, at higher doses intense stereotyped motor behavior is seen (head movements, sniffing, licking, and gnawing) at one location in the cage, undetected by the photocell beams. With all these measures it must be recognized that many physiological and environmental factors can influence levels of motor behavior and these must be controlled for. These include time of day, ambient temperature, noise levels, odors, familiarity with the environment, and estrus cycle. Modifications can be introduced to induce exploration of the environment. If the size of the arena is increased, the distribution of locomotor behavior reflects increased anxiety. Activity in the perimeter, including exploration of corners and walls, predominates. If the fear level is less, exploration of the center of the field is seen. Levels of defecation reflect these differences in fear level. Raising or lowering overhead illumination also influences the levels and distribution of activity. These behaviors can be more polarized in the light–dark box where the animals are given a free choice to spend time in the brightly lit or the dark side of the box. This principle was taken one step forward with the introduction of the elevated plus maze (see Chapter 14). Two opposite arms of the maze have no walls and are elevated well above the ground. The remaining two arms have walls and are darker. Again, the distribution of activity in the different arms is deemed to reflect fear levels, with less time spent on the open arms. The open field, the light–dark box, and the plus maze are all widely used in the evaluation of anxiolytic drugs (see Chapter 14).

Other unconditioned behaviors, such as feeding, drinking, and sexual and maternal behavior, are easily measured by observation in open-field arenas by recording the elements and sequences of naturalistic behavior. Again, internal and environmental factors influence the level and pattern of these behaviors. For example, when released from a holding cage into an arena containing unlimited food pellets, food-deprived rats eat, but they also repeatedly carry food back to the holding cage to be hoarded. In an operant chamber, it has been shown that food-deprived rats when lever pressing for dry food on an FI schedule also drink abnormally large amounts of water (schedule-induced polydipsia). The ascending dopamine pathways to the striatum are critical for the expression of these motivated behaviors.

Responses to Pain and Stress

The presentation of noxious stimuli also induces unconditioned behaviors that include the initial response to the stimulus followed by species-specific flight-or-fight behaviors. Electric shock and heat stimuli are the most commonly used noxious stimuli. A number of well-validated tests exist for measuring the acute response to nociceptive stimuli. These are key for the evaluation of drugs with analgesic properties, defined as a reduction of perceived pain without loss of consciousness (see Chapter 18). Manipulating stress levels also has powerful effects on simple and complex behavior. Unavoidable pain and stress disrupt behavior. *Tail suspension* and the *Porsolt forced swimming test* in rodents are examples. In the former, a rodent is suspended upside down by its tail. Initially, effort is made to regain the upright position, but this is quickly replaced by an immobile suspended posture. In the latter test, the rodent is placed in a small cylinder of water with no means of escape. The animal swims vigorously initially, but with time it performs the minimal activity required to keep its head above water. Both tests have played an important role in the assessment of drugs with antidepressant activity (see Chapter 14) and are described as forms of "learned helplessness." However, both tasks demand highly coordinated motor behavior, and although this may not be possible, one should not assume a loss of all aspects of behavioral control.

Conditioned Behavior

Spontaneous, unconditioned behaviors can be modified by manipulation of the environment, and this has proved particularly important in the development of animal models of anxiety and depression. Experimental psychologists spent a great deal of time and energy devising classical and operant conditioning paradigms, and many believed that the learning of associations was all that was necessary to understand the intelligence of organisms. However, there has been a growing realization that other cognitive processes, including attention, concept formation, and especially memory, are also critical for adaptive behavior to occur in complex and changing environments. Any such account needs to invoke a flexible mechanism of information input, storage, and retrieval. The tasks of a behavioral pharmacologist are to select portions of complex behavior defined by the principles described in the first section of this chapter, to understand how drugs lawfully modify those behaviors, and, increasingly, to contribute to our understanding of the neuroanatomical substrates mediating these different aspects of behavior. Powerful paradigms exist for evaluating the capacity for sensory discrimination in a number of species and across a wide range of modalities and for exploring the ability to generate concepts from those experienced stimuli. However, tests of learning and memory are extremely important for contemporary psychopharmacology.

There are different domains of knowledge that can be acquired. In simple terms, information can be acquired about the environment, the outcomes of behaving in that environment, and the emotional impact of those outcomes. We now conceive of three interacting forebrain systems orchestrating conditioned behavior: the acquisition and memory of environmental information depend on the cortex; motivation and reinforcement depend on the forebrain systems innervated by dopaminergic neurons; and emotional responsiveness depends on limbic structures, including the amygdala. It is not possible in conditioned behavioral tasks to isolate these processes, but tasks can be designed that put pressure on one rather than another aspect of information processing.

Psychologists have identified and characterized different aspects of human memory, and a variety of different terminologies have been used to describe these. The widely accepted taxonomy of human memory and the brain structures known to be critical for these functions is illustrated in Figure 3–7.

The classification broadly distinguishes two categories of long-term memory. *Declarative* memory (sometimes described as explicit) is under conscious control and ensures that information can be encoded, stored, and retrieved at a later time. It operates over timescales from minutes to hours or even longer. The first level of distinction is between declarative (explicit memory) and *nondeclarative* (sometimes described as implicit) memory that is not under conscious control. Both forms of memory can be divided further in terms of the kind of information handled. Within declarative memory, the ability to remember facts (often called *semantic*) is distinguished from the memory for personal experiences or events (often called *episodic*). Generally, in semantic memory facts are experienced time after time until well recalled. How to perform in a behavioral task and the grammatical rules of language fall into this category, sometimes referred to as *reference memory*. By contrast, episodic

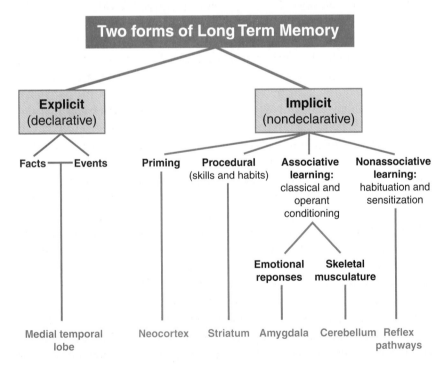

FIGURE 3–7. Taxonomy of different forms of memory. (Modified from Squire, 1987.)

memory enables an event presented in any modality to be recalled or recognized after a single presentation.

In parallel, a taxonomy of long-term memory has been developed from animal studies. Reading this literature is sometimes confusing because the studies on animals have often focused on the duration of memory rather than on the kind of information being remembered. This is reflected in the commonly used terms long- and short-term memory, suggesting different processes for what is almost certainly one process operating over a time range. It is therefore no longer a useful nomenclature. Rather, animal models of declarative memory that distinguish the memory for facts and rules as opposed to episodic memory for specific events are now in common use in behavioral pharmacology. Most of these capitalize on the remarkable ability of rats and mice to remember places they have visited, appearing to form spatial cognitive maps of their environment. The *Morris water maze* is the most widely used memory task drawing on this ability and tested in a complex spatial environment. Rats learn to swim in a large pool of water (made opaque with milk or dye) to find an unseen safe platform just below the surface. In each trial, swimming starts at a different point around the periphery. Since there are no local cues to guide the rat to the platform, it must learn the spatial location of the platform using distal landmarks around the room. The latency to escape onto the platform is measured, and using computer-controlled video tracking the swim path can be charted and its length measured. Task parameters vary from study to study, but usually several trials are given each day during the acquisition of the task. Then, at various delays after the final training trial, a single probe trial is given with the escape platform removed. The rats are allowed to swim for approximately 1 minute and the amount of time spent swimming within a short distance of the former location of the platform and in the opposite quadrant is recorded. The task has several advantages: (1) Learning is rapid, (2) the motivation is escape from the water so that the use of food or water reinforcement or electric shock is avoided, and (3) olfactory cues are eliminated (such cues can contaminate mazes). However, the experimenter loses the ability to vary the motivational level, and stress associated with water immersion may induce endocrine effects interacting with drug effects.

Rodent spatial memory has also been intensively studied in the *8-arm maze* (Fig. 3–8). Food rewards are placed at the end of each arm. Trial by trial, the rat is placed at the center and allowed to retrieve all the food rewards. The most efficient behavior follows the rule of entering the arms consecutively without returning to any previously visited arm. Within relatively few (approximately 20) trials, performance is virtually error free. To learn this task, the rat needs to use reference memory to acquire the general rules (i.e., leave the center and run into the baited arms only). However, it also requires memory for the series of responses being made. During each trial, the rat must also keep

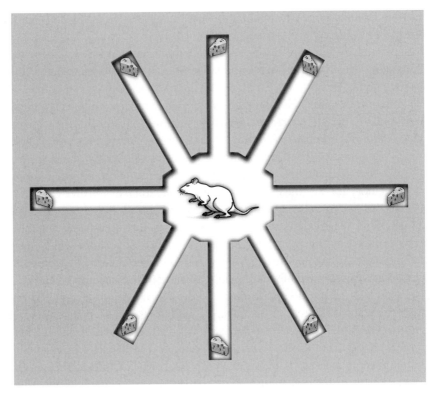

FIGURE 3–8. Radial-Arm Maze.
At the start of each trial food can be retrieved from the end of each of the eight arms. The rat is placed on the central platform and its task is to learn to visit each of the arms without repeating visits to any of them.

track of where it has already been so as not to reenter the arms where food has already been retrieved (sometimes termed *working memory*). Once all the arms have been visited, the rat can forget this particular sequence of behavior while retaining memory for the rule that will guide behavior on subsequent trials. With appropriate controls, it can be demonstrated that rats do not learn particular sequences of arm entry; they are not being guided by odor but use distal spatial cues to construct a map of the maze within which they demonstrate impressive spatial memory. In rats, the duration of this form of memory is long—approximately 4 hours. A number of modifications of this task have been used in order to invoke different aspects of memory. For example, if four arms are blocked and the rat has to remember which four are open for entry, then the task puts demands on long-term memory.

Under natural conditions, equally impressive spatial memory has been demonstrated in chimpanzees searching for food in a large arena after having watched the experimenter hide food in a number of locations. Other animals such as squirrels and certain species of birds hide food for later use and return to its location after months. We know from experimental studies in rats and humans that the hippocampus is critical for these remarkable levels of spatial memory.

Delayed matching to sample tasks have also proved useful in both rats and monkeys. In the rat version of this task, the animal is presented trial by trial with a retractable lever presented on either the right or the left of the test panel. The rat presses the lever, after which it is retracted. In the second part of the trial, a variable delay is introduced during which the rat is required to nose poke at another location, after which both levers appear and a response to the same lever that was presented in the first part of the trial is rewarded. Delay-dependent performance is observed. Drugs that specifically impair or enhance memory are expected to have an effect after long but not short delays. In monkeys, spatial or visual matching to sample can be tested with touch-screen technology. Typically, a trial starts with the presentation of a sample stimulus from a set (illuminated spatial location or visual pattern). After a delay during which the sample is no longer present, the animal is given a choice between the sample and one or more stimuli from the set. In each trial, a different stimulus from the set is used as the sample. The size of the sample set and the delay between the presentation of the sample and the choice stimuli can be varied to control for task difficulty.

Episodic memory proved much more difficult to measure in animals, and many early attempts involved reference memory for repeated facts—for example, discrete trial visual discrimination tasks in monkeys where the animal learns a rule that responding to one of a pair of visual stimuli, but not the other, is rewarded (Fig. 3–9). This associative rule learning may become habitual in nature and is not the counterpart of episodic memory. However, after much effort, episodic memory for objects or complex patterns seen only once was demonstrated in monkeys, and these tasks are described in more detail in Chapter 16.

In addition to long-term memory, there is another form of memory that enables us to hold and manipulate a number of related events. This was termed *working memory*. In comparison to long-term memory, this process was demonstrated to have limited capacity and to be of short duration. This process allows us to remember easily confused items of information, such as a telephone number after having looked it up in the directory. Its hallmark is that it holds information in temporary storage during the planning and execution of a task, often in the face of competing demands (i.e., distraction). This proved to be one of the most important advances in studies of human memory, although it was subsequently realized long after Baddeley's seminal studies that the equivalent tasks (delayed response and delayed alternation in a T or

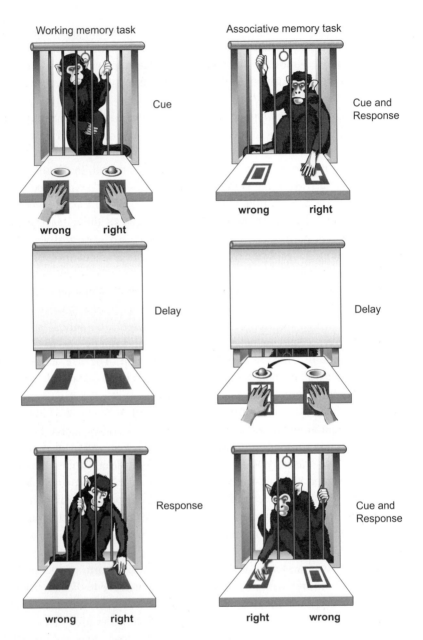

Working memory task

Cue

wrong   right

Delay

Response

wrong   right

Associative memory task

Cue and Response

wrong   right

Delay

Cue and Response

right   wrong

FIGURE 3–9. Tests of working and associative memory in monkeys, using the Wisconsin General Test Apparatus (WGTA). Delayed response tasks test prefrontal cortex function. In the working memory task (left), the monkey briefly views a target stimulus, in this case a piece of food being hidden by the experimenter in one of the food wells and then covered up. After a delay during which the food wells are not visible, the animal can retrieve the food. The experimenter randomly varies the location of the food from trial to trial so that each response tests the animal's short-term retention of visual and spatial information. In the

radial maze) had existed in the animal repertoire for decades and been shown to be dependent on the integrity of the dorsolateral frontal cortex. In monkeys, these tasks are normally tested by hand in the *Wisconsin General Test Apparatus*. On the delayed response task, the monkey faces a test board with two identical covered food wells to the left and right (Figure 3–9). The tester shows the monkey a food reward being hidden in one of the wells. A screen is lowered, obscuring the animal's view of the test board. After a delay, the screen is raised and the monkey is allowed to retrieve the food. From trial to trial, the reward is hidden randomly on the left or right. The monkey is dealing with two events occurring unpredictably. The correct response on a particular trial is of no value in guiding the next response. The monkey must remember only the most recent event and forget the rest (i.e., keep a running commentary in its memory of these two easily confused events). The *delayed alternation* task is similar in principle. Rewards alternate back and forth between the right and left food wells. There are no visual cues, and the task can only be solved in a given trial by accessing working memory (i.e., remembering where the previous response was made and going to the opposite side). Long-term and working memory are of much contemporary interest since they are impaired in a wide range of neuropsychiatric disorders.

The learning and memory of events of high emotional significance are also important. In a *passive avoidance task*, a rat is placed on a platform above a grid floor. Its instinct is to step down onto the floor, where it receives a foot shock. After a delay, the rat is returned to the platform and the latency to step down (a measure of memory) is recorded. Although simple to use, performance on this task is influenced by many factors (e.g., it contains elements of both classical and instrumental conditioning), thus requiring large numbers of experimental subjects to obtain reliable results. Conditioned fear is a simpler classical conditioning paradigm for quantifying the strength of emotional memory. The rat experiences several pairings of a tone/shock stimulus over a few minutes, separated by rest periods. Unconditioned freezing behavior is observed. After a delay of 24 hours, the rat is reintroduced to the chamber and the percentage of time spent freezing is measured as an index of fear memory. This is another form of conditioned emotional response that has been modified in the *fear-potentiated startle paradigm* where, after establishing an association between

---

associative memory task (right), in each trial the monkey views patterns covering food wells. In every trial the reward is to be found under one of the patterns (cross) and not under the other one (square). Between trials, the experimenter randomly switches the cross pattern between the two food wells, and after a minimal delay the screen is raised and the animal can retrieve the reward by reaching for the correct patterned cue. Here, the animal learns a reliable relationship between a visual pattern and reward. (From P. Goldman-Rakic, 1992.)

a light stimulus and shock, the light is presented with a loud noise. The normal startle response to the noise is greatly potentiated by the fear conditioning experience.

MODELS OF ABNORMAL BEHAVIOR

As previously discussed, behavior is under the control of a wide range of internal and external stimuli. When the animal no longer responds to these controlling stimuli in the usual way, we talk about maladaptive or abnormal behavior. However, there is a very fine and ambiguous line between normal and abnormal behavior, and often a behavior described as abnormal in one context is perfectly normal in another. Aggression is one such example. Aggression includes threat and attack and can be seen when an animal kills its prey. However, it can be induced equally well in a pigeon if reinforcement is suddenly terminated in an operant conditioning situation. Is this aggression normal or abnormal?

Historical View of Experimental Neurosis

Punishment provides the complementary force to reinforcement, and together these events largely determine behavioral output at any one time. If we speak anthropomorphically, behavior is considered to be motivated, on the one hand, by the seeking and expectancy of pleasing events and, on the other hand, by the experience or expectancy of an unpleasant one. Positive emotions are elicited by stimuli that denote food, safety, or comfort, whereas negative emotions are elicited by pain and lead to avoidance, escape, or protective responses. It could be claimed that the emotional state of the organism reflects at any one time the balance of these motivating forces. The elation after reinforcement or the depression of behavior consequent to punishment should not be considered abnormal, but clearly the response to such events can become abnormally accentuated and markedly disrupt ongoing behavior. In the clinical chapters, we consider a number of disorders characterized by abnormal responses to emotional stimuli and abnormal mood states. Emotions are conceived as transient responses to environmental, interoceptive, or cognitive stimuli, whereas mood is a predominant emotional state of an individual over time.

Model systems for studying abnormal behavior have been developed, to a great extent, by manipulating unpleasant events to induce marked change in the motivational and emotional state of animals. It was recognized that behavioral situations involving conflict between the aspirations of the animal and the state of the environment were useful for disrupting ongoing behavior. The term *experimental neurosis* was introduced to describe such paradigms in which operant responding is disrupted by Pavlovian responses. Whether experimental neurosis bears any resemblance to the neurosis common in everyday life is uncertain, and indeed neurosis was eliminated from the third edition of the *Diagnostic and Statistical Manual of Mental Disorders* and subsequent classifications of psychiatric symptoms. Conflict during classical conditioning was studied first in Pavlov's laboratory. Dogs were classically conditioned to salivate to a circle but not to an ellipse. Increasingly finer discrimination was required as the ellipse was made more circular, and at the point at which the dog could no longer discriminate, it became very excited and restless and so-called "neurotic" behavior emerged. Pavlov considered himself a physiologist, not a behaviorist, and interpreted neurosis in terms of a balance between excitation and inhibition in the nervous system, with little concern for behavioral responses.

Complementary results were obtained by Liddell and collaborators at Cornell in his classical studies of conditioned leg withdrawal in sheep and goats. The animals were placed in restraining harnesses, and front leg withdrawal was induced with electric shock. Leg withdrawal was conditioned to positive (S^D) and negative (S^Δ) stimuli, and a battery of physiological measures to assess respiration and cardiac function was taken as the animal responded. As the number of trials in a session was increased, aberrant behavior emerged. Persistent movement of the conditioned limb occurred between trials; the goat became unwilling to enter the laboratory, had to be forced onto the conditioning stand, and heartbeat and respiration became erratic. Liddell's studies extended over many years, and he followed the social history of his subjects, their recovery, and the remission of their neurotic behavior. He reported that heartbeat in neurotic sheep is irregular under normal conditions (e.g., while they sleep at night), and also that they show marked frustration when mildly disturbing noises occur. Such neurotic animals are also incapable of dealing with a situation of actual change in a realistic manner. When dogs invaded the flock, it was invariably a neurotic sheep that was the victim. The animal's neurosis so damages its herd instinct that while other members of the flock escape together in one direction, the neurotic animal flees in panic in another. Clearly, both Pavlov and Liddell believed that their work on neurosis was relevant to human psychopathology.

At approximately the same time, animal models of neurosis using conflict in operant conditioning situations were described. For example, cats trained to open a box puzzle for food reward subsequently received a strong puff of air or electric shock. Box opening is suppressed by this punishment procedure, and complex patterns of abnormal behaviors were seen in the animals. Masserman interpreted these behaviors from a psychoanalytical perspective and quantified them with a descriptive rating scale of enormous complexity that did not prove useful for dissociating the effects of drugs on neurosis. However, from this work emerged paradigms such as the Geller–Seifter conflict schedule for quantifying response suppression in an operant situation.

Model Systems for Studying Abnormal Behavior

Although it has been essential to understand the control of normal behavior before considering the abnormal, it is toward the abnormal that behavioral pharmacology turns since much of its concern centers on drugs that are used to modify abnormal behavioral responses in humans. Therefore, we emphasize that identification of well-controlled components of behavior in normal animals is critical to the development of animal models of human mental disorders. There is every reason to hypothesize that human behavior is controlled by the same basic contingencies as is behavior in the rat or pigeon. The difference in humans is that their interaction with the environment is far more complex, and the mosaic of controlling factors is accordingly much larger and more difficult to identify. However, progress can be made in understanding complex human behavior even by applying the comparatively simple principles gleaned from the pigeon's behavior. Ferster draws analogies of this kind and states, "Animal experiments do not tell us why a man acts but they do tell us where to look for factors of which his behavior is a function." Ferster maintains that when drugs are used to ameliorate mental illness, they do not induce normality by creating behavior missing from the repertoire. Drugs can only influence the existing repertoire, modulating the complex relationship between controlling stimuli and behavioral responses.

The following important determinants influence the effect of a drug on a particular pattern of behavior: (1) the ongoing behavior determined by the schedule of reinforcement and the nature of the reinforcer, (2) the rate of ongoing behavior manipulated with the use of multiple schedules, (3) the presence of discriminative stimuli both extero- and interoceptive, and (4) aversive stimuli as negative reinforcers or punishment. These principles have been investigated extensively by behavioral pharmacologists of the Skinnerian school, typified by the work of Dews and colleagues (reviewed by Barrett, 2006). However, other factors are more difficult to control for, such as (1) the context in which the behavior occurs, (2) the behavioral history of the animal or human, and (3) previous experience of the drug in different situations. Indeed, these factors may well be of particular significance for human psychopharmacology.

In discussing normal behavioral control, we have tried to stress the fact that the way reinforcing and punishing events are scheduled is more important for our understanding of behavior than the nature of the events. The same is true for behavior that appears to be abnormal. If such behavior is analyzed in sufficient detail, it is often possible to see that disordered behavior can be explained and that it has evolved from a particular combination and sequence of perfectly normal events.

With regard to mental illness and abnormal behavior in humans, there is a tendency to think that studies of social behavior, development, and maternal deprivation in animals are more relevant than the operant conditioning of simple responses. This may be so, but until we have identified more fully the spectrum of controlling stimuli for these aspects of complex behavior, they do not provide useful experimental baselines. It remains a fact that some of the simple techniques for manipulating behavior with aversive stimuli are the most useful for illustrating how, under certain conditions, stimuli may induce abnormal behavior and how drugs can modify this relationship.

SELECTED REFERENCES

Azrin, N. H. and W. C. Holtz (1966). "Punishment." In *Operant Behavior: Areas of Research and Application* (W. K. Honig, ed.). Appleton, New York, pp. 300–447.

Barrett, J. E. (2006). Behavioral determinants of drug action: The contributions of Peter B Dews. *J. Exp. Anal. Behav.* 86, 359–370.

Carlton, P. A. (1983). *A Primer of Behavioral Pharmacology*. Freeman, New York.

Ferster, C. B. (1966). Animal behavior and mental illness. *Psychol Rev.* 16, 345–356.

Geyer, M. and A. Markou (2002). The role of preclinical models in the development of psychotropic drugs. In: *Neuropsychopharmacology: The Fifth Generation of Progress* (K. Davis, D. Charney, J. Coyle, and C. Nemeroff, Eds.). Lippincott Williams & Wilkins, Philadelphia, pp. 446–455.

Iversen, S. D. and L. L. Iversen (1981). *Behavioral Pharmacology*. Oxford University Press, New York.

Kelleher, R. T. and W. H. Morse (1964). Escape behavior and punished behavior. *Fed. Proc.* 23, 808–817.

Schwartz, B, E. A. Wasserman, and S. J. Robbins (2002). *Psychology of Learning and Memory*. Norton, New York.

4

Receptors

Chemical signaling is the main mechanism by which biological function is controlled at all levels, from the single cell to the whole organism. Chemical recognition is the function of receptors, which, in addition to recognizing endogenous chemical signals, are the target of many important experimental and therapeutic drugs.

The concept that most drugs, hormones, and neurotransmitters produce their biological effects by interacting with receptor substances in cells is usually credited to the studies of Langley published in 1905. It was based on his observations of the extraordinary potency and specificity with which some drugs mimicked a biological response (*agonists*) while others prevented it (*antagonists*). However, a thorough review of the timeline for the concept of the receptor reveals that the concept actually arose earlier from Paul Ehrlich's rather than from Robert Langley's studies. The way Langley did his work with atropine, curare, and pilocarpine on denervated muscle has a good illustrative logic to it. The way Ehrlich did his was through selective cell staining and antibodies in 1890. The interested student can gain some insight from reviews by Rang and Maehle et al. as to how these divergent approaches led to the emergence and final acceptance of the drug receptor theory, which lies at the very heart of pharmacology. It was not until several decades later that Gaddum, Hill, and Clark independently described the quantitative characteristics of competitive antagonism between agonists and antagonists in combining with specific receptors in intact preparations. This receptor concept has been substantiated in the past decade by the actual isolation of macromolecular substances that fit all of the criteria of being receptors. To date, although not all have been cloned, receptors have been identified for all of the proven neurotransmitters as well as for histamine; a number of neuropeptides; and other cellular signal molecules such as prostaglandins, leukotrienes, and cannabinoids. In addition, as noted in Table 4–1, multiple receptors have been shown to exist for all of the biogenic amines, acetylcholine (ACh), γ-aminobutyric acid (GABA), histamine, opiates, and the amino acid transmitters. If receptors for all agents (e.g., hormones,

TABLE 4–1. Neurotransmitter Receptors

Adrenergic
   $\alpha_{1A}, \alpha_{1B}, \alpha_{1C}, \alpha_{1D}$
   $\alpha_{2A}, \alpha_{2B}, \alpha_{2C}, \alpha_{2D}$
   $\beta_1, \beta_2, \beta_3$
Dopaminergic
   D_1, D_2, D_3, D_4, D_5
GABAergic
   $GABA_A, GABA_{B1a}, GABA_{B1\gamma}, GABA_{B2}, GABA_C$
Glutaminergic
   NMDA, AMPA kainate, $mGluR_1, mGluR_2, mGluR_3, mGluR_4, mGluR_5, mGluR_6,$
      $mGluR_7$
Histaminergic
   H_1, H_2, H_3, H_4
Cholinergic
   Muscarinic: M_1, M_2, M_3, M_4, M_5
   Nicotinic: muscle, neuronal (α-bungarotoxin-insensitive),
      neuronal (α-bungarotoxin-sensitive)
Opioid
   $\mu_1, \mu_2, \mu_3, \delta_1, \delta_2, \kappa_1, \kappa_2, \kappa_3$
Serotonergic
   $5\text{-}HT_{1A}, 5\text{-}HT_{1B}, 5\text{-}HT_{1D}, 5\text{-}HT_{1E}, 5\text{-}HT_{1F}, 5\text{-}HT_{2A}, 5\text{-}HT_{2B}, 5\text{-}HT_{2C}, 5\text{-}HT_3, 5\text{-}HT_4,$
      $5\text{-}HT_5, 5\text{-}HT_6, 5\text{-}HT_7$
Glycinergic
   Glycine

GABA, γ-aminobutyric acid; NMDA, N-methyl-D-aspartate; AMPA, α-amino-3-hydroxy-5-methyl-4-isoxazole propionic acid; mGluR, metabotropic glutamate receptor; 5-HT, 5-hydroxytryptamine.
SOURCE: Watling, K. J. (Ed.) (2006). *The Sigma RBI Handbook of Receptor Classification and Signal Transduction,* 5th Edition, St. Louis, MO.

trophic factors, odorants, and peptides) in addition to the neurotransmitters were counted, a total of more than 1000 would not be surprising. This number would also include *orphan receptors*, which include cell surface receptors and nuclear receptors that have been cloned because of their similarity to known receptors but which have no known endogenous ligand.

Multiple receptors appear to proliferate at an uncontrollable rate, but this should be viewed skeptically until a physiological response to the ligand has been shown or a specific gene has been cloned and expressed. Some of the receptor subtypes have been identified only by binding techniques, which can lead to erroneous conclusions. All of the receptors for neurotransmitters and peptide hormones that have been studied, regardless of whether they have been isolated, are localized on the surface of the cell; only the receptors for steroid and thyroid hormones are intracellular.

After the discovery that the action of physostigmine (eserine) resulted from its anticholinesterase activity, it was assumed that most drugs acted by inhibiting an enzyme. However, it now appears that with few exceptions (an action on ion channels or transport proteins and some enzymes such as MAO and alcohol dehydrogenase), the mechanism of action of neuroactive drugs usually stems from their effect on specific receptors. Predictably, the current search for receptors is among the most intense areas in the neurosciences. This interest is not purely academic. The identification of adrenergic, dopaminergic, muscarinic, serotonergic, and histaminergic receptor subtypes has led to the synthesis of highly selective drugs that are considerably more specific than their prototypes, which were developed after general screening for activity. With advances in gene cloning and expression, increasingly more receptor subtypes are being identified, each presumably having its own function. This suggests that in the future drugs may be designed to fit a single receptor subtype, thus reducing the side effects associated with nonspecific drugs.

DEFINITION

In this rapidly developing field, considerable confusion has arisen as to what functional characteristics are required of an isolated, ligand-binding molecule to qualify as a receptor. This confusion, a semantic problem, developed after the successful isolation of macromolecules that exhibit selective binding properties, which made it mandatory to determine whether this material comprised both the binding element and the element that initiated a biological response or merely the former. Some investigators use the term *receptor* only when both binding and signal generation occur; they use the term *acceptor* if no biological response has been demonstrated. Others are content to ignore the bifunctional aspect and use *receptor* without specifications. In this chapter, we define a *receptor* as the binding or recognition component and refer to the element involved in the biological response as the *effector*, without specifying whether the receptor and effector reside in the same or separate units. The criteria for receptors will be dealt with soon; the biological response that is generated by the effector obviously has a wider range of complexity, from a simple one-step coupling to an unknown number of steps (Fig. 4–1).

ASSAYS

Basically, there are two ways to study the interaction of neurotransmitters, hormones, or drugs with cells. The first procedure (and until relatively recently

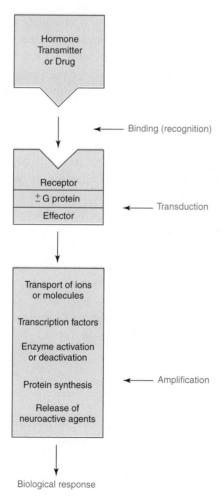

FIGURE 4–1. Schematic model of ligand–receptor interaction.

the only one) is to determine the biological response of an intact isolated organ, such as the guinea pig ileum, to applied agonists or antagonists. The disadvantage of this procedure is that one is obviously enmeshed in a cascade of events beginning with transport, distribution, and metabolism of the agent before it even interacts with a receptor, ranging through an unknown multiplicity of steps before the final biological response of the tissue is measured. Thus, although studies with agonists may be interpretable, it is not difficult to envision problems when antagonists are employed since these compounds may compete at a level different from receptor binding. Despite the not unusual problem of a nonlinear relationship between receptor occupancy and biological response, this approach has yielded a considerable amount of information. The second approach to studying receptors is by measuring ligand binding to a homogenate or slice preparation. This technique became feasible with the development of ligands of a high specific radioactivity and a high affinity for the receptor. Here, the direct method is to incubate labeled agonist or antagonist with the receptor preparation and then separate the receptor–ligand complex from free ligand by centrifugation, filtration, or precipitation. The indirect technique is to use equilibrium dialysis, where the receptor–ligand complex is determined by subtracting the ligand concentration in the bath from that in the dialysis sac.

It is also possible to apply an electrophysiological approach to identifying receptors. Intracellular stimulation and recording via microelectrodes inserted into a brain slice or neurons in culture, combined with the application of receptor agonists and antagonists, can functionally identify receptor subtypes.

Although not always appreciated, the advantage of using isolated tissues is that both the efficacy and the functional activity of an agonist are assessed, in contrast to binding procedures using broken cell preparations, where only affinity or a biochemical sequela of binding can be appraised. Ideally, both techniques should be used, but this is rarely done. It should be noted that efficacy and affinity are independent. To date, it appears that the drugs that exhibit high affinity but low efficacy have more efficient coupling to the effector than the reverse situation; therefore, these are the most potent and selective agents. For a detailed discussion of this topic, the review by Kenakin et al. (1992) is recommended.

IDENTIFICATION

In the midst of an intensive drive to isolate and characterize receptors, some zealous investigators have lost sight of the basic tenets that must be satisfied before it is certain that a receptor has indeed been isolated. Thus, occasionally, enzymes, transport proteins, and merely extraneous lipoproteins or proteolipids that exhibit binding properties have been mistakenly identified as receptors. Authentic receptors should have the following properties:

1. *Saturability*. The great majority of receptors are on the surface of a cell. Since there are a finite number of receptors per cell, it follows that a dose–response curve for the binding of a ligand should reveal saturability. In general, specific receptor binding is characterized by high affinity and low capacity, whereas nonspecific binding usually exhibits high capacity and low-affinity binding that is virtually nonsaturable.

2. *Specificity*. This is one of the most difficult and important criteria to fulfill because of the enormous mass of nonspecific binding sites compared with receptor sites in tissue. For this reason, in binding assays it is necessary to explore the displacement of the labeled ligand with a series of agonists and antagonists that represent both the same and different chemical structures and pharmacological properties as the binding ligand. One should also be aware of the avidity with which inert surfaces bind ligands. For example, substance P binds tenaciously to glass, and insulin can bind to talcum powder in the nanomolar range. With agents that exist as optical isomers, it is of obvious importance to show that the binding of the ligand is stereospecific. Even here, problems arise. With opiates it is the levorotatory enantiomorph that exerts the dominant pharmacological effect. Snyder, for example, has found glass fiber filters that selectively bind the levorotatory isomer. Specificity obviously means that one should find receptors only in cells known to respond to the particular transmitter or hormone under examination. Furthermore, a correlation should be evident between the binding affinity of a series of ligands and the biological response produced by this series. This correlation, the *sine qua non* for receptor identification, is unfortunately a criterion that is not often investigated.

3. *Reversibility*. Since transmitters, hormones, and most drugs act in a reversible manner, it follows that their binding to receptors should be reversible. Also, the ligand of a reversible receptor should be not only dissociable but also recoverable in its natural (i.e., nonmetabolized) form. This last dictum distinguishes receptor–agonist interactions but not receptor–antagonist binding from enzyme–substrate reactions.

4. *Restoration of function upon reconstitution*. Following the isolation and identification of the components of the receptor system, to "put Humpty Dumpty back together again" is the goal of all receptorologists.

5. *Molecular neurobiology*. The ultimate identification is to isolate the gene for a receptor, express it, and demonstrate the exact similarity of the cloned receptor to the natural one.

One method used to study the quantitative and spatial distribution of receptors utilizes autoradiography, but there can be several key problems. Where labeled ligands are employed to map neurotransmitter receptors in brain via light microscopy, a mismatch between neurotransmitter and receptor is often encountered. The following reasons are given for this problem: (1) Except for autoreceptors, neurotransmitters and receptors are located in different neurons; (2) in addition to the synapse, receptors and transmitters are found throughout the neuron and in glial cells; (3) ligands may label only a subunit of a receptor or only one state of the receptor; and (4) autoradiography is subject to quenching. With an alternative method, immunohistochemical peptide mapping, a possible problem is the recognition by the antibody of a prohormone or, alternatively, a fragment of a peptide hormone in addition to the well-recognized problem of cross-reactivity of the antibody with a physiologically different peptide.

Finally, all drugs do not necessarily act directly on a receptor. They could bind to a site that is adjacent to a receptor and thus influence the activity of the receptor.

As noted in Chapter 2, chemical synaptic transmission plays a fundamental role in the process of neuron-to-neuron and neuron-to-effector cell communication. The type of receptor present in the plasma membrane determines the response of a neuron or effector cell to a transmitter. The response elicited can be mediated through either direct opening of an ion channel (inotropic receptors) or alteration in the concentration of intracellular metabolites (metabotropic receptor). The magnitude of the response is determined by receptor number, the state of the receptors, and the amount of transmitter released. The response can be excitatory or inhibitory. The spatial or temporal summation of information conveyed by receptor activation determines whether the postsynaptic cell will generate an action potential or whether the effector cell (muscle) will contract.

SIGNAL TRANSDUCTION

Currently, there are four major groups of receptors known to be involved in signal transduction (Fig. 4–2), of which as mentioned above only two are *neurotransmitter-activated*.

The first group is referred to as *ligand-gated channels* or *ionotropic channels*. This group is composed of multiple subunits with a central pore, which, when activated, open to permit the passage of Na^+, K^+, Ca^{2+}, or Cl^+. Thus, depending on which ion is involved, the membrane potential may be either depolarized or hyperpolarized. Since no second messenger biochemical systems are involved, the effects of neurotransmitters on these cell surface

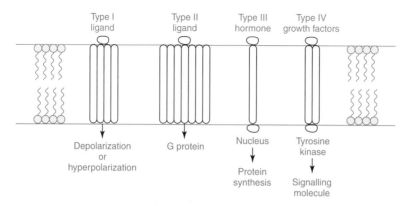

FIGURE 4–2. Type I is the ionotropic or ligand-gated receptor with a response time of milliseconds. An example is the nicotinic acetylcholine receptor. Type II is the metabotropic or G protein-linked receptor, generally modulatory, with a response time of minutes. Examples are the γ-aminobutyric acid$_B$ (GABA$_B$) and muscarinic receptors. Type III is the steroid receptor localized primarily on the nucleus rather than the cell membrane. The response time is usually minutes to hours, as exemplified by estrogen and thyroid hormones. Type IV represents the tyrosine kinase receptor, activated by insulin or growth factors, with a response time of minutes.

receptors are very fast, with excitatory and inhibitory responses occurring in milliseconds. Examples of these ionotropic receptors are the nicotinic ACh receptor, the *N*-methyl-D-aspartate receptor, the GABA$_A$ receptor, and the 5-hydroxytryptamine$_3$ (5-HT$_3$) receptor.

The second group of neurotransmitter-activated receptors that are also membrane localized are the G protein-coupled receptors, referred to as *metabotropic receptors*. These receptors mediate slower responses (seconds to minutes) that are generally modulatory, dampening, or enhancing the signal. All known G protein-coupled receptors contain seven hydrophobic transmembrane domains that are linked by hydrophilic groups. Examples of these receptors are muscarinic cholinergic, adrenergic, dopaminergic, serotonergic, metabotropic glutaminergic, opiate, peptidergic, and some purinergic receptors (*vida intra*). The structure of these receptors, as exemplified by the β$_2$-adrenergic receptor, is shown in Figure 4–3.

G proteins are a family of guanine nucleotide binding proteins with a heterotrimeric structure consisting of α, β, and γ subunits. When metabotropic receptors are activated, they bind a particular G protein to effect a response. To date, 22 different G protein α subunits and at least 5 β and 12 γ subunits have been identified. These proteins can be roughly classified into four groups: G$_s$, G$_i$, G$_q$, and G$_{12}$. Activation of the G$_s$ subunit family increases adenylyl cyclase activity, opens Ca^{2+} channels, and inhibits Na^1 channels. The G$_i$ subunit family opens K$^+$ channels, closes Ca^{2+} channels, inhibits adenylyl cyclase, and

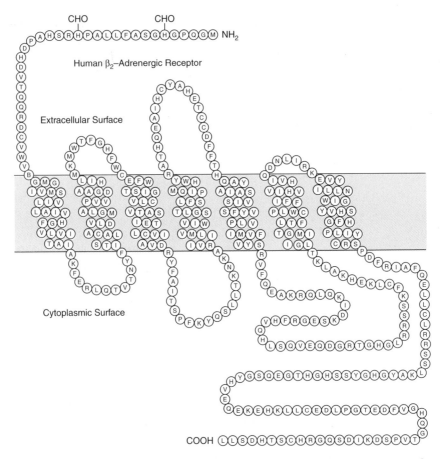

FIGURE 4–3. Topographical representation of the primary sequence of the human β_2-adrenergic receptor. The receptor protein is illustrated as possessing seven hydrophobic regions, each capable of spanning the plasma membrane, thus creating extracellular and intracellular loops as well as an extracellular terminus and a cytoplasmic C-terminal region. (From Lefkowitz et al., 1989.)

promotes cyclic guanosine monophosphate phosphodiesterase and probably phospholipase A_2. Increased phospholipase C is the effector for G_q, whereas with G_{12}, which activates Rho, a guanosine triphosphate (GTP)-binding protein, there is no other known function (a dysfunctional family?). Also recently recognized are a family of more than two dozen regulators of G protein signaling (RGS) that promote desensitization by activating GTPase. Of course, these RGS proteins, which may have other functions, are in turn regulated. To add to this bewildering complexity in neuronal signaling, in addition to the fact that a single receptor can activate multiple G proteins that may or may not interact, cloning studies have revealed multiple isoforms of adenylyl cyclase, phospholipase C, phospholipase A_2, and calcium and potassium channels.

An observation that has helped assign G proteins a role in signal transduction is that bacterial toxins catalyze the nicotinamide-adenine dinucleotide-dependent adenosine disphosphate ribosylation of the α subunit of many of the G proteins and inhibit their activity. Cholera toxin ribosylates G_s and G_t, whereas G_i and G_o are substrates for pertussis toxin. Some G proteins (unclassified) are resistant to both toxins.

The G protein-coupled receptors (GPCRs) are the largest class of cell surface receptors and are encoded by more than 1000 genes in the human genome. GPCRs are activated by a diverse array of endogenous ligands and transduce signals through a wide range of effectors. Thus, it is not surprising that these receptors modify a broad range of central nervous system activity, numerous diseases and disorders have been linked to mutations and polymorphisms in GPCRs, and they are targets of a large number of therapeutic agents. Their importance is indicated by the fact that approximately half of the drugs used in clinical practice directly or indirectly modify the actions of GPCRs.

Contrary to a large number of membrane proteins (e.g., tyrosine kinase receptors), GPCRs were initially considered to be monomeric entities, coupling to a single G protein heterotrimer with a 1:1 stoichiometry. However, in recent years much data have accumulated that challenged this view suggesting that some GPCRs can exist as dimers or higher-order oligomers. Until a few years ago, virtually all therapeutics directed toward GPCRs were designed using assays that presumed that these receptors were monomeric. The discovery that the functional GABA$_B$ receptor is an obligate heterodimer and the realization that a number of CPCRs form homo-oligomeric and hetero-oligomeric complexes have added a new dimension to rational drug design. Receptor–receptor interactions within receptor mosaics have had a significant impact on neuropsychopharmacology (Fuxe et al., 2008).

The third group are receptors for steroid hormones, thyroid hormones, vitamin D, and retinoic acids. These lipophilic ligands penetrate the cell, where they bind to the nuclear DNA to stimulate transcription. Response to hormones usually occurs in hours. Receptors for steroid hormones have previously been thought to be only intracellular since the hormones act on nuclear DNA to alter gene expression. This action is referred to as a *genomic* effect and usually takes hours to days to be observed. These genomic actions include the induction of neurotransmitter enzymes, receptors, and dendritic spines. However, evidence has accumulated that steroid receptors are also found on membranes. The hormone's *nongenomic* effects, occurring in seconds to minutes, act on the GABA$_A$ receptor to modulate chloride flux (see Chapter 6) and modulate a variety of other receptors (Fig. 4–4). The major players in this activity are progesterone and its metabolites, estrogens, testosterone, and adrenal steroids. The neuroactive steroids, some of which can be synthesized in the brain, may be sedative, anxiolytic, antidepressant, or anticonvulsant.

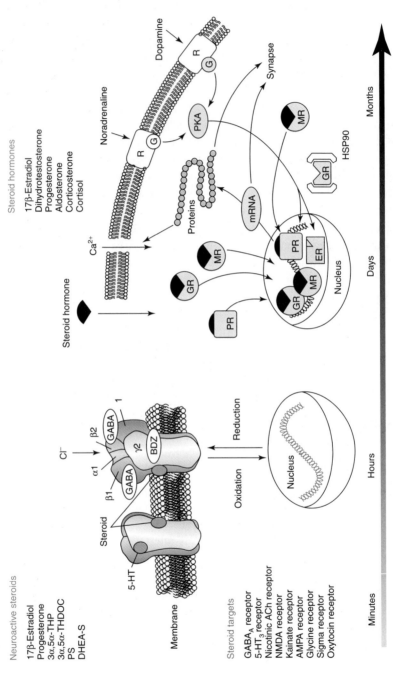

Neuroactive steroids

17β-Estradiol
Progesterone
3α,5α-THP
3α,5α-THDOC
PS
DHEA-S

Steroid targets

GABA$_A$ receptor
5-HT$_3$ receptor
Nicotinic ACh receptor
NMDA receptor
Kainate receptor
AMPA receptor
Glycine receptor
Sigma receptor
Oxytocin receptor

Steroid hormones

17β-Estradiol
Dihydrotestosterone
Progesterone
Aldosterone
Corticosterone
Cortisol

Membrane

5-HT

Steroid

β1

α1 β2

GABA

γ2

GABA 1

BDZ

Cl⁻

Nucleus

Oxidation

Reduction

Steroid hormone

Ca²⁺

Proteins

Dopamine

R

G

R

G

Noradrenaline

PKA

mRNA

Synapse

MR

HSP90

GR

PR

ER

MR

GR

MR

GR

PR

Nucleus

Minutes   Hours   Days   Months

Nongenomic effects   Genomic effects

The fourth group are the tyrosine kinase receptors, now numbering approximately 100, differing from other receptors in that the kinase activity is part of the receptor. Localized in the cell membrane, these receptors are activated by insulin and a number of growth factors, including nerve growth factor. In the presence of a ligand, the receptor dimerizes, activating the kinase to autophosphorylate. The subsequent phosphotyrosine residues provide acceptor sites for a variety of proteins.

Many neuroactive agents act on receptors that are coupled to the adenylyl cyclase system (Fig. 4–5). The components of this complex are the receptor, the catalytic portion of adenylyl cyclase that converts adenosine triphosphate (ATP) to cyclic adenosine monophosphate, and two G proteins referred to as G_s and G_i that are coupled to the catalytic unit of the enzyme. When the receptor is stimulated (e.g., a β_2-adrenergic receptor), the coupling protein is G_s. Conversely, when the receptor is inhibited (e.g., an α_2-adrenergic receptor), G_i is the coupling protein. Examples of adrenergic receptors whose activity is linked to the adenylate cyclase complex are the receptors α_2, β_1, and β_2 (but not α_1, which may be coupled to phosphatidyl inositide hydrolysis).

RECEPTOR DESENSITIZATION

Receptor desensitization is an important built-in mechanism, involving a complex series of events, for decreasing the cellular response to a given transmitter. For GPCRs there are two known mechanisms involved in desensitization. One rapid mechanism brought about by phosphorylation is a covalent modification of the receptor that occurs over a time frame of seconds to minutes. The other mechanism involves physical removal of the receptor by a process of

---

FIGURE 4–4. Nongenomic and genomic effects of neuroactive steroids. The term *neuroactive steroids* has been coined for steroids that interact with neurotransmitter receptors. Modulation of neuronal excitability by neuroactive steroids occurs over a very short (milliseconds to a few seconds) time period. The list on the top left-hand corner shows steroids that fulfill the criteria for neuroactive steroids; the bottom list gives neurotransmitter receptors that are targets for steroid modulation. The right-hand side of the figure describes the classical model of steroid hormone action via the steroid receptor cascade at the genomic level, which takes place over minutes to hours. The list on the right-hand side gives the names of typical steroid hormones. Certain steroids, such as 17β-estradiol and progesterone, have to be defined both as steroid hormones and as neuroactive steroids. BDZ, benzodiazepine; DHEAS, dehydroepiandrosterone sulfate; ER, estrogen receptor; G, G protein; GR, glucocorticoid receptor; HSP90, heat shock protein 90; MR, mineralocorticoid receptor; PKA, protein kinase A; PR, progesterone receptor; PS, pregnenolone sulfate; R, receptor; THDOC, tetrahydrodeoxycorticosterone; THP, tetrahydroprogesterone. (From Upprecht and Holsboer, 1999.)

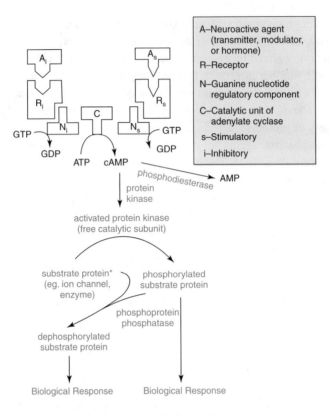

FIGURE 4–5. Components of a receptor-activated, cyclic nucleotide-linked system. (From Lefkowitz et al., 1984.)

receptor-mediated endocytosis and occurs over a longer time frame of minutes to hours. This latter process can be irreversible downregulation (degradation) or reversible sequestration (Kobilka, 1992).

Continued administration of agonists can cause many receptors to desensitize and downregulate. Desensitization, occurring on a timescale of minutes, is reflected by a decreased response of the cell and is often related to receptor phosphorylation. Downregulation of receptors is observed on a timescale of hours after prolonged agonist exposure when receptors are internalized and degraded. Conversely, and predictably, continued administration of receptor antagonists generally causes upregulation of receptors.

Finally, although not classified as receptors, another class of proteins that deserves mention is the transport proteins. With the exception of ACh, the action of all neurotransmitters that are released is terminated primarily by reuptake into their presynaptic terminals (amino acid transmitters can also be taken up by glial cells). ACh is hydrolyzed by acetylcholinesterase, and it is choline that is recaptured by the cholinergic terminal. Neurotransmitter transport proteins are relatively specific for each transmitter, are sodium dependent, exhibit high-affinity kinetics, and are dependent on the membrane potential of the neuronal terminal. The GABA and glutamate transporters have the ability to function in reverse, transporting the transmitters out of the cell. Cloned plasma membrane neurotransmitter transporters are categorized into two families—one that includes transporters for monoamines and GABA, containing 12 transmembrane domains, and one for glutamate and aspartate, whose topology is uncertain but likely to contain at least 8 transmembrane domains. As discussed in the chapters on each neurotransmitter, these reuptake systems are the basis of the mechanism of action of many neuropharmacological agents, particularly the antidepressant drugs and some drugs of abuse such as cocaine.

The transporters operate at the plasma membrane of terminals and are different from intracellular vesicular transporters, which accumulate transmitters into synaptic vesicles. Vesicular transporters, many of which have been cloned, operate via a vacuolar type H^+-pumping ATPase. This proton pump generates an H^+ electrochemical gradient whereby the efflux of H^+ is coupled to the reuptake of the transmitter into the vesicles.

MODULATION OF SYNAPTIC TRANSMISSION

Contrary to what one might assume, the more we learn about intercellular communication in the nervous system, the more complicated the situation appears. Until approximately the mid-1970s, synaptologists smugly focused on a straight point-to-point transmission, where a presynaptically released transmitter impinged on a postsynaptic cell. Gradually, situations emerged in which previously identified neurotransmitters were observed to not act in this manner but, rather, to modulate synaptic transmission. These departures from the previous norm and the continuing discovery of peptides and small molecules such as adenosine, which exhibited neuroactivity but did not appear to be transmitters in the classic sense, supported the broader view of modulation of synaptic transmission. In retrospect, it is a concept that should have been apparent early on since it imparts to neural circuitry an extraordinary degree of flexibility, which is necessary when considering the mechanisms of behavioral changes.

Definitions

Primarily via the activation of a receptor, synaptic transmission may be modulated either presynaptically or postsynaptically. With presynaptic modulation, regardless of the mechanism, the ultimate effect is a change in the amount of transmitter released. With postsynaptic modulation, the ultimate effect is a change in the firing pattern of the postsynaptic neuron or in the activity of a postsynaptic tissue (e.g., blood vessel, gland, and muscle). Because some confusion has arisen regarding the correct nomenclature of pre- and postsynaptic receptors, an explanation is in order. What may be classified as a presynaptic receptor on neuron B may be a postsynaptic receptor of neuron A that is making an axoaxonic contact with neuron B (see Fig. 2–3). Thus, depending on which neuron is being investigated, the receptor will be denoted as either pre- or postsynaptic.

Procedures to localize activity at the presynaptic receptor level in a terminal include (1) the use of synaptosomes; (2) the addition of tetrodotoxin to the preparation to block action potentials in neighboring interneurons; (3) patch clamping presynaptic terminals; (4) imaging techniques using appropriate dyes; or (5) where feasible, either chemical destruction of terminals or lesioning of the neuron and then demonstration by ligand binding of loss of the receptor. To complete the nomenclature on presynaptic receptors, an *autoreceptor* is located on the terminal or somatic–dendritic area of a neuron that is activated by the transmitter(s) released from that neuron. A *heteroreceptor* is a presynaptic receptor activated by a modulating agent that originates from a different neuron or cell. As discussed in Chapter 2, modulators differ from transmitters in that they have no intrinsic activity but modulate ongoing neural activity. However, a transmitter may modulate at a concentration that is subthreshold for transmitter activity. As we now detail, there exists an extraordinary number of possibilities for altering the point-to-point synaptic transmission mentioned previously.

Presynaptic Modulation

1. Receptor activation of a presynaptic neuron causing the following:

    a. A change in the firing frequency in the presynaptic neuron. This is probably the most common type of modulation, particularly in the central nervous system, where it can be assumed that the firing rate of virtually every neuron is governed by inputs on dendrites, soma, or axons. The firing rate determines the frequency of impulse conduction, hence the spread of action potentials into terminals or varicosities and the amount of transmitter that is liberated.

    b. A change in the transport or reuptake of a transmitter or precursor or in the synthesis, storage, release, or catabolism of a transmitter. All of these possibilities will result in a change in the concentration of a transmitter at the terminal. In practice, it has been shown that presynaptic activation of biogenic amine neurons promotes the phosphorylation of both tyrosine and tryptophan hydroxylase, which increases the synthesis of norepinephrine, dopamine, and serotonin. Curiously, phosphorylation of the pyruvate dehydrogenase complex causes a decrease in enzyme activity and in theory would decrease acetylcholine levels of (ACh) and the amino acid transmitters. To date, however, modulation of this enzyme activity by presynaptic receptor activation has not been observed.

c. An effect on ion conductances at the terminal. The three ions and their respective channels that one might focus on would be K^+, Ca^{2+}, and Cl^+. Endogenous neuroactive agents or drugs could alter transmitter release by opening or blocking the channels or changing the kinetics of channel open time via the possible mediation of protein phosphorylation or other second messengers.

2. A direct effect of neuropharmacological agents on some element of the release process. This could be an effect of the modulating agent on vesicular apposition to a terminal, fusion, or fission.

It is noteworthy that presynaptic inhibitory or facilitatory autoreceptors and heteroreceptors are targets for a large number of therapeutic agents (Langer, 2008).

Postsynaptic Modulation

1. A long-term change in the number of receptors. This is not observed under normal physiological conditions. It is, however, commonly noted pharmacologically where the administration of a receptor agonist for a period of time will result in downregulation of the receptor, and, conversely, treatment with a receptor antagonist increases receptor density.

2. A change in the affinity of a ligand for a receptor. The classic example is the salivary nerve of the cat, where both ACh and vasoactive intestinal peptide (VIP) are co-localized. When VIP is released upon electrical stimulation, it increases the affinity of ACh for the muscarinic receptor on the salivary gland up to 10,000-fold, with a consequent increase in salivation.

3. An effect on ionic conductances. As discussed previously, this is frequency modulation. It is a postsynaptic effect on the first neuron in a relay, but it would be classified as a presynaptic effect on the second neuron. References to many of the neurons and modulating agents that have been investigated are given in the reviews by Langer (2008) and Levitan and Kaczmarek (2002). These reviews can be summarized by stating that virtually every neuronal pathway is modulated, and virtually every endogenous neuroactive agent has been shown in one preparation or another to be capable of affecting synaptic transmission. All of this information is descriptive. Figure 4–6 depicts a major pathway for modulation of synaptic transmission. Rapidly accumulating

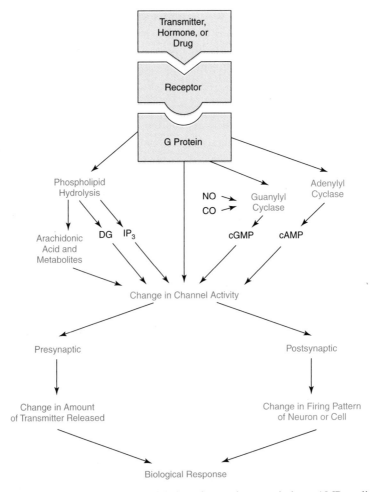

FIGURE 4–6. Major pathways for modulation of synaptic transmission. cAMP, cyclic adenosine monophosphate; cGMP, cyclic guanosine monophosphate; CO, carbon monoxide; DG, diacylglycerol; IP$_3$, inositol triphosphate; NO, nitric oxide.

evidence suggests that, in most cases of receptor-activated inhibitory presynaptic modulation, the ultimate effect is to open K channels. This hyperpolarizes terminals; less Ca^{2+} enters; and, as a consequence, less transmitter is released. Another major presynaptic mechanism is the inhibition of a calcium channel that would also decrease the evoked release of a transmitter. With the less common receptor-activated excitatory modulation, closing of a K channel has been implicated. A well-documented postsynaptic modulatory mechanism is that of a transmitter that inhibits a voltage-dependent K current, causing a subsequent depolarizing stimulus to produce an enhanced response.

Second Messenger Modulation

Second messenger systems play a major role in modulating synaptic transmission. Three major biochemical cascades (discussed here) and two gaseous messengers—nitric oxide and carbon monoxide (see Chapter 12)—have been described.

Protein Phosphorylation

Following the identification of cyclic nucleotides by Sutherland and associates and the implication that they act as a second messenger system preceded by an initial nerve impulse or hormonal signal, Krebs and colleagues demonstrated a multistep sequence of events that linked cyclic adenosine monophosphate (cAMP) generation in muscle to the regulation of carbohydrate metabolism. Since that time, the cyclic nucleotides have been shown to regulate an enormous diversity of processes ranging from axoplasmic transport to neuronal differentiation and including transmitter synthesis and release and the generation of postsynaptic potentials. All of these effects are attributable to the cAMP- or cyclic guanosine monophosphate (cGMP)-activating protein kinases and thus protein phosphorylation. Second messenger activity, achieved via protein phosphorylation, can be mediated by cAMP- and cGMP-dependent protein kinases as well as by calcium–calmodulin-dependent protein kinase and calcium–phosphatidylserine- or calcium–diacylglycerol-dependent protein kinase (protein kinase C). The phosphoryl acceptor in these proteins is the hydroxyl group of serine, threonine, or tyrosine, with the first two being the most prominent. All protein kinases can be autophosphorylated, a process that usually increases kinase activity. Although in most instances biological activity results from kinase-activated phosphorylation of a substrate protein, in some cases it is phosphatase-activated dephosphorylation of a phosphorylated protein that produces the biological response. Eight phosphoprotein phosphatases have been identified (protein phosphatase-2B is also referred to as calcineurin and is regulated by proteins referred to as immunophilins). Phosphatases are categorized into two broad classes: phosphoserine/phosphothreonine phosphatases and phosphotyrosine phosphatases.

Yet another level of regulation, noted previously, is suggested by the finding that protein phosphatase activity can be inhibited by other proteins, the most interesting of which is DARPP-32, found in D_1 dopaminoceptive neurons. DARPP-32 (dopamine- and cAMP-regulated phosphoprotein of 32 kDa), by acting as a protein phosphatase inhibitor when it is phosphorylated, can regulate the postsynaptic effects of dopamine in dopaminoceptive cells. Phosphorylated DARPP-32 is inactivated by protein phosphatase-2B. In some instances, Ca^{2+} acts as a second messenger without the participation of protein phosphorylation. The diversity of signals that are coupled to protein phosphorylation is

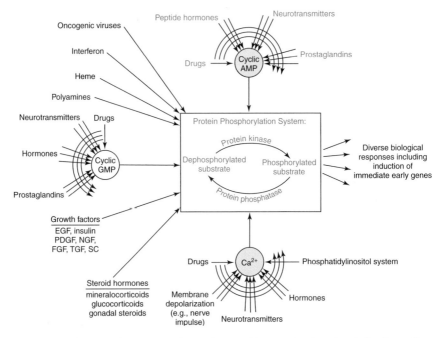

FIGURE 4–7. Schematic diagram of the role played by protein phosphorylation in mediating some of the biological effects of a variety of regulatory agents. Many of these agents regulate protein phosphorylation by altering intracellular levels of a second messenger, cyclic adenosine monophosphate (AMP), cyclic guanosine monophosphate (GMP), or Ca^{2+}. Other agents appear to regulate protein phosphorylation through mechanisms that do not involve these second messengers. Most drugs regulate protein phosphorylation by affecting the ability of first messengers to alter second messenger levels (curved arrows). A small number of drugs (e.g., phosphodiesterase inhibitors and Ca^{2+} channel blockers) regulate protein phosphorylation by directly altering second messenger levels (straight arrows). EGF, epidermal growth factor; FGF, fibroblast growth factor; NGF, nerve growth factor; PDGF, platelet-derived growth factor; SC, somatomedin C; TGF, transforming growth factor. (Modified from Nestler and Greengard, 1999.)

depicted in Figure 4–7. (For a molecular illustration of receptor coupling, see Fig. 4–3)

Despite the vast number of systems in which protein phosphorylation is implicated—more than 500—there are currently only approximately 20 cases in which direct evidence links this process to modulation of synaptic transmission, either pre- or postsynaptically. It is not known if the proteins that make up the channels are phosphorylated or if the phosphorylated proteins are morphologically associated with the channels. At any rate, with more than 100 proteins in the brain that are known to be phosphorylated (Table 4–2), the story is far from complete. Questions that remain to be answered include the regulation of the enormous number of steps in the cascade and the substrate specificity of the phosphodiesterases, protein kinases, and phosphoprotein phosphatases.

TABLE 4–2. Classes of Neuronal Proteins Regulated by Phosphorylation

Enzymes involved in neurotransmitter biosynthesis and degradation
    Tyrosine hydroxylase
    Tryptophan hydroxylase

Neurotransmitter receptors
    β-Adrenergic receptors
    α_2-Adrenergic receptors
    Muscarinic cholinergic receptors
    Opioid receptors
    $GABA_A$ receptor subunits
    NMDA glutamate receptor subunits
    Non-NMDA glutamate receptor subunits
    Nicotinic acetylcholine receptor subunits

Neurotransmitter transporters
    Monoamine reuptake transporters
    Monoamine vesicle transporters

Ion channels
    Voltage-dependent Na^+, K^+, Ca^{2+} channels
    Ligand-gated channels
    Ca^{2+}-dependent potassium channels

Enzymes and other proteins involved in the regulation of second messenger
    G proteins
    Phospholipases
    Adenylyl cyclases
    Guanylyl cyclases
    Phosphodiesterases
    IP_3 receptor

Protein kinases
    Autophosphorylated protein kinases (protein kinases phosphorylating themselves)
    Protein kinases phosphorylated by other protein kinases (many examples)

Protein phosphatase inhibitors
    DARPP-32
    Inhibitors 1 and 2

Cytoskeletal proteins involved in neuronal growth, shape, and motility
    Actin
    Tubulin
    Neurofilaments (and other intermediate filament proteins)
    Myosin
    Microtubule-associated proteins
    Actin-binding proteins

Synaptic vesicle proteins involved in neurotransmitter release
    Synapsins I and II
    Clathrin
    Synaptophysin
    Synaptobrevin

(Continued)

TABLE 4–2. Classes of Neuronal Proteins Regulated by Phosphorylation: Modified from Hyman and Nestler (1993) *(Continued)*

Transcription factors
  CREB family members
  Fos and Jun family members
  STATs
  Steroid and thyroid hormone receptors
  NE-κB–IKB family

Other proteins involved in DNA transcription or mRNA translation
  RNA polymerase
  Topoisomerase
  Histones and nonhistone nuclear proteins
  Ribosomal protein S6
  eIF
  eEF
  Other ribosomal proteins

Miscellaneous
  Myelin basic protein
  Rhodopsin
  Neural cell adhesion proteins
  MARCKS
  GAP-43

This list is not intended to be comprehensive but, instead, to indicate the wide array of neuronal proteins regulated by phosphorylation. Some of the proteins are specific to neurons, but most are present in many cell types in addition to neurons and are listed here because their multiple functions in the nervous system include the regulation of neuron-specific phenomena. Not included are the many phosphoproteins present in diverse tissues, including brain, that play a role in generalized cellular processes, such as intermediary metabolism, and that do not appear to play a role in neuron-specific phenomena. NMDA, N-methyl-D-aspartate: CREB, cAMP response element-binding protein; STAT, signal-transducing activator of transcription; GAP-43, growth-associated protein of 43 kDa; MARCKS, myristoylated alanine-rich C, kinase substrate; IP_3, inositol trisphosphate; DARPP-32, dopamine and cAMP-regulated phosphoprotein of 32-kDa; GABA, γ-aminobutyric acid; eIF, eukaryotic initiation factor; eEF, eukaryotic elongation factor.
SOURCE: Modified from Hyman and Nestler (1993).

What cannot be overemphasized is the involvement of phosphorylation in virtually every aspect of neuronal function, including transmitter release, synthesis, and reuptake; ion channel activity; regulation of receptors; cytoskeleton proteins; gene expression; and possibly short-term memory (Nestler and Duman, 2006).

Phosphoinositide Hydrolysis

In 1953, Hokin and Hokin showed that the incorporation of inorganic phosphate (P_i) into phosphatidylinositol (PI) and phosphatidic acid (PA) in pancreatic slices was stimulated by ACh and ultimately resulted in the release of amylase. This receptor-activated hydrolysis of phosphoinositides is referred to as the *phosphatidylinositol effect*. For nearly 30 years after this report, the literature on this effect was replete with the traditional scientific jargon "it is tempting to speculate that ...," with no one having solid evidence as to whether the phosphoinositides or the inositol phosphates were the message and, if so, exactly what was the medium for the exchange. That this situation has now dramatically improved is shown in Figure 4–8.

The signals that initiate this transduction process in neuronal systems include ACh, norepinephrine, serotonin, histamine, glutamate bradykinins, substance P, vasopressin, thyrotropin-releasing hormone, neurotensin, VIP, nerve growth factor, and angiotensin acting on brain, sympathetic ganglia, salivary glands, iris smooth muscle, adrenal cortex, and neuronal tumor cells. Specific receptors that have been implicated are muscarinic cholinergic receptors, α_1-adrenergic receptors, the H1 histaminergic receptor, substance P, and the V1 vasopressin receptor. In each case, Ca^{2+} appears to be the intracellular second messenger that activates phosphoinositide hydrolysis. Like the specific GTP-binding proteins that link receptors to the adenylate cyclase system discussed previously, a specific GTP-binding protein is also coupled to the phosphodiesterase that catalyzes the hydrolysis of phosphatidylinositol 4, 5-bisphosphate. In addition to the G protein-linked receptor, it is now known that a tyrosine kinase-linked receptor is coupled to a specific phosphodiesterase (phospholipase C), which yields inositol 1,4,5-trisphosphate ($InsP_3$) and diacylglycerol.

Thus, as noted in Figure 4–8, the key participants in the transduction process are a G protein-linked receptor, a tyrosine kinase-linked receptor, and phosphodiesterases, yielding two separate second messengers—the water-soluble $InsP_3$ and the lipid-soluble diacylglycerol. The former mobilizes calcium (released in a wave form; i.e., *oscillatory*), which can act through calmodulin to phosphorylate specific proteins. The latter, by activating protein kinase C, a calcium–phosphatidylserine-dependent family of protein kinases, also phosphorylates specific proteins. The $InsP_3$ receptor, associated with the smooth endoplasmic reticulum, is a tetramer of identical subunits that is regulated by ATP and cAMP. Since diacylglycerol can activate guanylate cyclase to produce cGMP, cGMP-dependent activity (protein kinase or otherwise) must be considered. With an assumed ambidexterity of neuronal cells, these two arms could function singly, cooperatively, or antagonistically, depending on the situation, thus providing subtle variations on the modulatory mechanism. In addition, as noted in Figure 4–8, calcium may produce a physiological response directly without invoking activation of calmodulin, so yet another control is indicated. On the subject of control, the activities of the various kinases, esterases, and phospholipases in the PI cycle would be expected to be vital control points. For example, five isoforms of phospholipase C have been

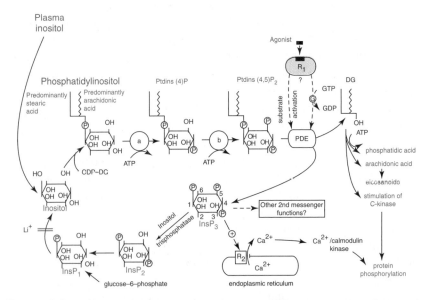

FIGURE 4–8. Receptor-activated phosphoinositide metabolism. The binding of an agonist to a receptor on the plasma membrane stimulates the hydrolysis of phosphatidylinositol 4,5-bis-phosphate [Ptdins (4,5)P$_2$] by a phosphodiesterase (PDE, phosphoinositidase, and phospholipase C), a specific phospholipase whose activity is controlled by a guanine nucleotide regulatory protein to form inositol 1,4,5-trisphosphate (InsP$_3$) and diacylglycerol (DG). The former binds to a receptor (R$_2$) on the endoplasmic reticulum to release calcium, which can directly produce a biological response or can activate calmodulin kinase to promote protein phosphorylation and a subsequent biological response. In some cells (e.g., mouse atria, neuroblastoma, and glioma hybrid NG108-15), receptor-activated production of InsP$_3$ requires extracellular Ca^{2+}.

The latter parallel arm of the cycle, diacylglycerol, can also promote a biological response via the production of prostaglandins, thromboxanes, and leukotrienes from released arachidonic acid (arachidonic acid has also been reported to stimulate guanylate cyclase to generate cyclic guanosine monophosphate) or via stimulation of protein kinase C (C-kinase) and subsequent protein phosphorylation. Diacylglycerol has also been reported to promote fusion of synaptic vesicles to terminal membrane. Diacylglycerol can also be generated from phosphatidylcholine via phospholipase D followed by phosphatidic acid phosphatase.

The phosphoinositides are synthesized from inositol with cytidine diphosphate:diacylglycerol (CDP-DG) as intermediary and the stepwise phosphorylation by kinases (a and b). As shown in the figure, lithium blocks the cycle by inhibiting inositol-1-phosphate. Although the antimanic activity of lithium has been ascribed to this inhibitory effect, the evidence is not compelling. ATP, adenosine triphosphate; GDP, guanosine diphosphate; GTP, guanosine triphosphate. (Modified from Berridge and Irvine, 1984.)

identified, of which some are enriched in specific brain areas. Free inositol in the brain must be derived from glycolysis since plasma inositol cannot pass the blood–brain barrier to any significant degree. Therefore, glycolysis would be another regulatory factor in the response mechanism.

Finally, although the origin of the mobilized calcium is now clear (it is released from endoplasmic reticulum and mitochondria), some controversy remains as to whether phosphoinositide hydrolysis releases only internal calcium or whether external calcium influx is also invoked. Evidence suggests that for neuronal modulation both or either may be involved, depending on the preparation. The same answer can also be given as to whether the PI effect is presynaptic or postsynaptic. A complication in the PI cycle that has recently surfaced is the finding that the inositol triphosphate that is produced is not always or only $Ins(1,4,5)P_3$ but may be $Ins(1,3,4)P_3$ as well as $InsP_4$, $InsP_5$, and $InsP_6$. The physiological role of these polyphosphate compounds is unknown, but they may function as phosphate donors.

Eicosanoids (Arachidonic Acid Metabolites)

Arachidonic acid, synthesized from dietary linoleic acid, derived on demand by either a G protein-regulated phospholipase A_2 or diglyceride lipase activation yields a bewildering array of bioactive metabolites. The three major groups are prostaglandins, thromboxanes, and leukotrienes (Fig. 4–9). These mediators act on a family of G protein-coupled receptors that display selectivity for the different prostanoids or leukotrienes.

Direct evidence has implicated arachidonic acid and lipoxygenases as second messengers. The cascade begins with the binding of a neuroactive agent to its receptor. Then, according to findings from the Axelrod laboratory, the receptor is coupled to G proteins, which may either activate or inhibit phospholipase A_2, although this has not been conclusively established for all neural tissues. The activated enzyme promotes the release of arachidonic acid, which will then act intracellularly as a second messenger. Arachidonic acid and its metabolites can also leave the cell to act extracellularly as first messengers on neighboring cells. Eicosanoids have been shown to mediate the somatostatin-induced opening of an M channel in hippocampal pyramidal cells and the release of VIP in mouse cerebral cortical slices. It is thus becoming clear, despite enormous technological difficulties in assaying eicosanoids, that these agents are major messengers. Before we leave the arachidonic acid story, we should mention that the endocannabinoids, anandamide and 2-arachidonyl-glycerol, are formed from arachidonic acid metabolites. Anandamide is synthesized by transfer of an arachidonic acid-containing phospholipid to the amine group of phosphatidylethanolamine to form n-arachidonoyl-phosphatidyletholamine followed by phospholipase hydrolysis to yield anandamide (see endocannabinoids, Chapter 12).

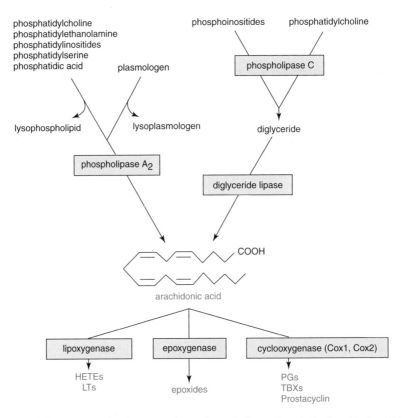

FIGURE 4–9. Pathways for the generation and metabolism of arachidonic acid. Arachido-nate can arise directly from phospholipids through the action of phospholipase A_2 or prior action of phospholipase C, followed by the action of diglyceride lipase. Alternatively, the diglyceride may be phosphorylated to phosphatidic acid by the action of diglyceride kinase, and arachidonate then can be released through the action of phospholipase A_2. The released arachidonate may then be metabolized by lipoxygenase, cyclooxygenase, or epoxygenase enzymes to form leukotrienes (LTs), hydroxyeicosatetraenoic acids (HETEs), prostaglan-dins (PGs), thromboxanes (TBXs), and epoxides. (Modified from Axelrod et al., 1988.)

Reflecting on the mechanisms available to nervous tissue to modulate syn-aptic transmission, one cannot fail to be overwhelmed by the almost infinite possibilities that provide the fine-tuning for behavioral changes. It may well turn out that the key player in this scenario is calcium. Since Ca^{2+} is released as a wave, its concentration as well as its translocation at discrete sites might dictate the modulatory effect of the attachment of a ligand to its receptor. It may also be the key to nonsynaptic cellular effects, such as cell movement or proliferation, gene expression, and metabolism, that involve second messen-ger systems. At any rate, one should be aware that the ultimate effect of cascades of second messenger systems, transcription factors, neurotrophic factors, transport factors, gene expression, or the endless numbers of signaling factors (irritatingly referred to by acronyms) is to cause a neuron to fire at a certain frequency or not to fire. It is that simple, except that a neuron may have 10,000 inputs dictating its ultimate effect on other neurons to which it is coupled.

It is hoped that one day it will be possible to understand the grand design in neuronal communication that leads to behavioral changes ranging from the subtle to the dramatic.

SELECTED REFERENCES

Axelrod, J. R. M. Burch, and C. L. Jelsema (1988). Receptor-mediated activation of phospholipase A$_2$ via GTP-binding proteins: Arachidonic acid and its metabolites as second messengers. *Trends Neurosci.* 11, 117.

Berridge, M. J., P. Lipp, and M. D. Bootman (2000). The versatility and unversatility of calcium signalling. *Nat. Rev. Mol. Cell. Biol.* 1, 11.

Bibb, J. A. and E. J. Nestler (2006). Serine and threonine phosphorylation. In *Basic Neurochemistry: Molecular, Cellular and Medical Aspects* (G. J. Siegel, R. W. Alpers, S. T. Brady, and D. L. Price, Eds.), 7th ed. Raven Press, New York, pp. 391–413.

Cooper, J. R., F. E. Bloom, and R. H. Roth (2002). *Biochemical Basis of Neuropharmacology*, 8th ed. Oxford University Press, New York.

Free, B. J., L. A. Hazelwood, Y. Namkung, M. L. Ranlin, E. B. Rex, and D. R. Sibley (2007). Synaptic transmission: Intracellular signaling. In *Handbook of Contemporary Neuropharmacology* (D. S. Sibley, I. Hanin, M. Kuhar, and P. Skolnick, Eds.). Wiley–Interscience, New York, pp. 59–106.

Fuxe, K., D. Marcellino, A. Rivera, S. Diaz-Cabiale, M. Filip, B. Gago, D. C. S. Roberts, U. Langel, S. Genedani, L. Ferraro, A. de la Calle, J. Narvaez, S. Tanganelli, A. Woods, and L. F. Agnati (2008). Receptor–receptor interactions within receptor mosaics. Impact on neuropsycopharmacology. *Brain Res. Rev.* 58(2), 415–452.

Groc, L. and D. Choquet (2008). Measurement and characteristics of neurotransmitter receptor surface trafficking. *Mol. Membr. Biol.* 25(4), 344–352.

Jonas, E. K. and L. K. Kaczmarek (1999). The inside story, subcellular mechanisms of neuromodulation. In *Beyond Neurotransmission* (P. S. Katz, Ed.). Oxford University Press, New York, p. 83.

Kenakin, T. (2004). Principles: Receptor theory in pharmacology. *Trends Pharmacol. Sci.* 25(4), 186–192.

Kenakin, T. P., R. A. Bond, and T. I. Bonner (1992). Definition of pharmacological receptors. *Pharmacol. Res.* 44, 351.

Kobilka, B. (1992). Adrenergic receptors as models for G-protein-coupled receptors. *Annu. Rev. Neurosci.* 15, 87–114.

Laduron, P. M. (1984). Criteria for receptor sites in binding studies. *Biochem. Pharmacol.* 33, 833.

Langer, S. Z. (2008). Therapeutic use of release-modifying drugs. *Handb. Exp. Pharmacol.* 184, 561–573.

Langley, J. N. (1905) On the reaction of cells and of nerve-endings to certain poisons, chiefly as regards the reaction of striated muscle to nicotine and curare. *J. Physiol.* 33, 374–413.

Leenders, A. G. M. and Z.-H. Sheng (2005). Modulation of neurotransmitter release by the second messenger-activated protein kinases: Implications for presynaptic plasticity. *Pharmacol. Ther.* 105, 69–84.

Lefkowitz, R. J., B. K. Kobilka, and M. G. Caron (1989). The new biology of drug receptors. *Biochem. Pharmacol.* 38, 2941.

Lefkowitz, R. J., M. G. Caron, and G. L. Stiles (1984). Mechanisms of membrane-receptor regulation. *N. Engl. J. Med.* 310, 1570.

Levitan, I. B. and L. K. Kaczmarek (2002). *The Neuron: Cell and Molecular Biology*, 2nd ed. Oxford University Press, New York.

Maehle, A.-H., C.-R. Prull, and R. F. Halliwell (2002). The emergence of the drug receptor theory. *Nat. Rev. Drug Discov.* 1(8), 637–641.

Milligan, G. and N. J. Smith (2007). Allosteric modulation of heterodimeric G-protein-coupled receptors. *Trends Pharmacol Sci.* 28(12), 616–620.

Nestler, E. J. and R. S. Duman (2006). G proteins. In *Basic Neurochemistry: Molecular, Cellular and Medical Aspects* (G. J. Siegel, R. W. Alpers, S. T. Brady, and D. L. Price, Eds.), 7th ed. Raven Press, New York, pp. 335–346.

Nestler, E. J. and P. Greengard (1999). Serine and threonine phosphorylation. In *Basic Neurochemistry: Molecular, Cellular and Medical Aspects* (G. J. Siegel et al., Eds.), 6th ed. Raven Press, New York, p. 471.

Peineau, S., C. Bradley, C. Taghibiglou, A. Doherty, Z. A. Bortolotto, Y. T. Wang, and G. L. Collingridge (2008). The role of GSK-3 in synaptic plasticity. *Br. J. Pharmacol.* 153, S428-S437.

Piomelli, D. (1994). Eicosanoids in synaptic transmission. *Crit. Rev. Neurobiol.* 8, 65–83.

Rang, H. P. (2006). The receptor concept: Pharmacology's big idea. *Br. J. Pharmacol.* 147, S9–S16.

Rupprecht, R. and A. F. Holsboer (1999). Neuroactive steroids: Mechanism of action and neuropsychopharmacological perspectives. *Trends Neurosci.* 22, 410.

Schimizu, T. and L. S. Wolfe (1990). Arachidonic cascade and signal transduction. *J. Neurochem.* 55, 1–15.

5

Amino Acid Neurotransmitters

On the basis of their functional actions, amino acid transmitters have been divided into two general categories: excitatory amino acid transmitters (glutamate [Glu], aspartate [Asp], cysteate, and homocysteate), which depolarize neurons in the mammalian central nervous system (CNS), and inhibitory amino acid transmitters (γ-aminobutyric acid [GABA], glycine [Gly], taurine, and β-alanine), which hyperpolarize mammalian neurons. A few amino acids have been demonstrated to fulfill most of the criteria for neurotransmitter candidates in the mammalian CNS. Among them are GABA, the major inhibitory transmitter in the brain; Glu, the major excitatory transmitter in the brain; and Gly, another important inhibitory transmitter in the brain stem, spinal cord, and hippocampus. This has not been an easy task since many amino acids are also involved in intermediary metabolism and obviously in protein synthesis, which makes it difficult to separate their biochemical role from their transmitter role. Agmatine, the decarboxylation product of arginine, has fulfilled many of these transmitter criteria and is the most recent addition to this family of transmitters. From a quantitative standpoint, the amino acids are probably the major transmitters in the mammalian CNS, whereas the better-known transmitters discussed in other chapters (acetylcholine, norepinephrine, dopamine, histamine, and 5-hydroxytryptamine) probably account for transmission at only a small percentage of central synaptic sites.

GLUTAMIC ACID

Long before a role for Glu in neurotransmission was established, it was recognized that certain amino acids, such as Glu and Asp, occur in uniquely high concentrations in the brain and that they can exert very powerful stimulatory effects on neuronal activity. Thus, if any amino acid is involved in the regulation of nerve cell activity, as an excitatory transmitter or otherwise, it seems unnecessary to look beyond these two candidates. The excitatory potency of Glu was first demonstrated in crustacean muscle and later by direct topical application to mammalian brain. However, except for the invertebrate model, where substantial evidence has accumulated to support a role for Glu as an excitatory neuromuscular transmitter, its status as a neurotransmitter in mammalian brain was uncertain for many years. This is probably in part explainable by the fact that Glu (and Asp) is a compound that is also intimately involved in intermediary metabolism in neural tissue. For example, it has an important function in the detoxification of ammonia in the brain, is an important building block in the synthesis of proteins and peptides including glutathione, and plays a role as a precursor for the inhibitory neurotransmitter GABA. Thus, it was extremely difficult to dissociate the role this amino acid plays in neuronal metabolism and as a precursor for GABA from its possible role as a transmitter substance. Transport of circulating Glu to the brain normally plays only a very minor role in regulating the levels of brain Glu. In fact, the influx of Glu from the blood across the blood–brain barrier is much lower than the efflux of Glu from the brain.

SYNTHESIS AND METABOLISM

In brain, L-Glu is synthesized in the nerve terminals from two sources: from glucose via the Krebs cycle and transamination of α-oxoglutatrate and from glutamine that is synthesized in glial cells, transported into nerve terminals, and locally converted by glutaminase into Glu (Fig. 5–1). In the Glu-containing nerve terminals, Glu is stored in synaptic vesicles and, upon depolarization of the nerve terminal, it is released by a calcium-dependent exocytotic process. The action of synaptic Glu is terminated by a high-affinity uptake process via the plasma membrane Glu transporter on the presynaptic nerve terminal and/or on glial cells. The Glu taken up into glial cells is converted by glutamine synthetase into glutamine, which is then transported via a low-affinity process into the neighboring nerve terminals, where it serves as a precursor for Glu. In astrocytes, glutamine can also be oxidized (via the Krebs cycle) into α-ketoglutarate, which can be actively transported into the neuron to replace the α-ketoglutarate lost during the synthesis of neuronal Glu. As noted

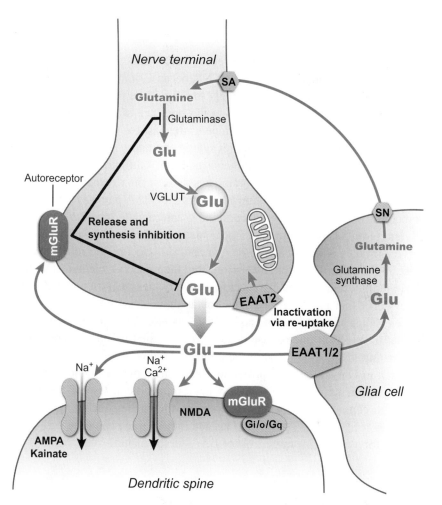

FIGURE 5–1. Glutamatergic axodendritic synapse illustrating pathways for glutamate utilization, metabolism, and signal transduction. Glutamate (Glu) released into the synaptic cleft is recaptured by neuronal-type excitatory amino acid (EAAT2) and glial-type (EAAT1/2) Na^+-coupled glutamate transporters. Glial Glu is converted to glutamine by the enzyme glutamine synthetase. Glutamine is transported out of glial cells by system N transporter (SN). Glutamine is present in high concentrations in the cerebral spinal fluid (approximately 0.5 mM) and can be transported into the neuron by the system A transporter (SA) to help replenish glutamate after hydrolysis by mitochondrial glutaminase. The postsynaptic dendrite contains both inotropic (AMPA and NMDA type) and metabotropic glutamate receptors (MGluR). AMPA, α-amino-3-hydroxy-5-methyl-4-isoxazole propinoic acid/glutamate receptor; NMDA, N-methyl-D aspartate/glutamate receptor; VGLUT, vesicular glutamate transporter.

later in this chapter, glutamine can replenish the transmitter pool of GABA via this pathway as well.

Although neuronal systems believed to utilize Glu or Asp as transmitter substances have been described in the CNS, because of their role in intermediary metabolism, it seems quite unlikely that it will be possible to map these systems accurately by simply tracking the presence of Glu or Asp or their synthesizing enzymes, as has been done in the past for the monoamines and GABA. The development of antibodies against excitatory amino acids (EAAs), especially antisera that can distinguish between Glu and Asp with a high degree of selectivity as well as antibodies against their receptors and transporters, has facilitated the anatomical mapping of EAA pathways. The development of reliable methods for combining anterograde labeling of primary afferent terminals with immunocytochemistry has helped to identify afferent nerve terminals enriched in Glu or Asp and to dissociate the role played by these amino acids in neurotransmission from their general role in metabolism. Nerve terminal enrichment in a specific EAA provides the most direct anatomical evidence that a pathway uses a particular amino acid as a neurotransmitter. The elegant studies of Rustioni and co-workers employing immunocytochemistry at the electron microscopic level have identified primary afferent fibers terminating in spinal laminae of the lumbar spinal cord with nerve terminals enriched in Glu and/or Asp, providing direct anatomical evidence that these primary afferents use these EAAs as neurotransmitters. Use of these techniques in conjunction with other less direct approaches, including mapping the EAA receptors by ligand-binding autoradiography, has provided strong support for a neurotransmitter role of EAAs in the mammalian CNS.

RELEASE

Although the status of Glu and Asp as neurotransmitters has suffered through many cycles of acceptability and nonacceptability in the past several decades, the rush to clone the Glu receptors and the extensive research on long-term potentiation demonstrating a function for Glu have stopped the doubters from speaking. Despite considerable evidence that Glu may be an excitatory transmitter in the CNS, little is known about the biosynthesis and release of the pool of releasable transmitter Glu. Utilizing the molecular layer of the dentate gyrus of the hippocampal formation to provide a definitive system in which the major input appears to be glutaminergic, Cotman and co-workers addressed these questions. Glu was shown to be released by depolarization from slices of the dentate gyrus in a Ca^{2+}-dependent manner, and lesions of the major input to the dentate gyrus originating from the entorhinal cortex diminished this release and the high-affinity uptake of Glu. Glu biosynthesis in the releasable pools was rapidly regulated by the activity of glutaminase and by uptake of glutamine. These properties are consistent with the properties expected of a neurotransmitter, and the observations strengthened the premise that Glu may be an important neurotransmitter in the molecular layer of the dentate gyrus. Furthermore, these studies demonstrated that the regulation of Glu synthesis and release share many properties with other transmitters. For example, similar to acetylcholine synthesis, Glu synthesis is regulated in part via the accumulation of its major precursor, glutamine, and newly synthesized Glu, like acetylcholine, is preferentially released. In addition, Glu synthesis is regulated by end-product inhibition. This is similar to the mechanism by which the rate-limiting enzyme in catecholamine synthesis, tyrosine hydroxylase, is regulated in catecholaminergic neurons by dopamine and norepinephrine. It is interesting that these similarities are demonstrable despite the involvement of Glu in general brain metabolism.

STORAGE

The vesicle hypothesis describing the quantal release of acetylcholine at the neuromuscular junction was introduced in the mid-1950s. Since then, the concept of vesicular storage and release of acetylcholine has become firmly established and has been extended to a number of other synapses and neurotransmitters. However, there was no direct experimental evidence for the participation of synaptic vesicles in the storage and release of EAA neurotransmitters until the late 1990s. At that time, the concept received strong support from the studies of Jahn and Ueda and co-workers on isolated synaptic vesicles from mammalian brain. These studies showed that vesicles are capable of Glu uptake and storage and that they have a specific carrier for L-Glu. This concept was finally validated with the cloning of the vesicular transporter for Glu. The difficulty in cloning this vesicular transporter is most likely due to the fact that it is unrelated to other known transmitter transporters, although it shares significant sequence homology with EAT-4, a worm protein implicated in glutamatergic transmission. The vesicular Glu transporter was identified as a protein that was previously suggested to mediate the sodium-dependent transport of inorganic phosphate across the membrane. It is found predominantly in axon terminals, particularly those that form asymmetric (excitatory) synapses. In contrast to the GABA transporter, for which Gly is also a substrate (see Release and Reuptake), the Glu vesicular transporter has a high specificity for Glu. This transporter has been extensively characterized biochemically and shown to play a key role in exocytosis. Three subtypes of vesicular glutamate transporter (VGLUT1, -2, and -3), consisting of approximately 600 amino acid residues, have been identified and appear to share more than 70% homology with one another. VGLUTs pack glutamate into synaptic vesicles so that they can be released into the synapse. VGLUT activity is dependent on a proton gradient that is created by hydrolyzing ATP. All the known subtypes of VGLUTs transport glutamate with an affinity that is 100- to 1000-fold lower than that of the excitatory amino transporters (EAATs) found in the plasma membrane (K_m approximately 1 mM versus K_m of 4–40 μm). Also in contrast to the EAATs, the VGLUTs do not appear to transport aspartate.

VGLUT subtypes are expressed differentially throughout the adult brain. VGLUT1 and -2 have a largely complementary distribution and are expressed in the terminals of all well-characterized glutamatergic synapses in brain and serve as a useful anatomical marker for their presence. VGLUT3, on the other hand, appears to be expressed in neuronal populations that release other classical neurotransmitters such as GABAergic interneurons in cortex and hippocampus, cholinergic neurons of the striatum, and in serotonin and catecholamine neurons. Unlike VGLUT1 and -2, it also has a distribution that is both axonal and somatodendritic.

PLASMA MEMBRANE GLU TRANSPORTERS

Most of the molecular biological research on EAA transmission has focused on receptors rather than the process of transmitter inactivation. Inactivation is an especially important process in EAA neurotransmission. The rapid removal of Glu from the synapse by high-affinity uptake not only serves to terminate the excitatory signal and recycle the Glu but also plays an important role in the maintenance of extracellular levels of Glu below those that could induce excitotoxic damage. Five distinct subtypes of EAAT have been identified, which together with the neutral amino acid transporters appear to be part of a novel gene family. These high-affinity, sodium-dependent EAATs exhibit distinct anatomical and cellular distributions and appear to have marked differences in pharmacological specificity (Table 5–1).

These Glu transporter genes share 50% sequence homology and exhibit minimal homology with other eukaryotic proteins, including the superfamily of neurotransmitter transporters that mediate the uptake of GABA, Gly, choline, and the biogenic amines. These Glu transporters have distinct brain distributions, and even the glial transporters exhibit regional and intracellular differences in expression, underscoring the heterogeneity of glia as well as neurons. All of the Glu transporters demonstrate a strong Na^+ dependence and are enantioselective (i.e., D-Asp, L-Asp, and L-Glu are substrates, whereas D-Glu is not). These transporters are also inhibited by well-characterized uptake blockers including β-threo-hydroxy-Asp, dihydrokainate, and L-*trans*-2,4-pyrrolidine decarboxylate. Preferential inhibition of several subtypes of EAAT can be achieved with several of the newer nonsubstrate antagonists.

TABLE 5–1. Distribution and Pharmacology of the Excitatory Amino Acid Transporters (EAATs)

SUBTYPE	PRIMARY LOCALIZATION	PHARMACOLOGICAL PROPERTIES
EAAT1 (GLAST1, rat)	Cerebellar glia	4-MG and L-SOS as substrates
EAAT2	Forebrain glia	DHK, MPDC, L-*trans*-2,3-PDC and 3-TMG as nontransportable inhibitors
EAAT3 (EAAC1, rabbit)	Cortical neurons	L-aspartate-β-hydroxamate as an inhibitor
EAAT4	Cerebellar Purkinje neurons	L-α-AA as a substrate
EAAT5	Retina	THA and L-*trans*-2,4-PDC as nontransportable inhibitors

4-MG, (2S,4R)-4-methylglutamate; L-SOS, L-serine-*O*-sulfate; DHK, dihydrokainic acid; 3-TMG, (±)-*threo*-3-methylglutamic acid; L-α-AA, L-α-aminoadipate; THA, β-*threo*-hydroxyaspartate; MPDC, L-anti-endo-3,4-methanopyrrolidine-3,4-dicarboxylate; PDC, pyrrolidine dicarboxylate; GLT1, glutamate transporter-L; EAAC1, excitatory amino acid carrier-L; GLAST1, glutamate-aspartate transporter.
SOURCE: Bridges (2001).

Neurons and glial cells appear to possess a similar plasma membrane glutamate uptake carrier that serves to terminate the postsynaptic action of neurotransmitter Glu and to maintain the extracellular Glu concentrations below levels that may damage neurons. The presence of certain Glu transporters on glial cells is consistent with the intricate interplay of glial and neuronal elements in the synthesis and fate of Glu. Because the Glu that is released from neurons is accumulated by glia and then metabolized to glutamine, there is an ultimate recycling of the released amino acid. The fate of Glu released from a neuron containing the neuronal Glu transporter is unclear. It has not been established if Glu released from a given neuron is taken up in part by a Glu transporter on that particular neuron or primarily by Glu transporters on other neurons or glia. Regardless, uptake appears to be the major process for terminating the action of released Glu. There does not appear to be any significant role for enzymatic inactivation of Glu similar to that observed with GABA, ACh, and the other classical neurotransmitters.

Based on abundant evidence, however, Glu appears to have satisfied four of the main criteria for classification as an excitatory neurotransmitter in the mammalian CNS: (1) It is localized presynaptically in specific neurons, where it is stored in and released from synaptic vesicles; (2) it is released by a Ca-dependent mechanism by physiologically relevant stimuli in amounts sufficient to elicit postsynaptic responses; (3) a mechanism (reuptake and specific transporters) exists that will rapidly terminate its transmitter action; and (4) it demonstrates pharmacological identity with the naturally occurring transmitter.

The most clear-cut evidence that EAAs can act physiologically as excitatory neurotransmitters at a given synapse comes from experiments in which intracellular recordings of pre- and postsynaptic events have been made. In studies of this nature, the criterion of identical and parallel change induced by antagonists on synaptic events elicited by stimulation and those elicited by the action of the exogenously administered putative transmitter substance is of critical importance in identifying the excitatory amino transmitter involved. In many situations, however, such studies are not feasible, so more indirect studies such as those summarized previously have been utilized.

Quite often at excitatory synapses the actual molecule acting at the postsynaptic receptor has not been definitively identified, even though pharmacological analysis indicates that the synaptic response is mediated by a particular EAA receptor. Thus, a critical link in establishing a neurotransmitter role for an EAA within a specific pathway is the demonstration and characterization of the EAA receptor that mediates synaptic transmission at that synapse.

EAA RECEPTORS

Our understanding of EAA transmitters and their function and regulation has been greatly enhanced by studies directed at the identification, characterization, localization, and isolation of receptors for these amino acids. In fact, progress on the definition of receptor subtypes and the availability of more selective agonists and antagonists has produced a quantum leap in knowledge about EAAs at synaptic sites throughout the vertebrate CNS. Furthermore, many aspects of Glu receptor dynamics have suggested an extraordinary degree of functional regulation.

Until the mid-1980s, neuropharmacologists were content with two major classes of EAA receptors, the NMDA receptors and the non-NMDA receptors, the latter composed at that time of kainate and quisqualate receptors. With the development of more selective agonists and antagonists, however, the classes of EAA receptors have expanded to at least five different types in the CNS—NMDA, kainate, α-amino-3-hydroxy-5-methylisoxazole-4-propionic acid (AMPA), 1,2-amino-4-phosphonobutyrate (AP-4), and 1-aminocyclopentane-1,3-dicarboxylic acid (ACPD)—each displaying distinct physiological characteristics. Three of these receptors have been defined by the depolarizing excitatory actions of select synthetic agonists (NMDA, kainate, and AMPA) and the blockade of the effects of these agonists by selective antagonists. A fourth, the AP-4 receptor, appears to represent an inhibitory autoreceptor. The fifth receptor, activated by ACPD, modifies inositol phosphate metabolism and has been called a metabotropic Glu receptor (mGluR). A summary of representative agonists and antagonists for each of these EAA receptor classes is given in Table 5–2.

Synaptic transmission in synapses using EAAs does not appear to follow the simple model of fast-acting synaptic transmission mediated by a single receptor class. In fact, individual synapses that use EAAs may not be restricted to distinct receptors but, rather, may have a combination of receptors and thereby exhibit different input/output properties and second messenger responses.

One specific subtype of EAA receptor, the NMDA receptor, has become a major focus of attention because of evidence that it may be involved in a wide range of both neurophysiological and pathological processes as important and diverse as memory acquisition (see Chapter 16), developmental plasticity, epilepsy (see Chapter 19), and the neurotoxic effects of brain ischemia.

NMDA RECEPTOR–IONOPHORE COMPLEX

The NMDA receptor is a ligand-gated ion channel composed of two different protein subunits, NMDAR1 and NMDAR2. NMDAR1 can exist in seven splice variants, and there are four different genes encoding variants of NMDAR2 (NMDAR2A, -B, -C, and -D). It is not clear how many NMDAR1 and NMDAR2 subunits are present in each functional NMDA receptor. This receptor complex has been extensively characterized physiologically and pharmacologically, and it is widely distributed in mammalian brain and spinal cord, with particularly high receptor densities found in hippocampus and cerebral cortex. NMDA receptors appear to have a pivotal role in long-term depression, long-term potentiation (LTP), and developmental plasticity. However, overactivation or prolonged stimulation of NMDA receptors can damage and eventually kill target neurons via a process referred to as excitotoxicity. Like the $GABA_A$ receptor, the NMDA receptor is a complex molecular entity endowed with a number of distinct recognition sites for endogenous and exogenous ligands, each with discrete binding domains. There appear to be at least six pharmacologically distinct sites through which compounds can alter the activity of this receptor (Fig. 5–2): (1) a transmitter binding site that binds L-glutamate and related agonists, promoting the opening of a high-conductance channel that permits entry of Na and Ca into target cells, with L-Glu being virtually ineffective unless the site that binds Gly, the strychnine-insensitive Gly modulatory site (2), is also occupied (this Gly site is distinct from the Gly binding site on the strychnine-sensitive Gly inhibitory receptor [see later discussion of Gly receptors]); (3) a site within the channel that binds phencyclidine (PCP) and related noncompetitive antagonists (MK-801 and ketamine), which act most

TABLE 5–2. Classification of Excitatory Amino Acid Receptors in the Mammalian Central Nervous System

| CURRENTLY ACCEPTED NAME | NMDA | | | AMPA | KAINATE | METABOTROPIC |
	GLUTAMATE SITE	GLYCINE SITE				
Subtype-selective agonists	NMDA	Glycine D-serine R(+)HA-966 (partial) L-687,414 (partial)		AMPA S(−)-5-Flu Quisqualic acid	Kainic acid Domoic acid	L-AP$_4$ ACPD L-CCG-I
Subtype-selective antagonists	D(−)-AP-5 D(−)-AP-7 CGS-19755 CGP-37849 CGP-40116 CPP, (±)-D-D-CPPene	7-Chlorokynurenic 5,7-Dichlorokvnurenic MNQX L-689,560		NBQX GYKI 52466		MCPG MTEP MPEP
Channel blockers	MK-801 Phencyclidine (PCP)					
Receptor-selective agonists	NMDA			AMPA	Kainic acid	L-AP-4
Receptor-selective antagonists	D(−)-AP-5			CNQX DNQX	CNQX DNQX	MCPG
Effector pathways	Na$^+$/K$^+$/Ca^{2+}			Na$^+$/K$^+$/Ca^{2+}	Na$^+$/K$^+$/Ca^{2+}	IP$_3$DAG

ACPD, 1-aminocyclopentane-1,3-dicarboxylic acid; AMPA, α-amino-3-hydroxy-5-methylisoxazole-4-propionic acid; AP-5, 2-amino-5-phosphonopentanoic acid; AP-7, amino-7 phosphonoheptanoic acid; CNQX, 6-cyano-7-nitroquinoxaline-2,3-dione; CPP, 3-(2-carboxypiperazin-4-yl)-propyl-1-phosphonic acid; DAG, diacylglycerol; D-CPPene, D-3-(2-carboxypiperazin-4-yl)-propyl-1-phosphonene; DNQX, 6,7-dinitroquinoxaline-2,3-dione; HA-966, 3-amino-1-hydroxypyrrolidone-2; IP$_3$, inositol trisphosphate; L-AP4, L-2-amino-4-phosphonobutanoic acid; L-687,414, R(+)-cis-β-methyl-3-amino-L-hydroxypyrrolid-2-one; L-CCG-I, (2S,3S,4S)-α-(carboxycyclopropyl) glycine; MCPG, α-methyl-4-carboxyphenyl-glycine; MNQX, 5,7-dinitroquinoxaline-2,3-dione; MPEP, 2-methyl-6-(phenylethynyl)-pyridine; MTEP, 3-((2-Methyl-1,3-thiazol-4-yl)ethynyl)pyridine, NBQX, 2,3-dihydro-6-nitro-7-sulfamoyl-benzof)quinoxaline; NMDA, N-methyl-D-aspartic acid; S(−)-5-Flu, S(−)-5-fluorowillardine.

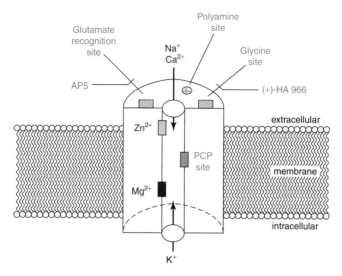

FIGURE 5–2. Schematic illustration of the NMDA receptor and the sites of action of different agents on the receptor. The NMDA receptor gates a cation channel that is permeable to Ca^{2+} and Na^+ and gated by Mg^{2+} in a voltage-dependent manner; K^+ is the counterion. The NMDA receptor channel is blocked by phencyclidine (PCP) and MK-801, and the complex is regulated at two modulatory sites by glycine and polyamines; 2-amino-5-phosphonopenta-noic acid (AP5) and 3-(2-carboxypiperazin-4-yl)-propyl-l-phosphonic acid are competitive antagonists at the NMDA site.

effectively when the receptor is activated (i.e., open channel block); (4) a voltage-dependent Mg^{2+} binding site; (5) an inhibitory divalent cation site near the mouth of the channel that binds Zn^{2+} to produce a voltage-independent block; and (6) a polyamine regulatory site whose activation by spermine and spermidine facilitates NMDA receptor-mediated transmission.

In addition, two distinct binding sites are apparently associated with the transmitter recognition site—one that preferentially binds agonists and one that preferentially binds antagonists. It is of interest that quinolinic acid, a metabolite of tryptophan and thus a natural brain constituent, may be a specific antagonist for a particular subtype of NMDA receptor since it shows regional variation in potency. A number of Gly agonists and antagonists have been identified for the Gly regulatory site.

The Gly modulatory site has attracted a great deal of interest as a potential site for the action of new antiepileptic drugs or agents that might be useful in preventing ischemic brain damage. D-Serine is a potent agonist at this site, and (+)HA-966 is a selective antagonist. Gly in submicromolar concentrations increases the frequency of the NMDA receptor channel opening in a strychnine-insensitive manner, and although brain and cerebrospinal fluid concentrations of

Gly are in the millimolar range, Gly is effective *in vivo*, indicating that the Gly site is not saturated. Thus, conditions that alter the extracellular concentration of Gly or compete with its binding site can dramatically alter NMDA receptor-mediated responses.

D-Serine is an endogenous ligand for the Gly site of the NMDA receptor found in high concentration in glia. It appears to be selectively localized in astrocytes containing its biosynthetic enzyme, serine racemase, which ensheath nerve terminals in brain areas enriched in NMDA receptors. Thus, D-serine has been suggested to play a role in the modulation of synaptic transmission at NMDA receptors, providing a mechanism by which astrocytes may play an active role in supporting synaptic transmission via the activation of NMDA receptors.

Polyamines such as spermine and spermidine function as allosteric modulators of NMDA receptors and potentiate NMDA currents in the presence of saturating concentrations of Glu and Gly. However, in contrast to Gly or D-serine, their presence is not a requirement for NMDA receptor activation. Under pathological conditions, such as brain ischemia or trauma, in which the production of polyamines is dramatically increased, polyamines may mediate or potentiate the excitotoxic mechanisms responsible for the neuronal damage produced. This idea is supported by findings that phenylethanolamines such as ifenprodil and eliprodil (SL820715), which are potent antagonists of the polyamine modulatory site of the NMDA receptor complex in a number of biochemical models, exhibit effective neuroprotective action in ischemia and trauma.

Kynurenate is a tryptophan metabolite that blocks the high-affinity Gly binding site. It can be thought of as an endogenous neuroprotective agent that is released from glial cells following the transamination of L-kynurenine. Manipulation of endogenous kynurenate formation may provide further insight into the role it plays in modulating the action of Gly on the NMDA receptor.

Quinolinic acid is an endogenous excitatory neurotoxin, synthesized from L-tryptophan via the kynurenine pathway, that has the potential of mediating NMDA-induced neurotoxicity and dysfunction. Its endogenous occurrence in normal brain is relatively low (approximately 50–100 pmol/g). Toxicity induced by exogenous quinolinic acid can be prevented or reversed by noncompetitive or competitive NMDA antagonists, suggesting that the neurotoxicity produced by locally administered quinolinic acid is mediated through the NMDA subtype of EAA receptors. Although quinolinic acid was first identified in the human brain in 1983, knowledge of the possible role played by this toxin in neuropathology was uncertain while speculation abounded. The observation by Heyes and co-workers in the late 1980s that quinolinate levels were dramatically elevated in acquired immunodeficiency syndrome (AIDS) was a major advance toward understanding the pathobiology of quinolinate. Further studies have demonstrated that the motor signs of AIDS dementia correlate strikingly with the levels of quinolinate in the cerebrospinal fluid. Treatment with the antiretroviral agent azidothymidine decreased the viremia and associated dementia and lowered the cerebrospinal fluid levels of quinolinate. Because cerebrospinal fluid levels of quinolinate are often higher than those found in blood, it has been argued that the origin of this neurotoxin may be via intracerebral synthesis, although this has not yet been documented. The highest reported levels of cerebrospinal fluid quinolinate are often obtained in AIDS patients with opportunistic infections. Elevated levels of cerebrospinal fluid quinolinate are found in human patients and in nonhuman primates with inflammatory neurological diseases, but it is unclear whether the mechanisms underlying the increased levels of quinolinate induced by bacterial and viral infection are similar. It also remains to be determined if the bacteria are actually involved in the synthesis of some of the increased quinolinate. No specific organism has been identified as responsible for elevating quinolinic acid since this neurotoxin is elevated in a variety of bacterial and viral infections. It has been suggested that astroglial apoptosis is the mechanism involved in the quinoline-induced neurocytotoxicity associated with several major inflammatory brain diseases such as AIDS dementia complex and other viral brain infections. The discovery of an effective inhibitor of quinolinic acid synthesis will help to elucidate the importance of this neurotoxin in inflammatory and infectious disease.

In addition to the multiple ligand binding and regulatory sites on the NMDA receptor for these relatively small molecules, the NMDA receptor exhibits an extremely high degree of interaction with many other membrane and cytoplasmic proteins. In fact, the complexity of the proteins with which this receptor has demonstrable interactions has established a new form of high-throughput molecular analysis combining the classical forms of two-dimensional gel chromatography with very sensitive methods of peptide sequence identification employing mass fragmentography. Using such "proteomic" methods, the NMDA receptor's known interacting partners increased from a single association with the intrinsic membrane protein PSD95, which was thought to be critical to anchor the receptor to the postsynaptic specialization site, to more than six dozen other proteins. Within this NMDA receptor protein complex, five main classes of proteins have been identified: neurotransmitter receptors (including other Glu receptors), cell adhesion proteins, adaptors, signaling enzymes, and cytoskeletal proteins.

NON-NMDA RECEPTORS

Both AMPA and kainic acid (KA) receptors mediate fast excitatory synaptic transmission and are associated primarily with voltage-independent channels that gate a depolarizing current primarily carried by the influx of Na^+ ions.

Although these receptors are easily distinguished from NMDA receptors, they are more difficult to distinguish from each other. Molecular biological studies have confirmed the existence of AMPA and KA classes of non-NMDA receptors but have revealed a considerable degree of heterogeneity within these two families. Some pharmacological discrimination can be achieved, with AMPA and quisqualate being the preferred agonists for AMPA receptors and domoate and kainate the preferred agonists for KA receptors. The most selective and potent non-NMDA antagonists available are a series of dihydroxyquinoxaline derivatives including 2,3-dihydro-6-nitro-7-sulfamoyl-benzo(F)quinoxaline (NBQX), 6-cyano-7-nitroquinoxaline-2,3-dione (CNQX), and 6,7-dinitroquinoxaline-2,3-dione (DNQX) (see Table 5–2)However, these agents competitively block both types of non-NMDA receptor, although NBQX appears to exhibit the best selectivity for AMPA receptors. Very few KA receptor-selective compounds have been identified. A new class of 2,3-benzodiazepine derivatives (most notably GYKI-52466) has been shown to block AMPA-induced responses noncompetitively and to attenuate ischemic neuronal damage effectively in animal models, highlighting the fact that non-NMDA receptors also play an important role in CNS pathology.

In studies of immature hippocampal neurons in culture, AMPA receptors were surprisingly found almost exclusively within the dendritic cytoplasm rather than in the dendritic membranes and spines. Using special constructs of the mRNA for the AMPA receptor coupled with green fluorescent protein, regular dynamic insertion and removal could be demonstrated for the receptors, which was accelerated by activity. This receptor cycling was quickly advanced as a mechanism for activating silent synapses by recruiting these receptors to the synaptic surfaces. However, whether this explanation would hold for mature neurons is dubious since such neurons exhibit abundant spine and synaptic AMPA receptors. Evidence suggests that in mature neurons, it may well be the NMDA receptors that are recruited to the cell surface during depolarizing events.

METABOTROPIC GLUTAMATE RECEPTORS

The metabotropic glutamate receptors (mGluRs) constitute a family of EAA receptors that are linked to G proteins and second messenger systems and are distinct from the ionotropic EAA receptors that form ion channels and are composed of the NMDA, AMPA, and kainate subtypes discussed previously. Whereas inotropic receptors are responsible for fast excitatory synaptic transmission, metabotropic glutamate receptors have an important role in synaptic modulation throughout the CNS. This more recently characterized group of receptors is coupled to a variety of signal transduction pathways via G proteins, producing alterations in intercellular second messengers and generating slow synaptic responses. This is in clear contrast to the ionotropic Glu receptors, which are directly coupled to cation-specific ion channels and mediate fast excitatory synaptic responses. *Metabotropic* is a term that was coined to indicate that these receptors, unlike the inotropic receptors that form ion channels, affect cellular metabolic processes. Unfortunately, this nomenclature is very misleading since mGluRs, similar to other G protein-coupled receptors, exert profound effects on neuronal function through the regulation of ion channels, protein phosphorylation, and second messenger cascades. The widespread distribution of metabotropic receptors in the CNS coupled with the prevalence of Glu as a neurotransmitter indicates that this system is a major modulator of second messengers in the mammalian CNS. Molecular cloning studies have revealed the existence of at least eight different subtypes of mGluR, $mGluR_1$ through $mGluR_8$, which have a common structure of a large extracellular domain preceded by the seven-member spanning domains.

Members of the mGluR family can be divided into three subgroups according to their sequence similarities, signal transduction properties, and pharmacological profiles to agonists (i.e., relative potencies when expressed in cell lines of Glu, quisqualate, ACPD, and AP-4). The first subgroup, composed of $mGluR_1$ and $mGluR_5$, is coupled to the stimulation of phosphatidylinositol hydrolysis/Ca^{2+} signal transduction. The second group, $mGluR_2$ and $mGluR_3$, is negatively coupled through adenylyl cyclase to cyclic adenosine monophosphate formation. The third group, consisting of $mGluR_4$, $mGluR_6$, $mGluR_7$, and $mGluR_8$, is also negatively linked to adenylyl cyclase activity but shows a different agonist preference from that of $mGluR_2$ and $mGluR_3$. As a group, the mGluRs are widely expressed throughout the brain, but the individual subtypes show some differential distribution. The pharmacology of the individual subtypes expressed in Chinese hamster ovary or in baby hamster kidney cells shows some interesting differences (see Table 5–2). LAP4 is a potent agonist of $mGluR_4$, $mGluR_6$, $mGluR_7$, and $mGluR_8$ but has little effect on the other receptor subtypes. LY404039 is a new, potent, and selective agonist that activates $mGluR_{2/3}$ at concentrations that have little or no effect on other mGluR subtypes.

In the past 5 years, substantial progress has been made in understanding the pharmacology and cellular actions of mGluRs, greatly facilitating appraisal of their potential use as therapeutic agents. The widespread distribution of mGluRs and their important role in synaptic modulation underscore their potential relevance in the pathophysiology of a wide range of neurologic and psychiatric disorders.

The discovery that phenylglycine derivatives are selective antagonists of $mGluR_5$ has permitted more rigorous testing of the physiological role of this receptor subclass in brain function and dysfunction. Data suggest a role in both synaptic transmission and synaptic plasticity. Several exciting new developments have occurred concerning the potential therapeutic use of groups I and II mGluR antagonists and agonists in several clinical disorders. Concerning mGluR$_5$, Conquet and collaborators and Bear and his group have reported new findings using knockout mice. Conquet's group found that mGluR$_5$ is an essential factor in cocaine self-administration and locomotor effects. Their studies showed that the reinforcing properties of cocaine are absent in mice lacking mGluR$_5$ and that a selective mGluR$_5$ antagonist, 2-methyl-6-(phenylethynyl)-pyridine, dose dependently decreased cocaine self-administration. Bear and his team found that a 50 percent reduction in mGluR$_5$ fixed multiple defects in the fragile X mice. His group also showed that in addition to correcting dendritic spines, reduced mGluR$_5$ improved altered brain development and memory, restored normal body growth, and reduced seizures in fragile X mice—many of the symptoms experienced by humans with fragile X syndrome. These finding should provide further incentive for the rapid development of more potent mGluR antagonists with greater subtype specificity and enhanced bioavailability. Interesting data on a subtype-specific mGluR agonists have also emerged. The discovery of a specific and potent agonist for mGlu$_{2/3}$ receptors that suppressed glutamatergic excitation in the limbic cortex and had antipsychotic activity in several animal models encouraged the study of this drug in schizophrenia. Promising clinical results against positive and negative symptoms in schizophrenia have been reported for this novel mGlu$_{2/3}$ receptor agonist.

With the availability of these new and additional subtype-selective antagonists and agonists, the near future holds promise for continued advances in our knowledge of the roles played by mGluRs in physiological and pathological processes and perhaps even several new treatments for neurological, psychiatric, and addictive disorders.

The function and distribution of the four classes of EAA receptors are summarized in Table 5–3. The NMDA receptor is an essential component in the generation of LTP. LTP results in an increase in synaptic efficacy that has been proposed as an underlying mechanism involved in memory and learning.

In addition to the roles that excitotoxic mechanisms may play in various chronic neurodegenerative disorders such as Huntington's disease and viral diseases such as AIDS, two chronic neurological syndromes have been linked to dietary consumption of amino acid toxins of plant origin. Neurolathyrism, a spastic disorder occurring in eastern Africa and southern Asia, is associated with dietary consumption of the chick pea *Lathyrus sativus*. β-*N*-Oxalylamino-L-alanine (L-BOAA) has been identified as the responsible toxin in this plant. This amino acid acts as an agonist at AMPA receptors. One of the primary effects of L-BOAA toxicity is the inhibition of mitochondrial complex 1 selectively in the motor cortex and lumbar spinal cord. Guam disease, also referred to as amyotrophic lateral sclerosis/parkinsonism/dementia, is thought to be

TABLE 5–3. Distribution and Function of Excitatory Amino Acid Receptors in the Mammalian Central Nervous System

RECEPTOR TYPE	DISTRIBUTION/FUNCTION
NMDA	Widely distributed in mammalian CNS (enriched in hippocampus, cerebral cortex). Demonstrated most easily by pharmacological antagonism under MG^{2+}-tree or depolarizing conditions or in binding experiments. Usually recognized as a slow component in repetitive activity generated primarily by non-NMDA receptors. Important in synaptic plasticity.
AMPA	Widespread in CNS; parallel distribution to NMDA receptors. Involved in the generation of fast component of EPSPs in many central excitatory pathways.
Kainate	Concentrated in a few specific areas of CNS, complementary to NMDA/AMPA distribution (e.g., stratum lucidum region of hippocampus). Difficult to distinguish from AMPA receptors pharmacologically due to nonspecificity of kainate in electrophysiological experiments. However, present specificity (in the absence of AMPA and NMDA receptors) on dorsal root C fibers.

Metabotropic (mGluRs)		Widespread in CNS, role in synaptic modulation
Group	Receptor	
I	mGluR1, mGluR5	Postsynaptic/Facilitates NMDA responses, Inc. in Neuronal plasticity, Promotion of LTP or LTD
II	mGluR2, mGluR3	Presynaptic/Inhibition of neurotransmitter release Decrease in neuronal excitability
III	mGluR4, mGluR7 mGluR8	Presynaptic terminal (active zone)/Inhibition of neurotransmitter release

NMDA, N-methyl-D-aspartate; AMPA, α-ainino-3-hydroxy-5-inethylisoxazole-4-propionic acid; EPSP, excitatory postsynaptic potential; IP_3 inositol-1,4,5-trisphosphate.
SOURCE: Modified from Watkins et al. (1990); Benarroch (2008).

related to the consumption of flour prepared from the seeds of the cycad *Cycas circinalis*, which contains the amino acid β-N-methyl-amino-L-alanine (BMAA). Although BMAA is a neutral amino acid that is not directly excitatory or toxic *in vitro*, in the presence of bicarbonate it becomes excitotoxic and acts as an agonist at AMPA and NMDA receptors.

Neurotoxicity has also been observed following ingestion of domoic acid. Domoic acid is an analog of KA that is approximately three times as potent. This substance is synthesized by marine algae and can be consumed in toxic amounts by eating mussels that have fed on such algae. An outbreak of domoic poisoning occurred in 1987 in Canada. Consumption of this neurotoxin by humans can damage the hippocampus and produce dementia.

With the availability of more specific pharmacological agents, it should be possible to evaluate in more detail the involvement of EAA pathways in normal brain function and in neuropathological conditions. The participation of NMDA receptors in LTP provides a strong link between these systems and the mechanisms of learning and memory. NMDA and other EAA receptors also appear to play a role in cell damage caused by hypoglycemia, hypoxia, seizures, and other disturbances associated with excess EEAs. Different subtypes of mGluRs regulate neuronal excitability, synaptic plasticity, neurotransmitter release, and glial function—processes that are important for brain development and mechanisms of learning, memory, neuroprotection, and injury. Thus, it is not surprising that mGluRs have been implicated in the pathophysiology of a number of neurological and psychiatric disorders, including epilepsy, fragile X syndrome, Parkinson's and Alzheimer's disease, anxiety, pain, depression, schizophrenia, and drug addiction.

THERAPEUTIC USE OF GLUTAMATERGIC DRUGS

NMDA receptor antagonists including dizocilpine(MK-801) have been extensively studied for use in treatment of diseases with excitotoxic components, such as stroke, traumatic brain injury, and neurodegenerative diseases such as Huntington's disease, Alzheimer's disease, and amyotrophic lateral sclerosis. However, NMDA antagonists such as dizocilpine have largely failed to show safety and effectiveness in clinical trials. Dizocilpine had a promising future as a neuroprotective agent until neurotoxic-like effects, called Olney's lesions, were seen in certain brain regions of test rats and Merck promptly dropped development of this compound.

A few nonselective glutamate receptor antagonists are still used clinically. Ketamine is a dissociative anesthetic used primarily in veterinary practice. However, it has been used as a pediatric anesthetic since children are less likely than adults to exhibit psychiatric side effects.

Memantine is a noncompetitive, low-affinity NMDA antagonist used to treat Alzheimer's disease (see Chapter 16).

Amantadine is another weak noncompetitive, low-affinity NMDA antagonist that also has dopamine-releasing properties. This drug is used to treat Parkinson's disease and as adjunctive therapy in the treatment of catatonic syndromes (see Chapter 17).

Riluzole is an NMDA receptor antagonist that also preferentially blocks TTA-S sodium channels and is used to treat amyotrophic lateral sclerosis.

The next glutamatergic drug to be registered may be the glutamate antagonist tezampanel for treatment of migraine, which is currently in phase III trials. Tezampanel is a non-NMDA competitive antagonist that blocks both AMPA and kainate receptors.

Rapid progress is being made in mGlu pharmacology and moving drug candidates toward the clinic, with particularly exciting new data on the use of mGlu$_{2/3}$ agonists in the treatment of schizophrenia. In a relatively short period of time (less than a decade), many highly potent, subtype-selective agents have become available and a few are already advancing to phase II clinical trials.

Although not yet approved for human therapeutics, mGluR$_5$ antagonists are entering into clinical trials for a broad range of psychiatric indications, including drug addiction, pain, and fragile X syndrome.

Optimized compounds and potentially clinically useful ligands have also been reported for mGlu$_1$ receptor antagonists for the treatment of pain and epilepsy.

GABA

Neurotransmitter Role in the Mammalian Central Nervous System

GABA was identified as the neurotransmitter for inhibitory neuromuscular junctions in the lobster. Since its discovery in 1950 by Roberts and Awarpara, numerous biochemical and neurophysiological observations have been made concerning brain GABA and GABA systems that make a strong case for its neurotransmitter role in mammalian brain.

Like other neurotransmitters or neurotransmitter candidates, GABA and its biosynthetic enzyme glutamic acid decarboxylase (GAD) have a discrete, nonuniform distribution in the brain. The brain contains a high-affinity, sodium-dependent transport system that serves to terminate GABA action. Storage of GABA can be demonstrated in selected synaptosomal populations, and a vesicular GABA transporter has been cloned and sequenced. Release of endogenous or radioactively labeled, exogenously accumulated GABA can be evoked by the appropriate experimental conditions. The presence of GABA-containing neurons has been verified, and the anatomical distribution of GABAergic neurons has been mapped out, using *in situ* hybridization for GAD mRNA and immunocytochemical detection of GAD. However, the most compelling evidence that GABA plays a neurotransmitter role in mammalian brain has emerged from intracellular recording studies, which show that GABA causes a hyperpolarization of neurons similar to that evoked by the naturally occurring transmitter substance and that these inhibitory actions of synthetic GABA and of GABA-containing pathways can be antagonized by drugs selective for the GABA receptor, such as bicuculline.

Distribution

Synthesized in 1883, GABA was known for many years as a product of microbial and plant metabolism. Not until 1950, however, did investigators identify

GABA as a normal constituent of the mammalian CNS. Moreover, no other mammalian tissue, with the exception of the retina, contains more than a mere trace of this material. Obviously, a substance with such an unusual enrichment in the brain must have some specific physiological effects that would make it important for the function of the CNS. Much evidence has accumulated in support of the hypothesis that the major share of GABA found in the brain functions as an inhibitory transmitter. The probability that GABA functions as an inhibitory transmitter in the brain has spurred a prodigious research effort to implicate GABA in the etiology of a host of neurological and psychiatric disorders. Although the current evidence is not overwhelming, GABA has been most convincingly implicated, both directly and indirectly, in the pathogenesis of epilepsy.

In mammals, GABA is found in high concentrations in the brain and spinal cord but is absent or present only in trace amounts in peripheral nerve tissue, such as sciatic nerve, splenic nerve, and sympathetic ganglia, or in any other peripheral tissue, such as liver, spleen, and heart. These findings provide some idea of the uniqueness of the occurrence of GABA in the mammalian CNS. Like the monoamines, GABA appears to have a discrete distribution within the CNS. However, unlike the monoamines, the concentration of GABA found in the CNS is on the order of millimoles per gram rather than nanomoles per gram. The brain also contains large amounts of glutamic acid (8–13 mmol/g), which is the main precursor of GABA and itself a neurotransmitter candidate (see Glutamic Acid).

Since GABA does not easily penetrate the blood–brain barrier, brain concentrations of GABA cannot be increased by systemic administration unless one opens the blood–brain barrier. GABA-lactam (2-pyrrolidinone), a less polar and more lipid-soluble compound, can reach the CNS but is not significantly hydrolyzed to GABA. A more successful approach has been use of the drug progabide, which not only penetrates the blood–brain barrier but also is subsequently metabolized into GABA.

Metabolism

Three primary enzymes are involved in the catabolism of GABA before its final metabolite, succinate, enters the Krebs cycle. The relative activity of enzymes involved in the degradation of GABA suggests that, as with monoamines, they play only a minor role in the termination of the action of any neurally released GABA.

Figure 5–3 outlines the metabolism of GABA and its relationship to the Krebs cycle and carbohydrate metabolism. As mentioned previously, GABA is formed by the α-decarboxylation of L-glutamic acid, a reaction catalyzed by GAD, an enzyme that occurs uniquely in the mammalian CNS

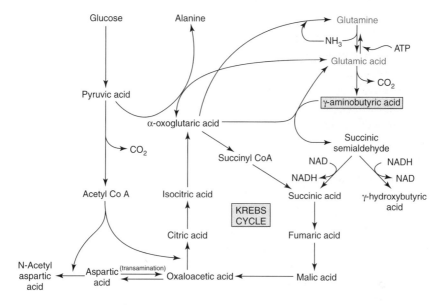

FIGURE 5–3. Interrelationship between GABA and carbohydrate metabolism.

and retinal tissue. The precursor of GABA, L-glutamic acid, can be formed from α-oxoglutarate by transamination or reaction with ammonia. GABA is intimately related to the oxidative metabolism of carbohydrates in the CNS by means of a "shunt," involving its production from glutamate; its transamination with α-oxoglutarate by GABA–α-oxoglutarate transaminase (GABA-T), yielding succinic semialdehyde and regenerating Glu; and, finally, its entry into the Krebs cycle as succinic acid via the oxidation of succinic semialdehyde by succinic semialdehyde dehydrogenase. In essence, then, the shunt bypasses the normal oxidative metabolism involving the enzymes α-oxoglutarate dehydrogenase and succinyl thiokinase.

Glutamic Acid Decarboxylase

GAD is the only synthetic enzyme responsible for the conversion of L-glutamic acid to GABA, and the reaction is irreversible. In mammals, this relatively specific decarboxylase is found primarily in the CNS, where it occurs in higher concentrations in the gray matter. In general, the localization of this enzyme in mammalian brain correlates quite well with the GABA content. The brain enzyme has been purified to homogeneity and its properties studied in detail. It has a pH optimum of approximately 6.5 and requires pyridoxal phosphate, a form of vitamin B_6, as a coenzyme. This purified enzyme is inhibited by structural analogs of Glu, carbonyl (pyridoxal phosphate [PLP])-trapping agents, sulfhydryl reagents, thiol compounds, and anions such as chloride. Two isoforms of GAD have been identified, which are encoded by two distinct genes. These two isoforms, designated GAD_{65} and GAD_{67} in accordance with their molecular weights, differ in amino acid sequence, antigenicity, cellular and subcellular location, and interaction with the GAD cofactor PLP. Their different intracellular distributions suggest that the two GAD forms may be regulated in different ways. GAD_{65} and GAD_{67} differ significantly in their affinity for the pyridoxal cofactor: GAD_{65} shows a relatively high affinity for the cofactor, whereas the larger GAD isoform does not. The affinity of GAD_{65} for the cofactor results in the ability of GAD_{65} enzyme activity to be efficiently and quickly regulated. In contrast, the activity of GAD_{67} is determined through induction of new enzyme protein rather than through posttranslational mechanisms.

GABA Transaminase

GABA-T, unlike the decarboxylase, has a wide tissue distribution. Therefore, although GABA cannot be formed to any extent outside the CNS, exogenous GABA can be rapidly metabolized by both central and peripheral tissue. However, since endogenous GABA is present only in nanomolar amounts in cerebrospinal fluid, it is unlikely that a significant amount of endogenous GABA leaves the brain intact. The brain transaminase has a pH optimum of 8.2 and requires PLP. It appears that the coenzyme is more tightly bound to this enzyme than it is to GAD. The brain ratio of GABA-T/GAD activity is almost always greater than 1. Sulfhydryl reagents tend to decrease GABA-T activity, suggesting that this enzyme requires the integrity of one or more sulfhydryl groups for optimal activity. Transamination of GABA catalyzed by GABA-T is a reversible reaction, so if a metabolic source of succinic semialdehyde were made available, it would be theoretically possible to form GABA by the reversal of this reaction. However, this does not appear to be the case *in vivo* under normal or experimental conditions.

Gabaculine is the most potent GABA-T inhibitor available. Similar to γ-acetylenic and γ-vinyl GABA, this agent is a catalytic inhibitor of GABA-T and, unfortunately, will inhibit GAD. However, gabaculine has a fair degree of specificity since it is approximately 1000-fold less effective as a GAD inhibitor than as a GABA-T inhibitor.

Succinic Semialdehyde Dehydrogenase

Brain succinic semialdehyde dehydrogenase (SSADH) has a high substrate specificity and can be distinguished from the nonspecific aldehyde dehydrogenase found in the brain. The enzyme purified from human brain has a pH optimum of approximately 9.2 and a K_m for succinic semialdehyde of 5.3×10^{-6} and a K_m for NAD of 3×10^{-5}. SSADH from rat brain has a similarly low K_m for succinic semialdehyde of 7.8×10^{-5} and for NAD of 5×10^{-5}. The high activity of this enzyme and the low Michaelis constant, which allow the enzyme to function effectively at low substrate concentrations, probably account for the fact that succinic semialdehyde has not even been detected as an endogenous metabolite in neural tissue, despite the active metabolism of GABA *in vivo*.

Alternate Metabolic Pathways

In addition to undergoing transamination and subsequently entering the Krebs cycle, GABA can apparently undergo various other transformations in the CNS, forming a number of compounds whose importance, and in some cases natural occurrence, has not been conclusively established. Figure 5–4 depicts a variety of derivatives for which GABA may serve as a precursor. Perhaps the simplest of these metabolic conversions is the reduction of succinic semialdehyde (a product of GABA transamination) to γ-hydroxybutyrate (GHB). The transformation of GABA to GHB has been demonstrated in rat brain both *in vivo* and *in vitro*. Studies have demonstrated that GHB administered in physiologically relevant concentrations can also be converted to GABA by transamination. GHB aciduria, a rare inborn error in the metabolism of GABA, has been reported in children and appears to be the result of a deficiency of SSADH, the enzyme that oxidizes succinic semialdehyde to succinic acid (see Fig. 5–3). GHB levels are increased in urine, plasma, and cerebrospinal fluid; however, it is unclear whether the main clinical symptoms of motor and mental retardation, muscular hypotonia, and ataxia are related to elevated levels of GHB.

GHB has achieved notoriety as a "date rape drug." Ingested in doses as low as 10 mg/kg, GHB, or its lactone precursor γ-butyrolactone, produces euphoria, impairment of judgment, anxiolysis, and amnestic deficits in short-term memory. Higher doses lead to unconsciousness, seizures, respiratory depression, and coma; several deaths have been attributed to GHB.

Storage

Like most classical neurotransmitters, GABA is packaged and stored in vesicles in the presynaptic terminals, from which it is released into the synaptic cleft. A vesicular transporter that accumulates GABA has been identified in GABAergic cells. This transporter was cloned on the basis of homology to *unc-47* in *Caenorhabditis elegans*, a strategy of moving from the worm to the mammalian species that has proven to be very useful for identifying a variety of mammalian transmitter-related genes. The vesicular GABA transporter

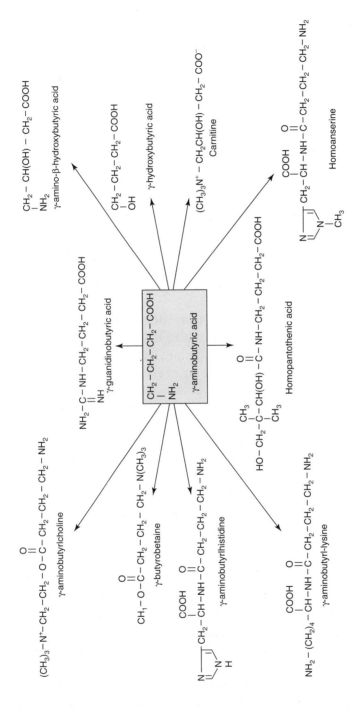

FIGURE 5–4. Possible alternate metabolic pathways for GABA.

(GAT) differs from the two vesicular monoamine transporters (VMATs; see Chapters 7 and 8) by having 10 rather than 12 presumptive transmembrane domains and a very large cytoplasmic N-terminus of approximately 130 amino acids. Like the vesicular Glu transporter, GAT is highly dependent on the electrical potential across the vesicular membrane and differs from VMATs in terms of this bioenergetic dependence. Specific inhibitors of the vesicular inhibitory GAT have not been identified.

However, the vesicular GAT shares with the VMATs a lack of substrate specificity and will transport the inhibitory transmitter glycine as well as GABA. Consistent with this pharmacology, the vesicular GAT has been found in glycine- as well as GABA-containing neurons. Accordingly, some have suggested that it can be more accurately designated a vesicular inhibitory amino acid transporter. Interestingly, a limited number of GABAergic neurons appear to lack this transporter, raising the suspicion that another (related) transporter may exist in these neurons or that this small population has an alternate mechanism of storage.

Release and Reuptake

The arrival of an action potential or other depolarizing stimulus in the presynaptic GABAergic terminal initiates a sequence of events that ultimately results in vesicular fusion and release of GABA into the synaptic cleft, as is presumed to be the case for all other neurotransmitters. After release, the action of GABA is terminated largely by removal from the synaptic cleft by the actions of several types of plasma membrane transporter. The uptake of several transmitters by both glia and neurons has been reported. This dual glial–neuronal reuptake is a common property in neurons using amino acid transmitters, probably because amino acids can play dual roles as both transmitters and metabolic intermediates.

The ability of glia to avidly accumulate GABA and other amino acids distinguishes amino acid transmitters from other classical transmitters. Reuptake is the primary mode of inactivation of GABA that is released from neurons. Molecular cloning techniques have suggested greater heterogeneity in the GATs than previously suspected, with genes for four distinct GATs being detected. At least three specific GAT proteins are expressed in the CNS. In addition, a betaine transporter that accumulates GABA has been cloned. All known GATs are expressed in both neurons and glia. There is no obvious answer to the question of why there are multiple transporters for GABA. GATs are expressed in both GABAergic neurons and non-GABAergic cells (presumably cells that receive GABA innervation) as well as glia. The presence of multiple transporter proteins for the same transmitter, localized in neurons as well as glia, differs from the situation for catecholamine transmitters, in which a single membrane-associated transporter protein with relatively selective substrate specificity is found in a neuron defining its chemical identity. One possibility is that the cloned GATs may be cotransporters for other amino acids. For example, no transporters for β-alanine and taurine have been cloned, but these amino acids are accumulated by GATs. Finally, it is possible that one or more of these transporters may have the ability to function in the outward direction, serving as a paradoxical mechanism for the release, rather than removal, of GABA.

The fact that the GATs transporters are not uniquely concentrated in the plasma membrane of the presynaptic GABA terminals has important functional ramifications. The GABA that is taken up in glia or non-GABAergic postsynaptic cells will not be available to recycle for another round of exocytotic release. This lost GABA will have to be replaced by *de novo* synthesis, placing enhanced demands on the synthetic capacity of the GABAergic neuron.

GABA Receptors

In vertebrate species, GABA receptors are found primarily in nerve cell membranes and are sufficiently widespread that most neurons in the CNS possess them. However, GABA receptors are not exclusively associated with neurons. They are also expressed by astrocytes, where they appear to be involved in the regulation of chloride channels. Interestingly, GABA receptors are also found outside the CNS on neurons of the autonomic nervous system.

In vertebrates, there are two major types of GABA receptors: the inotropic $GABA_A$ receptor and the metabotropic $GABA_B$ receptor. GABA receptors were initially subdivided into these two groups based on pharmacological evidence. However, the functional separation also extends to second messenger mechanisms, differences in the location of these receptor subtypes in the mammalian CNS, and their molecular composition. In addition, both receptor subtypes have pre- and postsynaptic locations and are thought to participate independently in synaptic transmission.

Autoreceptor Regulation of GABA Release

Pharmacological studies indicate that autoreceptor-mediated regulation of GABA neurons takes place predominantly through $GABA_B$ receptors located on GABAergic nerve terminals (see $GABA_B$ Receptor). Immunohistochemical studies have revealed that both $GABA_B$ and $GABA_A$ receptors are present on postsynaptic non-GABAergic neurons. Presumably, these $GABA_A$ postsynaptic receptors respond to GABA released from a presynaptic GABAergic neuron. An anatomical arrangement of one GABA neuron terminating on another GABA cell would have the same functional consequence as an autoreceptor (decreasing subsequent transmitter release), making it difficult to distinguish between true autoreceptor and heteroceptor regulation of GABA release.

GABA$_A$ Receptor

GABA$_A$ receptors are the major inhibitory neurotransmitter receptors in the brain and the site of action of many clinically important drugs (Fig. 5–5). These receptors are believed to be involved in mediating anxiolytic, sedative, anticonvulsant, muscle-relaxant, and amnesic activity.

The inotropic GABA$_A$ receptor is by far the most prevalent of the two known GABA receptor types in mammalian CNS and has been extensively studied and characterized. Like the nicotinic acetylcholine receptor (nAChR), the GABA$_A$ receptor is composed of four subunits comprising an integral transmembrane ion channel that is gated by the binding of two agonist molecules. However, unlike the nAChR, the receptor-associated GABA channel predominantly conducts chloride ions. Since the Cl$^-$ equilibrium potential is near the resting potential in most neurons, increasing chloride permeability hyperpolarizes the neuron and thereby decreases the depolarizing effects of an excitatory input, thus depressing excitability.

The GABA$_A$ receptor, a multisubunit receptor–channel complex, can be allosterically modulated by two important classes of drugs: the benzodiazepines and the barbiturates (see Chapter 14). The primary structure of the GABA$_A$ receptor, described in 1987, revealed that it is a member of a large superfamily

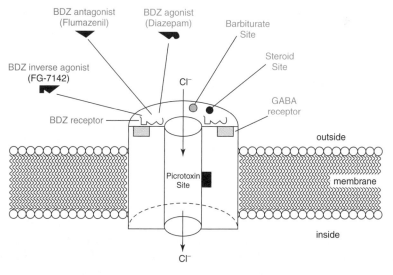

FIGURE 5–5. Schematic illustration of the GABA$_A$ receptor complex and the sites of action of different agents on the receptor. BDZ, benzodiazepine.

of ligand-gated ion channels that includes the nicotinic–cholinergic, inotropic Glu, Gly, and 5-hydroxytryptamine$_3$ (5HT$_3$) receptors. The GABA$_A$ receptor–ion channel complex is believed to be a heteropentameric glycoprotein of approximately 275 kDa composed of a combination of multiple polypeptide subunits (Fig. 5–6). Seven distinct classes of polypeptide subunits (α, β, γ, δ, ε, θ, and ρ) have been cloned, and multiple isoforms of each have been shown to exist so that the total number of identified subunits stands at 19. The existence of a large family of genes coding for diverse subunits ($\alpha_{1–6}$, $\beta_{1–4}$, $\gamma_{1–3}$, δ, ε, θ, and $\rho_{1–3}$) provides the basis for the extraordinary structural diversity of GABA$_A$ receptors.

The subunit composition of the GABA$_A$ receptors appears to vary from one brain region to another and even between neurons in a given region, but the exact composition of most native GABA$_A$ receptors is unknown. The distribution of mRNA in the CNS determined by *in situ* hybridization is very different for each subunit subtype. A cloned α subunit (α_6), which confers a unique pharmacology (binding of the partial inverse agonist RO-15-4513, a putative ethanol antagonist) to a recombinantly expressed GABA$_A$ receptor, is expressed in only a single type of neuron, the cerebellar granule neuron. Thus, it is becoming

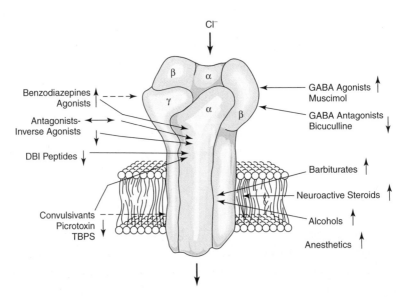

FIGURE 5–6. Schematic illustration of the GABA$_A$ receptor structure containing two α and β subunits and a single γ subunit to form an intrinsic Cl$^-$ ion channel. Putative ligands and drugs known to interact at one of the major sites associated with the GABA$_A$ receptors and to either positively or negatively modulate GABA-gated Cl$^-$ ion conductance are also illustrated. DBI, diazepam-binding inhibitor; TBPS, *t*-butylbicyclophosphothianate. (Modified From Paul, 1995.)

clear that the heterogeneity of the $GABA_A$ receptor subunit isoforms confers a diversity of pharmacological and perhaps physiological response characteristics upon the $GABA_A$ receptor. For example, coexpression of an additional γ subunit is necessary for the potentiation of GABA responses by benzodiazepines. In addition, coexpression of individual γ subunit variants ($γ_1$, $γ_2$, or $γ_3$) with α and β subunits results in varying degrees of modulation by benzodiazepine receptor ligands (agonist, antagonist, and inverse agonist). Photoaffinity-labeling studies have further suggested that the benzodiazepine binding site resides on the α subunit, whereas the GABA binding site resides on the β subunit. Finally, it appears that the α subunit heterogeneity determines the diversity of physiological and pharmacological response characteristics of native $GABA_A$ receptors, even though expression of the γ subunits is essential for conferring the modulatory actions of benzodiazepines on $GABA_A$ receptors. Thus, when coexpressed with $β_1$, the $α_1$ subunit yields a receptor with a relatively high affinity for GABA. By contrast, coexpression of the $α_2$ or $α_3$ subunit with the $β_1$ subunit results in $GABA_A$ receptors with far lower affinity for GABA. Thus, the subunit composition of a given receptor may actually determine the local response of the $GABA_A$ receptor to synaptically released GABA. These subtle differences in subunit organization may result in subpopulations of $GABA_A$ receptors that have different regional and cellular locations, each with differential sensitivity to GABA and allosteric modulators.

This extraordinary heterogeneity of $GABA_A$ receptors clearly provides a hitherto unexplored diversity in the function of receptor subtypes affecting their sensitivity to GABA, modulation by allosteric effectors, adaptation to stimulus conditions, distribution within a neuron and between neurons, ontogenetic development, and alterations in pathological states. An exciting new pharmacology is emerging from the recognition of the functional relevance of $GABA_A$ receptor subtypes, providing a rational basis for the development of subtype-specific ligands. Several studies have suggested that phosphorylation of the $GABA_A$ receptor channels may also be of importance for both short-term and long-term regulation of $GABA_A$ receptor function and expression. Currently, however, the physiological significance and specific consequences of the phosphorylation of $GABA_A$ receptor channels are unknown.

An increased understanding of the benzodiazepine GABA receptor chloride channel complex has led to the development of selective anxiolytic and anticonvulsant agents that lack significant sedative and muscle-relaxant action—properties that often limit the usefulness of traditional agents such as benzodiazepines and barbiturates. Conversely, some novel sleeping aids act as positive allosteric modulators of the benzodiazepine receptor (see Chapter 14). A better understanding of the molecular characteristics and regulation of the multiple allosteric sites of the supramolecular complex and the endogenous substances that may physiologically subserve these sites should not only contribute to our understanding of the possible etiology of anxiety and seizure disorders but also aid in the development of more effective and specific therapeutic agents. Once the functional properties of the $GABA_A$ subunits and their subtypes are more clearly defined, it should be possible to use this knowledge in the rational screening and/or design of new, clinically useful subtype-specific agents. The generation of animal models in which particular $GABA_A$ receptor subunits are either inactivated (knockout strategy) or selectively point mutated (knockin strategy) should help define the functional properties of $GABA_A$ subunits and their subtypes. These animals will also accelerate the recognition of the role of these receptor subtypes as potential drug targets.

$GABA_B$ Receptor

$GABA_B$ receptors belong to the superfamily of G protein-coupled receptors and are classified as metabotropic receptors. Their ligand-binding domain is not directly associated with their ion channel effector. As mentioned previously, the $GABA_B$ receptor is present at lower levels in the CNS than the $GABA_A$ receptor and is not linked to a chloride channel.

Since its pharmacological discovery in 1980, much progress has been made. Selective agonists and antagonists have been developed, and a functional role for this receptor as a mediator of slow inhibitory postsynaptic potentials in many brain regions has emerged. $GABA_B$ receptor activation also plays a role in attenuating the release of biogenic amines, acetylcholine, excitatory amino acids, neuropeptides, hormones, as well as GABA via an interaction with autoreceptors. Whereas $GABA_A$ receptors are directly associated with a Cl^- channel, $GABA_B$ receptors seem to be coupled to Ca^{2+} or K^+ channels via second messenger systems. The inhibitory hyperpolarizing action of $GABA_B$ receptor activation appears to be mediated through either increases in potassium conductance or decreases in calcium conductance.

Molecular cloning studies have revealed that $GABA_B$ receptors, like the mGluRs (see EAA Receptors), are members of the G protein-coupled receptor superfamily and contain seven presumptive transmembrane domains. Two major $GABA_B$ subunits have been cloned ($GABA_B$R1a and -R1b), and a novel $GABA_B$ receptor subunit has been identified ($GABA_B$R2). These G_i-coupled $GABA_B$ receptors are larger than most G protein-coupled receptors, being composed of 850–960 amino acids. The $GABA_B$ and mGluR receptors can be distinguished from most other G protein-coupled receptors (GPCR) by their large extracellular N-terminal domains. The functional $GABA_B$ receptor is an obligate heterodimer of the two subunits, making it an unusual GPCR.

$GABA_B$ receptors are expressed on both pre- and postsynaptic membranes, where, as mentioned previously, they decrease Ca^{2+} conductance, open K^+ channels, and inhibit adenylyl cyclase. In contrast to $GABA_A$ receptors, postsynaptic

GABA$_B$ receptors elicit a slower, longer-lasting form of inhibition—an effect that is attributed to the opening of inwardly rectifying K$^+$ channels. The GABA$_B$ receptor can be distinguished pharmacologically from the GABA$_A$ receptor by its selective affinity for the agonist baclofen and its lack of affinity for muscimol and bicuculline (see Table 5–4). The GABA$_B$ receptor is believed to be linked through GTP-sensitive proteins to a calcium channel. Activation of the GABA$_B$ presynaptic receptors by baclofen decreases calcium conductance and transmitter release. Postsynaptic GABA$_B$ receptors are indirectly coupled to K$^+$ channels via G proteins, and they mediate late inhibitory postsynaptic potentials. Unlike the GABA$_A$ receptor, the GABA$_B$ receptor is not modulated by the benzodiazepines or barbiturates. Pharmacological studies have demonstrated that blockade of GABA$_B$ receptors produces none of the profound behavioral sequelae observed following administration of GABA$_A$ antagonist (e.g., seizures). These observations suggest that unlike GABA$_A$ receptors, which are believed to be in a continuous tonically activated state, GABA$_B$ receptors may be activated only under certain physiological conditions.

With regard to the functions of the GABA$_B$ receptor in the brain, it seems premature to assign a physiological or pathological role. However, the discovery of selective GABA$_B$ antagonists that cross the blood–brain barrier has

TABLE 5–4. Subdivision of GABA Receptors

RECEPTOR CLASS	PHARMACOLOGY			CHANNELS	SECOND MESSENGERS
	AGONISTS	ANTAGONISTS	MODULATORS		
		Competitive			
GABA$_A$	GABA	Bicuculline	Benzodiazepines	Cl$^-$	None
		GABAzine			
		Non-competitive			
	Muscimol	Picrotoxin	Barbiturates		
	Isoguvacine	TBPS	Steroids		
			DBI peptides		
GABA$_B$	GABA	Phaclofen	None	↑ K$^+$	Adenyl cyclase
	R(+) Baclofen	CGP-36742 3-APPA		↓ Ca^{2+}	Phosphatidyl inositol turnover

DBI, diazepam-binding inhibitor; TBPS, t-butylbicyclophosphothianate; 3-APPA, 3-aminopropylphosphinic acid; CGP-36742 (SGS-742), 3-aminophopyl-n-butyl phosphinic acid.

aided in evaluating the functions of this receptor. With the development of a potent, orally effective $GABA_B$ antagonist, CGP-54626, it became possible to better evaluate the physiological role of this receptor. *In vivo* and *in vitro* studies clearly demonstrated that blockade of $GABA_B$ receptors with this agent increased neurotransmitter (GABA and Glu) release, reduced late inhibitory postsynaptic potentials of CA1 hippocampal pyramidal neurons, and led to an increase in neuronal excitability. Behavioral studies in several species have suggested that $GABA_B$ receptor blockade can improve cognition in rats (social learning), mice (passive avoidance), and rhesus monkeys (conditional spatial color test). However, baclofen is the only drug in clinical use that interacts with $GABA_B$ receptors. This drug is used as a muscle relaxant to decrease spasticity in a diversity of neurological disorders.

Pharmacology of GABAergic Neurons

Drugs can influence GABAergic function by interacting at many different sites, both pre- and postsynaptic (Fig. 5–7). Drugs can influence presynaptic events and modify the amount of GABA that ultimately reaches and interacts with postsynaptic GABA receptors. In most cases, presynaptic drug effects do not involve an interaction with GABA receptors. The most extensively studied presynaptic drug actions involved inhibitory effects exerted on enzymes involved in GABA synthesis (GAD) and degradation (GABA-T) and the neuronal reuptake of GABA. The major exception is the interaction of drugs with GABAergic autoreceptors to modulate both the physiological activity of GABA neurons and the release and synthesis of GABA in a manner analogous to the role played by dopamine autoreceptors in the regulation of dopaminergic function.

A great deal of emphasis has been directed to the study of drug interactions with GABA receptors. Drugs interacting at the level of GABA receptors can be classified into two general categories: GABA antagonists and GABA agonists. Figure 5–7 depicts possible sites of drug interaction in a hypothetical GABAergic synapse.

GABA Antagonists

The action of GABA at the receptor–ionophore complex may be antagonized by GABA antagonists either directly, by competition with GABA for its receptor, or indirectly, by modification of the receptor or inhibition of the GABA-activated ionophore. The two classic GABA antagonists (see Fig. 5–7), bicuculline and picrotoxin, appear to act by different means. Bicuculline acts as a direct competitive antagonist of GABA at the receptor level, whereas picrotoxin acts as a noncompetitive antagonist, presumably due to its ability to

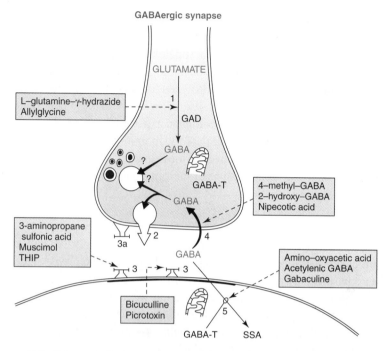

FIGURE 5–7. Schematic illustration of a GABAergic neuron indicating possible sites of drug delivery.

Site 1: *Enzymatic synthesis.* Glutamic acid decarboxylase (GAD-1) is inhibited by a number of various hydrazines. These agents appear to act primarily as pyridoxal antagonists and are therefore very nonspecific inhibitors. L-Glutamate-γ-hydrazide and allylglycine are more selective inhibitors of GAD-1, but these agents are also not entirely specific in their effects.

Site 2: *Release.* GABA release appears to be calcium dependent. No selective inhibitors of GABA release have been found.

Site 3: *Interaction with postsynaptic receptor.* Bicuculline and picrotoxin block the action of GABA at postsynaptic receptors. 3-Amonpropane sufonic acid and the hallucinogenic isoxazole derivative muscimol appear to be effective GABA agonists at postsynaptic receptors and autoreceptors. THIP, tetrahydroisoxazolopyridinol.

Site 3a: *Presynaptic autoreceptors.* Possible involvement in the control of GABA release.

Site 4: *Reuptake.* In the brain, GABA appears to be actively taken up into presynaptic endings by a sodium-dependent mechanism. A number of compounds will inhibit this uptake mechanism, such as 4-methyl-GABA and 2-hydroxy-GABA, but these agents are not GABA is metabolized primarily by transamination by GABA-T, which appears to be localized primarily in mitochondria. Amino-oxyacetic acid, gabaculline, and acetylenic GABA are effective inhibitors of GABA-T block GABA-activated ionophores. Although early studies raised some doubts about the usefulness of bicuculline as a selective GABA antagonist, this skepticism has been largely resolved and appears to be primarily related to the instability of bicuculline at 37°C and physiological pH. Under normal physiological conditions, bicuculline is hydrolyzed to bicucine, a relatively inactive GABA antagonist with a short half-life of several minutes. The quaternary salts now used for most electrophysiological experiments (bicuculline methiodide and bicuculline methochloride) are much more water-soluble and stable over a broad pH range of 2–8. However, these quaternary salts are not suitable for systemic administration because of their poor penetration into the CNS.

GABA Agonists

Electrophysiological studies have demonstrated a wide variety of compounds that are capable of directly activating bicuculline-sensitive GABA receptors. These agonists can be readily subdivided into two groups based on their ability to penetrate the blood–brain barrier, dictating whether they will be active or inactive following systemic administration. Agents such as 3-aminopropanesulfonic acid, β-guanidinoproprionic acid, 4-aminotetrolic acid, *trans*-4-aminocrotonic acid, and *trans*-3-aminocyclopentane-1-carboxylic acid are effective direct-acting GABA agonists. However, entry of these agents into the brain following systemic administration is minimal. In addition, compounds such as *trans*-4-aminotetrolic acid and 4-aminocrotonic acid also inhibit GABA-T and GABA uptake; therefore, their action is not totally attributable to their direct agonist properties.

In contrast to this class of direct-acting GABA agonists, other GABA agonists readily pass the blood–brain barrier and are active following systemic administration. Muscimol (3-hydroxy-5-aminomethylisoxazole) is the agent in this group that has been most extensively studied. Some other agents in this group include (5)-(2)-5-(1-aminoethyl)-3-isoxazole, tetrahydroisoxazolopyridinol (THIP; a bicyclic muscimol analog), SL-76002 (α[chloro-4-phenyl] fluro-5-hydroxy-2 benzilide-neamino-4H butyramide), and kojic amine (2-aminomethyl-3-hydroxy-4H-pyran-4-one). In addition, GABAergic substances may be further categorized as direct or indirect GABA receptor activators. For example, muscimol, isoguvacine, and THIP are GABA mimetic agents that interact directly with GABA receptors. Indirectly acting GABA mimetics facilitate GABAergic transmission by increasing the amount of endogenous GABA that reaches the receptor or by altering in some manner the coupling of the GABA receptor-mediated change in chloride permeability. Thus, many drugs often classified as indirect GABA agonists act presynaptically to modify GABA release and metabolism rather than by interacting directly with GABA receptors. For this reason, drugs such as gabaculine (a GABA-T inhibitor), nipecotic acid (a GABA uptake inhibitor), and baclofen (an agent that, in addition to many other actions, causes release of GABA from intracellular stores) are often classified incorrectly as GABA agonists. The benzodiazepines mentioned previously also appear to potentiate the action of tonically released GABA at the receptor by displacement of an endogenous inhibitor of GABA receptor binding, allowing more endogenous GABA to reach and bind receptors. Thus, benzodiazepines are sometimes also classified as GABA agonists. A GABA-like action can also be elicited by agents that bypass GABA receptors and influence GABA ionophores. It has been suggested that pentobarbital acts at the level of the GABA ionophore, but it is unclear whether its CNS-depressant effects are explained by this action.

The structures of some of the more potent and widely used direct-acting GABA agonists are illustrated in Figures 5–8 and 5–9. Included are muscimol, isoguvacine, THIP, and (1)-*trans*-3-aminocyclopentane carboxylic acid. Useful therapeutic effects have not been obtained by use of agents of this sort, which have direct GABA mimetic effects (e.g., muscimol), inhibit the active reuptake of GABA (e.g., nipecotic acid), or alter the rate of synthesis or degradation of GABA (e.g., amino-oxyacetic acid and gabaculine). However, useful therapeutic effects are achieved with the anxiolytic benzodiazepines (e.g., diazepam [Valium] and chlordiazepoxide [Librium]), which may exert their actions by facilitating GABAergic transmission via their positive allosteric agonist actions at $GABA_A$ receptors.

As the anatomical distribution and functional properties of $GABA_A$ receptor subtypes and subunits become clearly defined, this knowledge may enable the development of therapeutically useful subtype-specific agonists that can be directed to modify GABAergic function in selective brain areas.

Endogenous Modulators

The large number of recognition sites associated with $GABA_A$ receptors has led to speculation that a host of endogenous regulatory factors exist. A number of candidates have been identified, but with the exception of the neurosteroids and the endogenous diazepam-binding inhibitor, there is little compelling evidence that any play an important role in modulating $GABA_A$ receptor function *in vivo*.

Therapeutic Use of GABAergic Drugs

The GABA system is the main inhibitory neurotransmitter system in the brain and is the target for many clinically used drugs. $GABA_A$ receptors are the major molecular target for the action of many of the currently used GABAergic therapeutics (see Chapters 14 and 19).

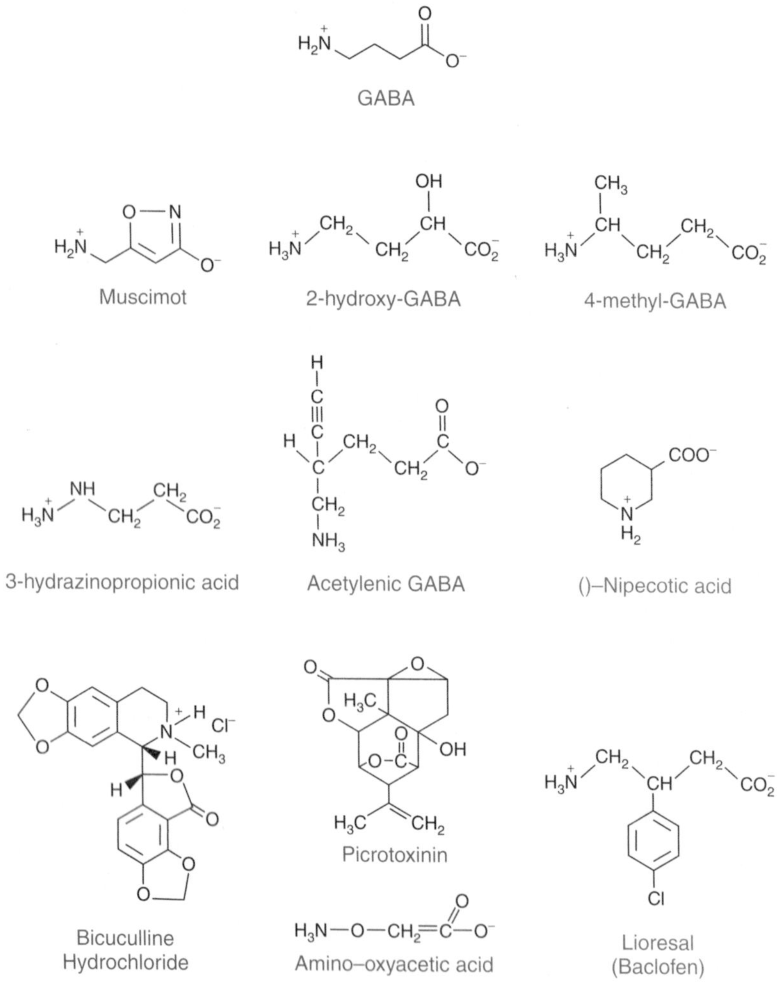

FIGURE 5–8. Structures of compounds that act at GABAergic synapses.

The enhancement or impairment of GABA-mediated synaptic transmission underlies the pharmacotherapy of various neurological diseases. $GABA_A$ receptors are thus targets for many clinically used neuroactive drugs, including classical benzodiazepines (BZ), mediating their anxiolytic, hypnotic, and anti-convulsant effects via the BZ site of $GABA_A$ receptors (see Fig. 5–5). Hypnotics such as Dalmane and Restoril and anxiolytics such as diazepam (Valium) and alprazolam (Xanax) act via the BZ site. The non-BZ $GABA_A$ positive allosteric modulators, three of which are approved in the United States for treatment of insomnia (eszopiclone [Lunesta], zaleplon [Sonata], and zolpidem [Ambien]), also act at the BZ site. Barbiturates used as sedatives, hypnotics,

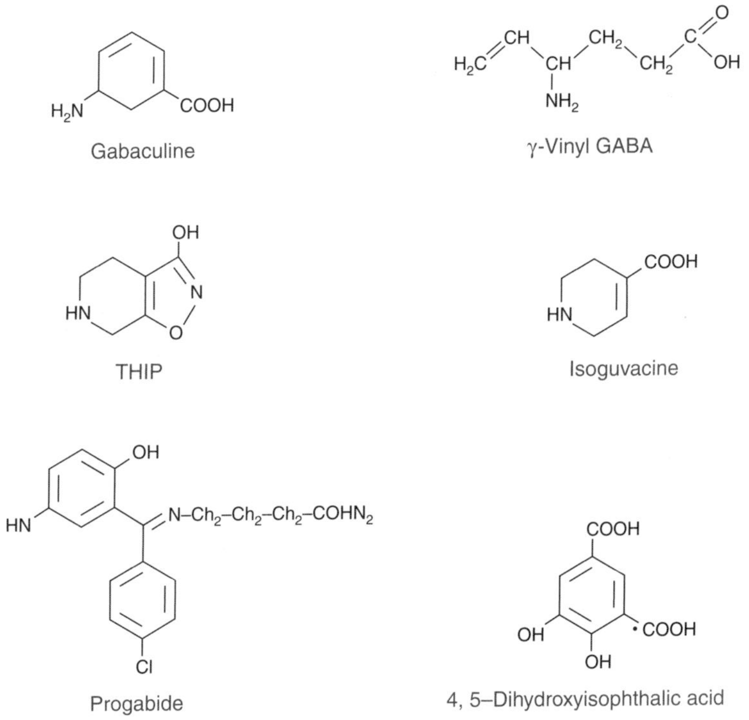

FIGURE 5–9. Structures of compounds that act at GABAergic synapses.

and anticonvulsants, such as amobarbital (Amytal), secobarbital (Seconal), and phenobarbital (Luminal), respectively, act at the barbiturate site of $GABA_A$ receptors. The synthetic steroid anesthetic alphaxalone is a potent modulator at the steroid site of $GABA_A$ receptors.

$GABA_B$ receptors have also been implicated in a wide variety of neurological and psychiatric disorders. However, only two $GABA_B$ drugs are on the market—baclofen (Lioresal) and GHB (Xyrem)—although several are under development and have shown promise in animal models. Lioresal acts as a muscle relaxant and is used to decrease spasticity in a variety of neurological disorders. It is used less frequently for the treatment of trigeminal neuralgia and neuropathic pain. Its use as a general analgesic is limited because of its sedative properties and rapid tolerance to its pain-relieving effects. Inhibition of glutamate release is believed to underlie its clinical efficacy. GHB (Xyrem) has been approved in a number of countries for general anesthesia and for the treatment of alcohol withdrawal and addiction. GHB is a controlled substance in the United States and approved by the Food and Drug Administration only for the treatment of narcolepsy; it is used by a small group of patients with narcolepsy who experience episodes of cataplexy.

GLYCINE

As an Inhibitory Transmitter

Structurally, Gly is the simplest amino acid. It is found in all mammalian body fluids and tissue proteins in substantial amounts. Although Gly is not an essential amino acid, it is an essential intermediate in the metabolism of protein, peptides, one-carbon fragments, nucleic acids, porphyrins, and bile salts. It is also considered to be an established inhibitory neurotransmitter, enriched in the medulla, spinal cord, and retina. Thus, Gly appears to have a more circumscribed function in the CNS than the more ubiquitously distributed GABA. As with the other major amino acid transmitters, numerous neurochemical studies have attempted to separate and distinguish between the general metabolic and transmitter functions of Gly within the CNS. Gly also appears to be an exclusively vertebrate transmitter, making it unique among the transmitter substances.

Glycinergic neurons appear to respond to activation as other chemically defined neurons do. Arrival of an action potential in the presynaptic nerve terminal initiates a calcium-dependent cascade of events, which ultimately involves fusion of the presynaptic membrane and release of Gly into the synaptic cleft. Gly is removed from the synaptic cleft by uptake transporters located on glial cells and on the presynaptic terminals of the glycinergic neurons. However, in the past several years, very little progress has been achieved in developing pharmacological tools that act selectively on Gly systems or in generating more information concerning Gly metabolism in neuronal tissue.

Uptake

In the spinal cord and brain stem, specific uptake of Gly has been demonstrated in regions exhibiting high densities of inhibitory Gly receptors. Two Gly transporter proteins have been cloned and shown to be expressed in brain as well as in peripheral tissues. Both are members of the large family of Na^+/Cl^--dependent neurotransmitter transporters (see Chapter 8) and share approximately 50% sequence identity with the GABA transporter. The Gly transporters have been named GLYT-1 and GLYT-2, in the order in which they were reported. These transporters have very similar kinetics and pharmacological properties but differ in the distribution of their transcripts, measured by *in situ* hybridization. The distribution of GLYT-1 and GLYT-2 mRNA suggests that GLYT-1 is primarily a glial transporter and GLYT-2 is associated primarily with neurons. GLYT-1 exists in three isoforms, which are probably generated by alternate splicing. These isoforms do not exhibit any known variation in their uptake properties but do possess distinct patterns of expression in the CNS.

GLYT-1 is expressed in both astrocytes and neurons, whereas GLYT-2 is localized on axons and the terminal boutons of neurons that contain vesicular Gly. Glycinergic neurotransmission is terminated by the uptake of glycine into glycinergic nerve terminals and neighboring glial cells. This uptake process is mediated by GLYT-1 and GLYT-2. GLYT-1, in addition to its role in glycinergic synapses, is thought to regulate the concentration of glycine at excitatory synapses containing NMDA receptors, which require glycine and/or D-serine as a co-agonist. Genetic studies in mice indicate that at glycinergic synapses, the glial transporter GLYT-1 catalyzes the removal of Gly from the synaptic cleft, whereas GLYT-2 is required for the reuptake of Gly into nerve terminals, thereby allowing for neurotransmitter reloading of synaptic vesicles. The GLYT-1 isoforms can be distinguished pharmacologically from GLYT-2 since they are sensitive to the effects of sarcosine, the N-methyl derivative of Gly, which is a natural amino acid found in muscle. A structurally and functionally distinct vesicular Gly transporter (VGAT/VIAAT), subject to inhibition by vigabatrin, is responsible for concentrating Gly (and GABA) within synaptic vesicles and storage in the nerve terminals.

Both GLYT-1 and GLYT-2 are expressed in the brain stem, spinal cord, and hippocampus—locations consistent with their role in terminating glycinergic transmission. However, GLYT-1 is also expressed in several regions of the forebrain that are devoid of glycinergic neurotransmission. Thus, GLYT-1 can regulate NMDA receptor function in these areas by controlling the levels of extracellular Gly available to allosterically modulate the activity of these receptors (see Glycine as a Modulator of NMDA Receptors). That being the case, GLYT-1 inhibitors may prove to be useful clinically to augment NMDA receptor function.

Glycine Receptors

The strychnine-sensitive glycine receptor(GlyR) was the first neurotransmitter receptor protein to be isolated from the mammalian CNS. GlyR has been cloned and expressed, and it appears to be structurally quite homologous to the multimeric subunits of other ligand-gated ion channels. Like $GABA_{A/C}$ receptors, GlyRs belong to the pentameric nAChR superfamily. Four different genes (called *Glra1–4*) encoding GlyR α subunits (α_{1-4}) and a single GlyR β subunit gene(*Glrb*) have been identified in mammals. Photoaffinity labeling reveals that both Gly- and strychnine-binding sites are located on the α subunit. Several GlyR α subunit variants have been shown to differ in their pharmacological properties and levels of expression. Expression of α_1 and α_2 subunits is developmentally regulated, with a switch from the neonatal α_2 subunit (strychnine-insensitive) to the adult α_1 form (strychnine-sensitive) approximately 2 weeks postnatally in the mouse. It is interesting that the timing of this switch corresponds with the development of spasticity in the mutant spastic mouse, prompting speculation that insufficient expression of the adult strychnine-sensitive isoform may underlie some forms of spasticity.

In addition to their presence in spinal cord and brain stem, electrophysiological, immunocytochemical, and *in situ* hybridization studies have shown that functional GlyRs are also present in other brain regions of developing and mature brain including the hippocampus, where they are expressed by CA1 pyramidal cells and interneurons. Studies demonstrating strychnine-sensitive, calcium-dependent, stimulus-induced release of glycine from nerve endings in the hippocampus suggest that glycine acts as an inhibitory transmitter here as well as in brain stem and spinal cord.

GlyRs play well-documented roles in motor control and sensory processing that are impaired in hyperekplexia, a rare neurological disease characterized by an exaggerated startle response. The fact that glycine illicits a potent tonic activation of hippocampal α_2 subunit of GlyRs and diminished synaptic transmission in CA1 pyrimidal cells indicates that GlyRs may play an important role in mediating inhibitory neurotransmission in the hippocampus.

Studies also implicate GlyRs in pain perception, the pathology of autism, human immunodeficiency virus-associated dementia, and generalized epilepsy. These broad roles indicate a significant clinical need for novel ligands that display high selectivity for and potency at GlyRs.

Release

Very little is known about the factors controlling the release of Gly from the spinal cord or hippocampus. Again, as with GABA, the efficient uptake process may explain why it is difficult to detect Gly release from the CNS. The main problem (as with GABA, Glu, etc.) is that there is no distinct neuronal pathway that may be isolated and stimulated; thus, all of the induced activity is very generalized, making the significance of any demonstrable release (metabolite or excess transmitter) very difficult to interpret.

Metabolism

Despite these well-characterized functional properties, our understanding of some aspects of the metabolism of Gly in nervous tissue remains rudimentary. For example, we still do not know whether biosynthesis is important for the maintenance of Gly levels in the spinal cord or whether the neurons depend on the uptake and accumulation of preformed Gly. As indicated in Figure 5–10, Gly can be formed from serine by a reversible folate-dependent reaction catalyzed by the enzyme serine *trans*-hydroxymethylase. Serine can also be formed in nerve tissue from glucose via the intermediates 3-phosphoglycerate and 3-phosphoserine. It is also conceivable that Gly might be formed from

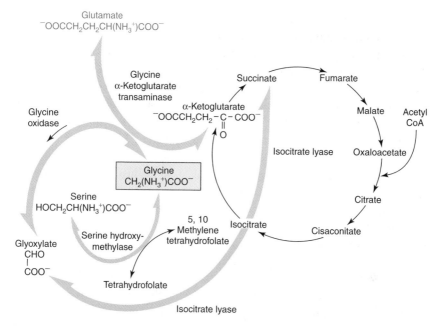

FIGURE 5–10. Possible metabolic routes for the formation and degradation of glycine by nervous tissue. (Modified from Roberts and Hammerschlag, 1972.)

glyoxylate via a transaminase reaction with Glu. Although not established definitively, it appears likely that serine serves as the major precursor of Gly in the CNS and that serine hydroxymethyltransferase and D-glycerate dehydrogenase are the best candidates for the rate-limiting enzymes involved in the biosynthesis of Gly. Not only is our knowledge of the metabolism of Gly in nervous tissue minimal but also only scanty information is available on the factors regulating the concentration of Gly in the CNS.

Glycine as a Modulator of NMDA Receptors

A new role has been proposed for Gly that is distinct from its established role as an inhibitory transmitter in lower brain stem areas, spinal cord, and, more recently, hippocampus mediated by a strychnine-sensitive chloride conductance. Several groups have shown that nanomolar concentrations of Gly increase the frequency of opening of one of the subsets of Glu receptors, namely the NMDA receptor channel. This effect of Gly is strychnine-insensitive, suggesting a mechanism involving allosteric regulation of the NMDA receptor complex through a distinct Gly binding site (see Fig. 5–2). This action can be mimicked with Gly agonists and blocked by other Gly antagonists, although not strychnine. This allosteric concept is supported by the existence of strychnine-insensitive Gly binding sites that have an anatomical distribution identical to that of the

NMDA receptor. Compared with the effects of benzodiazepines on the GABA receptor, the enhancement of NMDA responses observed with Gly is much greater. This suggests that the main effect of Gly is to prevent desensitization of the NMDA receptor during prolonged exposure to agonists. Gly appears to accomplish this by accelerating the recovery of the receptor from its desensitized state rather than by blocking the onset of desensitization. D-Serine has also been proposed to play a role as an important co-agonist for NMDA receptor activity. A surprising unique biosynthetic pathway for D-serine has been demonstrated, indicating the conservation of D-amino acid metabolism in mammals. D-Serine was originally thought to be exclusively made in astrocytes. However, data indicate that D-serine has a neuronal origin as well. There is a growing body of evidence indicating that D-serine, rather than glycine as originally thought, is the more important endogenous ligand for NMDA receptors in many brain structures. D-Serine is synthesized mainly in glial cells and it is released upon activation of glutamate receptors. Like glycine, D-serine concentration in the synaptic cleft controls the number of NMDA receptors available for activation by glutamate. Consequently, the glial environment of neurons and the extracellular level of co-agonist have a critical impact on the direction and magnitude of NMDA receptor-dependent synaptic plasticity. Since Gly and D-serine facilitation of synaptic responses mediated by NMDA receptors appears to be a common regulatory mechanism for excitatory synapses, transporters that regulate extracellular concentrations of these co-agonists in brain regions where NMDA receptors play a critical role in excitatory transmission provide novel targets for modulation of NMDA receptors. Accumulating evidence in animal models suggests that GlyT-1 inhibitors may be a potential therapeutic target for cognitive deficits in schizophrenia. It is noteworthy that double-blind, placebo-controlled studies of the endogenous Gly-T-1 inhibitor, N-methylglycine (sarcosine), demonstrated significant improvement in schizophrenic patients. Clinical studies with more potent bioavailable Gly-T-1 inhibitors are in progress.

Another interesting question is whether endogenous Gly antagonists (e.g., kynurenate) may also play a role in regulating neuronal function where NMDA receptors are involved in excitotoxic damage. However, clinical trials of a selective NMDA receptors Gly antagonist, previously reported to be neuroprotective in animal models of stroke, have shown no such efficacy when evaluated in the first 6 hours after a stroke.

SELECTED REFERENCES

Bear, M. F., G. Dolen, E. Osterweil, and N. Nagaarajan (2008). Fragile X: Translation in action. *Neuropsychopharmacology* 33, 84–87.

Benarroch, E. E. (2008). Metabotropic glutamate receptors: Synaptic modulators and therapeutic targets for neurological disease. *Neurology* 70, 964–968.

Betz, H. and B. Laube (2006). Glycine receptors: Recent insights into their structural organization and functional diversity. *J. Neurochem.* 97, 1600–1610.

Bowery, N. G. (2006). GABA$_B$ receptor: A site of therapeutic benefit. *Curr. Opin. Pharmacol.* 6(1), 37–43.

Bridges, R. J. (2001). The ins and outs of glutamate transporter pharmacology. *Tocris Rev.* 17, 1–5.

Conn, P. J., C. Tamminga, D. D. Schoepp, and C. Lindsley (2008). Schizophrenia: Moving beyond monoamine antagonists. *Mol. Interventions* 6, 18–23.

Cooper, J. R., F. E. Bloom, and R. H. Roth (2003). *The Biochemical Basis of Neuropharmacology*, 8th ed. Oxford University Press, New York.

Coyle, J. T., M. Leski, and J. H. Morrison (2004). The diverse roles of L-glutamic acid in brain signal transduction. In *Psychopharmacology: The Fifth Generation of Progress* (K. L. Davis, D. Charney, J. T. Coyle, and C. Nemeroff, Eds.). Lippincott Williams & Wilkins, Philadelphia, pp. 120–132.

Fell, M. J., K. A. Svensson, B. G. Johnson, and D. A. Schoepp (2008). Evidence for the role of mGlu2 not mGlu3 receptors in the preclinical antipsychotic pharmacology of the mGlu2/3 receptor agonist LY404039. *J. Pharmacol Exp. Ther.* 326(1), 209-217.

Javitt, D. C. (2008). Glycine transport inhibitors and the treatment of schizophrenia. *Biol. Psychiatry* 63, 6–8.

Oliet, S. H. R. and J.-P. Mothet (2008). Regulation of N-methyl-D-aspartate receptors by astrocytic D-serine. *Neuroscience*, in press.

Olsen, R. W. (2004). GABA. In *Psychopharmacology: The Fifth Generation of Progress* (K. L. Davis, D. Charney, J. T. Coyle, and C. Nemeroff, Eds.). Lippincott Williams & Wilkins, Philadelphia, pp. 120–132.

Paul, S. M. (1995). GABA and glycine. In *Psychopharmacology: The Fourth Generation of Progress* (F. E. Bloom and D. J. Kupfer, Eds.). Raven Press, New York, pp. 87–94.

Roberts, E. and R. Hammerschlag (1972). *Basic Neurochemistry*. Wiley, New York.

Rudolph, U. and H. Mohler (2006). GABA-based therapeutic approaches: GABA$_A$ receptor subtype functions. *Curr. Opin. Pharmacol.* 8(2), 99–107.

Shigeri, Y., R. P. Seal, and K. Shimamoto (2004). Molecular pharmacology of glutamate transporters, EAATs and VGLUTs. *Brain Res. Rev.* 45, 250–265.

Watling, K. J. (2006). *The Sigma-RBI Handbook of Receptor Classification and Signal Transduction,* 5th ed. Sigma, St. Louis.

Zhang, L.-H., N. Gong, D. Fei, L. Xu, and T.-L. Xu (2008). Glycine uptake regulates hippocampal network activity via glycine receptor-mediated tonic inhibition. *Neuropsychopharmacology* 33, 701–711.

Acetylcholine

The neurophysiological activity of acetylcholine (ACh) has been known since the early 19th century and its neurotransmitter role since the mid-1920s. With this long history, it is not surprising that students assume everything is already known about this transmitter. The main reason ACh assumed an early prominent role in guiding studies of neurotransmitters is the ease with which ACh can be studied. ACh is the transmitter at the neuromuscular junction, and thus both nerve terminal and its target can be readily accessed for experimental manipulations. Subsequent investigations also focused on the superior cervical ganglion, another peripheral site that was also easy to isolate and study. Lessons learned from experiments conducted on these peripheral tissues shaped our early approaches to defining the characteristics of neurotransmitters and neurotransmission. Unfortunately, the delay in developing sophisticated methods for determining where in the brain ACh was present in cholinergic tracts and terminals, which took decades to resolve, left this field far behind that of the biogenic amines. The following is the structural formula of ACh:

$$(CH_3)_3 \, N^+ - CH_2 \, CH_2 - O - C - CH_3$$
$$\underset{O}{\overset{\|}{}}$$

SYNTHESIS

ACh is synthesized in a single step by a reaction catalyzed by choline acetyl-transferase (ChAT):

$$\text{Acetyl CoA} + \text{choline} = \text{ACh} + \text{CoA}$$

Before entering into a discussion of ChAT, we should take note of Figure 6–1, which depicts the possible sources of acetyl coenzyme A (CoA) and choline. In brain slices, homogenates, acetone powder extracts, and preparations of nerve ending particles, glucose, or citrate are the best sources for ACh synthesis, with acetate rarely showing any activity. Regardless of its source, acetyl CoA is primarily synthesized in mitochondria. Since, as detailed later, ChAT appears to be in the synaptosomal cytoplasm, another still unsolved problem is how acetyl CoA is transported out of the mitochondria to participate in ACh synthesis. A probable carrier for acetyl CoA is citrate, which can diffuse into the cytosol and produce acetyl CoA via citrate lyase; a possible carrier is acetyl carnitine, and another possibility is Ca-induced leakage of acetyl CoA from mitochondria.

Choline is transported to the brain both free and in phospholipid form (possibly as phosphatidylcholine) by the blood. Following the hydrolysis of ACh, approximately 35–50% of the liberated choline is transported back

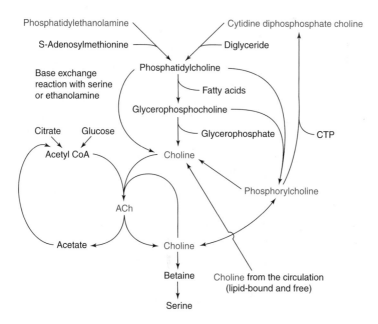

FIGURE 6–1. Acetylcholine (ACh) metabolism. CoA, coenzyme A; CTP, cytidine triphosphate.

into the presynaptic terminal by a sodium-dependent, high-affinity active transport system to be reutilized in ACh synthesis. As outlined in Figure 6–1, the remaining choline may be catabolized or become incorporated into phospholipids, which can again serve as a source of choline. A curious observation is that when brain cortical slices are incubated for 2 hours in a Krebs–Ringer medium, choline accumulates to approximately 10 times its original concentration. Similarly, a rapid postmortem increase in choline has been observed. The precise source of this choline is unknown; a probable candidate is phosphatidylcholine.

CHOLINE TRANSPORT

Choline crosses cell membranes by two processes, referred to as *high-affinity* and *low-affinity transport*. High-affinity transport, with a Michaelis constant (K_m) for choline of 1–5 μM, is saturable, carrier mediated, dependent on sodium, and stimulated by chloride. It is also dependent on the membrane potential of the cell or organelle so that any agent (e.g., K^+) that depolarizes the cell will concurrently inhibit high-affinity transport. Low-affinity choline transport, with a K_m of 40–80 μM, appears to operate by a passive diffusion process, to be linearly dependent on the concentration of choline, and to be virtually nonsaturable. In contrast to the other neurotransmitters, ACh is taken up in terminals only via low-affinity transport; it is only choline that exhibits high-affinity kinetics. Evidence suggests that the high-affinity transport of choline is specific for cholinergic terminals and is not present in aminergic nerve terminals. Furthermore, transport is kinetically (but not physically) coupled to ACh synthesis. Approximately 50–85% of the choline that is transported by the high-affinity process is utilized for ACh synthesis. Low-affinity transport, however, is found in cell bodies and in tissues such as the corneal epithelium, likely for the synthesis of choline-containing phospholipids. High-affinity choline transport that is coupled to phospholipid synthesis can also be found in tissues that do not synthesize ACh. Hemicholinium-3 is an extremely potent inhibitor of high-affinity transport (K_m of 0.05–1 μM) but a relatively weak inhibitor of low-affinity transport (K_m of 10–120 μM). There are three obvious mechanisms for regulating the level of ACh in cells: feedback inhibition by ACh on ChAT, mass action, and the availability of acetyl CoA and/or choline. Of these three possibilities, the major regulatory factor seems to be high-affinity choline transport. This view derives from early observations that choline is rate limiting in the synthesis of ACh coupled with findings in a number of laboratories. Using the septal–hippocampal pathway, a known cholinergic tract, Kuhar and associates showed that changes in impulse flow induced via electrical stimulation or pentylenetetrazol administration (both of which increase impulse flow) or via lesioning or the administration of pento-barbital (both of which decrease neuronal traffic) will alter high-affinity trans-port of choline into hippocampal synaptosomes. In their studies, procedures that activated impulse flow increased the maximal velocity (V_{max}) of choline transport, whereas agents that stopped neuronal activity decreased V_{max}. In neither situation was the K_m changed, a result to be expected since the concen-tration of choline outside the neuron (5–10 μM) normally exceeds the K_m for transport (1–5 μM). Recent evidence, however, suggests that this relationship between impulse traffic and choline transport does not occur in all brain areas (e.g., in the striatum, where cholinergic interneurons abound). In addition, the endogenous concentration of ACh is implicated in regulating the level of the transmitter in the brain. Thus, in several studies, an increase in choline uptake following depolarization of a preparation has been attributed to the release of endogenous ACh upon depolarization. Other studies, however, suggest that this increased choline uptake is not related to ACh release but, rather, to an increase in Na–K adenosine triphosphatase (ATPase) activity. The high-affinity choline transporter has been cloned by the Okuda group, who developed an antibody to map cholinergic neurons.

CHOLINE ACETYLTRANSFERASE

The synthetic enzyme ChAT is the definitive marker for the presence of cho-linergic neurons in brain. Multiple mRNAs encode ChAT, resulting from dif-ferential use of three promoters and alternative splicing of the 5′ noncoding region. In the rat, the different transcripts encode the same protein, but in humans they give rise to multiple forms of the enzyme, including both active and inactive forms. The functional significance of these different transcripts is uncertain.

Although ChAT is the sole enzyme in ACh synthesis, it is not the rate-liming step in ACh synthesis. The full enzymatic activity of ChAT is not expressed *in vivo*. The activity of ChAT measured *in vitro* is much greater that would be expected on the basis of ACh synthesis *in vivo*. It has been suggested that the reason for this discrepancy might be related to the requirement to transport acetyl CoA from the mitochondria to the cytoplasm, which may be the rate-limiting step in ACh synthesis. Alternatively, intracellular choline concentrations and choline transport may ultimately determine the rate of ACh synthesis. This latter speculation has led to the administration of choline precursors in an attempt to boost ACh synthesis in the brain of Alzheimer's patients in which there is a marked decrease in ACh in the cerebral cortex. Attempts to treat Alzheimer's disease by administration of choline precursors such as lecithin have been unsuccessful in diminishing dementia.

With respect to the cellular localization of ChAT, the highest activity is found in the interpeduncular nucleus, caudate nucleus, retina, corneal epithelium, and central spinal roots (3000–4000 mg ACh synthesized/g/hour⁻). In contrast, dorsal spinal roots contain only trace amounts of the enzyme, as does the cerebellum.

When highly purified from rat brain, ChAT has a molecular weight of 67–75 kDa: It has an apparent K_m for choline of 7.5×10^{-4} M and for acetyl CoA of 1.0×10^{-5} M. Recent estimates suggest an equilibrium constant of 13. The enzyme is activated by chloride and inhibited by sulfhydryl reagents. A variety of studies on the substrate specificity of the enzyme indicate that various acyl derivatives of both CoA and ethanolamine can be utilized. The major gap in our knowledge of ChAT is that we do not know of any useful (i.e., potent and specific) direct inhibitor. Styrylpyridine derivatives inhibit it but suffer from the fact that they are light sensitive, somewhat insoluble, and possess varying degrees of anticholinesterase activity. Hemicholinium inhibits the synthesis of ACh indirectly by preventing the transport of choline across cell membranes.

ACETYLCHOLINESTERASE

Everybody agrees that ACh is hydrolyzed by cholinesterases, but nobody is sure just how many cholinesterases exist in the body. All cholinesterases will hydrolyze not only ACh but also other esters. Conversely, hydrolytic enzymes such as arylesterases, trypsin, and chymotrypsin will not hydrolyze choline esters. The problem in determining the number of cholinesterases that exist is that different species and organs sometimes exhibit maximal activity with different substrates. For our purposes, we divide the enzymes into two rigidly defined classes: *acetylcholinesterase* (also called "true" or specific cholinesterase) and *butyrylcholinesterase* (also called "pseudo" or nonspecific cholinesterase; the term *propionylcholinesterase* is sometimes used since in some tissues propionylcholine is hydrolyzed more rapidly than butyrylcholine). Although their molecular forms are similar, the two enzymes are distinct entities, encoded by specific genes. Evidence suggests that in lower forms butyrylcholinesterase predominates, gradually giving way to acetylcholinesterase with evolution. The type of cholinesterase found in a tissue is often a reflection of the tissue. This fact is used as a discriminating index between cholinesterases. In general, neural tissue contains acetylcholinesterase, whereas glial cells and nonneural tissue usually contain butyrylcholinesterase. However, this is a generalization, and some neural tissue (e.g., autonomic ganglia) contains both esterases, as do some extraneural organs (e.g., liver and lung). Because of its ubiquity, cholinesterase activity cannot be used as the sole indicator of a cholinergic system in the absence of additional supporting evidence. To generalize on this point, until neuron-specific, transmitter-degrading enzymes are discovered, it is a neurochemical commandment that, to delineate a neuronal tract, one should always assay with an enzyme involved in the synthesis of a neurotransmitter and not one concerned with catabolism.

UPTAKE, SYNTHESIS, AND RELEASE OF ACH

Superior Cervical Ganglion, Brain, and Skeletal Muscle

The only major, thorough studies of ACh turnover in nervous tissue were done originally by MacIntosh and colleagues and subsequently by Collier using the superior cervical ganglion of the cat. Using one ganglion to assay the resting level of ACh and perfusing the contralateral organ, these investigators determined the amount of transmitter synthesized and released under a variety of experimental conditions, including electrical stimulation, addition of an anticholinesterase to the perfusion fluid, and perfusion media of varying ionic composition. Their results may be summarized as follows: During stimulation, ACh turns over at a rate of 8–10% of its resting content every minute (i.e., approximately 24–30 ng/minute). At rest, the turnover rate is approximately 0.5 ng/minute. Since there is no change in the ACh content of the ganglion during stimulation at physiological frequencies, it is evident that electrical stimulation not only releases the transmitter but also stimulates its synthesis. Choline is the rate-limiting factor in the synthesis of ACh. In the perfused ganglion, Na^+ is necessary for optimum synthesis and storage, and Ca^{2+} is necessary for release of the neurotransmitter. Newly synthesized ACh appears to be more readily released upon nerve stimulation than depot or stored ACh. Approximately half of the choline produced by cholinesterase activity is reutilized to make new ACh.

At least three separate stores of ACh in the ganglion are inferred from these studies: *surplus* ACh, considered to be intracellular, which accumulates only in an eserine-treated ganglion and is not released by nerve stimulation but is released by K depolarization; *depot* ACh, which is released by nerve impulses and accounts for approximately 85% of the original store; and *stationary* ACh, which constitutes the remaining 15% that is nonreleasable.

Choline analogs, such as triethylcholine, homocholine, and pyrrolcholine, are released by nerve stimulation only after they are acetylated in the ganglia. Increasing the choline supply in the plasma during perfusion of the ganglion only transiently increases the amount of ACh that is releasable with electrical stimulation, despite accumulation of the transmitter in the ganglion. The compound AH5183 (vesamicol) inhibits ACh transport into synaptic vesicles and blocks release of ACh from the stimulated ganglia.

Most of these characteristics, which were established decades ago, are recapitulated in the central nervous system (CNS).

ACh is synthesized via ChAT and, once formed, is transported into vesicles by the vesicular cholinergic transporter (VAChT). This transporter is distinct from the plasma membrane transporter that accumulates choline. ACh is not taken up into cholinergic terminals by a high-affinity transport system. However, as first described by Parsons' laboratory, ACh is transported into synaptic vesicles via a proton-pumping ATPase activity. A glycosylated ATPase pumps protons out of vesicles and drives ACh via a separate transporter into vesicles in exchange for the protons. VAChT was cloned on the basis of homology to a *Caenorhabditis elegans* gene(unc-17) that encodes a protein homologous with VMAT. VAChT is expressed in cholinergic neurons throughout the brain and is another useful marker in addition to ChAT for the presence of cholinergic neurons.

VAChT is present on chromosome 10, near the gene for ChAT, and is unique in that its entire coding region is contained in the first intron of the ChAT gene: Both genes are coordinately regulated.

Release

Following the discovery of presynaptically localized vesicles that contained ACh, the conclusion was almost unavoidable that these organelles are the source of the quantal release of transmitter as described in the neurophysiological experiments of Katz and collaborators. Thus, the obvious interpretation has been that as the nerve is depolarized, Ca^{2+} enters the terminal, vesicles in apposition to the terminal fuse with the presynaptic membrane, and ACh is released into the synaptic cleft to interact with receptors on the postsynaptic cell to change ion permeability. Synapsin I, a phosphoprotein that is localized in vesicles, may mediate the translocation of vesicles to the plasma membrane. It is of interest because botulinum toxin A binds to it and irreversibly degrades it, leading to a persistent blockade of neuromuscular transmission. The use of minute doses of locally injected botulinum toxin has found many medical uses (Chapter 17). Other vesicular proteins that have been implicated in the exocytotic process are the synaptotagmins, synaptophysins, and synaptobrevins (see Chapter 3). Synaptobrevin is the target for both tetanus toxin and botulinum toxin type B, which are zinc endopeptidases that inhibit ACh release by cleaving it. Synaptotagmin has been implicated as a Ca^{2+} sensor in the release process. The subsequent sequence of events is not clear, but in some manner the presynaptic membrane is pinocytotically recaptured and vesicles are resynthesized and simultaneously or subsequently repleted with ACh. This endocytotic event is apparently triggered by calcineurin, a Ca^{2+}-dependent protein phosphatase.

CHOLINERGIC PATHWAYS

The identification of cholinergic synapses in the peripheral nervous system has been relatively easy, and we have known for a long time that ACh is the transmitter at autonomic ganglia, at parasympathetic postganglionic synapses, and at the neuromuscular junction. In the CNS, however, until the late 1970s, technical difficulties limited our knowledge of cholinergic tracts to the motoneuron collaterals to Renshaw cells in the spinal cord. With respect to the aforementioned technical difficulties, the traditional approach has been to lesion a suspected tract and then assay for ACh, ChAT, or high-affinity choline uptake at the presumed terminal area. Problems with lesioning include making discrete, well-defined lesions and interrupting fibers of passage. This latter problem is illustrated by the discovery that a habenula–interpeduncular nucleus projection that, based on lesioning of the habenula, was always described as a cholinergic pathway is not: It turned out that what was lesioned were cholinergic fibers that passed through the habenula. Thus, although the interpeduncular nucleus has the highest choline uptake and ChAT activity of any area in the brain, the origin of this innervation remains largely unknown. A quantum leap in technology for tracing tracts in the CNS has occurred in the past several decades. Through the use of histochemical techniques (originally developed by Koelle and co-workers) that stain for regenerated acetylcholinesterase after DFP treatment (Butcher, Fibiger), autoradiography with muscarinic receptor antagonists (Rotter, Kuhar), immunohistochemical procedures with antibodies to ChAT (McGeer, Salvaterra, Cuello, Wainer), coupled with the employment of specific cholinotoxins, a clearer picture of cholinergic tracts in the CNS has emerged. The well-documented tracts are depicted in Figure 6–2. There is additional information that in the striatum and the nucleus accumbens septi, only cholinergic interneurons are found. Also, intrinsic cholinergic neurons have been reported to exist in the cerebral cortex, colocalized with vasoactive intestinal polypeptide and often in close proximity to blood vessels. Recent studies using electrophysiology, specific cholinotoxins, and molecular genetic techniques have enhanced our understanding of the roles played by acetylcholine in the CNS. Functional roles for CNS cholinergic neurons have been found in motivation and reward, sleep and arousal, and cognitive processes and stimulus processing. With respect to other neurotransmitter functions, ACh may participate in circuits involved with pain reception. Thus, the findings that nettles (*Urtica dioica*) contain ACh and histamine, that high concentrations of ACh injected into the brachial artery of humans result in intense pain, and that ACh applied to a blister produces a brief but severe pain indicate a relationship between ACh and pain. That ACh may act as a sensory transmitter in thermal receptors, taste fiber endings, and chemoreceptors has also been suggested, based on the excitatory activity of the compound on these sensory nerve endings.

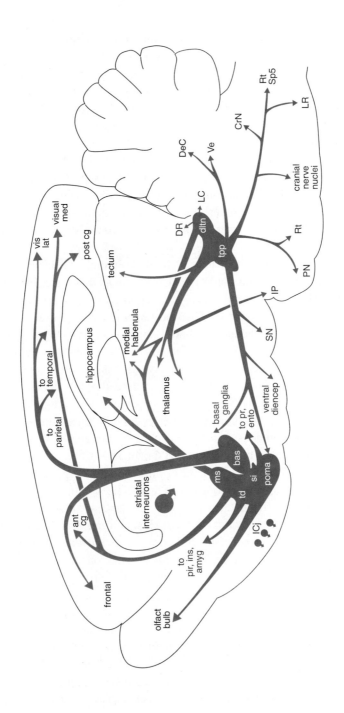

CHOLINERGIC RECEPTORS

Cholinergic receptors fall into two classes, muscarinic (Table 6–1) and nicotinic (Table 6–2). At last count, five muscarinic receptors (M_1–M_5) had been cloned. All of them exhibit a slow response time (100–250 milliseconds), are coupled to G proteins, and either act directly on ion channels or are linked to a variety of second messenger systems. M_1, M_3, and M_5 via G_q are coupled to phosphatidylinositol hydrolysis; M_2 and M_4 via G_i are coupled to cyclic adenosine monophosphate. When activated, the final effect can be to open or close K channels, Ca channels, or Cl channels, depending on the cell type. With this array of channel activity, therefore, stimulation of muscarinic receptors will lead to either depolarization or hyperpolarization. As noted in Table 6–1, second messenger systems have been described following activation of the muscarinic receptors. Knowing the messengers is fine, but it does not tell us anything about the message—that is, what the ultimate physiological effect is.

Cholinergic transmission in many of the most critical CNS circuits is mediated primarily by muscarinic acetylcholine receptors (mAChRs). Of the five identified mAChR subtypes (termed M_1–M_5), M_1 and M_4 are most heavily expressed in the CNS and are the most likely candidates for mediating the effects on cognition, attention, and sensory processing. In contrast, the most

---

FIGURE 6–2. Schematic representation of the major cholinergic systems in the mammalian brain. Central cholinergic neurons exhibit two basic organizational schemata: (1) local circuit cells (i.e., those that morphologically are arrayed wholly within the neural structure in which they are found), exemplified by the interneurons of the caudate putamen nucleus, nucleus accumbens, olfactory tubercle, and Islands of Calleja complex (ICj), and (2) projection neurons (i.e., those that connect two or more different regions). Of the cholinergic projection neurons that interconnect central structures, two major subconstellations have been identified: (1) the basal forebrain cholinergic complex composed of choline acetyltransferase (ChAT)-positive neurons in the medial septal nucleus (ms), diagonal band nuclei (td), substantia innominata (si), magnocellular preoptic field (poma), and nucleus basalis (bas) and projecting to the entire nonstriatal telencephalon and (2) the pontomesencephalotegmental cholinergic complex composed of ChAT-immunoreactive cells in the pendunuclopontine (tpp) and laterodorsal (dltn) tegmental nuclei and ascending to the thalamus and other diencephalic loci and descending to the pontine and medullary reticular formations (Rt), deep cerebellar (DeC) and vestibular (Ve) nuclei, and cranial nerve nuclei. Not shown are the somatic and parasympathetic cholinergic neurons of cranial nerves III–VII and IX–XII and the cholinergic α and γ motor and autonomic neurons of the spinal cord. amyg, amygdale; ant cg, anterior cingulate cortex; CrN, dorsal cranial nerve nuclei; diencep, diencephalon; DR, dorsal raphe nucleus; ento, entorhinal cortex; frontal, frontal cortex; IP, interpeduncular nucleus; ins, insular cortex; LC, locus ceruleus; LR, lateral reticular nucleus; olfact, olfactory; pir, piriform cortex; PN, pontine nuclei; pr, perirhinal cortex; parietal, parietal cortex; post cg, posterior cingulate cortex; SN, substantia nigra; Sp5, spinal nucleus of cranial nerve V. (Modified from Butcher and Woolf [1986] and Woolf and Butcher [1989].)

TABLE 6–1. Muscarinic Receptors

CURRENTLY ACCEPTED NAME	M1	M2	M3	M4	M5
Molecular biology classification	m1	m2	m3	m4	m5
Structural information	460 aa (human)	466 aa (human)	590 aa (human)	479 aa (human)	532 aa (human)
Subtype-selective agonists	McN-A343 (ganglion) Pilocarpine (relative to M3 and M5) L-689,660 Xanomeline TBPB (allosteric agonist)	Bethanechol (relative to M4)	L-689,660	McN-A343 (relative to M2) Xanomeline Vu10010 (allosteric potentiator)	None known
Subtype-selective antagonists	Pirenzepine Telenzepine	Methoctramine AF-DX-116 AF-DX-384 Gallamine (noncompetitive) Himbacine Tripitramine	Hexahydrosila-difenidol p-Fluorohexahydrosila-difenidol 4-DAMP	Tropicamide AF-DX-384	None known Himbacine

Receptor-selective agonists	Bethanechol	Bethanechol	Bethanechol	Bethanechol	Bethanechol
	Metoclopramide	Metoclopramide	Metoclopramide	Metoclopramide	Metoclopramide
	Muscarine	Muscarine	Muscarine	Muscarine	Muscarine
	Pilocarpine	Pilocarpine	Pilocarpine	Pilocarpine	Pilocarpine
	Oxotremorine M	Oxotremorine M	Oxotremorine M	Oxotremorine M	Oxotremorine M
Receptor-selective antagonists	Scopolamine	Scopolamine	Scopolamine	Scopolamine	Scopolamine
	QNB, (±)	QNB, (±)	QNB, (±)	QNB, (±)	QNB, (±)
	QNB, R(−)	QNB, R(−)	QNB, R(−)	QNB, R(−)	QNB, R(−)
	Atropine	Atropine	Atropine	Atropine	Atropine
Signal transduction mechanisms	$G_{q/11}$ (increase IP3/DAG)	G_i (cAMP modulation)	$G_{q/11}$ (increase IP3/DAG)	G_i (cAMP modulation)	$G_{q/11}$ (increase IP$_3$/DAG)
	NO	↑ K$^+$ (G)	NO	↑ K$^+$ (G)	NO
Radioligands of choice	[³H]-Pirenzepine	[³H]-AF-DX-384	[³H]-4-DAMP	[³H]-AF-DX-384	[³H]-QNB
	[³H]-Telenzepine	[³H]-QNB	[³H]-QNB	[³H]-QNB	[³H]-NMS
	[³H]-QNB				

AF-DX-116, 11-([2-[(Diethylamino)methyl]-1-piperidinyl]acetyl)-5,11-dihydro-6-pyridol[2,3-b][1,4]benzodiazepin-6-one; AF-DX-384, 5,11-dihydro-11-[2-[2-[N, N-dipropylaminomethyl)piperidin-1-yl]ethylamino]-carbony[6II-pyridol[2,3-b]I[1,4] benzodiazepin-6-one; 4-DAMP, 4-diphenylacetoxy-N-methylpiperidine methiodide; 1-689,660, 1-azabicyclo [2,2,2] octane, 3-(6-chloropyrazinyl)maleate; McN-A343, 4-(N-[3-chlorophenyl] carbamoyloxy)-2-butynyltrimethylammonium chloride; NMS, N-methylscopolamine; QNB, quinuclidinyl-α-hydroxydiphenylacetate (quinuclidinylbenzylate); NO, nitric oxide; IP$_3$/DAG, inositol triphosphate/diacylglycerol; cAMP, cyclic adenosine monophosphate.
Source: Modified from Watling (2006).

TABLE 6–2. Nicotinic Receptors

Currently used name	Neuronal (CNS) (α-bungarotoxin insensitive)	Neuronal (CNS) (α-bungarotoxin sensitive)	Neuronal (autonomic ganglia)	Muscular
Subunits (arranged as pentamers)	$\alpha_4\beta_2$ (major) $\alpha_3\beta_4$ $\alpha_2?\alpha_3?$	α_7 homomers $\alpha_8?$ $\alpha_9?$ α_9/α_{10}	α_7 homomers $\alpha_3\alpha_5\beta_4$ $\alpha_3\alpha_5\beta_2\beta_4$	$\alpha_1\beta_1\delta\gamma(\varepsilon)$
Receptor selective agonists	Cytisine RJR-2403 Epibatidine Anatoxin A ABT-418 A-85380	Anatoxin A DMAC GTS-21 AR-R-17779	Epibatidine SIB-1553A DMPP	Epibatidine Anatoxin A TMA
Receptor selective antagonists	Mecamylamine Dihydro-β-erythroidine Erysodine α-Conotoxin AuIB ($\alpha_3\beta_4$) α-Conotoxin MII ($\alpha_3\beta_2$) Chlorisondamine	Methllycaconitine α-Bungarotoxin α-Conotoxin IMI	Hexamethonium Chlorisondamine? Mecamylamine? κ-Bungarotoxin	α-Bungarotoxin

Signal transduction mechanisms	Modulation of cation channel conductance permeability properties	Modulation of cation channel conductance permeability properties	Modulation of cation channel conductance permeability properties	Modulation of cation channel conductance permeability properties
Radioligands of choice	[³H]-Nicotine [³H]-Epibatidine [³H]-Cytisine	[125I]-α-Bungarotoxin [³H]-Methyllycaconitine	[³H]-Epibatidine [125I]-α-Bungarotoxin [³H]-Methyllycaconitine	[125I]-α-Bungarotoxin

A-85380, 3-(2[S]-Azetidinylmethoxy)pyridine: ABT-418, (S)-3-methyl-5-(1-methyl-2-pyrrolidinyl)isoxazole: AR-R-17779, (−)-spiro1 [1-azabicyclo[2.2.2]octane-3,5′-oxazolidin-2′ one (4a); DMAC, 3-(4)-dimethylaminocinmamylidine anabaseine; DMPP, N,N-dimethyl-N′-phenyl-piperazinium iodide: GTS-21, [3-(2,4-dimethoxybenzylidene)-anabaseine; RJR-2403, N-methyl-4- (3-pyridinyl)-3-buten-1-amine: SIB-1553 A, 4-[[2-(1-methyl-2-pyrrolidinyl)ethyl]thio]phenyl hydrochloride; TMA, tetramethylammonium.
Source: Modified from Watling (2006).

prominent adverse effects of muscarinic cholinergic agents (bradycardia, gastrointestinal distress, salivation, and sweating) are mediated by activation of peripheral M_1, M_2, and M_3 mAChRs.

The pharmacological antagonists that have been used to define three of the muscarinic subtypes are pirenzepine, which has a high affinity for M_1; AFDX-116 and methoctramine with a high affinity for M_2; and 4-diphenylacetoxy-N-methylpiperidine methiodide, which exhibits the highest affinity for M_3. Most antagonists do not show more than a fivefold selectivity for one subtype over all other subtypes. The two classic muscarinic antagonists atropine and quinuclidinylbenzylate do not distinguish the subtypes but block all equally well.

The selectivity of classical muscarinic agonists among receptor subtypes is also very low due to the highly conserved nature of the orthosteric binding site among receptor subtypes. It would be a major advance if we knew whether each subtype subserved a specific function, such as bradycardia or smooth muscle contractibility. If this were the case (and it probably is), more specific drugs devoid of side effects could be developed. More selective muscarinic agonists that will define the various subtypes are clearly needed and several have recently emerged. A new, highly selective M_4 allosteric potentiator, VU10010, has been developed that potentiates the M_4 response to acetylcholine approximately 50-fold while having no activity at other mAChR subtypes. This compound and other positive allosteric modulators of M_4 do not activate the receptor directly but bind to an allosteric site on the receptor and increase affinity for ACh and coupling to G proteins. The discovery of a highly selective allosteric modulator of M_4 provides an unprecedented opportunity to selectively increase activity of this receptor and develop a more detailed understanding of the functional roles of M_4 in brain circuits that are heavily modulated by cholinergic innervation. One of the most important roles of cholinergic systems in the CNS is modulation of transmission through the hippocampal formation, a limbic cortical structure that has a critical role in learning and memory and is thought to be important for cholinergic regulation of cognitive function.

In addition to allosteric potentiators, a novel allosteric agonist termed TBPB has been characterized that is selective for the M_1 mAChR subtype. Unlike allosteric potentiators, allosteric agonists directly activate the receptor rather than potentiating the effects of ACh.

The development of novel ligands that are highly selective for individual mAChR subtypes promises to provide important information concerning the function these receptor subtypes subserve. The ultimate hope is that selective allosteric activation of M_1 and/or M_4 AChRs could lead to new treatments for psychiatric disorders associated with a component of cognitive dysfunction (i.e., schizophrenia, Alzheimer's disease, and Parkinson's disease).

Until relatively recently, the identification of nicotinic cholinergic receptors in the CNS was an enigma. Using labeled α-bungarotoxin, nicotine, mecamylamine, or dihydro-β-erythroidine, each investigation yielded mystifying results in which the antagonist could not be easily displaced by ACh or by unlabeled ganglionic or neuromuscular antagonists but occasionally was displaced by muscarinic agonists and antagonists. A major problem has been the low density of nicotinic compared to muscarinic receptors in the brain.

Conversely, much is known about the properties of the nicotinic cholinergic receptor of *Torpedo* and *Electrophorus electricus* organs. This reflects the abundance of the receptor in this tissue and the availability of two snake toxins, α-bungarotoxin and *Naja naja siamensis*, that specifically bind to the receptor and have facilitated its isolation and purification. In the past 15 years, however, research with monoclonal antibodies and cDNA has yielded considerable information about the mammalian nicotinic receptors (see Table 6–2).

As we enter the second century since the discovery of the nicotinic acetylcholine receptors (nAChRs) by Langley in 1905, we know a great deal about their subunit structure, channel function, and regulation. nAChRs are members of the Cys loop family of transmitter-gated ion channels that include the $5-HT_3$, $GABA_A$, and strychnine-sensitive glycine receptors. All nicotine receptors are formed as pentamers of subunits. Genes encoding a total of 17 subunits (α_{1-10}, β_{1-4}, δ, ε, and γ) have been identified to date. All these subunits are of mammalian origin with the exception of α_8, which is avian. The crucial physiological role of nicotine receptors in the autonomic nervous system is well established and their many potential roles in the CNS are becoming clearer. In autonomic and sensory ganglia that have been examined, $\alpha_3\beta_4$ receptors predominate. In the CNS, there are potentially a very large number of AChRs based on possible subunit combinations. In most brain regions, however, a relatively small number of subtypes appear to be represented. These include the homomeric α_7 receptor and several heteromeric receptors comprising the $\alpha_4\beta_2$ and the $\alpha_3\beta_4$ subtypes. Although all nAChRs share many pharmacological characteristics, especially the heteromeric subtypes, a number of ligands and a few drugs have emerged that can distinguish among the receptor subtypes. This is predominately seen between those containing β_2 and those containing β_4 subunits. The critical involvement of nAChRs in nicotine addiction makes them an important target for intervention in this disorder. In addition, because CNS nAChRs are strategically located to modulate the release of a number of important neurotransmitters, including glutamate, dopamine, GABA, norepinephrine, and ACh, they may influence a wide variety of CNS functions and pathways. Thus, it is not surprising that drug-targeting nAChR subtypes may have therapeutic potential in a number of conditions as diverse as neuropathic pain, Parkinson's disease, schizophrenia, Tourette's syndrome, attention deficit hyperactivity disorder (ADHD), as well as addiction to and dependence on nicotine.

In view of the previous discussion, it is no surprise that considerable attention is being devoted to nicotine despite the fact that use of nicotine or tobacco products is fraught with complications, including their highly addictive properties (see Chapter 26). This interest was sparked by the potential beneficial effect of nicotine in enhancing vigilance, improving memory and learning in animal models, as well as nicotine's antinociceptive properties suggesting potential use in the treatment of pain. Epidemiological studies indicating that smoking is associated with a lower incidence of Parkinson's disease further fueled the fire. In clinical studies, the finding that tobacco smoking reduces the incidence of cognitive dysfunction in Parkinson's and Alzheimer's disease encouraged testing of nicotine's efficacy in these disorders. Nicotine patches have been shown to improve cognition in Alzheimer's patients but to be ineffective in Parkinson's patients due in part to side effects. Increasing evidence, both preclinical and clinical, has demonstrated that α_7 nAChR agonists and partial agonists can lead to improvements in cognitive performance. Thus, the α_7 subtype of the nAChR has become a target of considerable interest in CNS drug discovery for disorders such as schizophrenia, Alzheimer's disease, and ADHD, which exhibit a component of cognitive dysfunction. In contrast to direct agonist activation, a novel approach to modulating α_7 nAChR function

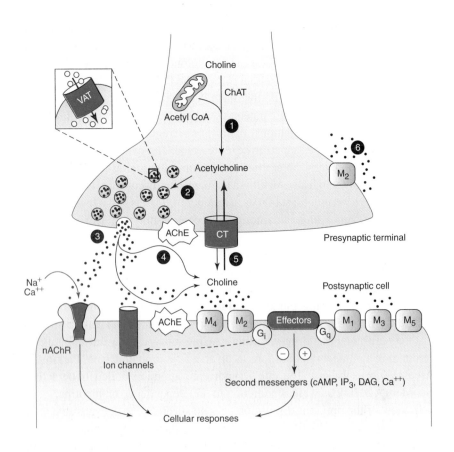

is to enhance the effects of the endogenous neurotransmitter ACh through positive allosteric modulation. Positive allosteric modulators are a class of compounds that selectively modulate the activity of ACh at α_7 nAChRs in a manner that avoids desensitization and may have significant advantages over indiscriminate and direct activation of nAChRs by nicotine/nicotinic agonists or by acetylcholinesterase inhibitors.

Another recent development is the discovery of a series of potent and selective $\alpha_4\beta_2$ nAChR partial agonists that exhibit dual agonist and antagonist activity in preclinical models. One of these agents, varenicline (Chantix), is

---

FIGURE 6–3. Model of an ACh synapse illustrating the presynaptic and postsynaptic molecular entities involved in the synthesis, storage, release, reuptake, and signaling of ACh. Choline is transported into the presynaptic terminal by an active uptake mechanism and converted to ACh by a single enzymatic step. The acetyl coenzyme A required for ACh synthesis is provided by presynaptic mitochondria. Muscarinic M_2 autoreceptors in the presynaptic terminal modulate the release of ACh. In contrast to monoamine synapses, the plasma membrane transporter of an ACh synapse does not return the neurotransmitter to the presynaptic terminal but, rather, recycles precursor choline. ACh is metabolized by ACh esterase (AChE) present on both pre- and postsynaptic membranes, which serves to terminate its action. Both G protein-coupled muscarinic receptors and ligand-gated ion channels (nicotinic receptors) may be present as depicted on the postsynaptic cell. Sites of drug action:

Site 1: ACh synthesis can be blocked by styrylpyridine derivatives such as NVP.

Site 2: ACh transport into vesicles is blocked by vesamicol (AH5183).

Site 3: Release is promoted by β-bungarotoxin, black widow spider venom, and La^{3+}. Release is blocked by botulinum toxin, cytochalasin B, collagenase pretreatment, and Mg^{2+}.

Site 4: Acetylcholinesterase is inhibited reversibly by physostigmine (eserine) or irreversibly by DFP, or soman.

Site 5: Choline uptake competitive blockers include hemicholinium-3, troxypyrrolium tosylate, or AF64A (noncompetitive).

Site 6: Presynaptic muscarinic receptors may be blocked by AFDX-116 (an M_2 antagonist), atropine, or quinuclidinyl benzilate. Muscarinic agonists (e.g., oxotremorine) will inhibit the evoked release of ACh by acting on these receptors.

Site 7: Postsynaptic receptors are activated by cholinomimetic drugs and anticholinesterases. Nicotinic receptors, at least in the peripheral nervous system, are blocked by rabies virus, curare, hexamethonium, or dihydro-β-erythroidine; n-methylcarbamylcholine and dimethylphenyl piperazinium are nicotinic agonists. Muscarinic receptors are blocked by atropine, pirenzepine, and quinuclidinyl benzilate.

AC, adenylyl cyclase; ChAT, choline acetyltransferase; CT, plasma membrane choline transporter; DAG, diacylglycerol; IP_3, inositol triphosphate; M, muscarinic receptors; nAChR, nicotinic acetylcholine receptors; PLC, phospholipase C; VAT, vesicular acetylcholine transporter (not yet isolated). (Modified from Nestler et al., 2001)

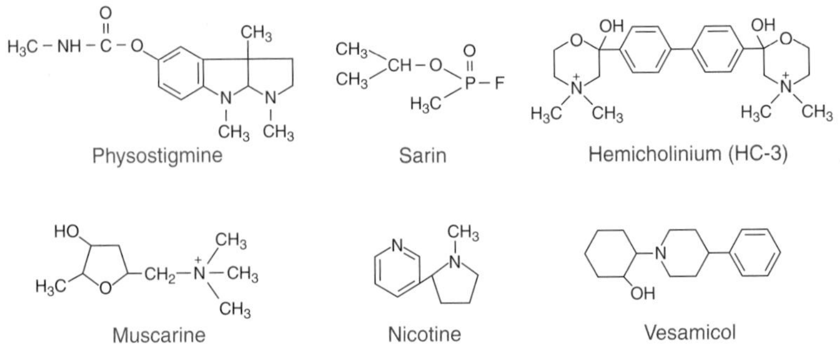

FIGURE 6–4. Structures of some drugs that affect the cholinergic nervous system.

now marketed for smoking cessation pharmacotherapy (see Chapter 26). The $\alpha_4\beta_2$ receptor has also been implicated in learning deficiencies. Finally, nicotine antagonists such as dihydro-β-erythroidine impair working memory. Obviously, pharmaceutical chemists have more than a casual interest in pursuing this interesting and potentially lucrative drug development area.

Figure 6–3 is a schematic model of an ACh synapse illustrating the presynaptic and postsynaptic molecular entities involved in the synthesis, storage, release, reuptake, and signaling of ACh and depicting potential sites of drug action. Structures of several protypic drugs that affect the cholinergic nervous system are illustrated in Figure 6–4.

ACETYLCHOLINE IN DISEASE STATES

Aside from myasthenia gravis and other autoimmune diseases, such as the Lambert–Eaton myasthenic syndrome (a presynaptic problem involving diminished release of ACh), the role of ACh in nervous system dysfunction is unclear. Certainly, a strong case can be made for familial dysautonomia, an autosomal recessive condition affecting Ashkenazi Jews that is diagnosed by a supersensitivity of the iris to methacholine. Huntington's disease, involving a degeneration of Golgi type 2 cholinergic interneurons in the striatum, is partially ameliorated by physostigmine, although this does not reverse the progressive disease. Administration of physostigmine to patients with tardive dyskinesia has produced mixed results.

Alzheimer's disease is characterized behaviorally by a severe impairment in cognitive function and neuropathologically by the appearance of neuritic plaques and neurofibrillary tangles (see Chapter 16). *In vivo* single photon emission computed tomography imaging of vesicular ACh transporter using [123I]-IBVM in early Alzheimer's disease strongly supports the belief that cholinergic degeneration occurs in the early stage of Alzheimer's disease and most likely is involved in the impairment of cognitive functions observed at this stage of the disease. The brain-penetrant anticholinesterase inhibitors are the current mainstays of symptomatic treatment for patients with early Alzheimer's disease (see Chapter 16).

CHOLINERGIC DRUGS

The enzymatic inactivation of ACh has been a fertile ground for the development of a large number of pharmaceutical agents. Anticholinesterase inhibitors such as tabun, VX, and sarin, initially developed for military use, are potent neurotoxins that have been used as nerve gases since World War II. Other anticholinesterases include organophosphates (e.g., parathion), which are widely used as insecticides. Whether the target is a tomato hornworm or human, anticholinesterases function in the same manner: Instead of the released ACh leading to discrete single depolarizations of muscle fibers, the accumulation of ACh at the neuromuscular junction leads to muscle fibrillations and, ultimately, depolarization inactivation of the muscle (i.e., the muscle is so excited that it stops contracting, resulting in flaccid paralysis). Anticholinesterases have a number of other less aggressive uses as well. Competitive neuromuscular blocking agents such as succinylcholine are occasionally used as an adjunct to anesthetics during surgery to increase muscle relaxation. Anticholinergic agents can be used to reverse muscle paralysis produced by succinylcholine. Cholinesterase inhibitors such as neostigmine and pyridostigmine are the mainstay in the treatment of myasthenia gravis, which as mentioned previously is a disorder of the neuromuscular junction that is usually marked by the presence of anti-nicotinic receptor antibodies. In terms of their useful CNS effects, the brain-penetrant cholinesterase inhibitors donepezil, galantamine, and rivastigmine are the current mainstays of symptomatic treatment for patients with early Alzheimer's disease. The target in this case is cortical brain ACh; *in vivo* imaging studies have demonstrated a significant decrease in cortical ACh in Alzheimer's patient. Unfortunately, the efficacy of these agents is limited and largely symptomatic.

Muscarinic cholinergic agonists are not currently used to treat CNS disorders but are used clinically to treat urinary retention and glaucoma. They are also effective in ameliorating the symptoms of Sjogren's syndrome, an autoimmune disorder characterized by degeneration of the salivary glands. However, as mentioned previously, several subtype-selective M_1 and M_4 mAChR allosteric agonists have become available, show efficacy in animal models, and are being tested for therapeutic effects in schizophrenia. Muscarinic antagonists such as benztropine and trihexyphenidyl are used to treat Parkinson's disease and the parkinsonian symptoms elicited by some antipsychotic drugs. Scopolamine, administered by a slow-release transdermal patch, is effective in preventing motion sickness.

In recent years, the most important therapeutic advance has been the development of nAChR-specific drugs. The clinical efficacy of the $\alpha_4\beta_2$ nAChR partial agonist varenicline (Chantix) for smoking cessation pharmacotherapy has been established (see Chapter 26). Chantix exhibits dual action by sufficiently stimulating $\alpha_4\beta_2$ nAChR-mediated dopamine release to reduce craving when quitting smoking and by inhibiting nicotine reinforcement when smoking. Since nAChRs in the CNS are strategically localized to modulate the function of numerous transmitters, there is no doubt that targeting nAChR subtypes will lead to the development of a number of useful CNS therapeutics in the near future.

SELECTED REFERENCES

Butcher, L. L. and N. J. Woolf (1986). Central cholinergic systems: Synopsis of anatomy and overview of physiology and pathology. In *The Biological Substrates of Alzheimer's Disease* (A. B. Scheibel and A. F. Wechsler, Eds.). Academic Press, New York, pp. 73–86.

Conn, P. J., C. Tamminga, D. D. Schoepp, and C. Lindsley (2008). Schizophrenia: Moving beyond monoamine antagonists. *Mol. Interventions* 6, 18–23.

Cooper, J. R., F. E. Bloom, and R. H. Roth (2002). *Biochemical Basis of Neuropharmacology*, 8th ed. Oxford University Press, New York.

Ellis, J. M. (2005). Cholinesterase inhibitors in the treatment of dementia. *J. Am. Osteropath. Assoc.* 105(3), 145-158.

Gotti, C. and F. Clementi (2004). Neuronal nicotinic receptors: From structure to pathology. *Prog. Neurobiol.* 74, 363–396.

Langley, J. N. (1907). On the contraction of muscle, chiefly in relation to the presence of "receptive" substances. *J. Physiol. (London)* 37, 347–384.

Mazere, J., C. Prunier, O. Barret, M. Guyot. C. Hommet, D. Guilloteau, J. F. Dartigues, S. Auriacombe, C. Fabrigoule, and M. Allard (2008). *In vivo* SPECT imaging of vesicular acetylcholine transporter using (^{123}I)-IBVM in early Alzheimer's disease. *NeuroImage* 40, 280–288.

Ng, H. J., E. R. Whittemore, M. B. Tran, D. J. Hogenkamp, R. S. Broide, T. B. Johnstone, L. Zheng, K. E. Stevens, and K. W. Gee (2007). Nootropic α_7 nicotinic receptor allosteric modulator derived from GABA$_A$ receptor modulators. *Proc. Natl. Acad. Sci. USA* 104, 8059–8064.

Nestler, E. J., S. E. Hyman, and R. C. Malenka (2001). *Molecular Neuropharmacology: A Foundation for Clinical Neuroscience*. McGraw-Hill, New York.

Picciotto, M. R., M. Alreja, and J. D. Jentsch (2002). Acetylcholine. In *Neuropsychopharmacology: The Fifth Generation of Progress* (K. L. Davis, D. Charney, J. T. Coleand, and C. Nemeroff, Eds.). Lippincott Williams & Wilkins, Philadelphia, pp. 3–14.

Roghani, A., J. Feldman, S. A. Kohan, A. Shirzadi, C. B. Gundersen, N. Brecha, and R. H. Edwards (1994). Molecular cloning of a putative vesicular transporter for acetylcholine. *Proc. Natl. Acad. Sci. USA* 91, 10620.

Rollema, H., J. W. Coe, L. K. Chambers, R. S. Hurst, S. M. Stahl, and K. E. Williams (2007). Rational, pharmacology and clinical efficacy of partial agonists of $\alpha_4\beta_2$ nACh receptors for smoking cessation. *Trends Pharmacol. Sci.* 28(7), 316–325.

Shirey, J. K., Z. Xiang, D. Orton, A. E. Brady, K. A. Johnson, R. Williams J. E. Ayala, A. L. Rodriguez, J. Wess, D. Weaver, C. M. Niswender, and P. J. Conn (2008). An allosteric potentiator of M_4 mAChR modulates hippocampal synaptic transmission. *Nature Chem. Biol.* 4, 42–50.

Taylor, P. and J. H. Brown (2006). Acetylcholine. In *Basic Neurochemistry*, (G. C. Siegel, R. W. Albers, S. Brady, and D. L. Price, Eds.), 7th ed. Elsevier, San Diego.

Watling, K. J. (2006). *The Sigma-RBI Handbook of Receptor Classification and Signal Transduction*, 5th ed. Sigma-RBI, Natick, MA.

Woolf, N. J. and L. L. Butcher (1989). Cholinergic systems: Synopsis of anatomy and overview of physiology and pathology. In *The Biological Substrates of Alzheimer's Disease* (A. B. Scheibel and A. F. Wechsler, Eds.). Academic Press, New York, pp. 73–86.

Catecholamines

NOREPINEPHRINE AND EPINEPHRINE

Norepinephrine (NE) and epinephrine (E) are chemically catecholamines. The term *catecholamine* refers generically to all organic compounds that contain a catechol nucleus (a benzene ring with two adjacent hydroxyl substituents) and an amine group (Fig. 7–1). In practice, the term usually means dihydroxyphenylethylamine (dopamine; DA) and its metabolic products NE and E. Major advances in the understanding of the biochemistry, physiology, and pharmacology of these compounds have come mainly through the development of sensitive assay techniques and methods for visualizing catecholamine neurons, their connections, and their metabolic enzymes and receptors *in vivo* and *in vitro*.

In 1946, it was demonstrated by von Euler in Sweden, and soon thereafter by Holtz in Germany, that mammalian peripheral sympathetic nerves use NE as a transmitter instead of E (which is the sympathetic transmitter in the frog). With only minimal evidence based on tissue content, von Euler predicted that NE was highly concentrated in the nerve terminal region from which it was released to act as a neurotransmitter. This prediction was conclusively documented approximately 10 years later with the development of techniques for visualizing catecholamines in freeze-dried tissue sections, which helped to define the anatomy of the peripheral NE neuron.

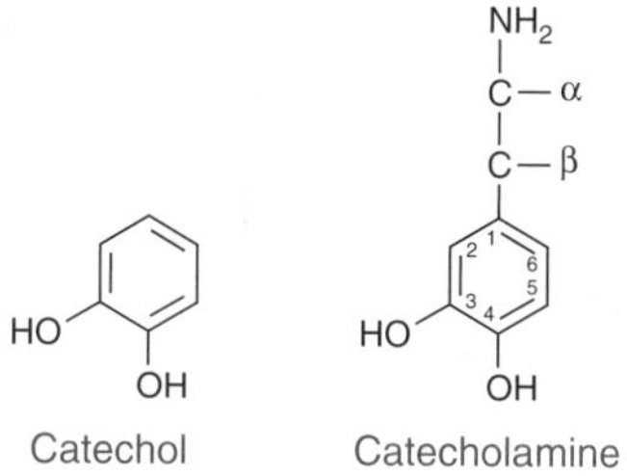

FIGURE 7–1. Catechol and catecholamine structures.

Soon after NE was established as the neurotransmitter substance of sympathetic nerves in the peripheral nervous system, Holtz identified it as a normal constituent of mammalian brain. For some years, however, it was thought that the presence of NE in the mammalian brain only reflected vasomotor innervation to the cerebral blood vessels. In 1954, Vogt demonstrated that NE was not uniformly distributed in the central nervous system (CNS) and that this non-uniform distribution did not in any way coincide with the density of blood vessels found in a given brain region. This regional localization within the mammalian brain suggested that NE might subserve some specialized function, perhaps as a central neurotransmitter. The relative regional distribution of NE in the brain is quite similar in most mammalian species.

Morphology of the Catecholamine Neuron

The morphology of the peripheral NE neuron became clear following the development by Falck and Hillarp of the fluorescent histochemical method for the visualization of catecholamines by condensation with dry formaldehyde vapor at 60–80°C. Under the fluorescent microscope, all parts of the NE neuron can be visualized (cell bodies, dendrites, axons, and nerve terminals), but the highest concentration of NE and the strongest fluorescence are found in the nerve terminal varicosities. A diffuse, widespread innervation pattern is characteristic of the sympathetic nervous system and its NE nerves. A single neuron can give rise to nerve terminal branches with lengths on the order of 10–20 cm, possessing several thousand nerve terminal varicosities. The localization of catecholamines and their precursors within morphologically recognizable microscopic structures by fluorescence and electron microscopy has been a great advantage for investigators studying NE mechanisms where fluorescence intensity, vesicle contents, and amine content correlate. The lack of a suitable histochemical technique for the visualization of acetylcholine has been a serious handicap by comparison for those interested in cholinergic mechanisms (see Chapter 6).

With the development in the 1960s of completely different histological techniques based on the presence of a given type of transmitter substance or on specific synthetic enzymes involved in the formation of a given transmitter, it became possible to map chemically defined neuronal systems in the CNS of many species. By the time such techniques had been employed for several years, it became clear that the distribution of these chemically defined mono-amine neuronal systems did not necessarily correspond to that of systems described earlier with the classic techniques.

However, it was really not until the mid-1960s that the histochemical fluo-rescent technique of Falck and Hillarp was applied to brain tissue and the anatomy of the monoamine-containing neuronal systems was described. By a variety of pharmacological and chemical methods, it has subsequently been possible to discriminate between NE-, E-, and DA-containing neurons and to describe in detail the distribution of these catecholamine-containing neurons in the mammalian CNS. Several thorough surveys of these systems are avail-able using multiple histochemical measures, including mapping of mRNAs, immunodetection of synthetic proteins, and ligand binding to receptors and transporters.

Figure 7–2 provides a schematic illustration of a central NE-containing neuron as observed by fluorescence and electron microscopy. The cell bodies contain relatively low concentrations of amine (approximately 10–100 μg/g), whereas the terminal varicosities contain a very high concentration (approxi-mately 1000–3000 μg/g). The axons, however, consist of highly branched, largely unmyelinated fibers that have such a low concentration of amine that they are barely visible in untreated adult animals. With the electron microscope, depending on the type of fixation, it is possible to observe small granular vesi-cles that are thought to represent the subcellular storage sites containing the catecholamines. These granular vesicles are concentrated in the terminal vari-cosities of the central NE neuron, just as they are observed in the peripheral sympathetic neuron.

Dopamine is also present in the mammalian CNS, and its distribution dif-fers markedly from that of NE, an early indication that DA functions as more than a precursor of NE in the CNS (see the section on dopamine). DA is also present in the carotid body and superior cervical ganglion, where it also likely plays a role independent of NE. The superior cervical ganglion appears to have at least three distinct populations of neurons: cholinergic neurons, NE neurons, and, small, intensely fluorescent cells that contain DA but whose functional significance is unclear.

The endogenous occurrence of E in the mammalian CNS at relatively low levels (approximately 5–10% by bioassay of the NE content) was reported in the early 1960s. Many investigators suggested that these original estimates are subject to error and in the past have discounted the importance of E in the

Electron microscope   Fluorescence microscope

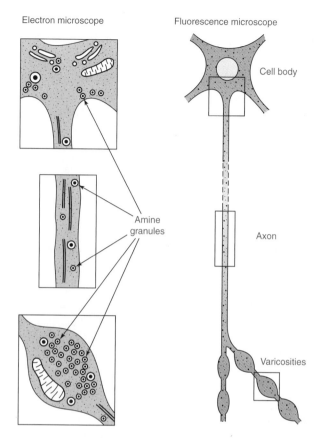

FIGURE 7–2. Schematic illustration of a central monoamine-containing neuron. The right side depicts the general appearance and intraneuronal distribution of monoamines based on fluorescence microscopy. Cell bodies contain a relatively low concentration of catecholamine (approximately 10–100 μg/g), whereas the terminal varicosities contain a very high concentration (1000–3000 μg/g). Preterminal axons contain very low concentrations of amine. At the electron microscopic level (left), dense core granules can be observed in the cell bodies and axons but appear to be highly concentrated in the terminal varicosities. (Modified from Fuxe and Hökfelt, 1971.)

mammalian brain. However, its presence has been documented by more sophisticated analytical techniques, such as gas chromatography–mass spectrometry and liquid chromatography coupled with electrochemical detection, and confirmed by immunohistochemical techniques.

The detailed topographical survey of brain catecholamines at different levels of organization within the CNS has provided a framework for organizing and conducting logical experiments concerning the possible functions of these amines. The anatomy, biochemistry, and pharmacology of CNS NE, E, and DA systems are discussed in detail later in this chapter.

Life Cycle of the Catecholamines

Biosynthesis

Catecholamines are formed in the brain, chromaffin cells, sympathetic nerves, and sympathetic ganglia from their amino acid precursor tyrosine by a sequence of enzymatic steps first postulated by Blaschko in 1939. This pathway was confirmed in 1964 by Nagatsu and co-workers, who demonstrated that tyrosine hydroxylase (TH) converts L-tyrosine to 3,4-dihydroxyphenylalanine (DOPA). Tyrosine is normally present in the circulation at a concentration of approximately 5×10^{-5} M. It is taken up from the bloodstream and concentrated within the brain and presumably in other sympathetically innervated tissue by an active transport mechanism. Once inside the peripheral neuron, tyrosine undergoes a series of chemical transformations, resulting in the formation of NE or, in the brain or chromaffin cell, NE, DA, or E, depending on the availability of the required downstream synthetic enzymes (see Fig. 7–3). Both phenylalanine and tyrosine are normal constituents of the mammalian brain, present in a free form at a concentration of approximately 5×10^{-5} M. However, NE biosynthesis is usually considered to begin with tyrosine, which represents a branch point for many important biosynthetic processes in animal tissues. The percentage of tyrosine used for catecholamine biosynthesis as opposed to other biochemical pathways is minimal (<2%).

Tyrosine hydroxylase

The first enzyme in the biosynthetic pathway, TH, was the last enzyme in this series of reactions to be identified. It was demonstrated by Udenfriend and colleagues in 1964, and its properties have been reviewed repeatedly. It is present in the adrenal medulla, brain, and all sympathetically innervated tissues as a unique constituent of catecholamine-containing neurons and chromaffin cells. The enzyme is stereospecific; requires molecular O^2, Fe^{2+}, and a tetrahydropteridine cofactor; and shows a fairly high degree of substrate specificity for L-tyrosine and, to a smaller extent, L-phenylalanine. The single human gene for TH has been cloned and found to encode multiple mRNAs that are heterogeneous at the $5'$ end of the coding region. The functional significance of the variant messages remains to be determined. Tyrosine hydroxylation is the rate-limiting step in the biosynthesis of NE in the peripheral nervous system and of NE and DA in the brain. In most sympathetically innervated tissues, including the brain, the activity of DOPA decarboxylase and that of dopamine-β-hydroxylase have a magnitude 100–1000 times that of TH. Further proof that this enzyme is the rate-limiting step in catecholamine biosynthesis is that pharmacological intervention at this step reduces NE biosynthesis, whereas blockade of the last two steps in the synthesis of NE does not. Inhibitors of TH

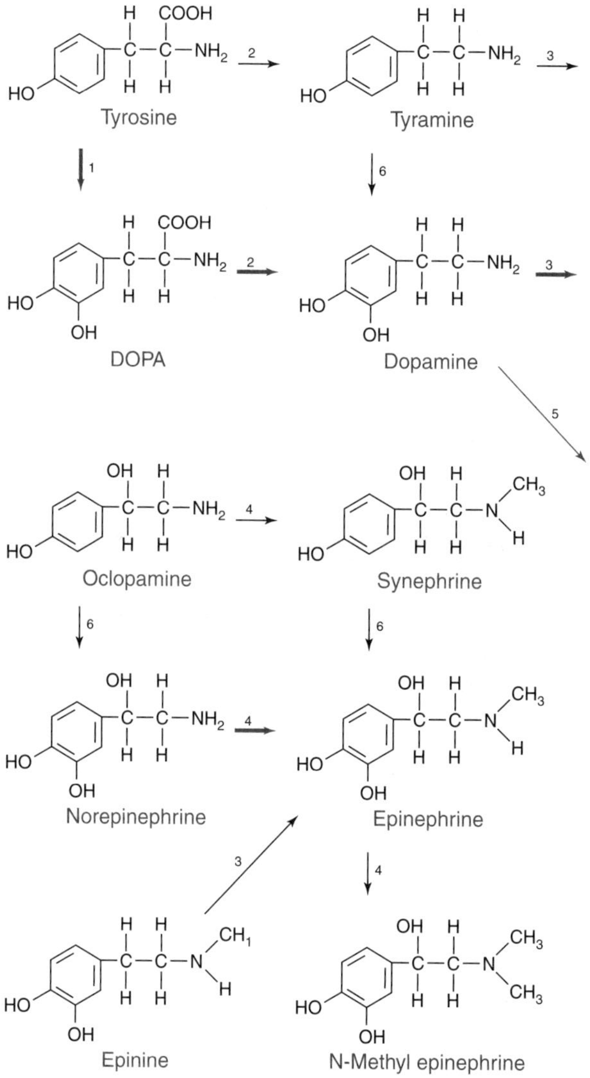

Figure 7–3. Primary and alternative pathways in the formation of catecholamine: (1) tyrosine hydroxylase; (2) aromatic amino acid decarboxylase; (3) dopamine-β-hydroxylase; (4) phenylethanolamine-N-methyltransferase; (5) nonspecific N-methyltransferase in lung and folate-dependent N-methyltransferase in brain; and (6) catechol-forming enzyme.

markedly reduce endogenous NE and DA in the brain and NE in the heart, spleen, and other sympathetically innervated tissues. Effective inhibitors of this enzymatic step can be categorized into four main groups: (1) amino acid analogues, (2) catechol derivatives, (3) tropolones, and (4) selective iron chelators. Some effective amino acid analogues include α-methyl-p-tyrosine and its ester, α-methyl-3-iodotyrosine, 3-iodotyrosine, and α-methyl-5-hydroxytryptophan. In general, α-methyl-amino acids are more potent than the unmethylated analogues, and a marked increase in activity in the case of the tyrosine analogues can also be produced by substituting a halogen at the 3 position of the benzene ring. Most of the agents in this category act as competitive inhibitors of the substrate tyrosine. α-Methyl-*p*-tyrosine and its methyl ester have been the inhibitors most widely used to demonstrate the effects of exercise, stress, and various drugs on the turnover of catecholamines and to lower NE formation in patients with pheochromocytoma and malignant hypertension.

Dihydropteridine reductase

Although not directly involved in catecholamine biosynthesis, dihydropteridine reductase is intimately linked to the TH step. This enzyme catalyzes the reduction of the quinonoid dihydropterin, which has been oxidized during the hydroxylation of tyrosine to DOPA. Since reduced pteridines are essential for tyrosine hydroxylation, alterations in the activity of dihydropteridine reductase affect the activity of TH. Dihydropteridines with amine substitution at positions 2 and 4 are effective inhibitors of this enzyme, whereas folic acid antagonists such as aminopterin and methotrexate are relatively ineffective. The distribution of dihydropteridine reductase is quite widespread, with the highest activity being found in the liver, brain, and adrenal gland. The distribution of this enzyme activity in the brain extends well beyond catecholamine or serotonin innervation, suggesting that reduced pterins most likely participate in other reactions besides the hydroxylation of tyrosine and tryptophan. In fact, reduced pteridines are critical for nitric oxide synthetase.

Dihydroxyphenylalanine decarboxylase

The second enzyme involved in catecholamine biosynthesis is DOPA-decarboxylase, which was actually the first catecholamine synthesis enzyme to be discovered. Although originally believed to remove carboxyl groups only from L-DOPA, a study of purified enzyme preparations and specific inhibitors demonstrated that this DOPA-decarboxylase acts on all naturally occurring aromatic L-amino acids, including histidine, tyrosine, tryptophan, and phenylalanine, as well as both DOPA and 5-hydroxytryptophan. Therefore, this enzyme is more appropriately referred to as "L-aromatic amino acid decarboxylase." DOPA-decarboxylase is, relative to other enzymes in the biosynthetic pathway for NE formation, very active and requires pyridoxal phosphate (vitamin B_6) as a cofactor. The apparent K_m value for this enzyme is 4×10^{-4} M. The high activity of this enzyme may explain why it has been difficult to detect endogenous DOPA in sympathetically innervated tissue and brain. It is rather ubiquitous in nature, occurring in the cytoplasm of most tissues, including the liver, stomach, brain, and kidney in high levels, suggesting that its function in metabolism is not limited solely to catecholamine biosynthesis. Although decarboxylase activity can be reduced by vitamin B_6 deficiency in animals, this does not usually result in significant reduction of tissue catecholamines, although it appears to interfere with the rate of repletion of adrenal catecholamines after insulin depletion. In addition, potent decarboxylase inhibitors have very little effect on endogenous levels of NE in tissue. However, these inhibitors have been useful as pharmacological tools (e.g., DOPA accumulation following administration of a decarboxylase inhibitor as an *in vivo* index of tyrosine hydroxylation).

Dopamine-β-hydroxylase

Although it has been known for many years that the brain, sympathetically innervated tissue, sympathetic ganglia, and adrenal medulla can transform DA into NE, it was not until 1960 that the enzyme responsible for this conversion was isolated from the adrenal medulla. This enzyme, called dopamine-β-hydroxylase, is, like TH, a mixed-function oxidase. It requires molecular oxygen and utilizes ascorbic acid as a cofactor. Its K_m for its substrate DA is approximately 5×10^{-3} M. The mRNA is expressed only in NE neurons or adrenal chromaffin tissue. Dopamine-β-hydroxylase does not show a high degree of substrate specificity and acts *in vitro* on a variety of substrates besides DA, oxidizing almost any phenylethylamine to its corresponding phenylethanolamine (i.e., tyramine to octopamine and α-methyldopamine to α-methylnorepinephrine). A number of the resultant structurally analogous metabolites can replace NE at the NE nerve endings and function as "false" neurotransmitters.

Dopamine-β-hydroxylase can be inhibited by a variety of compounds, including the copper chelators: D-cysteine and L-cysteine, glutathione, mercaptoethanol, and coenzyme A. Inhibition can be reversed by addition of N-ethylmaleimide, which reacts with sulfydryl groups and interferes with the chelating properties of these substances. Copper-chelating agents such as diethyldithiocarbamate(disulfuram) and bis(1-methyl-4-homopiperazinyl-thiocarbonyl)-disulfide (FLA-63) have proved to be effective inhibitors both *in vivo* and *in vitro*. Thus, it has been possible to treat animals with these agents and produce a reduction in brain NE and an elevation of brain DA.

Phenylethanolamine-N-methyltransferase

In the adrenal medulla, NE is *N*-methylated by the enzyme phenylethanolamine-*N*-methyltransferase (PNMT) to form E. This enzyme is largely restricted to the adrenal medulla, although low levels of activity exist in heart and mammalian brain. Like the decarboxylase, this enzyme appears in the supernatant of homogenates. Demonstration of activity requires the presence of the methyl donor S-adenosylmethionine. Interest in the biosynthetic pathway for catecholamines has also led to the cloning of a single PNMT gene with three exons. The transcript is present in the adrenal medulla, heart, and brain stem, and PNMT is found in these tissues. Regulation of this enzyme in the brain has not been extensively studied, but glucocorticoids are known to regulate the activity of PNMT in the adrenal gland.

Synthesis regulation

It has been known for a long time that the degree of sympathetic activity does not influence the endogenous levels of tissue NE, and it has been speculated that there must be some homeostatic mechanism whereby the level of transmitter is maintained relatively constant in the sympathetic nerve endings despite the additional losses assumed to occur during enhanced sympathetic activity.

More than 45 years ago, von Euler hypothesized, on the basis of experiments carried out in the adrenal medulla, that during periods of increased functional activity, the sympathetic neuron must also increase the synthesis of its transmitter substance NE to meet the increased demands placed on the neuron. If the sympathetic neuron had the ability to increase transmitter synthesis, this would enable the neuron to maintain a constant steady-state level of transmitter despite substantial changes in transmitter utilization. Some years later, experiments carried out by several laboratories on peripheral sympathetically innervated tissues as well as brain directly demonstrated that this was, in fact, the case. Electrical stimulation of sympathetic nerves, median forebrain bundle, or locus ceruleus both *in vivo* and *in vitro* resulted in increased formation of NE in the tissues innervated by these NE neurons. Further studies demonstrated that the observed acceleration of NE biosynthesis produced by enhanced noradrenergic activity was due to an increase in the activity of the rate-limiting enzyme involved in catecholamine biosynthesis, TH. Emphasis then shifted toward defining the mechanisms by which impulse flow changed enzyme activity. It is now well appreciated that the function of TH is determined by two major factors: changes in enzyme activity (the rate at which the enzyme converts the precursor into its product) and changes in the amount of enzyme protein. The most recent studies favor the involvement of Ca^{2+}–calmodulin-dependent phosphorylation in the impulse-dependent activation process (Fig. 7–4). α_2-NE or D_2 dopaminergic autoreceptor-mediated reduction of TH may also be achieved via regulation of the cAMP or Ca^{2+}–calmodulin-dependent protein phosphatases.

A second means of regulating the activity of the enzyme is through end-product inhibition: Catecholamines can inhibit the activity of TH through competition for a required pterin cofactor for the enzyme. Finally, the amount of reduced pteridine cofactor (tetrahydrobiopterin, BH_4) can also influence TH activity because the levels of the cofactor are not saturating under basal conditions.

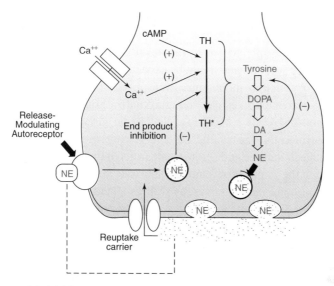

FIGURE 7–4. Model illustrating mechanisms for regulation of transmitter synthesis in norepinephrine neurons. DA, dopamine; DOPA, 3,4-dihydroxyphenylalanine; NE, norepinephrine; TH, tyrosine hydroxylase.

In general, very rapid, short-term upregulation of TH occurs primarily by these posttranslational changes, whereas longer-term changes in TH occur through transcriptional upregulation of the TH gene. However, the degree to which increases in catecholamine synthesis depend on *de novo* synthesis of new enzyme protein or changes in enzymatic activity appears to differ between CNS NE and dopaminergic neurons. For example, increased synthetic demand in NE neurons of the brain stem nucleus locus ceruleus appears to be accomplished primarily by increasing TH gene expression. In contrast, the same conditions and treatments that increase TH gene expression in brain stem NE neurons fail to increase TH mRNA levels in DA-containing neurons of the midbrain. In these dopaminergic neurons, it appears that synthesis is regulated primarily by altering the activity of TH—that is, by phosphorylation (see the section on dopamine).

Storage

A great conceptual advance made in the study of catecholamines more than 45 years ago was the recognition that in almost all tissues a large percentage of the NE present is located within highly specialized subcellular particles (later shown to be synaptic vesicles but colloquially referred to as "granules") in sympathetic nerve endings and chromaffin cells. Much of the NE in the CNS is also located within similar vesicles. These granules contain adenosine triphosphate (ATP) in a molar ratio of catecholamine to ATP of approximately 4:1.

Some complex of the amines with ATP and protein is probable since the intra-vesicular concentration of amines, at least in the adrenal chromaffin granules and probably in the splenic nerve granules (0.3–1.1 M), would be hypertonic if present in free solution and might be expected to lead to osmotic lysis of the vesicles. Two vesicular monoamine transporters (VMATs) localized to the membranes of synaptic vesicles and chromaffin granules have been cloned (VMAT-1 and VMAT-2). VMAT-1 is found in the adrenal medulla, in the adrenal chromaffin cells that synthesize and release monoamines. VMAT-2 is present in catecholamine and serotonin neurons in the CNS. VMAT-2, the isoform found in the brain, shows modest substrate specificity and can transport catecholamines and indoleamines, as well as histamine, into vesicles. These VMATs define another new family of transporter proteins that display the common motif of 12 hydrophobic, putative transmembrane domains and move transmitters into acidic intracellular compartments such as neurotransmitter vesicles. These transporters display no significant sequence homology with the plasma membrane Na^+/Cl^--coupled family, but they do resemble bacterial drug-resistance transporters. VMATs can also be distinguished from plasma membrane transporters by their use of transmembrane H^+ gradients instead of Na^+. All of the amine storage vesicles studied in brain and adrenal chromaffin cells contain a vascular-type H^+-pumping ATPase similar to that found in lysosomes and Golgi membranes. The significant homology of these vesicular transporters to a group of bacterial drug-resistance transporters suggests that VMATs may play a role in detoxification. VMAT enables vesicles to sequester toxins and reduce their cellular toxicity. For example, mice heterozygous for one knockout copy of VMAT-2 show increased toxicity of DA neurons to the DA neurotoxin 1-methyl-4-phenyl-1,2,3,6-tetrahydropyridine. Loss of VMAT means less sequestration of the toxin, which can then exert its toxic action by targeting mitochondrial respiration (see the section on dopamine).

Release

The release of NE, similar to the release of acetylcholine (ACh), is Ca^{2+} dependent and appears to occur by the same Ca^{2+}-dependent process (exocytosis) that has been described for other transmitters (see Chapter 2). Exocytosis requires that the entire content of the granular vesicle be released (i.e., catecholamine, ATP, and soluble protein). Since the nerve terminal region, as far as we know, cannot synthesize any protein, high rates of axonal flow from the nerve cell body would be required to replenish the protein lost during exocytosis. Alternatively, one might propose a "protein reuptake" mechanism to recapture the protein released during synaptic transmission. In peripheral nerves, release of NE is frequency dependent within a physiological range of frequencies. Evidence has also been presented that newly synthesized NE may be released preferentially. This preferential release is additional evidence to support the contention that NE exists in more than one pool within the sympathetic neuron.

It has been a great deal more difficult to demonstrate NE release from its nerve endings in the CNS. However, with the independent development of the push–pull cannula, microdialysis techniques, and electrochemical detectors, catecholamines can be detected extracellularly from certain deep nuclear masses of the CNS or measured directly by *in vivo* voltammetry. NE release determined by the previously discussed techniques is Ca^{2+} dependent and influenced by the functional activity of the NE neuron.

Regulation of release

The major homeostatic mechanism for regulation of catecholamine release in both central and peripheral catecholamine neurons involves interaction of the released catecholamine with specific presynaptic receptors (autoreceptors), which are located on the nerve terminals.

In most catecholamine-containing systems, administration of catecholamine agonists attenuates stimulus-induced release, whereas administration of catecholamine receptor blockers augments release. These pharmacological studies have established the concept that presynaptic receptors modulate release by responding to the concentration of catecholamine in the synapse (high concentrations inhibiting release and low concentrations augmenting release). Presynaptic autoreceptors have also been implicated in the regulation of DA synthesis (see the section on dopamine).

Several types of presynaptic receptors are involved in the inhibition of transmitter release from NE nerves. These include α_2-NE autoreceptors as well as muscarinic, opiate, and DA receptors. Different presynaptic receptors are linked to facilitation of NE release, including β_2-NE adrenoceptors, nicotinic cholinergic receptors, and angiotensin II receptors. The precise mechanism by which autoreceptors influence neurotransmitter release from NE neurons varies depending on their location on the neuron. Activation of α_2-adrenoceptors inhibits NE release by several possible mechanisms, including (1) attenuation of the rate of Ca^{2+} entry through inhibition of voltage-gated Ca^{2+} channels; (2) opening of K channels, leading to hyperpolarization of the neuron terminals; and (3) inhibition of adenylate cyclase, resulting in a decrease of intracellular cAMP and Ca^{2+} concentration.

Presynaptic β-NE receptors are also present in some sympathetic tissues. These autoreceptors are usually believed to be of the β_2 subtype. The β_2-adrenoceptor-mediated facilitation of NE release may be due to stimulation of adenylate cyclase, leading to an increase in cAMP and a subsequent increase in intracellular Ca^{2+} concentrations. Alternatively, it has been suggested that the facilitation may be due to a transsynaptic signal involving a local renin–angiotensin response. This hypothesis posits that β-adrenoceptor agonists activate postsynaptic β_2-adrenoceptors in the vascular wall. This activation results in the synthesis of angiotensin II, which diffuses across the synaptic cleft to activate presynaptic angiotensin II receptors that facilitate NE release.

The presence of presynaptic facilitatory and inhibitory NE receptors on the same nerve terminals may provide for a fine-tuning control of stimulus-evoked NE release. Since the affinity of E for β_2-adrenoceptors is much greater than that of NE, this subset of adrenoceptors is more likely to be activated by endogenous E than NE. Thus, low synaptic concentrations of E could activate presynaptic β_2-adrenoceptors preferentially, leading to an increase in NE release. At higher concentrations of E or NE, activation of α_2-adrenoceptors would predominate and NE release would be diminished rather than enhanced.

Prostaglandins of the E series are also potent inhibitors of neurally induced release of NE in a great number of tissues, and their action appears to be dissociated from any interaction with presynaptic receptors. These substances are released from sympathetically innervated tissues, and most evidence indicates that inhibition of local prostaglandin production is associated with an increase in the release of NE and subsequent effector responses induced by neuronal activity. The control of NE release by this prostaglandin-mediated feedback mechanism appears to operate through restriction of calcium availability for the NE release process and to be most efficient within the physiological frequency range of nerve impulses.

Metabolism

The metabolism of exogenously administered or endogenous catecholamines is markedly slower than that of ACh by the ACh–ACh-esterase system. The major mammalian enzymes of importance in the metabolic degradation of catecholamines are monoamine oxidase (MAO) and catechol-*O*-methyltransferase (COMT) (Fig. 7–5). MAO is an enzyme that converts catecholamines to their corresponding aldehydes. This aldehyde intermediate is rapidly metabolized, usually by oxidation by the enzyme aldehyde dehydrogenase to the corresponding acid. In some circumstances, the aldehyde is reduced to the alcohol or glycol by aldehyde reductase. In the case of brain NE, reduction of the aldehyde metabolite appears to be the favored route of metabolism. MAO is a particle-bound protein, localized largely in the outer membrane of mitochondria, although partial microsomal localization cannot be excluded. There is also evidence for a riboflavin-like material in MAO isolated from liver mitochondria. MAO is usually considered to be an intraneuronal enzyme, but it occurs in abundance extraneuronally. In fact, most experiments indicate that chronic denervation of a sympathetic end organ leads only to a relatively small reduction in MAO, suggesting that the greater proportion of this enzyme is extraneuronal. However, it is the intraneuronal enzyme that seems to be important in catecholamine metabolism. MAO present in human and rat brain exists

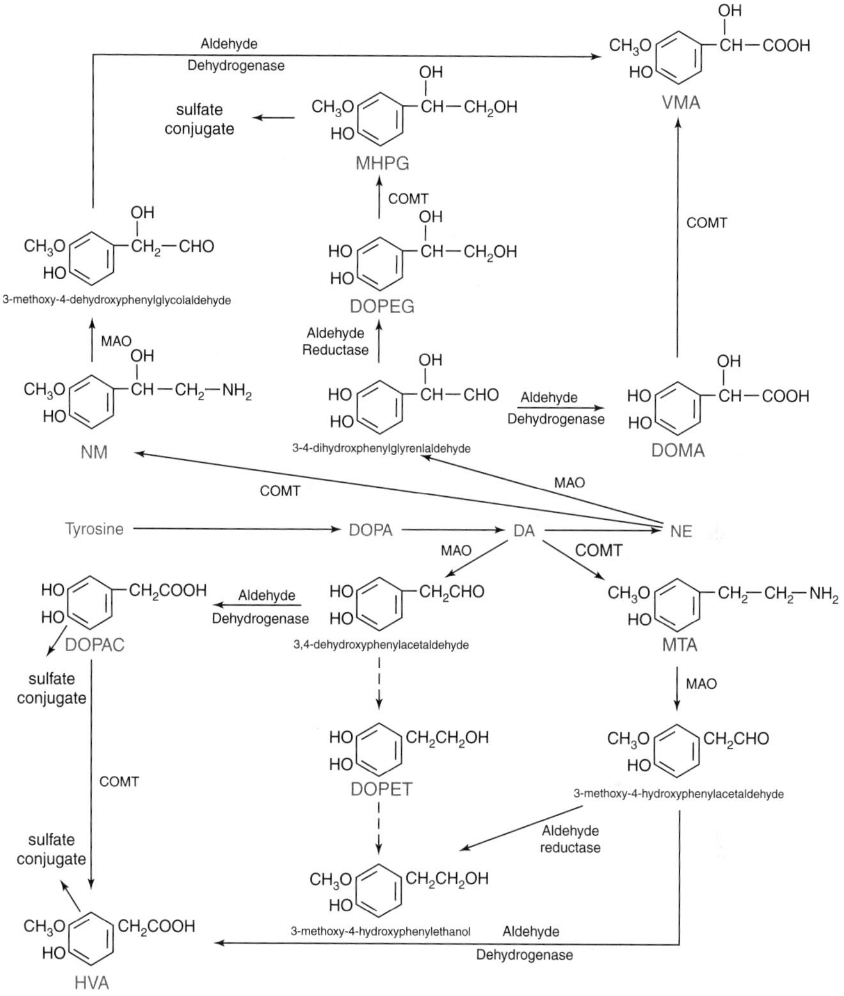

FIGURE 7–5. Dopamine and norepinephrine metabolism. Dashed arrows indicate steps that have been firmly established. COMT, catechol-*O*-methyltransferase; DA, dopamine; DOMA, 3,4-dihydroxymandelic acid; DOPA, 3,4-dihydroxyphenylalanine; DOPAC, 3,4-dihydroxyphenylacetic acid; DOPEG, 3,4-dihydroxyphenylglycol; DOPET, 3,4-dihydroxyphenylethanol; HVA, homovanillic acid; MAO, monoamine oxidase; MHPG, 3-methoxy-4-hydroxyphenylglycol; MTA, 3-methoxytyramine; NE, norepinephrine; NM, normetanephrine; VMA, 3-methoxy-4-hydroxymandelic acid.

in at least two different forms, designated MAO-A and MAO-B based on substrate specificity and sensitivity to inhibition by selected inhibitors.

Clorgyline is a specific inhibitor of MAO-A, which has a substrate preference for NE and serotonin. Deprenyl is a selective inhibitor of MAO-B, which has a substrate preference for β-phenylethylamine and benzylamine as substrates.

DA, tyramine, and tryptamine appear to be equally good substrates for both forms of the enzyme. MAO-A and -B arise from distinct genes on chromosome X and are expressed in different regions of the nervous system. The differential expression of the two forms of MAO in biogenic amine neurons is noteworthy. MAO-A mRNA appears to be the main form of the enzyme expressed in peripheral and central NE neurons, whereas MAO-B mRNA is found primarily in serotonergic neurons in the midbrain raphe and histaminergic neurons in the hypothalamus. Neither mRNA appears to be expressed in midbrain dopaminergic neurons, although this remains a matter of controversy.

The role and relative importance of these two types of MAO in physiological and pathological states is unknown, but this is an important area for further research. It has been speculated that in certain circumstances MAO could regulate NE biosynthesis by controlling the amount of substrate DA available to the enzyme dopamine-β-hydroxylase. MAO is not an exclusive catabolic enzyme for the catecholamines since it also oxidatively deaminates other biogenic amines, such as 5-hydroxytryptamine, tryptamine, and tyramine. The intraneuronal localization of MAO in mitochondria or other structures suggests that this would limit its action to amines that are present in a free (unbound) form in the axoplasm. Here, MAO can act on amines that have been taken up by the axon before they are sequestered by VMAT or even on amines that are released from the VMAT before they pass out through the axonal membrane. Interestingly, the latter possibility seems of minor physiological importance since MAO inhibition does not potentiate the effects of peripheral sympathetic nerve stimulation.

The second enzyme of importance in the catabolism of catecholamines is COMT, discovered by Axelrod in 1957. COMT is a relatively nonspecific enzyme that catalyzes the transfer of methyl groups from S-adenosylmethionine to the m-hydroxyl group of catecholamines and various other catechol compounds. COMT is found in the cytoplasm of most animal tissue, being particularly abundant in kidney and liver. A substantial amount is also found in the CNS and in various sympathetically innervated organs. The precise cellular localization of COMT has not been determined, although it has been suggested that it functions extraneuronally. The purified enzyme requires S-adenosylmethionine and Mg^{2+} ions for activity. As with MAO, inhibition of COMT activity does not markedly potentiate the effects of sympathetic nerve stimulation, although in some tissues it tends to prolong the duration of the response to stimulation. Therefore, neither MAO nor COMT seems to be the primary mechanism for terminating the action of NE liberated at sympathetic nerve terminals. It may be, however, that these enzymes play a more important role in terminating transmitter action and regulating catecholamine function in the CNS. In fact, data suggest that COMT may play an important role in the regulation of synaptic DA in the prefrontal cortex (see the section on dopamine), in contrast to its minimal action in the mesoaccumbens and meso-striatal DA systems. In the peripheral nervous system and CNS, the aldehyde intermediate produced by the action of MAO on NE and normetanephrine can be oxidized to the corresponding acid or reduced to the corresponding glycol. In contrast to the CNS, in the symphatic nervous system oxidation usually exceeds reduction and, quantitatively, vanilylmandelic acid (VMA) is the major metabolite of NE and is readily detectable in the urine. In fact, urinary levels of VMA are routinely measured in clinical laboratories to provide an index of peripheral sympathetic nerve function as well as to diagnose the pres-ence of catecholamine-secreting tumors such as pheochromocytomas and neuroblastomas. In the CNS, however, reduction of the intermediate aldehyde formed by the action of MAO on catecholamines or catecholamine metabo-lites predominates, and a major metabolite of NE found in the brain is the gly-col derivative 3-methoxy-4-hydroxy-phenethyleneglycol (MHPG). Very little, if any, VMA is found in the brain.

In many species, a large fraction of the MHPG formed in the brain is sulfate conjugated. However, in primates, MHPG exists primarily in an unconjugated "free" form in the brain. Some normetanephrine is also found in the brain and spinal cord. Destruction of NE neurons in the brain or spinal cord causes a reduction in the endogenous levels of these metabolites, although not as marked as the corresponding reduction in endogenous NE. Direct electrical stimula-tion of the locus ceruleus or severe stress produces an increase in the turnover of NE as well as an increase in the accumulation of the sulfate conjugate of MHPG in the rat cerebral cortex. These effects are completely abolished by ablation of the locus ceruleus or by transection of the dorsal pathway, suggest-ing that the accumulation of MHPG-sulfate in the brain may reflect the func-tional activity of central NE neurons. Since MHPG-sulfate readily diffuses from the brain into the cerebrospinal fluid (CSF) or general circulation, esti-mates of its concentration in the CSF or in urine are thought to reflect the activity of NE neurons in the brain. Although MHPG is proportionately a minor metabolite of NE in the peripheral sympathetic nervous system, a fairly large portion of MHPG in the urine still derives from the periphery. It has been estimated that in rodents the brain provides a minor contribution (25–30%) to urinary MHPG, whereas in primates the brain contribution is quite large (60%). Thus, at least in rodents, it is quite probable that relatively large changes in the formation of MHPG by the brain are necessary to produce detectable changes in urinary MHPG. For example, in rats, destruction of the majority of NE-containing neurons in the brain by treatment with 6-hydroxy-dopamine leads to only an approximately 25% decrease in urinary MHPG levels. Nevertheless, measurement of urinary changes in MHPG is still a rea-sonable strategy for obtaining some insight into possible alterations of brain NE metabolism in patients with psychiatric illnesses. Measurement of CSF levels of MHPG also provides another possible approach to assessing central NE function in human subjects. Studies have suggested that plasma levels of MHPG might provide a reflection of central NE activity. In these studies, stimulation of the locus ceruleus in the rat was shown to result in a significant increase in the levels of plasma MHPG. Also, administration of drugs that are known to alter NE activity in rodents has predictably changed plasma levels and venous–arterial differences in MHPG in nonhuman primates. Changes in urinary, plasma, and CSF levels of MHPG and their relationship to central NE function have to be interpreted with considerable caution.

Reuptake

When sympathetic postganglionic nerves are stimulated at frequencies low enough to be comparable to those encountered physiologically, very little intact NE overflows into the circulation, suggesting that local inactivation is very efficient. This local inactivation is not significantly altered when COMT, MAO, or both are inhibited; it is believed to involve mainly reuptake of the transmitter by sympathetic neurons. Much attention has been focused on the role of tissue-uptake mechanisms in the physiological inactivation of catecholamines, but only in the past decade has this concept received direct experimental support via isolation of the NE transporter and the cloning of its gene. This uptake process is a saturable membrane transport process dependent on temperature and requiring energy. The stereochemically preferred substrate is L-NE; furthermore, NE is taken up more efficiently than its N-substituted derivatives. It is now appreciated that neuronal reuptake of catecholamines is a major means of inactivation of the released transmitter in the brain and peripheral nervous system. The reuptake process conserves transmitter and allows intracellular enzymes that degrade catecholamines to act, thus bolstering the actions of extracellular enzymes. Neuronal reuptake of catecholamines, and indeed of all transmitters for which a reuptake process has been identified, has several characteristics. The reuptake process is energy dependent, saturable, and depends on Na^+ cotransport. In addition, extracellular Cl^- is necessary for transport. Because reuptake depends on coupling to the Na^+ gradient across the neuronal membrane, toxins that inhibit Na^+,K^+-ATPase also inhibit reuptake. These plasma membrane transporters, in contrast to the monoamine transporters associated with neuronal vesicles, are not Mg^{2+} dependent and not inhibited by reserpine. A DNA clone encoding a human NE transporter has been isolated. The isolated cDNA sequence predicts a protein of 617 amino acids with the typical transporter motif of 12 highly hydrophobic regions, probable membrane-spanning domains. Expression of the cDNA clone in transfected HeLa cells indicates that the NE transport activity is sodium dependent and sensitive to NE transport inhibitors. Striking sequence homology is notable between the NE transporter and the rat and human γ-aminobutyric acid (GABA) transporters, suggesting a new transporter gene family.

The plasma membrane transporters have been intensively studied at the biochemical, pharmacological, and molecular levels. It has become clear that these Na^+- and Cl^--coupled transporters represent a group of integral membrane proteins encoded by a closely related family of genes that includes the transporters of monoamines, GABA, glycine, and choline. A different class of plasma membrane transporters is represented by the glutamate transporter (see Chapter 6). Plasma membrane transporters can be classified into families and subfamilies based on ion dependence, topology, and sequence relatedness. The NE transporters (NETs) are members of the Na^+/Cl^--dependent neurotransmitter transporter family, which includes the DA transporter (DAT) and the serotonin transporter (SERT). Expression of NET, SERT, and DAT in nonneuronal cells has established model systems for analysis of the structural basis of transporter specificity for transmitters and transporter-specific antagonists. The catecholamine transporters, NET and DAT, are not very specific, with each accumulating both DA and NE. In fact, the NET has a higher affinity for DA than for NE and, under certain conditions, can play a role in the modulation of DA transmission. No specific transporter for E-containing neurons has been found in mammalian species, but one has been identified in the frog. The catecholamine transporters are important targets of many drugs. Amphetamine and cocaine increase extracellular levels of catecholamine by blocking catecholamine transporters. In particular, cocaine shows a very high affinity for DAT; amphetamine is a less potent inhibitor but also induces "release" (via transporter reversal) of both catecholamines. Drugs used clinically in the treatment of attention deficit disorder, including amphetamine, methylphenidate, and atomoxetine, also act by blocking catecholamine transporters. NET is the molecular target of atomoxetine and tricyclic antidepressant drugs, which potently inhibit NE reuptake (see Fig. 7–6 and Chapter 14).

The availability of pure transporter proteins has facilitated the development of transporter-specific antibodies and nucleic acid probes and stimulated renewed interest in the endogenous control mechanisms acutely regulating monoamine transport *in vivo*. Also, the availability of human cDNA encoding the NET offers the opportunity to determine whether alterations in transporter genes could have important etiological implications for major depression or affective disorder. NET exerts a fine-regulated control over NE-mediated behavioral and physiological effects, including mood, depression, cognition, feeding behavior, and regulation of blood pressure and heart rate. As noted previously, NET is a target of several drugs that are therapeutically used in the treatment or diagnosis of disorders, among which depression, attention deficit hyperactivity disorder, and feeding disturbances are the most common. Thus, the potential involvement of the NET in the pathophysiology and treatment of attention deficit hyperactivity disorder, substance abuse, neurodegenerative disorders (e.g., Alzheimer's disease and Parkinson's disease), and depression has long been recognized. It is noteworthy that many of these important findings have resulted from studies *in vitro* using postmortem tissues.

Individual genetic variations in the gene encoding the human NET (hNET), located at chromosome 16q12.2, may contribute to the pathogenesis of some of these disorders. An increasing number of studies on the identification of single nucleotide polymorphisms in the hNET gene and their potential association with disease, as well as the functional investigation of naturally occurring or induced amino acid variations in hNET, have contributed to a better understanding of NET function, regulation, and genetic contribution to disorders.

Several studies suggest that a novel T-182C polymorphism in the promoter region of the NET gene is associated with major depression. A mutation in the hNET, causing diminished function, has also been associated with postural orthostatic tachycardia syndrome in a large Swedish American family. An epigenetic mechanism (hypermethylation of CpG islands in the NET gene promoter region) that results in reduced expression of the noradrenaline transporter and consequently a phenotype of diminished neuronal reuptake of noradrenaline has been implicated in both postural orthostatic tachycardia syndrome and panic disorder. However, no association of NET gene polymorphisms and bipolar disorder or attention deficit hyperactivity disorder in adults has been observed.

Since many aspects of NE neurotransmission, including synthesis and release, are tightly regulated, it would not be unexpected to find that the NET is also subject to regulatory control. In fact, more than 40 years ago, Schneider and Gillis noted that following stimulation of the sympathetic input to the heart, a rapid increase in the retention of NE occurred in the cat atrium. A number of similar observations have been made during the past four decades, suggesting that NE reuptake increases in parallel with an increased rate of sympathetic discharge and NE release. Although the mechanism responsible for the increase in NET activity remains to be determined, the presence of serine/threonine phosphorylation sites on human NET raises the possibility that this effect might be mediated by protein phosphorylation. The role of protein phosphorylation or other posttranslational modifications in regulating transporter function in the CNS is only beginning to be evaluated. However, the fact that NET proteins can now be visualized suggests that this should be a fertile area for future investigations. Little is known about promoter regions and other regulatory elements involved in the transcriptional regulation of the NET and SERT genes. However, rats treated chronically with antidepressant drugs exhibit a decrease in SERT mRNA levels and a reduction in NET using [^{3}H]nisoxetine autoradiography.

The availability of cDNAs encoding transporter proteins has facilitated the development of sensitive screening techniques to help develop new and selective agents that target specific neurotransmitter transporters. Although this screening technology has not yet led to the development of uniquely selective inhibitors of the monoamine transporters, a number of selective inhibitors of NE uptake are available, several of which are used clinically in the treatment of affective disorders (see Chapter 14) and attention deficit hyperactivity disorder (see Chapter 16). Several protype selective NE-uptake blockers are illustrated in Figure 7–6).

NE receptors

When catecholamines are released from either NE nerve terminals or the adrenal medulla, they are recognized by and bind to specific receptor molecules on the plasma membrane of the neuroeffector cells that transduce catecholamine interactions with the cell into a physiological response. Depending on the nature of the receptor, this interaction sets off a cascade of membrane and intracellular events, which cause the cell to carry out its specialized function. Classically, peripheral and central NE receptors have been divided into two distinct classes, called $\alpha\beta$ and β receptors. The development of synthetic compounds active at NE receptors has allowed further differentiation of NE receptors into α_1, α_2, β_1, and β_2 subtypes. Genes for these subtypes of NE receptor have been cloned; this has shown that these receptors are members of a larger family of hormone receptors that mediate their activity through interaction with one of a series of guanine nucleotide-binding regulatory proteins

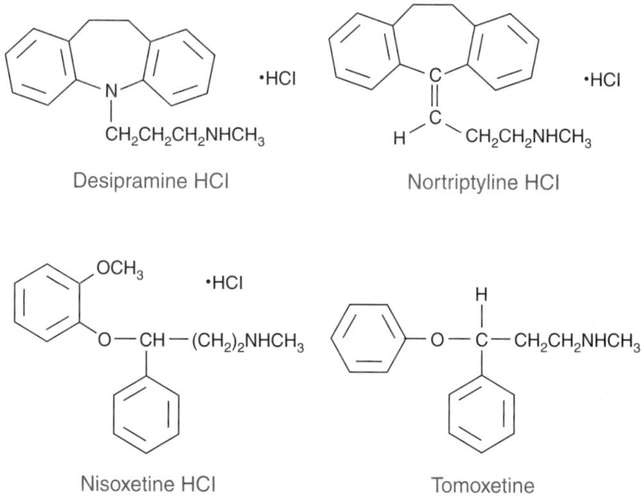

FIGURE 7–6. Representative compounds that selectively inhibit norepinephrine reuptake.

(G proteins). In addition to traditional classification based on their pharmacological profile, NE receptors can be divided into three major classes by their differential coupling to G proteins (Table 7–1). β-NE receptors activate G_s to stimulate adenylate cyclase. α_2-NE receptors decrease adenylyl cyclase activity through coupling to G_i. α_1-NE receptors stimulate phospholipase C action through a still ill-defined G_q. As schematically illustrated in Figure 7–7, β-adrenoceptor signals are transmitted through the effector cell membrane via the adenylyl cyclase system. Occupation of the β adrenoceptor by the catecholamines stimulates adenylyl cyclase to generate cAMP by a series of intramembrane events (see Chapter 4). Initially, the receptor interacts with a guanosine triphosphate (GTP)-dependent protein, G_s. G_s is linked to a catalytic unit, which generates cAMP upon activation by G_s; the catalytic unit then converts adenosine monophosphate (AMP) to cAMP. The latter compound triggers a series of intracellular events involving protein kinases. The protein kinases activate further unknown biochemical changes to generate the final biological response to the transmitter.

The interaction of NE agents with their receptors is saturable, stereospecific, and reversible. Prolonged exposure of β adrenoceptors to endogenous or exogenous agonists often reduces the responsiveness of these receptors (desensitization). Desensitization can also be caused by uncoupling of β receptors from the adenylyl cyclase and by a decrease in the number of receptors (downregulation). Depriving the β adrenoceptors of catecholamine (by chemical or surgical denervation) increases their responsiveness.

The α_1 adrenoceptor appears to be associated with calcium mobilization (see Fig. 7–7), possibly via stimulation of phospholipase C and phospholipase A_1. The α_1 receptor is distinguished from the α_2 adrenoceptor by its inhibition by the selective α_1-blocking agent prazosin. The α_2-NE receptor is negatively linked to the adenylyl cyclase complex via an inhibitory G protein (G_i). Like G_s, G_i is activated by GTP, but in this case it inhibits the generation of AMP by the catalytic unit. In the peripheral sympathetic nervous system, the α_2 receptor is localized mainly on presynaptic nerve terminals, where it modulates NE release. Stimulation of this receptor by catecholamines inhibits impulse-dependent release of transmitter; blockade of this receptor facilitates release.

Although it is clear that activation of α_2 adrenoceptors inhibits adenylyl cyclase activity (see Fig. 7–7) mediated through an inhibitory G protein, this may not in all cases represent the signal transduction mechanism responsible for the effects associated with receptor activation. For example, the α_2-mediated inhibition of neurotransmitter release is generally insensitive to inactivation of inhibitory G proteins by pertussis toxin, suggesting the involvement of another as yet undetected signal transduction mechanism.

TABLE 7–1. Characterization of Adrenergic Receptor Subtypes

RECEPTOR SUBTYPE	Receptor-Specific Agents		TISSUE DISTRIBUTION	MAJOR G PROTEIN	EFFECTOR SYSTEM
	AGONIST	ANTAGONIST			
$\alpha_1 A$	⎧ Cirazoline	⎧ Corynanthine	Vas deferens, brain	G_q	↑ Phospholipase C
$\alpha_1 B$	⎨ Methoxamine	⎨	Liver, brain		↑ Ca^{2+} channel
$\alpha_1 C$	⎩ Phenylephrine	⎨ Indoramin	Olfactory bulb		↑ Phospholipase A_2
$\alpha_1 D$		⎩ Prazosin	Vas deferens, brain		↑ Phospholipase D
					↑ Adenylylate cyclase
$\alpha_2 A$	⎧ Guanabenz	⎧ RX 821002	Aorta, brain	G_i	↑ $K^+ \downarrow Ca^{2+}$
$\alpha_2 \beta$	⎨ p-Aminoclonidine	⎨ Yohimbine	Liver, kidney		↑ Na^+ –H^+ exchange
$\alpha_2 C$	⎩ BHT-920	⎩ SKF 86426	Brain		↑ Phospholipases C, A_1
β_1	Isoproterenol	Alprenolol	Heart, brain, pineal	G_s	↑ Adenylylate cyclase
β_2		Propranolol	Lung, prostate		
β_3		Pindolol			↑ Ca^{2+} channel

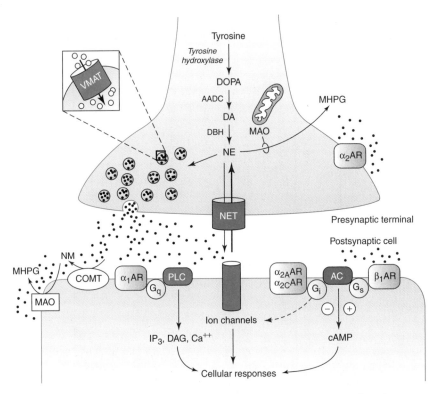

FIGURE 7–7. Model of a norepinephrine synapse illustrating the presynaptic and postsynaptic molecular entities involved in the synthesis, storage, release, reuptake, and signaling of norepinephrine. Tyrosine is transported into the presynaptic terminal by an active uptake mechanism and converted to NE by a series of enzymatic steps. NE is taken up from the axoplasm and stored by the VMAT. Once released, NE can interact with two categories of adrenergic receptors, α and β. α_2 autoreceptors localized in the nerve terminals modulate the synthesis and release of NE, whereas cell body and dendritic α_2 autoreceptors modulate impulse flow. The majority of G protein-coupled adrenergic receptors are localized postsynaptically where they mediate the cellular responses of the postsynaptic neuron. NE is metabolized by MAO and COMT, giving rise to MHPG, a major brain NE metabolite. The synaptic action of NE is terminated by reuptake into the presynaptic terminal by NET. AC, adenylyl cyclase; AR adrenergic receptor; DAG, diacylglycerol; IP$_3$, inositol triphosphate; MHPG, 3-methoxy-4-hydroxy phenethylene glycol; NET, plasma membrane norepinephrine transporter; NM, normetanephrine; PLC, phospholipase C; VMAT, vesicular monoamine transporter. (Modified from Nesther et al., 2001)

Norepinephrine Pathways in the Central Nervous System

Detailed analysis of catecholamine pathways in the CNS has been greatly accelerated by improvements in the application of fluorescence histochemistry, such as the use of glyoxylic acid as the fluorogen, and by the application of numerous auxiliary mapping methods mentioned previously. Extensive progress in the functional analysis of these systems has also been made possible by evaluation with microelectrodes of the effects produced by selective electrical stimulation of the catecholamine (especially NE) cell body groups. From such studies, it is clear that the systems can be characterized in simple terms only by ignoring large amounts of detailed cytological and functional data and that the earlier catecholamine wiring diagrams are no longer tenable. Furthermore, anatomic details for monoamine systems in rodents seem to bear only rudimentary homology to their detailed selective anatomic configurations in human and nonhuman primates. There are two major clusterings of NE cell bodies from which axonal systems arise to innervate targets throughout the entire neuraxis.

Locus Ceruleus

This compact cell group within the caudal pontine central gray is named for the pigment the cells bear in humans and some higher primates; in the rat, the nucleus contains approximately 1500 neurons on each side of the brain. In humans, the locus ceruleus is composed of approximately 12,000 large neurons on each side of the brain. The axons of these neurons form extensive collateral branches, which project widely along well-defined tracts. At the electron microscope level, terminals of these axons exhibit, under appropriate fixation methods, the same type of small granular vesicles seen in the peripheral sympathetic nerves.

Fibers from the locus ceruleus form five major NE tracts (Fig. 7–8), including the central tegmental tract (or dorsal bundle described by Ungerstedt), a central gray dorsal longitudinal fasciculus tract, and a ventral tegmental–medial forebrain bundle tract. These tracts remain largely ipsilateral, although there is a crossing over in some species of up to 25% of the fibers. These three ascending tracts then follow other major vascular and fascicular routes to innervate all cortices, specific thalamic and hypothalamic nuclei, and the olfactory bulb. Another major fascicle ascends in the superior cerebellar peduncle to innervate the cerebellar cortex. The fifth major tract descends into the mesencephalon and spinal cord, where the fibers course in the ventral–lateral column. At their terminals, the locus ceruleus fibers form a plexiform network in which the incoming fibers gain access to a cortical region by passing through the major myelinated tracts, turning vertically toward the outer cortical surface, and then forming characteristic T-shaped branches, which run parallel to the surface in the molecular layer; this pattern is seen in the cerebellar, hippocampal, and cerebral cortices.

Virtually all of the NE pathways that have been studied physiologically to date are efferent pathways of the locus ceruleus neurons; in cerebellum, hippocampus, and cerebral cortex, the major effect of activating this pathway is to inhibit spontaneous discharge. This effect has been associated with the slow type of synaptic transmission, in which the hyperpolarizing response of the

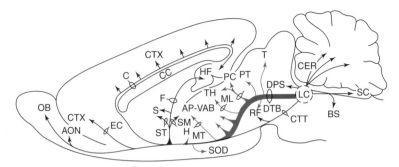

FIGURE 7–8. Diagram of the projections of the locus ceruleus viewed in the sagittal plane. AON, anterior olfactory nucleus; AP-VAB, ansa peduncularis–ventral amygdaloid bundle system; BS, brain stem nuclei; C, cingulum; CC, corpus callosum; CER, cerebellum; CTT, central tegmental tract; CTX, cerebral neocortex; DPS, dorsal periventricular system; DTB, dorsal catecholamine bundle; EC, external capsule; F, fornix; H, hypothalamus; HF, hippocampal formation; LC, locus ceruleus; ML, medial lemniscus; MT, mammillothalamic tract; OB, olfactory bulb; PC, posterior commissure; PT, pretectal area; RF, reticular formation; S, septal area; SC, spinal cord; SM, stria medullaris; SOD, supraoptic decussations; ST, stria terminalis; T, tectum; TH, thalamus. (Diagram compiled by R. Y. Moore, from the observations of Lindvall and Björklund, 1974; Jones and Moore, 1977.)

target cell is accompanied by increased membrane resistance. The mechanism of this action has been experimentally related to the second messenger scheme in which the NE receptor elicits its characteristic action on the target cells by activating the synthesis of cAMP in or on the postsynaptic membrane. Pharmacologically and cytochemically, target cells responding to NE or the locus ceruleus projection in these cortical areas exhibit β-NE receptors.

Lateral tegmental norepinephrine neurons

A large number of NE neurons lie outside of the locus ceruleus, where they are more loosely scattered throughout the lateral ventral tegmental fields. In general, the fibers from these neurons intermingle with those arising from the locus ceruleus, with those from the more posterior tegmental levels contributing mainly descending fibers within the mesencephalon and spinal cord and those from the more anterior tegmental levels contributing to the innervation of the forebrain and diencephalon. Because of the complex intermingling of the fibers from the various NE cell body sources, the physiological and pharmacological analysis of the effects of brain lesions becomes extremely difficult. Nevertheless, NE neurons in this tract have been implicated in behavioral functions relevant to psychiatric disorders. The strong ascending projections of the NE cells in this tract to forebrain areas such as nucleus accumbens, amygdala, hypothalamus, and bed nucleus of the stria terminalis have been shown to be important in affective and cognitive processes. Studies have provided compelling evidence for the importance of this NE system in addiction and stress-induced anxiety.

Epinephrine Neurons

In the sympathetic nervous system and the adrenal medulla, E shares with NE the role of final neurotransmitter, with the proportion of this sharing being a species-dependent, hormonally modified arrangement. Until method refinement, however, little evidence could be gathered to document the existence of E in the CNS because the chemical methods for analyzing E levels or for detecting activity attributable to the synthesizing enzyme PNMT were unable to provide unequivocal data. With the development of sensitive immunoassays for PNMT and their application in immunohistochemistry and with the application of gas chromatography–mass fragmentography and high-performance liquid chromatography with electrochemical detection to brain neurotransmitter measurements, the necessary data were rapidly acquired and the existence of E-containing neurons in the CNS was confirmed. By immunohistochemistry, E-containing neurons are defined as those that are positively stained (in serial sections) with antibodies to TH, dopamine-β-hydroxylase, and PNMT. These cells are found largely in two groups: One, called C1 (Hokfelt et al., 1984), is intermingled with NE cells of the lateral tegmental system; the other, called C2, is found in the regions in which the NE cells of the dorsal medulla are also found. The axons of these two E systems ascend to the hypothalamus with the central tegmental tract, then via the ventral periventricular system into the hypothalamus. A third group of cells (C3) in the midline (medial longitudinal fascicle) has also been described (Fig. 7–9). Within the mesencephalon, the E-containing fibers innervate the nuclei of visceral efferent and afferent systems, especially the dorsal motor nucleus of the vagus nerve. In addition, E fibers innervate the locus ceruleus, the intermediolateral cell columns of the spinal cord, and the periventricular regions of the fourth ventricle.

Although there are considerably fewer E than DA and NE neurons in the brain, they appear to have a discrete anatomic distribution and are believed to subserve physiological functions discrete from other catecholamines. Selective plasma membrane transporters have been described for DA and NE, and these transporters have been extensively studied both *in vivo* and *in vitro*. However, little attention has been given to the hypothetical E transporter, and a specific transporter for E has not been isolated from mammalian brain nor have drugs that selectively block E reuptake been described. All of the pharmacological agents that have been shown to block the NET (see Fig. 7–6) selectively are also effective inhibitors of E uptake. Thus, it remains uncertain whether a selective transporter for E actually exists in the mammalian CNS or peripheral nervous system. The cloning and expression of the E transporter

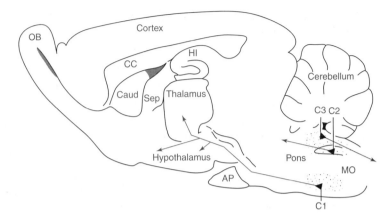

FIGURE 7–9. Schematic illustration of the distribution of the main central neuronal pathways containing epinephrine. The C1 group represents a rostral continuation of the noradrenergic cell group in the ventrolateral medulla oblongata. The dorsal C2 group of cells is located mainly in the dorsal vagal complex, with the vast majority of cell bodies in the solitary tract nucleus. A C3 group of cells in the midline (medial longitudinal fascicle) has also been described. The ventral group of epinephrine-containing neurons gives rise to both ascending and descending pathways, innervating largely periventricular regions such as the periaqueductal central gray and various hypothalamic nuclei and the lateral sympathetic column in the spinal cord. AP, ansa peduncularis; CAUD, caudate; CC, corpus callosum; HI, hippocampus; MO, medulla oblongata; OB, olfactory bulb; SEP, septum. (Data from Hokfelt et al., 1984.)

might permit a search for selective inhibitors, which, if discovered, could provide valuable pharmacological tools for elucidating the functional role of central E-containing neurons.

Except for tests of E in the locus ceruleus (where it inhibits firing), no other tests of the cellular physiology of this system have been reported. Our understanding concerning the function of E-containing neurons in the brain is very limited, but based on the distribution of E in specific brain regions, attention has been directed to their possible role in neuroendocrine mechanisms and blood pressure control.

Pharmacology of Central Catecholamine-Containing Neurons

A great deal of information has become available concerning the anatomy, biochemistry, and functional organization of CNS catecholamine systems. This has fostered knowledge concerning the mechanisms and sites of action of many psychotropic drugs. It is now appreciated that drugs can influence the output of catecholamine systems by interacting at several distinct sites. For example, drugs can influence the output of NE systems by (1) acting presynaptically to alter the life cycle of the transmitter (i.e., synthesis, storage, and release, etc. [see Figs. 7–8 and 7–10]), (2) acting postsynaptically to mimic or block the action of the transmitter at the level of postsynaptic receptors, and (3) acting at the level of cell body autoreceptors to influence the physiological activity of NE neurons. The activity of NE neurons can also be influenced by postsynaptic receptors via negative neuronal feedback loops. In the latter two actions, drugs appear to exert their influence by interacting with noradrenergic receptors. Figure 7–11 illustrates the various neuronal pathways and local mechanisms regulating synaptic homeostasis in central NE neurons. In general, catecholamine receptors can be subdivided into two broad categories: those that are localized directly on catecholamine neurons (often referred to as *presynaptic receptors*) and those on other cell types, often termed simply *postsynaptic receptors* since they are postsynaptic to the catecholamine neurons, the source of the endogenous ligand. When it became appreciated that catecholamine neurons, in addition to possessing receptors on the nerve terminals, appear to have receptors distributed over all parts of the neurons (i.e., soma, dendrites, and preterminal axons), the term *presynaptic receptors* really became inappropriate as a description for all of these receptors. In 1975, Carlsson suggested that *autoreceptor* was a more appropriate term to describe these receptors since the sensitivity of these catecholamine receptors to the neuron's own transmitter seemed more significant than their location relative to the synapse. The term autoreceptor achieved rapid acceptance, and pharmacological research in the succeeding years resulted in the detection and description of autoreceptors on neurons in almost all chemically defined neuronal systems.

The presence of autoreceptors on some neurons may turn out to be only of pharmacological interest since they may never encounter effective concentrations of the appropriate endogenous agonist *in vivo*. Others, however, in addition to their pharmacological responsiveness, may play a very important physiological role in the regulation of presynaptic events. This certainly appears to be the case for DA autoreceptors (see the section on dopamine).

The pharmacology of central and peripheral NE neurons is quite similar (see Fig. 7–10). The main differences seem to be related primarily to drug delivery and the greater complexity of the neuronal pathways regulating synaptic homeostasis of the central NE systems.

Physiological functions of central norepinephrine neurons

Many functions have been proposed for the central NE neurons and their several sets of synaptic connections. Among the hypotheses that have the most supportive data are those concerning their role in affective psychoses, learning and memory, reinforcement, sleep–wake cycle regulation, and the anxiety–nociception hypothesis. It has also been suggested that a major function of central NE neurons is not on neuronal activity and related behavioral phenomena at all but, rather, a more general role in cerebral blood flow and metabolism. However, available data fit better into a more general proposal: The main function of the locus ceruleus and its projections is to determine the brain's global orientation concerning events in the external world and within the viscera. Such a hypothesis of central NE neuron function has been generated by observations of locus ceruleus unit discharge in untreated, awake, behaviorally responsive rats and monkeys. These studies reveal the locus ceruleus units to be highly responsive to a variety of nonnoxious sensory stimuli and that the responsiveness of these units varies as a function of the animal's level of behavioral vigilance. Increased neuronal activity in the locus ceruleus is associated with unexpected sensory events in the subject's external environment, whereas decreased NE activity is associated with behaviors that mediate tonic vegetative behaviors. Such a global-orienting function can also incorporate other aspects of presumptive function expressed by earlier data, but none of those more discrete functions can be documented as necessary or sufficient explanations of locus ceruleus function.

Pharmacology of epinephrine neurons

Limited experiments have suggested that the pharmacology of central E neurons is similar to that of central NE neurons. Agents that block TH,

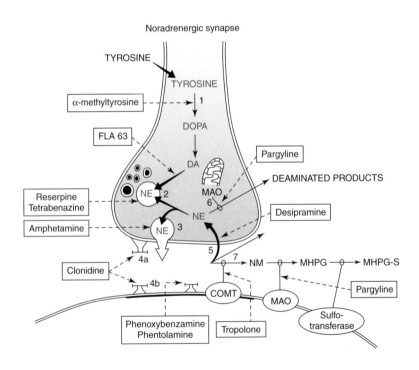

DOPA-decarboxylase, and dopamine-β-hydroxylase lead to a reduction of both NE and E in the brain. Depleting agents such as reserpine, which cause release of NE and DA, are also effective at releasing E. MAO inhibitors cause an elevation of NE, DA, and E; but inhibitors of MAO-A are much more effective at elevating E. In fact, most of the pharmacological data are consistent with the hypothesis that, at least in the rat hypothalamus, oxidative deamination is an important metabolic process by which E is degraded and that MAO-A is

FIGURE 7–10. Schematic model of central noradrenergic neuron indicating possible sites of drug action.

Site 1: *Enzymatic synthesis:*

a. Tyrosine hydroxylase reaction blocked by the competitive inhibitor, α-methyltyrosine.
b. Dopamine-β-hydroxylase reaction blocked by a dithiocarbamate derivative, Fla-63-bis-(1-methyl-4-homopiperazinyl-thiocarbonyl)-disulfide (FLA 63).

Site 2: *Storage:* Reserpine and tetrabenazine interfere with the uptake–storage mechanism of the amine granules. Depletion of norepinephrine (NE) produced by reserpine is long-lasting, and the storage granules are irreversibly damaged. Tetrabenazine also interferes with the uptake–storage mechanism of the granules, except the effects of this drug are of a shorter duration and do not appear to be irreversible.

Site 3: *Release:* A mechanism by which amphetamine causes release is by its ability to effectively block the reuptake mechanism.

Site 4: *Receptor interaction:*
a. Presynaptic α_2 autoreceptors
b. Postsynaptic α_2 receptors

Clonidine appears to be a very potent autoreceptor-stimulating drug. At higher doses, clonidine will also stimulate postsynaptic receptors. Phenoxybenzamine and phenotolamine are effective α receptor-blocking agents. These drugs may also have some presynaptic α_2 receptor-blocking action. However, yohimbine and piperoxane are more selective as α_2 receptor-blocking agents.

Site 5: *Reuptake:* NE has its action terminated by being taken up into the presynaptic terminal. The tricyclic drug desipramine is an example of a potent inhibitor of this uptake mechanism.

Site 6: *Monoamine oxidase (MAO):* NE or dopamine (DA) present in a free state within the presynaptic terminal can be degraded by the enzyme MAO, which appears to be located in the outer membrane of mitochondria. Pargyline is an effective inhibitor of MAO.

Site 7: *Catechol-O-methyltransferase (COMT):* NE can be inactivated by the enzyme COMT, which is believed to be localized outside the presynaptic neuron. Tropolone is an inhibitor of COMT. The normetanephrine (NM) formed by the action of COMT on NE can be further metabolized by MAO and aldehyde reductase to 3-methoxy-4-hydroxyphenylglycol (MHPG). The MHPG formed can be further metabolized to MHPG-sulfate (MHPG-S) by the action of a sulfotransferase found in the brain. Although MHPG-S is the predominant form of this metabolite found in rodent brain, the free unconjugated MHPG is the major form found in primate brain.

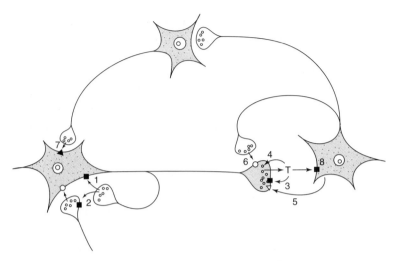

FIGURE 7–11. Neural pathways regulating synaptic homeostasis of locus ceruleus neurons. Influence of locus ceruleus neuron (shaded) on its target cells can be regulated both by modulation of transmitter release (*1–7*) and by amplification of signal provided by that release (*8*). This involves a large variety of cell surface receptors, including receptors that respond to norepinephrine (solid square) as well as receptors responding to other chemical signals (solid triangle and open circle, square, and triangle). Principal pathways for regulating norepinephrine release: *1*, direct action of recurrent collaterals onto soma; *2*, indirect action of recurrent collaterals, mediated via influence on presynaptic afferents; *3*, direct action of norepinephrine on presynaptic terminals; *4*, alterations in rate of norepinephrine reuptake; *5*, humoral signals generated by target; *6*, neural signals providing short-loop negative feedback from target; *7*, neural signals providing long-loop negative feedback from target; *8*, extent to which signal is amplified can be modulated by short-term modification of the sensitivity of the target, by long-term changes in number of receptors, and by other means such as release of cotransmitter. (Modified from Stricker and Zigmond, 1986.)

predominantly involved in this degradation. Similar to observations made in central NE neurons, α_2 agonists such as clonidine decrease E formation and α_2 antagonists increase E turnover. These data are also consistent with the possibility that α_2 receptors are involved in the regulation of synthesis and release of E and perhaps in the control of the functional activity of NE neurons.

DOPAMINE

Dopamine is the most recently discovered catecholamine transmitter in the mammalian brain. Until the mid-1950s, it was exclusively considered to be an intermediate in the biosynthesis of the catecholamines NE and E. Significant tissue levels of DA were first demonstrated in peripheral organs of ruminant species. A short time later, Montagu, Carlsson, and co-workers found that DA was also present in the brain in approximately equal concentrations to those of NE but with a quite different distribution. The very marked differences in regional distribution of the catecholamines DA and NE, both within the CNS and in bovine peripheral tissue, led Swedish investigators to propose a biological role for DA independent of its function as a precursor for NE biosynthesis. Studies demonstrating that most brain DA is confined to the basal ganglia led to the hypothesis that it might be involved in motor control and that decreased striatal DA could be the cause of extrapyramidal symptoms in Parkinson's disease. The discovery of profound depletions of DA in the striatum of parkinsonian patients and the demonstration that L-DOPA has beneficial effects in these patients substantiated the clinical relevance of this theory. These and other largely pharmacological studies were the impetus for the almost explosive developments in DA research during the past four decades. With the development of histochemical methods for the visualization of DA or its main synthetic enzyme in brain tissue, the anatomy of brain DA systems could also be described, paving the way for more direct studies on this neurotransmitter. This research culminated in the award of the Nobel Prize in 2000 to three scientists—Carlsson, Greengard, and Kandel—for their seminal contributions to this field.

Dopaminergic Systems

The central DA-containing systems are considerably more complex in their organization than the NE and E systems. Not only are there many more DA cells (the number of mesencephalic DA cells has been estimated to be approximately 15,000–20,000 on each side, whereas the number of NE neurons in the entire brain stem is reported to be approximately 5000 on each side) but also there are several major DA-containing nuclei. From anatomical studies of the DA systems in the 1970s (Fig. 7–12), these systems have been divided into three major categories based on the length of the efferent dopamine fibers:

1. *Ultrashort systems.* Among the ultrashort systems are the *interplexiform amacrine-like neurons*, which link the inner and outer plexiform layers of the retina, and the *periglomerular dopamine cells* of the olfactory bulb, which link together mitral cell dendrites in separated adjacent glomeruli. These neurons make extremely localized connections.

2. *Intermediate-length systems.* The intermediate-length systems include (1) the *tuberohypophysial dopamine cells*, which project from arcuate and periventricular nuclei into the intermediate lobe of the pituitary and into the median eminence (often referred to as the *tuberoinfundibular system*); (2) the *incertohypothalamic neurons*, which link the dorsal and posterior hypothalamus with the dorsal anterior hypothalamus and lateral septal nuclei; and

(3) the *medullary periventricular group*, which includes those DA cells in the perimeter of the dorsal motor nucleus of the vagus nerve, the nucleus tractus solitarius, and the cells scattered in the tegmental radiation of the periaqueductal gray matter.

3. *Long systems.* The long systems are the long projections linking the ventral tegmental (A8 and A10) and substantia nigra (A9) DA cells with three principal sets of targets: the neostriatum (principally the caudate and putamen), the limbic cortex (medial prefrontal, cingulate, and entorhinal areas), and other limbic structures (the regions of the septum, olfactory tubercle, nucleus accumbens septi, amygdaloid complex, and piriform cortex). These latter two groups have frequently been termed the *mesocortical* and *mesolimbic dopamine projections*, respectively. Under certain conditions, these limbic target systems, compared to the nigrostriatal system, exhibit some unique pharmacological properties, which are discussed in detail later. When DA systems were first visualized in the CNS, it was thought that all DA cells within the zona compacta of the substantia nigra projected to the caudate putamen nucleus. Dopamine cells in the ventral tegmental area surrounding the interpeduncular nucleus were believed to project exclusively to parts of the limbic system. This beautiful simplicity lasted a relatively short time. Soon, DA inputs to the cortex were discovered, and within a few years, primarily through the use of retrograde tracing techniques, it became apparent that DA cells within the A8, A9, and A10 areas form an anatomically heterogeneous population in terms of their projection areas (Björklund and Lindvall, 1984). Retrograde tracing techniques also led to the important discovery that DA cells project topographically to the areas that they innervate. Thus, although there is some overlap, DA cells that are near each other in a given area are more likely to innervate a common region than are DA cells distant from each other.

The anatomical studies described previously were carried out in the albino rat. Subsequent work in primates has suggested that the anatomy of the DA systems, although similar, is more complex, exhibiting a number of important differences noted later.

Of course, the larger primate brain has more DA neurons than the smaller rodent brain. Thus, vervet and rhesus monkeys have approximately 20 times as many midbrain DA neurons as the rat, and the human brain possesses approximately twice as many as that of the monkey. Some distinct differences in the organization of DA systems are seen between primate and rodent brain, which are expanded upon next.

The A9 cells of substantia nigra pars compacta exist in two tiers. The ventral tier of TH-positive neurons contains groups of cells that are more densely packed than those in the dorsal tier. In the primate, the ventral tier

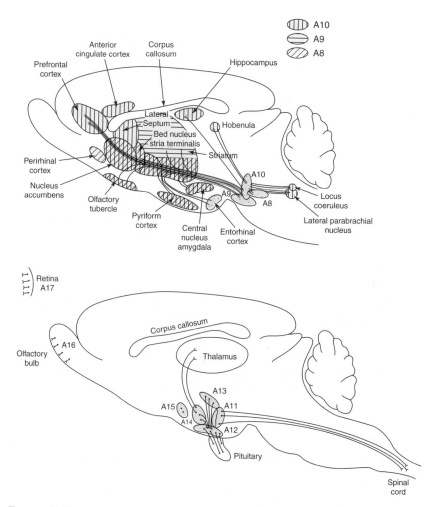

FIGURE 7–12. Schematic diagram illustrating the distribution of the main central neuronal pathways containing DA. Stippled regions indicate major nerve terminal areas and their cell groups of origin. Cell groups are named according to the nomenclature of Dahlström and Fuxe (1964).

cells do not form a continuous band dorsal to the substantia nigra pars reticulata, as in the rodent. Instead, groups of tightly packed cells penetrate deep into the pars reticulata in fingerlike extensions or in isolated clusters. In addition to the relatively distinct A8–A10 populations, there are diffusely arranged DA cell bodies throughout the tegmentum, and these are particularly numerous in primates compared to rodents. Midbrain DA neurons in the primate are distinguished from those in other species by the marked age-dependent accumulation of neuromelanin, a pigment responsible for the dark coloration of the substantia nigra; these melanized DA neurons are preferentially lost in

Parkinson's disease. In fact, in primates but not rodents, there is a normal age-dependent decrease in the number of midbrain DA cells, which may be exaggerated in Parkinson's disease. Another difference occurs in the A15 population, in which in primates, but not in rodents, abundant DA cells belonging to this group are located in the supraoptic nucleus.

In primates, the DA innervation of cortical areas is more extensive than in rodents, with the dense DA innervation of primate motor cortices being a notable difference. Another striking difference is that in the rodent the meso-cortical DA neurons originate almost exclusively in the A10, but in the primate DA afferents to the frontal lobes arise from the dorsal aspects of all three mesencephalic DA cell groups (A8–A10). In contrast to the rodent brain, the coexistence of DA with neurotensin or cholecystokinin in particular mesence-phalic DA neurons is low or nonexistent in primate brain.

Function

The different locations of the various DA systems in the brain dictate that they have different afferent and efferent connections, which in turn determine the roles they play in brain function. These are reviewed here. It should also be appreciated that it is not possible to completely segregate the motor, motivational, and cognitive behaviors that are often attributed to the nigrostriatal, mesolimbic, and mesocortical DA systems, respectively.

Nigrostriatal system

Dopaminergic innervation of the basal ganglia plays an essential role in many aspects of motor control, cognition, and emotion. The striatum is one of the principal input structures of the basal ganglia. The importance of the DA input to the striatum is evident from the motor abnormalities (e.g., bradykinesia, rigidity, and tremor) exhibited by patients with Parkinson's disease, which is characterized by a marked loss of nigrostriatal DA neurons (see Chapter 17). DA innervations to limbic and cortical regions are also affected in Parkinson's disease but to a lesser extent than the striatal input. DA release in the striatum modulates activity in two striatopallidal circuits ("direct" and "indirect"), which in turn exert control over thalamocortical circuits essential for voluntary control of movement. The signs of Parkinson's disease do not appear until a large majority (approximately 80%) of nigrostriatal DA neurons have been lost because surviving DA neurons efficiently increase their activity to compensate for the damage. It is now apparent that nigrostriatal DA neurons do not merely allow motor behavior to occur but that they also play an important role in the selection and initiation of actions and establishing motor skills and habits. Current treatments for Parkinson's disease typically involve administration of the DA precursor L-DOPA or DA receptor agonists (see Chapter 17).

Future treatments are likely to include restoration of dopaminergic tone by transplantation of fetal DA neurons or stem cells or by gene therapy.

Mesolimbic system

The function of the mesolimbic dopaminergic system, in particular the projection from the VTA to the nucleus accumbens, has been strongly implicated in goal-oriented (motivated) behaviors, in addition to reward, attention, and pharmacologically induced locomotion. Enhancement of DA transmission in this system has been linked with the addicting, reinforcing, and sensitizing effects of repeated exposure to psychostimulant drugs of abuse. Furthermore, the therapeutic effects of antipsychotic drugs used in the treatment of schizophrenia may depend on the inhibition of mesolimbic DA neuron activity that these drugs induce. The ability of antipsychotic drugs to block DA receptors and thereby reduce DA transmission is central to the 40-year-old DA hypothesis of schizophrenia, which posits that the disease is related to excessive central DA activity. Imaging studies in patients have provided support for the existence of disrupted DA transmission in schizophrenia. A revision to the hypothesis is the concept of underactivity in cortically projecting DA neurons together with overactivity in subcortical DA systems. Persuasive evidence implicates developmental, functional, and structural abnormalities in schizophrenia involving other transmitter systems besides DA, such as glutamate and GABA.

Mesocortical system

The prefrontal cortex has rich connections with other neocortical regions, limbic regions, and other subcortical regions. The prefrontal cortex has been implicated in a wide variety of cognitive functions, and it particularly appears to be involved in directing appropriate attention, prioritizing the significance of stimuli, monitoring the temporal sequence of stimuli, referencing stimuli to internal representations or cues, and devising abstract concepts. The well-defined DA projection to the prefrontal cortex has been suggested to be involved in short-term and "working" memory. It has been hypothesized that the mesoprefrontal DA system is involved in the pathophysiology of schizophrenia and that defects in this system, or its associated neuronal connections, may be responsible for the negative and cognitive deficits that characterize the disorder. Evidence suggests that an abnormally reduced activity of prefrontal DA neurons may lead to enhanced DA neurotransmission in the striatum and nucleus accumbens, and it has been speculated that such a dysfunction may play a significant role in ADHD and Tourette syndrome.

Diencephalon systems

DA neurons in the posterior dorsal hypothalamus and periventricular gray of central thalamus (A11) project to the spinal cord, and they appear to have a role in sensory and nociceptive processing and sensory integration. Tuber-oinfundibular DA neurons (A12) are located in the arcuate nucleus and peri-ventricular nucleus of mediobasal hypothalamus and project to the external layer of the median eminence. They play an important role in inhibiting the release of prolactin from the anterior lobe of the pituitary. Incertohypotha-lamic DA neurons (A13) reside in the rostral portion of the medial zona inserta, and they terminate in the central nucleus of the amygdala, the horizontal diag-onal band of Broca, and the paraventricular nucleus of the hypothalamus. Their functions are not clear but probably involve integration of autonomic and neuroendocrine responses to sensory stimuli. Two subpopulations of A14 neurons have been distinguished. The periventricular–hypophyseal (tuberohy-pophyseal) DA neurons terminate in the intermediate lobe of the posterior pituitary and inhibit secretion of α-MSH and proopiomelanocortin-derived peptides. The other defined group of A14 DA neurons is located in the peri-ventricular hypothalamic nucleus. Fibers of these neurons extend into the medial preoptic nucleus and anterior hypothalamus. Females possess a greater number of these neurons than do males, and they are believed to play a role in gonadotrophin secretion in females and reproductive behavior in males. DA neurons in the ventrolateral hypothalamic comprise the A15 cell group, and they extend processes to the lateral hypothalamus and caudal supraoptic.

Life Cycle of Dopamine

It has become apparent that midbrain DA neurons are quite heterogeneous in terms of their biochemistry, physiology, pharmacology, and regulatory prop-erties compared to the prototypic nigrostriatal system, on which most early studies were performed. Although midbrain DA neurons differ in a number of important ways, their functional organization generally reflects features of transmitter dynamics that are shared by all DA neurons. These features have been most thoroughly studied in the nigrostriatal pathway and are summa-rized here (see Fig. 7–13).

Dopamine synthesis

Dopamine synthesis originates from tyrosine, and its rate-limiting step is the conversion of L-tyrosine to L-DOPA by the enzyme TH. DOPA is subse-quently converted to DA by L-aromatic amino acid decarboxylase at rates so rapid that DOPA levels in the brain are negligible under normal conditions. Because endogenous levels of DOPA are normally low in the brain, the forma-tion of DA can be enhanced dramatically by providing this enzyme with increased amounts of L-DOPA. Since the levels of tyrosine in the brain are rel-atively high and above the K_m for TH, under normal conditions it is not feasi-ble to augment DA synthesis significantly by increasing brain levels of this

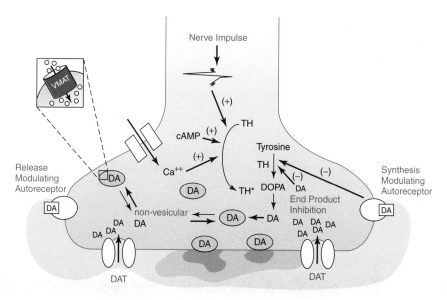

FIGURE 7-13. Schematic model of a prototypic dopaminergic nerve terminal illustrating the life cycle of DA and the mechanisms that modulate its synthesis, release, and storage. Invasion of the terminal by a nerve impulse results in Ca^{2+}-dependent release of DA. This release process is attenuated by release-modulating autoreceptors. Increased impulse flow also stimulates tyrosine hydroxylation. This appears to involve the phosphorylation of TH, resulting in conversion to an activated form with greater affinity for tetrahydrobiopterin cofactor and reduced affinity for the end-product inhibitor DA. The rate of tyrosine hydroxylation can be attenuated by (1) activation of synthesis-modulating autoreceptors, which may function by reversing the kinetic activation of TH, and (2) end-product inhibition by intraneuronal DA, which competes with cofactor for a binding site on TH. Release- and synthesis-modulating autoreceptors may represent distinct receptor sites. Alternatively, one site may regulate both functions through distinct transduction mechanisms. The plasma membrane DA transporter is a unique component of the DA terminal that serves an important physiological role in the inactivation and recycling of DA release into the synaptic cleft. The vesicular monoamine transporter (VAT) transports cytoplasmic DA into storage vesicles, decreasing the cytoplasmic concentration of DA and preventing metabolism by monoamine oxidase. VAT modulates the concentration of free DA in the nerve terminals.

amino acid. Endogenous mechanisms for regulating the rate of DA synthesis in DA neurons primarily involve modulation of TH activity through four major regulatory influences:

1. Dopamine and other catecholamines function as end-product inhibitors of TH by competing with a tetrahydrobiopterin (BH_4) cofactor for a binding site on the enzyme.

2. The availability of BH_4 may also play a role in regulating TH activity. Since endogenous levels of BH_4 are controlled by GTP cyclohydrolase activity, this

rate-limiting enzyme in BH_4 synthesis can indirectly influence tyrosine hydroxylation. TH can exist in two kinetic forms, which exhibit different affinities for BH_4. Conversion from low- to high-affinity forms is thought to involve direct phosphorylation of the enzyme, and the proportion of TH molecules in the high-affinity state appears to be a function of the state of neuronal firing.

3. Presynaptic DA receptors also modulate the rate of tyrosine hydroxylation. These receptors are activated by DA released from the nerve terminal, resulting in feedback inhibition of DA synthesis. Autoreceptors can modulate both synthesis and release of DA and represent important sites for the pharmacological manipulation of dopaminergic function by DA agonists and antagonists.

4. Dopamine synthesis in the striatum also depends on the rate of impulse flow in the nigrostriatal pathway. During periods of increased impulse flow, the rate of tyrosine hydroxylation is increased primarily through kinetic activation of TH, which increases its affinity for BH_4 and decreases its affinity for the normal end-product inhibitor DA. Under conditions of increased impulse flow, tyrosine hydroxylation is also more susceptible to precursor regulation by tyrosine availability.

Calcium-dependent release of DA from the nerve terminal is thought to occur in response to invasion of the terminal by an action potential. The extent of DA release appears to be a function of the rate and pattern of firing. The burst-firing mode leads to enhanced release of DA. Dopamine release is also modulated by presynaptic release-modulating autoreceptors. In general, DA agonists inhibit while DA antagonists enhance the evoked release of DA.

Dopamine uptake and the dopamine transporter

Dopamine nerve terminals possess high-affinity DA uptake sites, which are important in terminating transmitter action and maintaining transmitter homeostasis. Uptake is accomplished by a membrane carrier, the DAT, which can transport DA into and out of the terminal depending on the existing concentration gradient. Substantial progress in the 1980s led to the development of a new class of very potent and selective DA uptake inhibitors, the GBR series (Fig. 7–14). With these drugs, the stage was set for the isolation and molecular characterization of the DAT, successfully achieved in 1991 by several groups.

The DNA encoding the rat DAT exhibits high sequence similarity with the previously cloned NE and GABA transporters. The DAT is a 619-amino acid protein with 12 putative hydrophobic membrane-spanning domains and is a member of the family of Na^+/Cl^--dependent plasma membrane transporters. Using the energy provided by the Na^+ gradient generated by the Na^+/K^+-transporting adenosine triphosphatase (ATPase), the DAT recaptures DA soon after its release, thereby modulating its concentration in the synapse and its time-dependent interaction with both pre- and postsynaptic receptors.

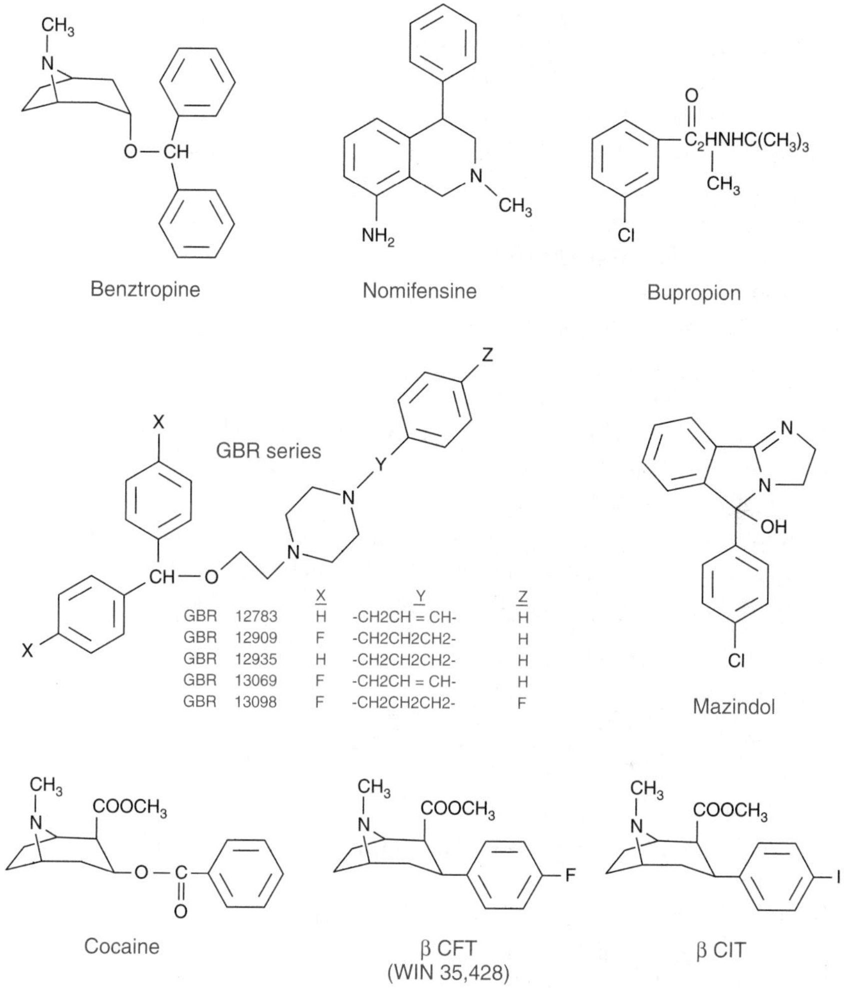

FIGURE 7–14. Chemical structures of some DA uptake inhibitors.

Molecular characterization and cloning of rat, bovine, and human DATs have shown that these proteins are highly conserved between species, with similar orientation in the plasma membrane and potential sites of glycosylation and phosphorylation.

A number of studies have suggested that DAT is a useful phenotypic marker for DA neurons and their nerve terminals and perhaps even better in some cases than TH. Nevertheless, caution should be exercised in the use of this DAT marker since its expression varies significantly among DA cell groups. The tuberoinfundibular DA neurons (A12), which release DA into the pituitary portal blood system, lack demonstrable DAT mRNA and protein. Because

DA released from tuberoinfundibular neurons is carried away rapidly in the vascular system, the existence of a transporter protein on these DA neurons seems superfluous.

During development, embryonic midbrain DA neurons express DA and TH well before they express DAT. Although the catecholamine transporters have highly similar molecular features, they exhibit important differences in their selectivity for their catecholamines and for neurotoxins such as 1-methyl-4-phenylpyridinium (MPP^+) and also very distinct pharmacologies (cf. Figs. 7–14 and 7–6).

Immunohistochemical studies of the subcellular localization of these transporters led to an unexpected finding. The use of antibodies generated against DAT revealed that the transporter is typically expressed outside of the synapse, in the extrasynaptic region of the axon terminal. This suggests that the transporter may be used to inactivate (accumulate) DA that has escaped from the synaptic cleft and, thus, that diffusion is the initial process by which DA is removed from the synapse. This is consistent with *in situ* studies indicating that perisynaptic concentrations of DA can reach approximately 1.0 mM. Receptors for DA and many other transmitters are also found extrasynaptically (indeed, along the length of axons); this observation, coupled with the presence of catecholamine transporters in extrasynaptic regions, suggests that extrasynaptic ("paracrine" or "volume") neurotransmission may be of considerable importance for catecholaminergic signaling.

Mesolimbic DA neurons are implicated in the reinforcing properties of a variety of drugs of abuse, including psychomotor stimulants such as cocaine and amphetamine. Cocaine and related drugs bind to DAT and prevent DA transport in a manner that correlates well with their behavioral reinforcing and psychomotor-stimulating properties. In fact, DATs have often been referred to as the brain's principal "cocaine receptors."

Receptor binding studies have demonstrated that compounds that bind to the DAT also inhibit DA uptake, with a rank order of potency proportional to the affinity demonstrated in binding studies. This relationship of uptake inhibitory potency and binding potency suggests that the two processes may be intimately linked and that any compound that binds to DAT will also block DA transport. However, point mutation studies of the cloned DAT indicate that reuptake inhibition and binding potency may be distinct processes that, under certain conditions, are separable, not inextricably linked. These and other studies on chimeric DAT proteins have revealed that the cocaine binding site on DAT is distinct from the substrate recognition site. These observations suggest that it may be possible to develop agents that can prevent binding of stimulants such as cocaine to the DAT while still allowing normal DA transport to ensue, thus supporting the feasibility of developing cocaine antagonists for the treatment of drug overdose, withdrawal, or addiction.

The DAT has also assumed importance in the study of 1-methyl-4-phenyl-1,2,3,6-tetrahydropyridine (MPTP)-induced and idiopathic Parkinson's disease. The selectivity of DA neurotoxins such as MPTP seems to depend on their high affinity for the DAT. In primates, MPTP toxicity can be prevented by pretreatment with DAT inhibitors, but once transported into the neuron, the toxin destroys the DA neurons, ultimately producing parkinsonism (see Chapter 17). Expression of the cloned DAT in COS cells confers sensitivity to MPP^+ toxicity, whereas expression of a vesicular transporter clone confers resistance to MPP^+ in sensitive Chinese hamster ovary cells. Thus, the levels of vesicular transporter and DAT expression in combination could conceivably dictate the response to exogenous or endogenously generated neurotoxins. Interestingly, regional differences in the levels of DAT expression appear to correlate with the extent of DA cell loss after MPTP treatment or in Parkinson's disease.

Dopamine metabolism

Dopamine can be metabolized in the brain by the same enzymatic reactions that catabolize norepinephrine, summarized in Figure 7–5. The major mammalian enzymes of importance in the metabolic degradation of catecholamines are MAO and COMT. MAO converts catecholamines to their corresponding aldehydes. This aldehyde intermediate is rapidly metabolized, usually by oxidation by the enzyme aldehyde dehydrogenase to the corresponding acid. In some circumstances, the aldehyde is reduced by aldehyde reductase. MAO is located on the outer membranes of mitochondria and thus, in brain, is present primarily in nerve terminals and glia. Separate genes encode two isoforms of MAO (types A and B), which can be distinguished by substrate specificity and sensitivity to the irreversible selective inhibitors. In brain, MAO-A is preferentially located in dopaminergic and NE neurons, whereas MAO-B appears to be the major form present in serotonergic neurons and glia. MAO is a particle-bound protein localized largely in the outer membrane of mitochondria. Usually considered to be an interneuronal enzyme, it also occurs in abundance extraneuronally.

The second enzyme of importance in catabolism of catecholamines is COMT, discovered by Julius Axelrod in 1957. This is a relatively nonspecific enzyme that catalyzes the transfer of methyl groups from S-adenosylmethionine to the m-hydroxyl group of catecholamines and various other catechol compounds. There are two isoforms of COMT—a membrane-bound form and a soluble form. Membrane-bound COMT is the major form found in the CNS, has a higher affinity for catecholamines, and is located principally in neurons. The soluble form has a lower affinity for catecholamines and is the major form expressed in the periphery, but it is also present in CNS glia. The membrane-bound isoform of COMT, which has a high affinity for DA, is expressed at neuronal dendritic processes in cortex and striatum, but the expression and activity of COMT are higher in frontal cortex than in striatum. Relevant to this is evidence that in the prefrontal cortex DAT is rarely expressed within synapses and exerts minimal influence on DA flux in the prefrontal cortex. Thus, in the frontal cortex, COMT activity appears to have a more important function in regulating DA neurotransmission than in other regions. In fact, it has been estimated that the flux of DA through the COMT pathway exceeds 60% in the prefrontal cortex but only 15% in the striatum, where DAT is the chief mechanism for terminating the action of DA. The importance of COMT to the actions of DA in the prefrontal cortex is strongly supported by the finding that compared with wild-type mice, COMT knockout mice have increased DA levels in prefrontal cortex but not in striatum, and such mice perform better on prefrontal cortex-dependent behavioral tasks. Another interesting facet to the role of COMT in frontal cortex is the finding that the COMT gene contains a polymorphism (Val158Met) that affects the *in vivo* activity of the enzyme. Met158 homozygotes have approximately one-third less COMT enzyme activity in prefrontal cortex than Val158 homozygotes. Consistent with its role in modulating prefrontal cortex DA levels, the Val158Met polymorphism is associated with performance on tests of working memory and executive function, which depend on prefrontal cortex function. Thus, the high-activity Val158 allele is linked with relatively poorer performance on such tasks, relative to the Met158 allele, presumably as a result of increased DA metabolism. The COMT polymorphism has been implicated in a number of neuropsychiatric phenotypes. In particular, there is evidence to support an association between COMT allele frequency and the genetic risk of schizophrenia. Working memory is highly dependent on DA function in the prefrontal cortex, and working memory dysfunction is a cardinal feature of schizophrenia.

The major DA metabolites found in brain differ, depending on the species under study. In general, however, acidic, rather than neutral, metabolites predominate. In rodents, the primary metabolites of DA found in the CNS are 3,4-dihydroxyphenylacetic acid (DOPAC) and homovanillic acid (HVA) and a small amount of 3-methoxytramine. DOPAC usually predominates. In addition, a considerable proportion of these metabolites in rodent brain are found in the form of conjugates. In both human and nonhuman primates, however, the major DA metabolite is HVA, and only a small amount is found in the conjugate form. It is well documented that in the rat, short-term fluctuations in DOPAC and HVA concentrations in the striatum, nucleus accumbens, and prefrontal cortex provide a useful index, respectively, of alterations in impulse flow in the nigrostriatal, mesolimbic, and mesocortical DA pathways. For example, electrical stimulation or pharmacologic treatments that alter impulse flow in these DA-containing neurons produce predictable changes in DA metabolite levels in the area of the brain innervated by these neurons. Studies of DA metabolism in primate brain have also revealed that (similar to observations made in rodents) antipsychotic drugs (DA receptor-blocking agents) and phencyclidine administered acutely produce major changes in brain levels of HVA, and in the case of antipsychotic drugs, these changes are paralleled by alterations in levels of HVA found in cerebral spinal fluid.

Functional Regulation

The synthesis and release of DA are clearly influenced by the activity of dopaminergic neurons, but these neurons behave differently from peripheral or central NE neurons; indeed, differences exist between DA neurons. Increased impulse flow in the nigrostriatal or mesolimbic DA system does lead to both an increase in DA synthesis and turnover and a frequency-dependent increase in the accumulation of DA metabolites in the striatum and olfactory tubercle. This parallels other monoamine systems, in which an increase in impulse flow causes an increase in the synthesis and turnover of transmitter.

Short-term stimulation of central dopaminergic neurons increases tyrosine hydroxylation by kinetic alterations in TH, with an increased affinity for pteridine cofactor and a decreased affinity for the natural end-product inhibitor DA. As in central NE systems, it seems that a finite period of time is necessary for this activation to occur and that, once activated, the enzyme remains in this altered physical state for a short period after the stimulation ends. The activation appears to involve TH phosphorylation.

However, if impulse flow is interrupted in the nigrostriatal or mesolimbic DA system, either mechanically or pharmacologically by treatment with γ-hydroxybutyrate, the neurons respond in a rather peculiar manner by rapidly increasing the concentration of DA in the nerve terminals of the respective DA systems. Not only do the terminals accumulate DA by reducing release but also there is a dramatic increase in the rate of DA synthesis. This increase occurs despite the steadily increasing concentration of endogenous DA within the nerve terminal.

The actual mechanisms whereby a cessation of impulse flow initiates changes in the properties of TH are unclear, although they may involve a decrease in the availability of intracellular calcium. Similar changes in the activity or properties of TH are not observed in central NE neurons or in other DA neurons (e.g., the mesoprefrontal DA neurons) lacking synthesis-modulating autoreceptors. Currently, the physiological significance of this paradoxical response to a cessation of impulse flow is unclear. However, it is conceivable that these neurons achieve some operational advantage by increasing their supply of transmitter rapidly during periods of quiescence.

Potential Sites of Drug Action on Dopaminergic Neurons

There are many sites at which drugs can influence the function of DA neurons. The potential sites for modulation are illustrated in Figure 7–15 and summarized in Table 7–2. For the purpose of this discussion, drug effects can be divided into three broad categories:

1. Nonreceptor-mediated effects on presynaptic function
2. Dopamine receptor-mediated effects
3. Effects mediated indirectly as a result of drug interaction with other neurotransmitter systems that interact with DA neurons

The relative importance of each of these potential sites of drug action will vary among different DA systems, depending on factors such as the presence or absence of autoreceptors, the efficiency of postsynaptic receptor-mediated neuronal feedback pathways, and the nature of the afferent inputs impinging on the DA neurons in question.

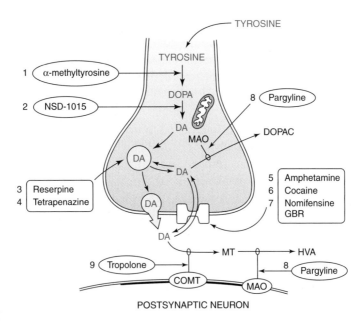

Figure 7–15. Schematic model of striatal dopaminergic nerve terminal. Drugs that alter the DA life cycle include (1) α-methyltyrosine, a competitive inhibitor of tyrosine hydroxylase; (2) NSD-1015, an inhibitor of DOPA decarboxylase; (3) reserpine, which irreversibly damages DA uptake/storage mechanisms and produces long-lasting depletion of DA; (4) tetrabenazine, which also interferes with DA uptake/storage but the effects are of shorter duration than those of reserpine and do not appear to be irreversible; (5), amphetamine, which increases synaptic DA through a number of mechanisms, including induction of release of DA and blockade of DA reuptake; (6) cocaine, which also blocks DA reuptake and induces DA release; (7) nomifensine and GBR, which also block DA reuptake but lack DA-releasing ability; (8) pargyline, an inhibitor of MAO; and (9) tropolone, an inhibitor of COMT. HVA, homovanillic acid; MT, 3-methoxytyramine; DOPAC, dihydrophenylacetic acid.

TABLE 7–2. Potential Sites for Modulating Dopaminergic Function

SITE	CONSEQUENCES
Modulatory effects at DA receptors	
1. Stimulate postsynaptic DA receptors	A. Enhance dopaminergic transmission
	B. Enhance function of neuronal feedback loops
Block postsynaptic DA receptors	A. Block dopaminergic transmission
	B. Interfere with function of neuronal feedback loops
2. Stimulate presynaptic DA autoreceptors	A. Decrease DA synthesis and release
	B. Decrease firing rate and diminish DA output from nerve terminal
Block presynaptic DA autoreceptors	A. Increase DA synthesis and release
	B. Decrease somatodendritic DA turnover (?)
3. Stimulate somatodendritic DA autoreceptors	A. Interfere with feedback regulation of firing rate and DA output from terminal
Block somatodendritic DA autoreceptors	B. Interfere with feedback regulation of somatodendritic DA turnover
Modulatory effects at non-DA receptors on DA neurons	
4. Modify afferent input to cell body (i.e., block or mimic effects of transmitter released by afferent terminal)	A. Alter firing rate of DA cell and thus alter DA output from nerve terminal
	B. Alter somatodendritic turnover of DA (and co-localized peptides?)
5. Modify afferent input to nerve terminal	A. Alter release from nerve terminal of DA (and co-localized peptides?)

Nonreceptor-mediated effects

There are several stages in the life cycle of DA (synthesis, storage, and release) in which drugs can influence transmitter dynamics, as illustrated in Figure 7–15. There are many useful pharmacological tools for modifying dopaminergic activity and manipulating dopaminergic function at these sites, but most of these agents are not very selective for dopaminergic synapses and will interact with other catecholamine (NE and E) systems (in some cases, with other monoamine [5-hydroxytryptamine] systems as well). Some drugs that interact with the plasma membrane transporter do not have a high degree of specificity. For example, amphetamine, cocaine, benztropine, and nomifensine interact with the plasma membrane transporter that normally functions in the reuptake of released DA. However, these drugs also have an appreciable affinity for NE (and in some cases serotonergic) uptake sites.

Nevertheless, drugs that are highly selective for the DA transport complex have been developed and employed as valuable experimental tools for visualization of the integrity of DA systems *in vivo*. In fact, striking results have been obtained with several new cocaine derivatives, such as 3β-(4-fluorophenyl)tropane-2β-carboxylate (CFT) and 3β-(4-iodo-phenyl)tropane-2β-carboxylate (β-CIT), which exhibit high affinity for the DAT (see Figure 7–14). These agents have been used in autoradiographic experiments and in positron emission tomography (PET) and single photon emission computed tomography (SPECT) studies to image the striatal DAT in both normal and parkinsonian monkeys and humans. These studies have demonstrated (1) loss of striatal DAT in both experimental and idiopathic Parkinson's disease and (2) restoration of DAT density and improvement of behavioral functions following nigral grafts in the caudate of transplanted MPTP monkeys. DAT ligands used for *in vivo* imaging in the future may be routinely employed in the diagnosis of certain diseases such as parkinsonism and for following the progression of the disease and the response to treatment. Imaging of DAT may also prove very useful for monitoring the viability of DA grafts and their outgrowth once transplanted into parkinsonian recipients.

Dopamine receptor-mediated effects

Originally, it was thought that all drugs that affect DA activity, including the neuroleptics, worked through nonreceptor-mediated mechanisms such as those described previously. However, it is now clear that many therapeutically important drugs interact with DA receptors. Drugs that affect DA receptors can be classified into two groups (Table 7–3):

1. Receptors on nondopamine cell types, which are usually referred to as "postsynaptic" receptors since they are postsynaptic to a DA-releasing cell

2. Receptors on DA cells, which are referred to as "autoreceptors" to indicate their sensitivity to the neuron's own transmitter

Postsynaptic Dopamine Receptors. Postsynaptic DA receptors can be classified as either D1 or D2, based on the functional and pharmacological criteria described here. Both types of receptor have been found in the projection areas of midbrain DA neurons, although it is unclear whether they are located on distinct subsets of DA-receptive cells in various projection fields. In the striatum, postsynaptic DA receptors regulate the activity of neuronal feedback pathways by which striatal neurons can communicate with DA cell bodies in the substantia nigra. This enables DA-innervated cells in the striatum to modulate the physiological activity of nigrostriatal DA neurons. In general, increased postsynaptic receptor stimulation results in decreased nigrostriatal DA activity.

TABLE 7–3. Biochemistry, Physiology, and Pharmacology of D_1 and D_2 Dopamine
Receptors

Biochemical Manifestations Induced by Receptor Stimulation			
D_1 RECEPTORS (INCREASE IN cAMP FORMATION, PHOSPHORYLATION OF DARPP-32)		D_2 RECEPTORS (DECREASE IN cAMP FORMATION OR NO CHANGE)	
LOCATION	FUNCTION	LOCATION	FUNCTION
CNS: postsynaptic to DA neuron terminals dendrites (striatum, nuc. acc., olf. tub., SN, etc.)	Enabling effect on behavioral and electrophysiological effect elicited by stimulation of D_2 receptors; function uncertain	Striatum and nuc. acc., DA nerve terminals	Autoreceptors inhibit DA synthesis and release and modulate turnover
		Retina	Mediate light-adaptive response of photoreceptors (↑ blink)
Bovine parathyroid gland	Increases parathyroid hormone release	SN and VTA: soma dendrites	Inhibits DA cell firing
Vascular smooth muscle (canine renal and mesenteric bed most used model system)	Vascular relaxation	Striatum: cholinergic interneurons	Inhibits acetylcholine release
Vertebrate retina: in teleost, localized specifically to horizontal cells	Mediates responses of horizontal cells	Pituitary gland: anterior lobe	Inhibits cAMP and prolactin release; may also regulate Ca^{2+} channels
		Pituitary gland: intermediate lobe melano-trophs	Inhibits cAMP and α-MSH release
		Chemosensitive trigger zone	Emesis
		Carotid body	Depresses spontaneous chemosensory discharge

(Continued)

TABLE 7–3. Biochemistry, Physiology, and Pharmacology of D_1 and D_2 Dopamine Receptors *(Continued)*

Biochemical Manifestations Induced by Receptor Stimulation

D_1 RECEPTORS (INCREASE IN cAMP FORMATION, PHOSPHORYLATION OF DARPP-32)		D_2 RECEPTORS (DECREASE IN cAMP FORMATION OR NO CHANGE)	
LOCATION	FUNCTION	LOCATION	FUNCTION
		Sympathetic nerve terminals (numerous tissues)	Inhibits norepinephrine release
Pharmacology			
Selective agonists	SKF-38393 (partial agonist), dihydrexidine (full agonist), SKF-82526 (fenoldopam)	LY-171555 (quinpirole), RU-24926, [+]PHNO, EMD-23-448 (autoreceptor-selective)	
Selective antagonists	SCH-23390, SKF-83566, SCH-39166	(−)-Sulpiride, YM-09151-2, domperidone, raclopride	

cAMP, cyclic adenosine monophosphate;, CNS, Central nervous system; DARPP-32, dopamine and cAMP-regulated phosphoprotein of 32 kDa; MSH, melanocytc-stimulating hormone; nuc. ace, nucleus accumbens; olf. tub., olfactory tubercle; SN, substantia nigra; VTA, ventral tegmental area.

Following chronic exposure to DA agonists or antagonists, postsynaptic DA receptors exhibit adaptive changes. For example, chronic exposure to DA antagonists or chemical denervation with 6-hydroxydopamine (6-OHDA) produces an increase in the number of DA binding sites measured in receptor binding assays. This may be related to the behavioral supersensitivity to DA agonists that also develops as a result of chronic antagonist administration or denervation. Conversely, repeated administration of DA agonists decreases the number of DA binding sites and produces subsensitivity to subsequent administration of DA agonists in behavioral as well as biochemical and electrophysiological models. Changes such as these may be relevant to understanding the state of DA receptors in diseases believed to involve chronic dopaminergic hyper- or hypoactivity.

Autoreceptors. Autoreceptors can exist on most portions of DA cells, including the soma, dendrites, and nerve terminals. Stimulation of DA autoreceptors in the somatodendritic region slows the firing rate of DA neurons, whereas stimulation of autoreceptors on the nerve terminals inhibits DA synthesis and release. Thus, somatodendritic and nerve terminal autoreceptors work in concept to exert feedback on dopaminergic transmission. Both somatodendritic and nerve terminal autoreceptors can be classified as D2 receptors and exhibit similar pharmacological properties. Like postsynaptic receptors, somatodendritic and nerve terminal autoreceptors develop supersensitivity after chronic antagonist treatment or prolonged decreases in DA release and desensitize in response to repeated administration of DA agonists. Interestingly, the autoreceptors are more readily desensitized than postsynaptic DA receptors. This has been suggested to play a role in the "on–off" effects observed during chronic L-DOPA therapy in Parkinson's disease.

Dopamine autoreceptors can be defined functionally in terms of the events they regulate and are therefore divided into three categories: synthesis-modulating, release-modulating, and impulse-modulating autoreceptors. However, it is not known whether distinct receptor proteins modulate each of these functions or whether the same receptor protein is coupled to each function through distinct transduction mechanisms. It is clear, however, that autoreceptor-mediated pathways for the regulation of DA release from the nerve terminal are distinct from autoreceptor-mediated pathways for the regulation of DA synthesis since DA terminals in the prefrontal and cingulate cortices possess autoreceptors that regulate release but lack functional synthesis-modulating autoreceptors.

Autoreceptors Versus Postsynaptic Receptors: Pharmacological and Functional Considerations.   Autoreceptors and postsynaptic DA receptors differ in several ways. The most clear-cut difference is that autoreceptors are 5–10 times more sensitive to the effects of DA and apomorphine than postsynaptic DA receptors in behavioral, biochemical, and electrophysiological models. In the low-dose range, therefore, autoreceptor-mediated effects of DA agonists predominate, resulting in diminished dopaminergic function, whereas higher doses also stimulate postsynaptic receptors, leading to enhanced dopaminergic function.

Autoreceptors also differ from postsynaptic receptors in their pharmacological profile. Dopamine agonists that are relatively selective for autoreceptors have been synthesized. As would be predicted, autoreceptor-selective agonists inhibit DA release, synthesis, and impulse flow in DA neurons and elicit behavioral responses associated with diminished dopaminergic function. These agonists are very useful experimental probes for studying DA receptor function and may prove useful in diseases thought to involve excessive dopaminergic activity. Dopamine antagonists that selectively block autoreceptors have also been synthesized. By blocking DA autoreceptors, they enhance DA function. Some of these agents appear to have a built-in ceiling on their response since as the dose is increased, they exert an antagonistic action on postsynaptic DA receptors.

Dopamine agonists and antagonists may act on several types of DA receptor to elicit biochemical changes in DA metabolism and alter the functional output of dopaminergic systems (see Table 7–3). A drug's net effect on dopaminergic activity will depend on both its pre- and postsynaptic effects and the selectivity with which it acts at these different sites.

Drug Interactions at D_1 and D_2 Receptors

In the preceding discussion, DA receptors were broadly divided into presynaptic and postsynaptic categories. A second popular DA receptor classification that received increasing attention in the 1980s is based on the presence or absence of positive coupling between the receptor and adenylate cyclase activity. On the basis of biochemical, physiological, and pharmacological studies, it is well established that DA can act on at least two types of brain receptors, termed D_1 and D_2 receptors (see Table 7–3). These two classes of receptors are clearly distinguished by their biochemical characteristics. D_1 receptors mediate the DA-stimulated increase of adenylate cyclase activity. D_2 receptors are thought to mediate effects that are independent of D_1-mediated effects and to exert an opposing influence on adenylate cyclase activity. The D_2 site is further characterized by picomolar affinity for antagonist, whereas the D_1 site is characterized by millimolar affinity for antagonist.

With the development of D_1- and D_2-selective agonists and antagonists, however, it has become common to rely on pharmacological characteristics when determining whether an effect is mediated by D_1 or D_2 receptors. The distinction between pharmacological and functional definitions is important because it is becoming clear that DA receptors with the same pharmacological characteristics do not necessarily have the same functional characteristics. For example, DA receptors with D_2 pharmacology are present in both the striatum and the nucleus accumbens but are coupled to inhibition of adenylate cyclase only in the striatum. Regional differences in coupling between DA receptors and GTP-binding proteins have also been reported. Furthermore, DA receptors can influence cellular function through mechanisms other than stimulating or inhibiting adenylate cyclase (see Table 7–4). These may include direct effects on potassium and calcium channels as well as modulation of inositol phosphate production. It therefore seems unrealistic to expect equivalence between pharmacological and biochemical classifications of DA receptor subtypes.

Dopamine Signaling

Although D_1 and D_2 receptors can have opposite effects on adenylate cyclase activity, it is apparent that the physiological significance of their interaction is more complex. While D_1 and D_2 agonists can have opposite effects on oral

TABLE 7–4 Signal-Transduction Mechanisms Associated with Dopamine Receptors

D_2 RECEPTORS	D_1 RECEPTORS
Inhibition of adenylate cyclase	Stimulation of adenylate cyclase
Inhibition of Ca^{2+} entry through voltage-sensitive Ca^{2+} channels	Stimulation of phosphoinositide turnover
Enhancement of K^+ conductance	
Modulation of phosphoinositide metabolism	

movements, they also produce a synergistic increase in locomotor activity and behavioral stereotypes in certain circumstances. Electrophysiological experiments have suggested that D_1 receptor activation is required for full postsynaptic expression of D_2 effects. The interaction of the D_1 receptor with other neurotransmitter systems is still being explored. Despite widespread interest in DA signaling, little was known until recently about the molecular and cellular basis for the action of DA on its target cells. A phosphoprotein named DARPP-32 (dopamine and cAMP-regulated phosphoprotein of 32 kDa) plays a key role in the biology of dopaminoceptive neurons (Fig. 7–16). By acting on the D_1 receptors, DA stimulates adenylyl cyclase via a G protein to increase cAMP formation and the activity of cAMP-dependent protein kinase (protein kinase A; PKA), leading to phosphorylation of DARPP-32 on a single threonine residue. Phosphorylation converts this phosphoprotein into a potent inhibitor of protein phosphatase-1. At least two intracellular pathways that decrease DARPP-32 phosphorylation are involved in the modulation of DA signaling via D_2 receptors. One mechanism involves inhibition of adenylyl cyclase, a decrease in cAMP, a decrease in the activity of PKA, and a decrease in DARPP-32 phosphorylation. The other D_2-mediated effect involves an increase in intracellular calcium and activation of calcineurin. One of the actions of calcineurin is to dephosphorylate DARPP-32 and thus relieve the inhibition of protein phosphatase-1. Striatonigral neurons receive glutamate input from the cerebral cortex as well as a rich DA innervation from the substantia nigra. In these neurons, glutamate acting on N-methyl-D-aspartate (NMDA) receptors also gives rise to a large influx of calcium (see Fig. 7–16). Thus, in this system, stimulation of NMDA receptors also results in activation of calcineurin and enhanced dephosphorylation of DARPP-32, producing an effect very similar to the stimulation of D_2 receptors.

Dynamics of Dopamine Receptors

Destruction of the nigrostriatal DA systems has clear and reproducible behavioral consequences. Unilateral lesions of this system produce rotational behavior.

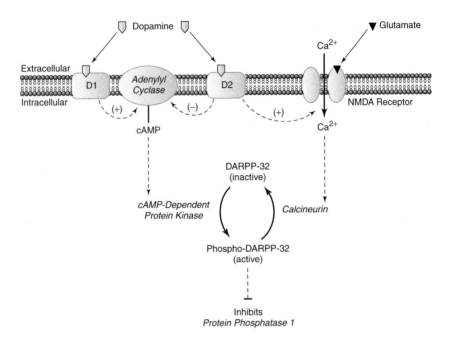

FIGURE 7–16. Postulated pathways by which DA and glutamate may regulate DA and DARPP-32 phosphorylation. Dopamine, by acting on the D_1 class of receptors, stimulates adenylyl cyclase via a G protein to increase cAMP formation and the activity of cAMP-dependent protein kinase (PKA), leading to phosphorylation of DARPP-32. Phosphorylation converts this phosphoprotein into a potent inhibitor of protein phosphatase-1. Inhibition of protein phosphatase-1 increases the phosphorylation state of numerous phosphoproteins involved in the regulation of important physiological processes. Dopamine, via D_2 receptors, decreases DARPP-32 phosphorylation by two intracellular signaling pathways. One mechanism involves inhibition of adenylyl cyclase, a decrease in cAMP, a decrease in the activity of PKA, and decreased phosphorylation of DARPP-32. The other D_2-mediated effect involves an increase in intracellular calcium, activation of calcineurin, and increased dephosphorylation of phospho-DARPP-32. Glutamate acting on NMDA receptors also gives rise to a large influx of calcium. Thus, stimulation of NMDA receptors can also lead to activation of calcineurin and enhanced dephosphorylation of DARPP-32, producing an effect very similar to stimulation of D_2 receptors.

Behavioral studies in lesioned rats indicate that DA receptors in the denervated striatum are supersensitive. Administration of DA agonists (e.g., apomorphine) that selectively stimulate DA receptors produces rotational behavior in rats with unilateral lesions of the nigrostriatal DA neurons. The degree of receptor sensitivity can be quantified by measuring the amount of rotational behavior. The number of DA receptors in the striatum ipsilateral to the lesion increases markedly, and this increase appears to correlate with the extent of the behavioral supersensitivity reflected by the rotational behavior. Thus, an increase in DA receptor density appears to be related to the behavioral supersensitivity observed following unilateral destruction of the nigrostriatal DA system.

Changes in the number of DA receptors are also observed in the striatum following chronic administration of DA antagonists. This led to the speculation that serious side effects, such as tardive dyskinesia, following chronic treatment with a neuroleptic drug might be due to supersensitivity of DA receptors that have been chronically blocked.

Dopamine receptors have been observed to change in disease states. In schizophrenia, the density of the DAT and of the D_1 dopamine receptor is normal. However, the D_2 receptor density is consistently elevated in postmortem studies of brain regions such as caudate and putamen, even in tissue obtained from neuroleptic-free individuals. Some preliminary evidence indicating abnormal D_2 structure as well as reduced linkage between D_1 and D_2 receptors is available, warranting a detailed study of the genes for these two receptors in schizophrenia. Loss of midbrain DA in Parkinson's disease is accompanied by a matching loss of the DAT and a rise in density of both D_1 and D_2 receptors. These alterations are found in the caudate nucleus and putamen tissues from unmedicated patients. Long-term treatment with L-DOPA appears to revert the receptor densities back toward normal levels. D_1 and D_2 receptors are decreased in the striatum of patients with Huntington's chorea, and there appears to be reduced or absent linkage between them.

Molecular Biology of Dopamine Receptors

D_1 and D_2 receptors are distinct molecular entities, utilize different transducing units (see Table 7–3), and have a different distribution in the brain (see Table 7–2).

Developments in molecular biology, including cloning of the cDNA and/or genes for several members of the large family of G protein-coupled receptors, have revealed that heterogeneity in the biochemical characteristics or pharmacology of individual receptors often indicates the presence of previously unsuspected molecular subtypes (see Chapter 10). For DA systems, even though the D_1/D_2 receptor classification is widely accepted, biochemical, pharmacological, and behavioral approaches have produced data that are increasingly difficult to reconcile with the existence of only two DA receptor subtypes and suggested the presence of several novel subtypes of both receptor types. Cloning studies have identified four subtypes of the D_2 receptor and two subtypes of the D_1 receptor (Table 7–5).

Two forms of the D_2 receptor, $D_{2(short)}$ and $D_{2(long)}$, were identified by gene cloning and shown to be derived from alternative splicing of a common gene. These two subtypes appear to have an identical pharmacology. A third subtype of the D_2 receptor, the D_3 receptor, was isolated by screening rat brain cDNA and genomic libraries by reverse-transcriptase polymerase chain reaction. This new D_3 receptor exhibits several novel characteristics. It has a different

TABLE 7-5. Comparison of Dopamine Receptor Subtypes

RECEPTOR ISOFORMS	D_1	D_2(SHORT)	D_2(LONG)	D_3	D_4	D_5
Chromosome	$5_q35.1$	11_q22-23		$3_q13.3$	$11_p15.5$	4_p15-16
Brain regions enriched	C/P	C/P	C/P	OT	FCX	TH
	OT	OT	OT	NA	Midbrain	Hi
	NA	NA	NA	IC	AMG	Hyp
Posterior pituitary	Absent	Present	Present	Absent	?	Absent
Nigral dopamine cells	No	Yes	Yes	Yes	No	No
GTP regulation	Yes	Yes	Yes	Yes	Yes	No
Adenylylate cyclase	Stimulates	Inhibits	Inhibits	Inhibits	Inhibits	Stimulates
Affinity for dopamine	Micromolar	Micromolar	Micromolar	Nanomolar	Submicromolar	Submicromolar
Characteristic agonist	SKF-38393	Bromocriptine	Bromocriptine	7-OH-DPAT	CP-226269 PD, 168, 077, A-412997	SKF-38393
Characteristic antagonist	SCH-23390	Sulpiride	Sulpiride	UH-232	Clozapine, NGD-94-1, U-101387	SCH-23390
Amino acids						
Rat	446	415	444	446	185	475
Human	446	414	443	400	387	477
Amino acid sequence homology in transmembrane vs. $D_{2(long)}$ (%)	44	100	100	75	53	47

C/P, caudate/putamen; OT, olfactory tubercle; NA, nucleus accumbens; IC, islands of Calleja; FCX, frontal cortex; AMG, amygdala; TH, thalamus; Hi, hippocampus; Hyp, hypothalamus; GTP, guanosine triphosphate.

anatomical distribution, with the highest levels found in limbic brain structures, and its pharmacological profile, although similar to the $D_{2(short)}$ and $D_{2(long)}$ forms, shows some distinct differences; the D_3 receptor exhibits an approximately 100-fold increase in affinity for the DA agonist quinpirol.

The fourth subtype of the D_2 receptor, the D_4 receptor gene, which was cloned in 1991, has high homology to the human D_2 and D_3 receptor genes. The pharmacological profile of this receptor resembles that of the D_2 and D_3 receptors, but its affinity for the atypical antipsychotic drug clozapine is an order of magnitude higher. The D_4 RNA has an interesting regional distribution in monkey brain, with high levels observed in the frontal cortex, midbrain, amygdala, and medulla and lower levels detected in the basal ganglia. The function of these D_2 receptor subtypes is unknown. All known varieties of the D_2 receptor have seven membrane-spanning domains, similar to the structure originally proposed for β-NE receptors. Differences in ligand binding and transduction mechanisms are presumably related to variations in the sequence of the receptor. The D_1 receptor of humans and rats has also been cloned, expressed, and characterized by several laboratories; this work in conjunction with other studies is consistent with the idea that other D_1 receptor subtypes may also exist. In fact, a gene encoding a 477-amino acid protein has been cloned that has a striking homology to the cloned D_1 receptor. This D_1 receptor subtype, called D_5, has a pharmacological profile similar to that of the cloned D_1 receptor but displays a 10-fold higher affinity for the endogenous agonist DA. Similar to the D_1 receptor, the D_5 receptor stimulates adenylate cyclase activity. This receptor is neuron specific and located primarily in the limbic areas of the brain but is absent from the parathyroid, kidney, and adrenal gland.

Pharmacology of Dopamine Receptor Subtypes

No selective ligands have been developed that can distinguish between D_1 and D_5 receptors. Pharmacologically, the only characteristic that distinguishes D_1 from D_5 receptors is the increased affinity of the D_5 receptor for DA. Most neuroleptic drugs exhibit a higher affinity for D_2 receptors than for D_3 or D_4 receptors. Uniquely among the subtypes, D_4 receptors respond to low concentrations of NE and E as well as to DA. The most interesting feature of the human D_4 receptor is its apparent high affinity for clozapine (an atypical neuroleptic) and its unique distribution in primate brain (frontal cortex > midbrain > amygdala > striatum), differing markedly from D_2 and D_3 receptor mRNA. This interesting pharmacology and unique distribution in brain has generated a great deal of excitement, particularly from a clinical standpoint. The possibility that clozapine exerts its therapeutic effects via a D_4 receptor mechanism was seen immediately as offering a new and rational target for drug development. Seeman and colleagues provided tantalizing evidence that there may be an increase in the number of D_4 receptors in schizophrenic patients, further fueling the impetus to develop D_4-selective antagonists as potential antipsychotic drugs. However, this provocative, albeit indirect, study has not been replicated using more direct measures to assess D_4 receptor numbers in brains of normal and schizophrenic subjects. Also, the significance of this finding, even if replicated, would still be uncertain. The neuroleptics taken by patients throughout the course of their disease could modify DA receptor density, and the overabundance of D_4 receptors observed in the autopsied brains of schizophrenic patients could be a result of drug treatment rather than a cause of the disease. Future clinical research efforts might profitably be directed to the use of *in vivo* imaging techniques (i.e., SPECT and PET) to evaluate DA receptor subtypes in schizophrenia as appropriate D_4- and D_3-selective ligands become available. However, the low density of these receptors, especially D_4 receptors, may present an insurmountable obstacle.

The identification of novel DA receptor subtypes has already had a dramatic impact on our understanding of dopaminergic systems. Studies of the human D_4 receptor indicate that its DNA sequence is highly polymorphic at both the DNA and the amino acid levels, exhibiting at least 25 alleles. A novel polymorphism of the D_4 receptor was observed within the putative third cytoplasmic loop of the protein, suggesting that some polymorphic variants may display different pharmacological properties. This high frequency of variation in the coding region of a functional receptor protein is unprecedented and could confer differences in efficacy of drug treatment and/or predispose an individual to the development of DA -dependent neuropsychiatric disorders. In fact, the D_4 receptor gene (*DRD4*) has been implicated in the pathophysiology of several common neuropsychiatric disorders, including mood disorders, ADHD, Parkinson's disease, and specific personality traits. The evidence is particularly strong for ADHD.

The availability of receptor clones, receptor antibodies, and expressed receptor proteins has permitted gene mapping as well as in-depth studies of the circuitry of the dopaminergic systems and the mechanisms regulating them at both genomic and cytoplasmic levels. It has also allowed the physical structure of the receptors to be ascertained and facilitated the design and development of highly specific ligands. It was hoped that these new selective agents would be helpful not only in studying the function of DA systems in normal and pathological states but also in the therapeutic management of disorders associated with malfunction of specific dopaminergic systems. Strides toward this goal had already begun with the successful development of selective D_4 antagonists by several pharmaceutical companies a decade ago. However, these D_4 antagonists have not provided the magic bullet for the treatment of schizophrenia. Nevertheless, these agents have been useful in studying the localization and function of D_4 receptors in animals, including monkeys and humans, and may someday find a therapeutic use in the treatment of specific DA-dysregulated states.

Pharmacology of Dopaminergic Systems

Nigrostriatal and mesolimbic dopamine systems

The nigrostriatal and mesolimbic DA neurons appear to respond in a similar manner to drug administration. Acute administration of DA agonists (DA receptor stimulators) decreases DA cell activity, turnover, and catabolism. Acute administration of antipsychotic drugs (DA receptor blockers) increases dopaminergic cell activity, turnover, catabolism, and biosynthesis. The increase in DA biosynthesis occurs at the TH step and is in part a result of the ability of antipsychotic drugs to block postsynaptic receptors and to increase dopaminergic activity via a neuronal feedback mechanism. Also, some of the observed effects are enhanced as a result of interaction with nerve terminal autoreceptors. Blockade of nerve terminal autoreceptors increases both the synthesis and the release of DA. These systems respond to MAO inhibitors with an increase in DA and a decrease in DA synthesis, as do the other DA systems discussed later.

Long-term treatment with antipsychotic drugs produces a different spectrum of effects on central dopaminergic neurons. For example, following long-term treatment with haloperidol, nigrostriatal DA neurons in the rat become quiescent, and DA metabolite levels and DA synthesis and turnover in the striatum return to normal limits. The kinetic activation of striatal TH, which occurs following an acute dose of an antipsychotic drug, also subsides following long-term treatment. These results are usually interpreted as indicative of the development of tolerance in the nigrostriatal DA system. In contrast, tolerance to the biochemical effects observed following acute administration of antipsychotic drugs does not appear to develop in the mesoprefrontal and mesocingulate cortical DA pathways after chronic administration.

Mesocortical dopamine system

The response of the mesocortical DA systems to dopaminergic drugs in most instances is qualitatively similar to that of the nigrostriatal and mesolimbic systems, although some notable exceptions have been observed. The mesotelencephalic DA neurons, which were once believed to be three relatively simple and homogeneous systems, have been found to be an anatomically, biochemically, and electrophysiologically heterogeneous population of cells with differing pharmacological responsiveness. For example, although a great majority of midbrain DA neurons appear to possess autoreceptors on their cell bodies, dendrites, and nerve terminals, DA cells that project to the prefrontal and cingulate cortices appear either to have a greatly diminished number of these receptors or to lack them entirely. The absence (or insensitivity) of impulse-regulating somatodendritic as well as synthesis-modulating nerve terminal autoreceptors on the mesoprefrontal and mesocingulate cortical DA neurons may, in part, explain some of the unique biochemical, physiological, and pharmacological properties of these two subpopulations of midbrain DA neurons (Table 7–6). For example, the mesoprefrontal and mesocingulate DA neurons appear to have a faster firing rate and a more rapid turnover of transmitter than the nigrostriatal, mesolimbic, and mesopiriform DA neurons. Transmitter synthesis is also more readily influenced by altered availability of precursor tyrosine in midbrain DA neurons lacking autoreceptors (mesoprefrontal and mesocingulate) than in those possessing autoreceptors. This may be related to the enhanced rate of physiological activity in this subpopulation of midbrain DA neurons, making them more responsive to precursor regulation. Mesoprefrontal and mesocingulate DA neurons also show diminished biochemical and electrophysiological responsiveness to DA agonists and antagonists. Low doses of apomorphine or autoreceptor-selective DA agonists, in contrast to their inhibitory effect on other midbrain DA neurons, are ineffective at decreasing the activity or DA metabolite levels in these two cortical DA projections. Dopamine receptor-blocking drugs, such as haloperidol, produce large increases in the synthesis and accumulation of DA metabolites in nigrostriatal, mesolimbic, and mesopiriform DA neurons but have only a modest effect in mesoprefrontal and mesocingulate DA neurons.

Heterogeneity among midbrain DA neurons is also found when one studies the effects of chronic antipsychotic drug administration. When classic antipsychotic drugs are administered repeatedly over time, the great majority of DA cells cease to fire due to the development of a state of depolarization

TABLE 7–6. Unique Characteristics of Mesotelencephalic Dopamine Systems Lacking Autoreceptors (Mesoprefrontal and Mesocingulate) Compared to Those Possessing Autoreceptors (Mesopiriform, Mesolimbic, and Nigrostriatal)

1. A higher rate of physiological activity (firing) and a different pattern of activity (more bursting).
2. A higher turnover rate and metabolism of transmitter DA.
3. Greatly diminished biochemical and electrophysiological responsiveness to DA agonists and antagonists.
4. Lack of biochemical tolerance development following chronic antipsychotic drug administration.
5. Resistance to the development of depolarization-induced inactivation following chronic treatment with antipsychotic drugs.
6. Transmitter synthesis more readily influenced by altered availability of precursor tyrosine.

inactivation. However, some midbrain DA cells appear to be unaffected by repeated antipsychotic drug administration. These DA cells are the neurons projecting to the prefrontal and cingulate cortices. Parallel observations have been made biochemically. Following chronic administration of antipsychotic drugs, tolerance develops to the metabolite-elevating effects of these agents in the midbrain DA systems that possess autoreceptors but not in the systems that lack autoreceptors. When the atypical antipsychotic drug clozapine (which possesses therapeutic efficacy but lacks Parkinson-like side effects and an ability to produce tardive dyskinesia) is administered repeatedly, DA neurons in the ventral tegmental area develop depolarization inactivation but neurons in the substantia nigra do not. The reason for this differential effect is unknown. Foot shock, swim stress, and conditioned fear cause selective (benzodiazepine-reversible) metabolic activation of mesoprefrontal DA neurons without causing a marked or consistent effect on other midbrain DA neurons, including the mesocingulate DA neurons. Thus, this selective activation does not appear to be due solely to the absence of autoreceptors. The anxiogenic benzodiazepine receptor ligands, such as the β-carbolines, also produce a selective dose-dependent activation of mesoprefrontal DA neurons without increasing DA metabolism in other midbrain DA neurons.

In summary, certain mesotelencephalic DA systems, namely the mesoprefrontal and mesocingulate DA neurons, possess many unique characteristics compared to the nigrostriatal, mesolimbic, and mesopiriform DA systems (see Table 7–6). Many of these unique characteristics may be the consequence of a lack of impulse-regulating somatodendrite and synthesis-modulating nerve terminal DA autoreceptors. However, some, such as the response to stress and the anxiogenic β-carbolines, are clearly dependent on other regulatory influences and not solely related to the absence of autoreceptors. These findings suggest that DA action at autoreceptors may be one of the more critical ways in which DA cells modulate their function. If valid, how do midbrain DA systems that lack autoreceptors regulate themselves? Perhaps it is through afferent systems by neuronal feedback. Some studies have suggested that a substance P/substance K innervation of the ventral tegmental area (A10) may influence the functional activity of mesocortical and mesolimbic DA neurons.

A number of studies have demonstrated the importance of NMDA receptors and of the glutamatergic input to the ventral tegmental area in the regulatory control of mesoprefrontal DA neurons. This input is believed to be at least partially responsible for converting pacemaker-like firing in DA cells into burst-firing patterns. NMDA receptors in the ventral tegmental area appear to modulate differentially the DA projections to the prefrontal cortex and nucleus accumbens. The NMDA receptor is selectively activated by NMDA and regulated at several pharmacologically distinct sites, including a high-affinity, strychnine-insensitive glycine binding site (see Chapter 6). Competitive antagonists of this strychnine-insensitive glycine site, which cross the blood–brain barrier, have made possible the *in vivo* pharmacological modulation of the NMDA receptor via this site. In behavioral paradigms (restraint stress and conditioned fear) that cause metabolic activation of meso-prefrontal and mesaccumbens DA neurons, these agents (e.g., [+]-HA-966) selectively abolish the activation of mesoprefrontal DA neurons. The stress-induced activation of serotonin neurons in the prefrontal cortex and the dopa-minergic activation of the nucleus accumbens are not altered by (+)-HA-966. Activation of mesoprefrontal DA neurons elicited by acute administration of phencyclidine and/or Δ-9-tetrahydrocannabinol, the active ingredient in mari-juana, is also attenuated by HA-966. These data indicate that under certain perturbed states the NMDA receptor complex and the associated glycine-modulatory site play an important role in the afferent control of the DA neu-rons in the prefrontal cortex and provide a potential target for pharmacological regulation of this important DA projection.

The observation that central DA systems are quite heterogeneous from both a biochemical and a functional standpoint holds promise that it will soon be possible to develop drugs targeted to modify or restore function to selective DA systems that are abnormal in various behavioral or pathological states. Some progress has already been achieved in developing agents that appear to

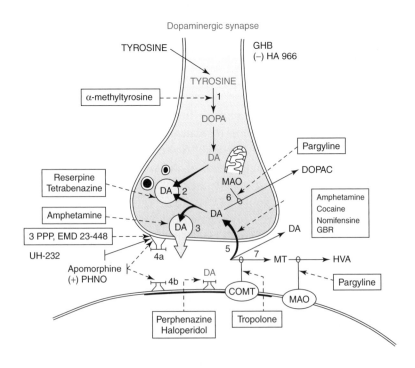

act at selective DA receptor sites (see Fig. 7–6). Whether these agents will be useful in selectively modifying the function of subsets of midbrain DA neurons remains to be determined.

Many classes of psychotropic drugs interact in one way or another with catecholamine-containing neurons. Figures 7–10 and 7–17 outline the life cycle of CNS catecholamines in NE and dopaminergic neurons, respectively, indicating possible sites at which drugs may intervene in this cycle. This schematic model also provides examples of drugs or chemical agents that interfere at the various sites within the life cycle of the transmitter substances. Although the pharmacology of NE and that of dopaminergic neurons exhibit a number of similarities, some selectivity in modulating function can be achieved by targeting specific pre- and postsynaptic receptors and plasma membrane transporters.

FIGURE 7–17. Schematic model of a central dopaminergic neuron indicating possible sites of drug action.

Site 1: *Enzymatic synthesis:* Tyrosine hydroxylase reaction blocked by the competitive inhibitor α-methyltyrosine and other tyrosine hydroxylase inhibitors.

Site 2: *Storage:* Reserpine and tetrabenazine interfere with the uptake–storage mechanism of the amine granules. The depletion of DA produced by reserpine is long-lasting, and the storage granules appear to be irreversibly damaged. Tetrabenazine also interferes with the uptake–storage mechanism of the granules, except that the effects of this drug do not appear to be irreversible.

Site 3: *Release:* γ-Hydroxybutyrate and HA-966 effectively block the release of DA by blocking impulse flow in dopaminergic neurons. Amphetamine administered in high doses releases DA, but most of the releasing ability of amphetamine appears to be related to its ability to effectively block DA reuptake.

Site 4: *Receptor interaction:* Apomorphine is an effective DA receptor-stimulating drug, with both pre- and postsynaptic sites of action. Both 3-PPP and EMD-23-448 (an indolebutylamine) are autoreceptor agonists. Perphenazine and haloperidol are effective DA receptor-blocking drugs.

Site 5: *Reuptake:* DA has its action terminated by being taken up into the presynaptic terminal. Amphetamine as well as benztropine, the anticholinergic drug, are potent inhibitors of this uptake mechanism.

Site 6: *Monoamine oxidase (MAO):* DA present in a free state within the presynaptic terminal can be degraded by the enzyme MAO, which appears to be located in the outer membrane of mitochondria. DOPAC is a product of the action of MAO and aldehyde oxidase on DA. Pargyline is an effective inhibitor of MAO. Some MAO is also present outside the dopaminergic neuron.

Site 7: *Catechol-O-methyltransferase (COMT):* DA can be inactivated by the enzyme COMT, which is believed to be localized outside the presynaptic neuron. Tropolone is an inhibitor of COMT.

Imaging Dopamine Transmission and Integrity in Neurological and Psychiatric Disorders

Advances in neuroimaging techniques have made it possible to visualize DA transmission in neuropsychiatric disorders. Radiotracer imaging with PET and SPECT can be used to measure pre-, post-, and intrasynaptic aspects of dopaminergic transmission. Presynaptic sites can be labeled with radiotracers for the DAT, VMAT, or the synthetic enzyme aromatic L-amino acid decarboxylase. Postsynaptic sites can be labeled with radiotracers for the D_1 or D_2 receptor. Estimates of synaptic endogenous DA release can be made indirectly by measuring the displacement of receptor tracers by endogenous DA. Pharmacological agents that either release (i.e., amphetamine) or deplete (α-methyl-p-tyrosine) DA tissue stores are used to assess alterations in synaptic DA in normal and disease states.

SELECTED REFERENCES

Aston-Jones, G. (2004). Norepinephrine. In *Psychopharmacology: The Fifth Generation of Progress* (K. L. Davis, D. Charney, J. T. Cole, and C. Nemeroff, Eds.). Lippincott Williams & Wilkins, Philadelphia, pp. 47–58.

Björklund, A. and S. B. Dunnett (2007). Dopamine neuron systems in the brain: An update. *Trends Neurosci.* 30, 194–202.

Bönisch, H. and M. Brüss (2006). The norepinephrine transporter in physiology and disease. *Handb. Exp. Pharmacol.* 175, 485–524.

Cooper, J. R., F. E. Bloom, and R. H. Roth (2003). *The Biochemical Basis of Neuropharmacology*, 8th ed. Oxford University Press, New York.

Dahlström, A. and A. Carlsson (1986). Making visible the invisible. In *Discoveries in Pharmacology. Pharmacology Methods, Receptors and Chemotherapy* (M. J. Parnham and J. Bruinvels, Eds.), Vol. 3. Elsevier, Amsterdam, pp. 97–125.

Dahlström, A. and K. Fuxe (1964). Evidence for the existence of monoamine-containing neurons in the central nervous system. I: Demonstration of monoamines in the cell bodies of brain stem neurones. *Acta Physiol. Scand.* 62(Suppl. 232), 1–55.

Deutch, A. Y. and R. H. Roth (2008). Neurotransmitters. In *Fundamental Neuroscience* (L. Squire, D. Berg, F. E. Bloom, S. du Lac, A. Ghosh, and N. C. Spitzer, Eds.), 3rd ed. Academic Press, New York, pp. 133–154.

Elsworth, J. and R. Roth (2007). Dopamine: Neurotransmission and neuromodulation. In *Elsevier's Encyclopedia of Neuroscience* (L. Squires, T. Albright, F. Bloom, F. Gage, and N. Spitzer, Eds.). Elsevier, New York.

Esler, M., M. Alvarenga, C. Pier, J. Richards, A. El-Osta, D. Barton, D. Haikerwal, D. Kaye, M. Schlaich, L. Guo, G. Jennings, F. Socratous, and G. Lambert (2006). The neuronal noradrenaline transporter, anxiety and cardiovascular disease. *J. Psychopharmacol.* 20, 60–66.

Fuxe, K. and T. Hokfelt (1971). Histochemical fluorescence detection of changes in central monoamine neurons provoked by drugs acting on the CNS. *Triangle* 10(3): 73-84.

Grace, A. A. (2004). Dopamine. In *Psychopharmacology: The Fifth Generation of Progress* (K. L. Davis, D. Charney, J. T. Coyle, and C. Nemeroff, Eds.). Lippincott Williams & Wilkins, Philadelphia, pp. 120–132.

Greengard, P., P. B. Allen, and A. C. Nairn (1999). Beyond the dopamine receptor: The DARPP-32/protein phosphatase-1 cascade. *Neuron* 23, 435–447.

Jones, B. E. and R. Y. Moore (1977). Ascending projections of the locus coeruleus in the rat. II Autoradiographic study. *Brain Res.* 127, 25–53.

Kozisek, M. E. and D. B. Bylund (2007). Norepinephrine/epinephrine. In *Handbook of Contemporary Neuropharmacology* (D. R. Sibley, I. Hanin, M. Kuhar, and P. Slolnick, Eds.). Wiley, New York.

Lammel, S., A. Hetzel, O. Hackel, I. Jones, B. Liss, and J. Roeper (2008). Unique properties of mesoprefrontal neurons within a dual mesocorticolimbic dopamine system. *Neuron* 57, 760–773.

Lindvall, O. and A. Björklund (1974). The organization of the ascending catecholamine neuron systems in the rat brain as revealed by the glyoxylic acid fluorescence method. *Acta Physiol. Scand.* 412, 1–47.

Missale, C., S. R. Nash, S. W. Robinson, M. Jaber, and M. G. Caron (1998). Dopamine receptors: From structure to function. *Physiol. Rev.* 78, 189–225.

Munafo, M. R., B. Yalcin, S. A. Willis-Owen, and J. Flint (2008). Association of the dopamine D4 receptor (DRD4) gene and approach-related personality traits: Meta-analysis and new data. *Biol. Psychiatry* 63, 197–206.

Nestler, E. J., S. E. Hyman, and R. C. Malenka (2001). *Molecular Neuropharmacology: A Foundation for Clinical Neuroscience.* McGraw-Hill, New York.

Nikolaus, S., C. Antke, K. Kley, T. D. Poeppel, H. Hautzel, D. Schmidt, and H. W. Muller (2007). Investigating the dopaminergic synapse *in vivo*. I: Molecular imaging studies in humans. *Rev. Neurosci.* 18, 439–472.

Robbins, T. W. and B. J. Everitt (1995). Central norepinephrine neurons and behavior. In *Psychopharmacology: The Fourth Generation of Progress* (F. E. Bloom and D. J. Kupfer, Eds.). Raven Press, New York, pp. 363–372.

Stricker, E. M. and M. J. Zigmond (1986). *In Handbook of Physiology: The Nervous System IV* (P. Bloom, ed.). pp. 677–700. American Physiological Society, Bethesda, Maryland.

Tunbridge, E. M., P. J. Harrison, and D. R. Weinberger (2006). Catechol-O-methyltransferase, cognition, and psychosis: Val158Met and beyond. *Biol. Psychiatry* 60, 141–151.

von Euler, U. S. (1956). *Noradrenaline.* Charles C. Thomas, Springfield, IL.

Watling, K. J. (2006). *The Sigma-RBI Handbook of Receptor Classification and Signal Transduction*, 5th ed. Sigma–Aldrich, St. Louis.

8

Serotonin

Of all the neurotransmitters discussed in this book, serotonin remains historically the most intimately involved with neuropsychopharmacology. From the mid-19th century, scientists had been aware that a substance found in serum caused powerful contraction of smooth muscle organs, but more than 100 years passed before scientists at the Cleveland Clinic succeeded in isolating this substance as a possible cause of high blood pressure.

At the same time, investigators in Italy were characterizing a substance found in high concentrations in chromaffin cells of the intestinal mucosa. This material also constricted smooth muscular elements, particularly those of the gut. The material isolated from the bloodstream was given the name *serotonin*, whereas that from the intestinal tract was called *enteramine*. Subsequently, both materials were purified, crystallized, and shown to be 5-hydroxytryptamine (5-HT), which could then be prepared synthetically and shown to possess all of the biological features of the natural substance. The indole nature of this molecule bore many resemblances to the psychedelic drug lysergic acid diethylamide (LSD), with which it could be shown to interact on smooth muscle preparations *in vitro*. 5-HT is also structurally related to other psychotropic agents (Fig. 8–1).

When 5-HT was first found within the mammalian central nervous system (CNS), the theory arose that various forms of mental illness could be due to biochemical abnormalities in its synthesis. This line of thought was extended when

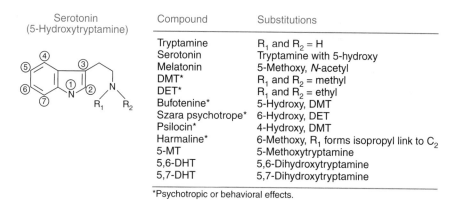

Serotonin (5-Hydroxytryptamine)	Compound	Substitutions
	Tryptamine	R_1 and R_2 = H
	Serotonin	Tryptamine with 5-hydroxy
	Melatonin	5-Methoxy, N-acetyl
	DMT*	R_1 and R_2 = methyl
	DET*	R_1 and R_2 = ethyl
	Bufotenine*	5-Hydroxy, DMT
	Szara psychotrope*	6-Hydroxy, DET
	Psilocin*	4-Hydroxy, DMT
	Harmaline*	6-Methoxy, R_1 forms isopropyl link to C_2
	5-MT	5-Methoxytryptamine
	5,6-DHT	5,6-Dihydroxytryptamine
	5,7-DHT	5,7-Dihydroxytryptamine

*Psychotropic or behavioral effects.

FIGURE 8–1. Structural relationships of the various indolealkyl amines.

the tranquilizing substance reserpine was observed to deplete brain 5-HT; throughout the duration of the depletion, profound behavioral depression occurred. As we shall see, many of these ideas are still maintained, although we now have much more evidence with which to evaluate them.

BIOSYNTHESIS AND METABOLISM OF SEROTONIN

Serotonin is found in many cells that are not neurons, such as platelets, mast cells, and the enterochromaffin cells mentioned previously. In fact, only approximately 1% to 2% of the serotonin in the whole body is found in the brain. Nevertheless, because 5-HT cannot cross the blood–brain barrier, brain cells must synthesize their own.

For brain cells, the first important step is uptake of the amino acid tryptophan, which is the primary substrate for synthesis. Plasma tryptophan arises primarily from the diet, and unlike the catecholamine precursor tyrosine, elimination of dietary tryptophan can profoundly lower the levels of brain serotonin. In addition, an active uptake process is known to facilitate the entry of tryptophan into the brain, and this carrier process is open to competition from large neutral amino acids, including the aromatic amino acids (tyrosine and phenylalanine), the branched-chain amino acids (leucine, isoleucine, and valine), and others (e.g., methionine and histidine). The competitive nature of the large neutral amino acid carrier means that brain levels of tryptophan will be determined not only by the plasma concentration of tryptophan but also by the plasma concentration of competing neutral amino acids. Thus, dietary protein and carbohydrate content can specifically influence brain tryptophan and serotonin levels by effects on plasma amino acid patterns. Because plasma tryptophan has a daily rhythmic variation in its concentration, it seems likely that this concentration variation could also profoundly influence the rate and synthesis of brain serotonin.

The first step in the synthetic pathway is hydroxylation of tryptophan at the 5 position (Fig. 8–2) to form 5-hydroxytryptophan (5-HTP). The enzyme responsible for this reaction, tryptophan hydroxylase, occurs in low concentrations in most tissues, including the brain; and it was very difficult to isolate for study. After purifying the enzyme from mast cell tumors and determining the characteristic cofactors, however, it became possible to characterize this enzyme in the brain. (Students should investigate the ingenious methods used for the initial assays of this extremely minute enzyme activity.) As isolated from brain, the enzyme appears to have an absolute requirement for molecular oxygen, for reduced pteridine cofactor, and for a sulfhydryl-stabilizing substance, such as mercaptoethanol, to preserve activity *in vitro*. With this fortified assay system, there is sufficient activity in the brain to synthesize 1 mg of 5-HTP per gram

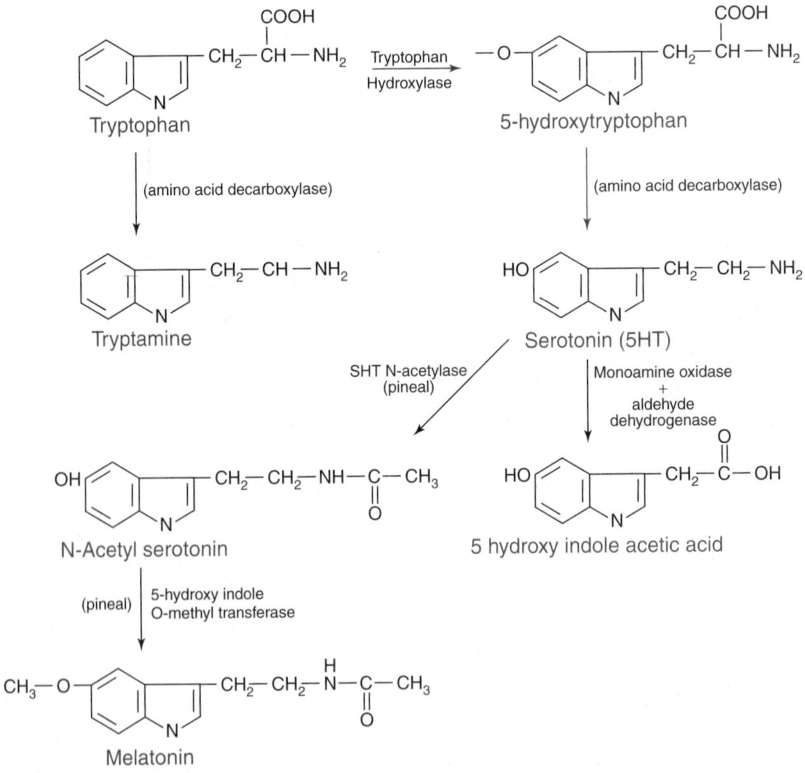

FIGURE 8–2. The metabolic pathways available for the synthesis and metabolism of serotonin.

of brain stem in 1 hour. The pH optimum is approximately 7.2, and the K_m for tryptophan is 3×10^{-4} M. Additional research on the nature of the endogenous cofactor tetrahydrobiopterin yielded a K_m for tryptophan of 5×10^{-5} M, which is still above normal tryptophan concentrations. Thus, the normal plasma tryptophan content and the resultant uptake into brain leave the enzyme normally unsaturated with available substrate.

Purified tryptophan hydroxylase has a molecular weight of 52–60 kDa. It is a multimer of identical subunits that can be activated by phosphorylation, Ca^{2+} phospholipids, and partial proteolysis.

Cloning and sequencing of cDNAs for tryptophan hydroxylase have been accomplished. Comparison of the rabbit tryptophan hydroxylase sequence with the sequences of phenylalanine hydroxylase and tyrosine hydroxylase demonstrates that these three pterin-dependent aromatic amino acid hydroxylases are highly homologous, reflecting a common evolutionary origin from a single primordial genetic locus. The pattern of sequence homology supports the hypothesis that the C-terminal two-thirds of the molecules constitute the enzymatic activity cores and the N-terminal one-third constitutes domains for substrate specificity.

Tryptophan hydroxylation, like tyrosine hydroxylation, is the rate-limiting step in serotonin synthesis. Tryptophan hydroxylation is catalyzed by two enzymes coded by the two genes THP1 and THP2. These two genes are expressed in a tissue-specific manner. THP1 is predominantly expressed in peripheral organs, whereas THP2 is the major isoform expressed in brain and controls serotonin synthesis in the mammalian CNS. The human gene is located on the long arm of chromosome 12 and several polymorphisms in the gene coding for THP2 have associated with susceptibility to affective disorders. Most recently, genetic variations in this gene have been shown to be associated with response to antidepressant treatment.

The tryptophan hydroxylase step in the synthesis of 5-HT can be specifically blocked by p-chlorophenylalanine, which competes directly with the tryptophan and binds irreversibly to the enzyme. Therefore, recovery from tryptophan hydroxylase inhibition with p-chlorophenylalanine appears to require the synthesis of new enzyme molecules. In the rat, a single intraperitoneal injection of 300 mg/kg of this inhibitor lowers the brain serotonin content to less than 20% within 3 days, and complete recovery does not occur for almost 2 weeks.

Considerable attention has been directed to the overall regulation of this first enzymatic step of serotonin synthesis, especially in animals and humans treated with psychoactive drugs alleged to affect the serotonin systems as a primary mode of action. These studies have made an important general point that seems to apply to the brain's response to drug exposure in many other cell systems as well as to serotonin: Because transmitter synthesis, storage, release, and response are dynamic processes, the acute imbalances produced initially by drug treatments are soon counteracted by the built-in feedback nature of synthesis regulation. Thus, if a drug reduces tryptophan hydroxylase activity, the nerve cells may respond by increasing their synthesis of the enzyme and transporting increased amounts to the nerve terminals.

Decarboxylation

Once synthesized from tryptophan, 5-HTP is almost immediately decarboxylated to yield serotonin. The enzyme responsible for this conversion is identical to the enzyme that decarboxylates dihydroxyphenylalanine (DOPA; i.e., aromatic amino acid decarboxylase, AADC [EC 4.1.128], or DOPA-decarboxylase). Since this decarboxylation reaction occurs so rapidly and since its K_m (5×10^{-6} M) requires less substrate than the preceding steps, tryptophan hydroxylase is the rate-limiting step in the synthesis of serotonin. Because of this kinetic relationship, drug-induced inhibition of serotonin by interference with the decarboxylation step is not feasible.

It is possible to increase serotonin formation by administering 5-HTP and bypassing the rate-limiting tryptophan hydroxylase step. AADC is widespread in distribution; it is found in the peripheral and central nervous systems associated with catecholamine- and serotonin-containing neurons and in the adrenal and pineal glands. It is also found in the kidney, liver, and various other tissues in which little or no monoamine transmitter is normally produced. Thus, unlike tryptophan administration, which can result in a selective increase in serotonin in serotonin-containing neurons, 5-HTP administration will result in the nonspecific formation of serotonin at all sites containing AADC, including the catecholamine-containing neurons. Despite this, 5-HTP is legally marketed as a means of "boosting the body's serotonin levels."

Catabolism

The only effective route of continued metabolism for serotonin is deamination by monoamine oxidase. The product of this reaction, 5-hydroxyindoleacetaldehyde, can be further oxidized to 5-hydroxyindoleacetic acid (5-HIAA) or reduced to 5-hydroxytryptophol, depending on the ratio of the oxidized to the reduced form of nicotinamide adenine dinucleotide (NAD^+/NADH) in the tissue. In the pineal gland, serotonin can be further metabolized by acetylation and O-methylation to form melatonin (see Fig. 8–2). Melatonin acts in the suprachiasmatic nucleus to regulate circadian rhythms and has been suggested as an alternative therapy for insomnia. Melatonin is available for over-the-counter use as a hypnotic agent to induce sleep, but research has not established efficacy for melatonin in the treatment of this phase of insomnia.

However, ramelteon, a melatonin agonist that acts on MT1 and MT2 receptors, is a marketed hypnotic that has been shown to have some efficacy in improving sleep onset but is ineffective in sleep maintenance. Ramelteon can be a useful agent to induce natural sleep in subjects who mostly suffer from initial insomnia (see Chapter 14).

Control of Serotonin Synthesis and Catabolism

Several mechanisms have been postulated for the physiological regulation of tryptophan hydroxylase induced by alterations in neuronal activity within serotonergic neurons. The majority of evidence supports the involvement of calcium-dependent phosphorylation in this impulse-coupled regulatory process.

Serotonin Uptake and the Serotonin Transporter

As with the catecholamine-containing neurons, reuptake serves as a major mechanism for the termination of the action of synaptic serotonin. Serotonin nerve terminals possess high-affinity serotonin uptake sites that play an important role in terminating transmitter action and in maintaining transmitter homeostasis. This reuptake of released serotonin is accomplished by a plasma membrane carrier that is capable of transporting serotonin in either direction, depending on the concentration gradient. Although the involvement of transporters in norepinephrine (NE) and serotonin clearance has been appreciated for several decades (see Chapter 7), progress in understanding transporter structure and regulation was initially slow, mainly because of difficulties associated with transporter protein purification. However, this changed dramatically with the successful expression and homology-based cloning of the monoamine transporters (NE, dopamine, and serotonin) and the realization that they are members of a large gene family composed of carriers for other transmitters, including γ-aminobutyric acid (GABA) and glycine (see Chapter 5). Expression of these transporters in nonneuronal cells has established useful model systems for analyzing the structural basis of transporter specificity for transmitters and antagonists. The availability of transporter protein has also enhanced the feasibility of obtaining transporter-specific antibodies and nucleic acid probes. Antibodies raised against the cloned serotonin transporter (SERT) as well as DNA and RNA probes derived from it have enabled the localization and expression of SERT in the CNS. The SERT protein is ubiquitous in the CNS, which is consistent with its transport to the nerve terminals of the extensive projections of the serotonin neurons throughout the brain and spinal cord. This is in contrast to SERT mRNA expression, which occurs almost exclusively in the serotonergic cell bodies in the raphe nuclei; especially high levels are found in the median and dorsal raphe.

SERT mRNA expression is absent from other brain stem nuclei, including the substantia nigra and locus ceruleus. The availability of transporter-specific antibodies and nucleic acid probes has made it feasible to investigate the endogenous mechanism that acutely regulates monoamine transporters *in vivo* and to determine whether chronic alterations in transporter genes underlie neuropsychiatric disorders. The gene that encodes the serotonin transporter is called solute carrier family 6 neurotransmitter transporter, serotonin, member 4 (SLC6A4). In humans, the gene maps to chromosome 17q11.2 and is composed of 14 exons that span approximately 40 kilobases. The sequence of transcripts predicts a protein made up of 630 amino acids with 12 membrane domains. Multiple RNA species due to alternative promoters, differential splicing, and untranslated region variability likely regulate expression of this gene in humans. The transcriptional activity of SLC6A4 is modulated by variation in the length of the serotonin transporter gene-linked polymorphic region, short and long repeats, together with two single nucleotide polymorphisms in this region.

A polymorphism in the regulatory region of the serotonin transporter gene is associated with anxiety and depression-related personality traits, and preliminary studies suggest that it also influences the risk of developing affective disorders, alcohol dependence, and late-onset dementias. Evidence shows a significant relationship between a promoter region polymorphism in the serotonin transporter gene and antidepressant response. To date, however, the cloning of SERT has not had as large an impact on the field, in terms of novel drug design, as the cloning of serotonin receptor subtypes.

SERTs are subject to multiple levels of posttranslational regulation that can rapidly alter serotonin uptake and clearance rates. SERT uptake capacity (V_{max}) is regulated by kinase-linked pathways, particularly those involving protein kinase C (PKC), resulting in transporter phosphorylation and sequestration. Ligand occupancy of the transporter significantly impacts both SERT phosphorylation and sequestration. Emerging evidence indicates that regulation of transporter function and surface expression can be rapidly modulated by "intrinsic" transporter activity. Antidepressant drugs and psychomotor stimulants that block monoamine transport have a profound effect on transporter regulation. Specific cell surface receptors are known to regulate SERT trafficking and/or catalytic function via pathways activating PKC, protein kinase G, and p38 mitogen-activated protein kinase.

Localizing Brain Serotonin to Nerve Cells

Serotonin-containing neurons are restricted to clusters of cells lying in or near the midline or raphe regions of the pons and upper brain stem (Fig. 8–3). In addition to the nine 5-HT nuclei (B1–B9) originally described by Dahlström and Fuxe, the immunocytochemical localization of 5-HT, by formation of a

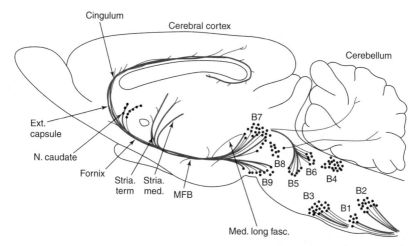

FIGURE 8–3. Schematic diagram illustrating the distribution of the main serotonin-containing pathways in the rat central nervous system. (Modified from Breese, 1975)

fluorescent product after condensation with formaldehyde, has detected reactive cells in the area postrema and the caudal locus ceruleus, as well as in and around the interpeduncular nucleus. The more caudal groups, studied by electrolytic or chemically induced lesions, project largely to the medulla and spinal cord. The more rostral 5-HT cell groups (raphe dorsalis, raphe medianus, and centralis superior, or B7–B9 [see Fig. 8–3]) are thought to provide the extensive 5-HT innervation of the telencephalon and diencephalon. The intermediate groups may project into both ascending and descending groups, but since lesions here also interrupt fibers of passage, discrete mapping has required analysis of the orthograde and retrograde methods. Immunocytochemical studies have also revealed a far more extensive innervation of the cerebral cortex, which, unlike the noradrenergic cortical fibers, is quite patternless in general.

In part, these studies could be viewed as disappointing in that most raphe neurons appear to innervate overlapping terminal fields and thus are more NE-like than dopamine-like in their lack of obvious topography. Exceptions to this generalization are that the B8 group (raphe medianus) appears to furnish a very large component of the 5-HT innervation of the limbic system, whereas B7 (or dorsal raphe) projects with greater density to the neostriatum, cerebral and cerebellar cortices, and thalamus (see Fig. 8–3).

Immunohistochemical techniques have revealed that the cerebral cortex in many mammals is innervated by two morphologically distinct types of 5-HT axon terminal. Fine axons with small varicosities originate from the dorsal raphe nuclei, and beaded axons with large spherical varicosities arise from the median raphe nuclei. These two types of 5-HT-containing axon have different regional and laminar distributions and appear to be differentially sensitive to the neurotoxic effects of certain amphetamine derivatives, including 3,4-methylenedioxymethamphetamine (MDMA), referred to more commonly as "Ecstasy." The fine axons are much more sensitive to the neurotoxic effects than the beaded axons, and the loss of fine axons lasts for months and may be permanent. Beaded axons appear to be resistant and remain unaffected following neurotoxic treatment with MDMA. This finding may be relevant to human studies, which have indicated that individuals using MDMA as a recreational drug may be exposed to dosages approximating those shown to exhibit serotonin neurotoxicity in nonhuman primates. A 26% decrease in the serotonin metabolite 5-HIAA was observed in the cerebrospinal fluid of MDMA users. This indirect evidence of a decrease in serotonin turnover in the brain perhaps reflects destruction or compromised function of this fine serotonin-containing axon system. Further studies of MDMA users seem warranted and could provide important information on the effects of selective loss of this fine axon system in humans (see Chapter 21). Currently, the functional roles played by the fine and beaded axon systems and whether the functions are distinct or similar remain unclear. In serial section analysis of 5-HT terminals in the primate visual cortex, the fine and fat boutons appeared to coexist in the same axon, arguing against distinct 5-HT innervation of this brain region.

5-HT Receptors

It has been more than 50 years since Gaddum and Picarelli (1957), basing their work on the pharmacological properties of serotonin agonists and antagonists, reported evidence for two separate serotonin receptors in peripheral smooth muscle preparations studied *in vitro*. One they named the *D* receptor because it was blocked by dibenzyline, and the other they called the *M* receptor because the indirect contractile response to 5-HT mediated by the release of acetylcholine from cholinergic nerves in the myenteric plexus could be antagonized by morphine. The advent of receptor binding studies in the 1970s revealed the existence of multiple binding sites, but whereas a correlation existed between the pharmacological profile of the 5-HT_2 binding site and the D receptor, no such correlation existed between the 5-HT_1 receptor subtypes identified by receptor binding techniques and the M receptor. Since the M receptor originally described in the nerves of the guinea pig ileum is pharmacologically distinct from the 5-HT_1 and 5-HT_2 receptors and their numerous subtypes, it was renamed the 5-HT_3 receptor. With the introduction of several extremely potent and highly selective 5-HT_3 antagonists, attention has shifted to this receptor and its possible functions in both the periphery and the CNS, as well as the therapeutic potential for these newly developed 5-HT_3 compounds.

At least eight subtypes of serotonin receptor in brain tissue have been defined and characterized, based on radioligand binding studies. As noted in Chapter 4, it is premature to characterize as a receptor a binding site defined in this manner. Nevertheless, the majority of the original speculations about serotonergic receptor subtypes generated from radioligand binding experiments appear to have been substantiated by many other types of experiments, including, most recently, the cloning of three of these subtypes. Table 8–1 lists the characteristics of these 5-HT receptor subtypes.

TABLE 8–1. Characteristics of 5-HT Receptor Subtypes

	5-HT$_1$ Receptors		
	5-HT$_{1A}$	5-HT$_{1B}$	5-HT$_{1D}$
High-density regions	Raphe nuclei Hippocampus	SN GP	GP SN BG
Selective agonists	R(1)8-OH DPAT 5-CAT	5-CAT	Sumatriptan 5-CAT
Selective antagonists	Spiperone S(2)-Pindolol WAY-100135	Isamoltane	Isamoltane GR-127935
Membrane effects	Hyperpolar via opening K channels	?	?
Other functional correlates	Basilar artery Thermoregulation Hypotension Sexual behavior 5-HT syndrome (somatodendritic autoreceptor)	Autoreceptor (Release Mod.)	Autoreceptor (Release Mod.)

	5-HT$_2$ Receptors		
	5-HT$_{2A}$	5-HT$_{2B}$	5-HT$_{2D}$
High-density regions	Layer IV Cortex Hippocampus FMN	Stomach Fundus Cortex	Choroid plexus Medulla Hippocampus
Selective agonists	DOI DOB α-Me5-HT	DOI	DOB α-Me-5-HT
Selective antagonists	MDL-100,907 Ketanserin Ritanserin Spiperone	Ketanserin	Ketanserin Spiperone Metergoline

(Continued)

TABLE 8–1. Characteristics of 5-HT Receptor Subtypes (*Continued*)

	5-HT$_2$ Receptors		
	5-HT$_{2A}$	5-HT$_{2B}$	5-HT$_{2D}$
Membrane effects	Depolarization	Depolarization	Depolarization via opening of Ca^{2+} channel
Other functional correlates	?	Vas. cont. Platelet aggregation Paw edema Head twitches	

	Other 5-HT Receptor Subtypes		
5-HT$_3$	5-HT$_4$	5-HT$_6$	5-HT$_7$
PN	Hippocampus	Striatum	Thalamus
EC	Colliculi	Accumbens	Hypothalmus
Area postrema	Ileum	Cortex	Amygdala Heart
α-Me-5-HT	SC-53116	5-CAT LSD	LSD
Zacopride	SDZ-205557	Lisuride	Clozapine
Odansetron Granisetron Depolarization		Clozapine	Amitriptyline
Transmitter release	Smooth muscle relaxation	Cognition enhancement	Thermoregulation Sleep Mood
von Bezold- Jarisch reflex	Ionotropic		

α-Me-5-HT, α-methyl-5-hydroxytryptamine; BG, basal ganglia; DOB, 2,5-dimethoxy-4-bromoamphetainine; DOI, 2,5-dimethoxy-4-odoamphetamine; EC, entorhinal cortex; 5-CAT, 5-carboxamidotryptamine; FMN, facial motor neurons; GP, globus pallidus; PN, peripheral neurons; SN, substantia nigra; 5-HT, 5-hydroxytryptamine; LSD, lysergic acid diethylamide; Rel. Mod., release modulation; Vas. cont., vascular contraction.

Molecular Biology

Since the mid-1980s, a vast amount of new information has become available concerning the various 5-HT receptor subtypes and their functional and structural characteristics. This derives from two main research approaches—operational pharmacology employing selective agonists and antagonists and molecular biology. With the advent of the latter technique, the field of 5-HT receptors has experienced exceptionally rapid growth during the past 10 years and the existence of multiple 5-HT receptors has been unequivocally confirmed. Because medicinal chemistry has lagged behind molecular biology in 5-HT neuropharmacology, there are very few highly selective receptor agonists and antagonists for the individual 5-HT receptor subtypes.

Serotonin receptors are highly heterogeneous, and cloning not only has led to the discovery and recognition of previously unknown receptors but also has greatly facilitated their classification. There are at least 15 molecularly identified 5-HT receptors, some with splice variants and others with isoforms created by mRNA editing. The majority of the 5-HT receptors belong to the large family of receptors interacting with G proteins, except for the 5-HT_3 receptors, which are ligand-gated ion channel receptors (Table 8–2). The 5-HT receptors belonging

TABLE 8–2. Mammalian 5-HT Receptor Subtypes and Their Signal Transduction Pathways

G PROTEIN-COUPLED RECEPTORS	RECEPTOR SUBTYPE	G PROTEIN	EFFECTOR PATHWAY
5-HT_1 family	5-HT_{1A}	G_i	Inhibition of adenylate cyclase
		G_i	Opening of K^+ channel
		G_o	Closing of Ca^{2+} channel
	5-HT_{1B}	G_i	Inhibition of adenylate cyclase
	5-HT_{1D}	G_i	Inhibition of adenylate cyclase
	5-HT_{1F}	G_i	Inhibition of adenylate cyclase
5-HT_2 family	5-HT_{2A}	G_q	Phosphoinositide hydrolysis
	5-HT_{2B}		Phosphoinositide hydrolysis
	5-HT_{2C}		Phosphoinositide hydrolysis
Others	5-HT_4	G_s	Activation of adenylate cyclase
	$5\text{-HT}_{5A,}\ 5\text{-HT}_{5B}$	?	Unknown coupling mechanism
	5-HT_6	G_s	Activation of adenylate cyclase
	5-HT_7	G_s	Activation of adenylate cyclase
Ligand-gated ion channels	5-HT_3	None	Ligand-gated ion channel

to the G protein receptor superfamily are characterized by the presence of seven transmembrane domains and the ability to alter G protein-dependent processes. The amino acid sequence of the membrane-spanning domains shows the least amount of variability compared with other cloned biogenic amine receptors.

This group of 5-HT receptors can be divided into distinct families based on their coupling to second messengers and their amino acid sequence homology. The 5-HT$_1$ family contains receptors that are negatively coupled to adenylyl cyclase. The 5-HT$_2$ family contains three receptors that have striking amino acid homology and the same coupling with second messenger—that is, activation of phospholipase C. The 5-HT receptors that are positively coupled to adenylyl cyclase are a heterogeneous group, including the 5-HT$_4$, 5-HT$_6$, and 5-HT$_7$ subtypes. The 5-HT$_5$ group contains two types, 5-HT$_{5A}$ and 5-HT$_{5B}$, and represents a new family of 5-HT receptors that do not resemble receptors of the 5-HT$_1$ and 5-HT$_2$ families in terms of amino acid sequence, pharmacological profile, and transduction system. They are probably coupled to a different effector system. In contrast to the G protein-coupled 5-HT receptors that modulate cell activities via second messenger systems, 5-HT$_3$ receptors directly activate a 5-HT-gated cation channel that rapidly and transiently depolarizes a variety of neurons. Like other ligand-gated ion channels, the 5-HT$_3$ receptor consists of four transmembrane segments and a large extracellular N-terminal region incorporating a cysteine–cysteine loop and potential N-glycosylation sites. Other members of this molecular receptor family include GABA, glutamate, glycine, and the nicotinic cholinergic receptors.

A third major molecular recognition site for 5-HT is the transporter proteins. These transporter proteins consist of 12 membrane-spanning proteins and represent a large gene family encoding Na$^+$ and Cl$^-$-dependent transport proteins. The first 5-HT transporter was identified in rat brain, but 5-HT transporters have been characterized in other tissues, including platelets, placenta, lung, and basophilic leukemia cells. A number of selective 5-HT uptake blockers have been developed, such as fluoxetine, sertraline, citalopram, and paroxetine (see Fig. 8–4), and several have exhibited clinical utility in the treatment of depression and obsessive–compulsive disorders (see Chapter 14).

The careful categorization of old and new subtypes of 5-HT receptors should be an important foundation for defining their function. The development of selective agents targeting these receptors, coupled with the molecular approaches highlighted in Chapter 3, such as antisense oligonucleotides to decrease steady-state levels of target proteins and transgenic animals in which specific receptors have been "knocked out," will undoubtedly continue to enhance our understanding of the function of central serotonergic systems. The existence of a large number of receptors with distinct signaling properties and expression patterns might enable a single substance such as 5-HT to generate simultaneously a large array of effects in many discrete brain structures.

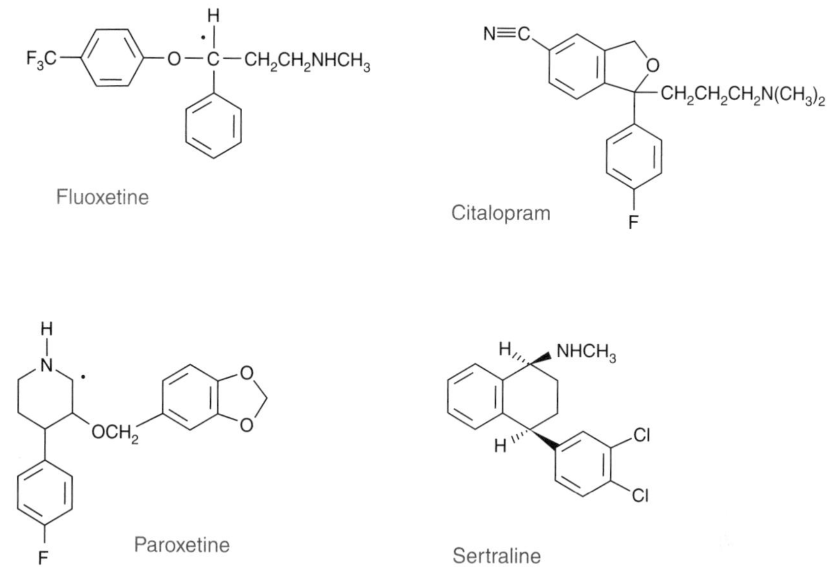

Fluoxetine

Citalopram

Paroxetine

Sertraline

FIGURE 8–4. Selective inhibitors of the serotonin transporter

Signal Transduction Pathways

In general, two major 5-HT receptor-linked signal transduction pathways exist: direct regulation of ion channels and a multistep enzyme-mediated pathway. Both pathways require a guanine nucleotide triphosphate (GTP)-binding protein (G protein) to link the receptor to the effector molecule. The 5-HT$_1$ family of receptors is negatively coupled to adenylyl cyclase via the G$_i$ family of G proteins. The 5-HT$_{1A}$ receptor is the best characterized of this family. This receptor, in addition to coupling with adenylyl cyclase, is linked directly to voltage-sensitive K$^+$ channels via G$_i$-like proteins. This direct coupling with both adenylyl cyclase and the K$^+$ channel is a recognized characteristic of G$_i$-linked receptors. Direct coupling to L-type Ca^{2+} channels has also been described as an additional transduction pathway for the G$_i$-linked family of receptors. The other members of the 5-HT$_1$ family of receptors have also been shown to be negatively coupled to adenylyl cyclase (see Table 8–2). The 5-HT$_2$ family of receptors, in contrast to the 5-HT$_1$ family, is coupled to phospholipase C. The G protein involved has not been identified but is assumed to be a member of the G$_q$ family. Phospholipase C activation induces diverse changes in the cell, leading to regulation of numerous cellular processes. All members of this family appear to be coupled primarily to phospholipase C, leading to phosphoinositide hydrolysis. Although stimulation of adenylyl cyclase was the first signal transduction pathway to be linked to 5-HT, the specific receptors mediating activation of adenylyl cyclase—the 5-HT$_4$, 5-HT$_6$, and 5-HT$_7$

receptors—were identified only recently. The 5-HT$_4$ receptor is found in rodent brain (hippocampus) and peripheral tissue, including the guinea pig ileum and human atrium. The 5-HT$_7$ receptor is also found in the brain and heart (see Table 8–1). Another novel receptor, 5-HT$_6$, is the most recent serotonin receptor to be identified by molecular cloning. The 5-HT$_6$ receptor has also been shown conclusively to couple positively to adenylyl cyclase and to have a high affinity for tricyclic antidepressant drugs. The interesting distribution of this receptor in the brain coupled with its high affinity for atypical antipsychotic and tricyclic antidepressant drugs has led to significant efforts to learn more about its function and possible role in psychiatric disorders. Although our knowledge is far from complete, emerging data suggest that 5-HT$_6$ receptors regulate cholinergic neurotransmission in the brain rather than the anticipated modulation of dopaminergic function.

The 5-HT$_3$ receptor differs from other 5-HT receptors by forming an ion channel that regulates ion flux in a G protein-independent manner. This receptor is a member of a large family of ligand-gated ion channels and thus shares more similarities with the nicotinic cholinergic receptor, which is the prototype of this superfamily, than with the 5-HT$_1$ and 5-HT$_2$ receptor families. The 5-HT$_3$ receptors were first found on peripheral sensory, autonomic, and enteric neurons, where they mediate excitation. The direct demonstration that 5-HT$_3$ receptors in the guinea pig submucosal plexus are ligand-gated ion channels implies a role for 5-HT as a "fast" synaptic transmitter and fits with their function in the periphery. Molecular studies indicated that the cloned 5-HT$_3$ receptor protein forms a homomeric subunit, which regulates the gating of cations and thus presumably mediates the rapid and transient depolarization that occurs following 5-HT$_3$ receptor activation. Immunocytochemical studies have revealed that 5-HT$_3$ receptor-immunoreactive neurons are broadly distributed throughout the rat brain and spinal cord and suggest that this receptor can subserve significant participation in CNS neurotransmission. However, the neuronal circuits in which this receptor might participate and the functions subserved by it remain to be established.

In general, the pharmacological and electrophysiological characteristics of the cloned receptor are largely consistent with the properties of the native receptors. Despite this consistency, however, a number of biochemical, pharmacological, and electrophysiological studies have suggested that CNS 5-HT$_3$ receptors exhibit heterogeneity with respect to subtypes and intracellular signal transduction mechanisms. Due to the pharmacological similarities between the 5-HT M receptors and the 5-HT$_3$ receptors, there are numerous pharmacological agents that exert specific effects on 5-HT$_3$ receptors, and many studies using these agents have addressed the possible functions of 5-HT$_3$ receptors. Results from *in vivo* studies have also suggested the presence of multiple 5-HT$_3$-like receptors, spurring on the search for other subunit proteins that might explain this pharmacological heterogeneity. The possibility should be entertained that 5-HT$_3$ receptors are analogous to the glutamate receptors, which were first characterized as inotropic receptors and later shown to exist also as G protein-linked metabotropic receptors. Clearly, additional studies are required to determine whether the 5-HT$_3$ receptor heterogeneity can be explained by subtypes of 5-HT$_3$ receptor from both inotropic and metabotropic superfamilies. The discovery of multiple subtypes of 5-HT$_3$ may help to clarify the electrophysiological observation that 5-HT$_3$-like receptors in the prefrontal cortex elicit a slow depression of cell firing rather than the fast activation expected for a ligand-gated 5-HT$_3$ receptor.

Data suggest that 5-HT$_3$ receptors are coupled to an ion channel, probably a calcium channel. Thus, they share more similarities with the nicotinic cholinergic receptor than with the 5-HT$_1$ or 5-HT$_2$ receptors. The direct demonstration that 5-HT$_3$ receptors in guinea pig submucosal plexus are ligand-gated ion channels implies a role for 5-HT (and perhaps for other biogenic amines) as a "fast" synaptic transmitter.

Adaptive Regulation

5-HT$_{2A}$ and 5-HT$_{2C}$ receptors adapt to chronic activation by reducing response sensitivity or receptor density as expected, but chronic inactivation does not elicit the opposite adaptive response. Central 5-HT$_2$ and 5-HT$_{2C}$ receptors seem to be relatively resistant to upregulation. For example, 5-HT$_{2A}$ receptors are not upregulated after denervation of 5-HT neurons or chronic administration of 5-HT antagonists. Instead, chronic administration of 5-HT antagonists results in a paradoxical downregulation of both 5-HT$_{2A}$ and 5-HT$_{2C}$ receptors.

Physiology

Neurophysiological and behavioral studies have benefited from the development and characterization of selective agents for 5-HT receptors. Electrophysiological studies have clearly demonstrated that 5-HT$_{1A}$ receptors mediate inhibition of the raphe nuclei. The firing of serotonergic neurons is tightly regulated by intrinsic ionic mechanisms (e.g., calcium-activated potassium conductance), which accounts for the well-known tonic pacemaker pattern of activity of these cells. The intrinsic pacemaker is modulated by at least two neurotransmitters: (1) NE acting through adrenergic receptors accelerates the pacemaker, and (2) 5-HT acting through somatodendritic 5-HT$_{1A}$ autoreceptors slows the pacemaker. In the hippocampus, which is another anatomical structure containing a high density of 5-HT$_{1A}$ sites, 5-HT$_{1A}$ agonists hyperpolarize CA1 pyramidal cells by opening potassium channels via a pertussis toxin-sensitive G protein. Electrophysiological studies carried out in *Xenopus* oocytes, which express the 5-HT$_{1C}$ receptor, revealed that application of 5-HT causes a detectable inward current that is blocked by mianserin. Activation of the 5-HT$_{1C}$ receptor apparently liberates inositol phosphates, raising intracellular Ca^{2+} levels and leading to the opening of Ca^{2+}-dependent chloride channels. In mammalian systems, two specific neurophysiological effects have been attributed to activation of the $5\text{-}HT_2$ receptor. 5-HT facilitates the excitatory effects of glutamate in the facial motor nucleus, an action that is antagonized by $5\text{-}HT_2$ antagonists. Similar data were obtained from intracellular studies that showed that activation of 5-HT receptors caused a slow depolarization of facial motor neurons and increased input resistance, leading to increased excitability of the cell, probably through a decrease in resting membrane conductance to potassium. These data suggest that $5\text{-}HT_2$ receptors mediate the 5-HT-induced excitation of facial motor neurons.

It has also been shown that 5-HT causes a slow depolarization of cortical neurons that is associated with decreased conductance. The effect can be desensitized by repeated applications of 5-HT and blocked by the selective $5\text{-}HT_2$ antagonist ritanserin. Thus, the effects of 5-HT on cortical pyramidal neurons share many similarities to the depolarizing effects observed in the facial motor nucleus and appear to be mediated by $5\text{-}HT_2$ receptors.

$5\text{-}HT_3$ receptors in peripheral nervous tissue mediate excitatory responses to 5-HT and are involved in modulating transmitter release. These receptors are also found in the CNS, where they are present in high density in the entorhinal cortex and area postrema. Release of endogenous dopamine by stimulation of $5\text{-}HT_3$ receptors in the striatum occurs in a calcium-dependent manner. Although the physiological function of $5\text{-}HT_3$ receptors in the CNS is unclear, the observation that selective $5\text{-}HT_3$ antagonists possess central activity in rats and primates in anxiolytic and antidopaminergic-like behavioral models has generated considerable excitement and speculation about the potential therapeutic use of $5\text{-}HT_3$ antagonists and agonists. From animal experiments, it has been speculated that these compounds may be useful in treating schizophrenia, pain, anxiety, drug dependence, and cytotoxic drug-induced emesis; to date, however, only the analgesic and antiemetic effects have been demonstrated in humans.

Electrophysiology of 5-HT Receptors

Knowledge of the molecular biology of 5-HT receptors has revolutionized electrophysiological approaches to investigating the 5-HT systems in brain since studies can now be directed toward neurons that express specific 5-HT receptor subtypes based on *in situ* hybridization maps of receptor mRNA expression. This has enabled the diverse electrophysiological actions of 5-HT in the CNS to be categorized according to receptor subtypes and their respective effects or mechanisms of action. The following are a few generalizations from these studies: (1) Inhibitory effects of 5-HT are mediated by $5\text{-}HT_1$ receptors linked to the opening of K^+ channels or to the closing of Ca^{2+} channels, both via pertussis toxin-sensitive G proteins; (2) facilitative effects of 5-HT that are mediated by $5\text{-}HT_2$ receptors and involve the closing of K^+ channels can be modulated by the phosphatidylinositol second messenger system and protein kinase C acting as a negative feedback loop; (3) other facilitative effects of 5-HT appear to be mediated by 5-HT_4 and 5-HT_7 receptors by a reduction in certain voltage-dependent K^+ currents mediated through the protein kinase A phosphorylation pathway and thus involving positive coupling of the 5-HT response to adenylyl cyclase; and (4) fast excitations are mediated by 5-HT_3 receptors through a ligand-gated cationic ion channel that does not require coupling with a G protein or a second messenger. Thus, it is clear that the electrophysiological actions of 5-HT encompass the two major neurotransmitter gene superfamilies—the G protein-coupled receptors and the ligand-gated cationic channels. The end effects are determined by the receptor subtype and its anatomical location (Fig. 8–5).

Pharmacology of Serotonin Receptors

The large number of serotonin receptors (see Table 8–1) has made it more difficult to design subtype-specific agonists and antagonists. However, despite the lack of agents that are highly selective for a single serotonin receptor subtype, numerous drugs that bind to serotonin receptors have clinical applications.

The 5-HT_{1A} partial agonists buspirone and gepirone are used with minimal effectiveness to treat general anxiety disorder (see Chapter 14). Sumatriptan, a somewhat selective 5-HT_{1D} agonist, was the first agent of this class to be used to treat migraine headaches. Since its introduction in 1993, a number of other orally effective triptan derivatives have become available (see Chapter 18).

Many of the atypical antipsychotic drugs, such as clozapine, risperidone, quetiapine, olanzapine, and ziprasidone, exert potent antagonistic activity at 5-HT_{2A} receptors in addition to their D_2 antagonistic properties (see Chapter 15).

The potent 5-HT_3 receptor antagonists granisetron, tropisetron, and ondansetron are used clinically to control nausea and emesis in patients undergoing cancer chemotherapy or radiation treatment.

The 5-HT_4 agonist metaclopramide, which is also a potent D_2 antagonist, is also a useful antiemetic.

Tricyclic antidepressants such as amitriptyline, whose ability to block norepinephrine and serotonin transporters is well established, also antagonize 5-HT_6 and 5-HT_7 receptors. Whether action at these receptors contributes to the antidepressant or antinociceptive properties of these drugs is not known. Similarly, the selective serotonin reuptake inhibitor (SSRI) fluoxetine has been shown to antagonize 5-HT_{2C} receptors.

These discoveries, although interesting, are humbling since they complicate our understanding of the action of antidepressant drugs. However, they may suggest new targets for agents used to treat depression or the selection of multiple targets to enhance efficacy.

SSRI antidepressants currently in use are fluoxetine, sertraline, fluvoxamine, paroxetine, citalopram, and escitalopram (see Chapter 14).

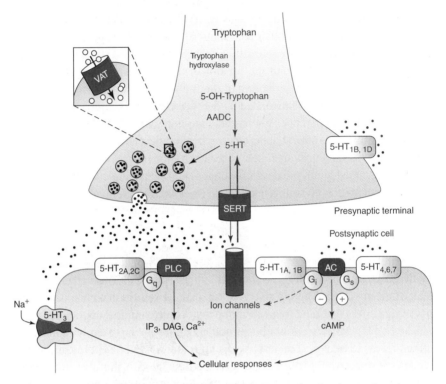

FIGURE 8–5. Model of a serotonin (5-HT) synapse. Tryptophan is taken up into the neuron by an active transport mechanism and converted to 5-OH tryptophan (5-HTP) by the rate-limiting enzyme tryptophan hydroxylase. Aromatic amino acid decarboxylase (AADC) converts 5-HTP to 5-HT. 5-HT is taken up and stored by the VMAT. Once released, 5-HT can interact with as many as 15 different receptors. 5-HT autoreceptors (5-HT$_{1B}$ rodent, and 5-HT$_{1D}$ human), which modulate the stimulus-induced release of 5-HT, are located on the presynaptic terminals. 5-HT$_{1A}$ autoreceptors are located on the 5-HT cell bodies and dendrites, where they modulate impulse flow. A number of G protein-coupled 5-HT receptors are located postsynaptically. The 5-HT$_3$ receptor is also localized postsynaptically but in contrast to the other 5-HT receptors is a ligand-gated ion channel similar to the cholinergic nicotinic receptor. The action of 5-HT is terminated by reuptake into the neuron by SERT. AC, adenylyl, cyclase; DAG, diacylglycerol; IP$_3$, inositol triphosphate; PLC, phospholipase C; SERT, plasma membrane serotonin transporter; VMAT, vesicular monoamine transporter. (Modified from Nesther et al., *Molecular Neuropharmacology.* 2001)

BEHAVIORAL ASPECTS OF SEROTONIN FUNCTION

5-HT neurons in the brain stem raphe nuclei exhibit spontaneous monotonic activity, discharging in a clocklike manner with an intrinsic frequency of 1–5 spikes/second. In the rodent, these monotonic properties are manifested early in development (3 or 4 days before birth). The 5-HT neurons appear to possess a negative feedback mechanism that limits their neuronal activity. As the physiological activity of the 5-HT neuron increases, the local release of 5-HT from dendrites or axonal collaterals acts on somatodendritic 5-HT autoreceptors to inhibit neuronal activity. This autoregulatory mechanism seems to function only under physiological conditions and to be inoperative during periods of low-level activity, but it becomes functional as neuronal activity increases. Dysfunction of this autoregulatory mechanism has been implicated in some forms of human neuropathology, so autoreceptors have become a potentially important site for drug-targeted therapeutic intervention. The combined use of 5-HT$_{1B}$ autoreceptor antagonists and selective 5-HT uptake blockers holds some promise.

In view of the extraordinarily widespread projections and highly regulated pacemaker pattern of activity that is characteristic of serotonin neurons, a broad homeostatic function has been suggested for serotonergic systems. By exerting simultaneous modulatory effects on neuronal excitability in diverse regions of the brain and spinal cord, the serotonergic system is in a strategic position to coordinate complex sensory and motor patterns during varied behavioral states. Single-unit electrophysiological recordings from serotonergic neurons in unanesthetized animals have shown that serotonergic activity is highest during periods of waking arousal, reduced in quiet waking, reduced further in slow-wave sleep, and absent during rapid eye movement sleep. An increase in tonic activity of serotonergic neurons during waking arousal would enhance motor neuron excitability via descending projections to the ventral horn of the spinal cord. Conversely, suppression of sensory input would screen out distracting sensory cues. Cessation of serotonergic neuronal activity during rapid eye movement sleep would tend to impede motor function in this paradoxical state in which internal arousal is associated with diminished motor output. Altered function of serotonergic systems has been reported in several psychopathological conditions, including affective illness, hyperaggressive states, and schizophrenia. There is increasing evidence for impaired serotonergic function in major depressive illness and suicidal behavior. In this connection, several effective antidepressant drugs appear to act by enhancing serotonergic transmission.

The pathophysiology of major affective illness is poorly understood, but several lines of clinical and preclinical evidence indicate that enhancement of 5-HT-mediated neurotransmission might underlie the therapeutic response to different types of antidepressant treatment (see Chapter 14). Table 8–3 shows the effects of long-term administration of different types of antidepressants on the 5-HT system assessed with electrophysiological techniques. Treatment with all of these drugs appears to cause a net increase in 5-HT neurotransmission. Several clinical observations have also provided strong evidence of a pivotal role for 5-HT neurotransmission in depression. For example, inhibition of 5-HT synthesis in drug-remitted depressed patients, using either the tryptophan hydroxylase inhibitor p-chlorophenylalanine or the tryptophan depletion paradigm, produces a rapid relapse of depression. In the latter paradigm, the symptomatology reactivated by the tryptophan depletion was nearly identical to that present before the response to the antidepressant treatment, suggesting a causal relationship.

TABLE 8–3. Effects of Long-Term Administration of Antidepressant Drugs and Electroconvulsive Therapy on the 5-HT System Assessed Using Electrophysiological Techniques

ANTIDEPRESSANT TAREATMENT	RESPONSIVENESS OF SOMATODENDRITIC 5-HT$_{1A}$ AUTORECEPTORS[a]	FUNCTION OF TERMINAL 5-HT AUTORECEPTORS	FUNCTION OF TERMINAL α_2 ADRENOCEPTORS	RESPONSIVENESS OF POSTSYNAPTIC 5-HT RECEPTORS[b]	NET 5-HT NEUROTRANSMISSION
Selective 5-HT reuptake inhibitors	Decrease	Decrease	n.c.	n.c.	Increase
Monoamine oxidase inhibitors	Decrease	n.c.	Decrease	n.c. Or decrease	Increase
5-Ht$_{1a}$ receptor agonists	Decrease	n.c.	n.c.	n.c.	Increase
Tricyclic antidepressants	n.c.	n.c.	n.d.	Increase	Increase
Electroconvulsive shocks	n.c.	n.c.	n.c.	Increase	Increase

n.c. no change; n.d., not determined.
[a] Assessed by microiontophoresis or systemic injection of 5-HT receptor agonists.
[b] Determined from the firing activity of the presynaptic neurons and the effect of stimulating the ascending pathway on postsynaptic neurons.
SOURCE: Modified from Blier and deMontigny (1994).

Relevance to Clinical Disorders and Drug Actions

The diversity of receptors and transduction pathways that underlie the actions of 5-HT, together with the differential expression of 5-HT receptor subtypes in different neuronal and effector cell populations, helps to explain how it is possible for a single transmitter to be linked to such a large array of behaviors, clinical conditions, and drug actions. Alterations in 5-HT function have been implicated in a host of clinical states, including affective disorder, obsessive–compulsive disorder, schizophrenia, anxiety states, phobic disorders, eating disorders, migraine, and sleep disorders (Table 8–4). There is also a wide range of psychotropic drugs that affect 5-HT neurotransmission, including antidepressants (selective 5-HT uptake blockers; e.g., fluoxetine [see Fig. 8–4]), hallucinogens (e.g., LSD and psilocin [see Fig. 8–1]), anxiolytics (e.g., buspirone), atypical antipsychotics (e.g., clozapine), antiemetics (e.g., ondansetron), appetite suppressants (e.g., fenfluramine), and antimigraine drugs (e.g., sumatriptan).

Figure 8–6 summarizes possible sites of drug interaction in a hypothetical serotonin synapse in the CNS.

In this chapter, we have encountered one of the more striking examples of an intensively studied brain biogenic amine, and there is every reason to believe that it is an important synaptic transmitter. Still to be determined are the precise synaptic connections at which this substance transmits information and the functional role these connections play in the overall operation of the brain with respect to both effective and other multicellular interneuronal operations. The central pharmacology of serotonin, however, remains poorly resolved. Specific inhibition of uptake and synthesis are possible, but truly effective and selective postsynaptic antagonists remain to be developed.

TABLE 8–4. Clinical Conditions Influenced by Altered Serotonin Function

Affective disorders	Neuroendocrine regulation
Aging and neurodegenerative disorders	Obsessive–compulsive disorder
Anxiety disorders	Pain sensitivity
Carcinoid syndrome	Premenstrual syndrome
Circadian rhythm regulation	Posttraumatic stress syndrome
Developmental disorders	Schizophrenia
Eating disorders	Sexual disorders
Emesis	Sleep disorders
Migraine	Stress disorders
Myoclonus	Substance abuse

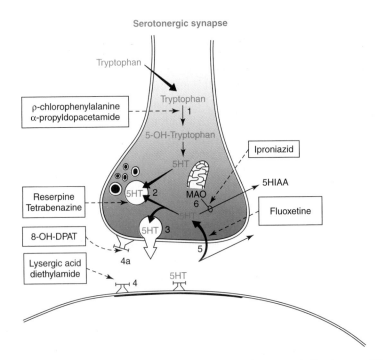

Serotonergic synapse

FIGURE 8–6. Schematic model of a central serotonergic neuron indicating possible sites of drug action.

Site 1: *Enzymatic synthesis:* Tryptophan is taken up into the serotonin-containing neuron and converted to 5-OH-tryptophan by the enzyme tryptophan hydroxylase. This enzyme can be effectively inhibited by *p*-chlorophenylalanine and α-propyldopacetamide. The next synthetic step involves the decarboxylation of 5-OH-tryptophan to form serotonin (5-HT).

Site 2: *Storage:* Reserpine and tetrabenazine interfere with the uptake–storage mechanism of the amine granules, causing a marked depletion of serotonin.

Site 3: *Release:* Currently, there is no drug available that selectively blocks the release of serotonin. However, LSD, because of its ability to block or inhibit the firing of serotonin neurons, causes a reduction in the release of serotonin from the nerve terminals.

Site 4: *Receptor interaction:* LSD acts as a partial agonist at serotonergic synapses in the CNS. A number of compounds have also been suggested to act as receptor-blocking agents at serotonergic synapses, but direct proof of these claims is lacking.

Site 5: *Reuptake:* Considerable evidence suggests that serotonin may have its action terminated by being taken up into presynaptic terminals. The tricyclic drugs with a tertiary nitrogen, such as imipramine and amitriptyline, appear to be potent inhibitors of this uptake mechanism.

Site 6: *Monoamine oxidase (MAO):* Serotonin present in a free state within the presynaptic terminal can be degraded by the enzyme MAO, which appears to be located in the outer membrane of mitochondria. Iproniazid and clorgyline are effective inhibitors of MAO. 5-HIAA, 5-hydroxyindoleacetic acid.

SELECTED REFERENCES

Aghajanian, G. K. and E. Sanders-Bush (2002). Serotonin. In *Neuropsychopharmacology: The Fifth Generation of Progress* (K. L. Davis, D. Charney, J. T. Cole and C. Nemeroff, Eds.). Lippincott Williams & Wilkins, Philadelphia, pp. 15–34.

Bach-Mizrachi, H., M. D. Underwood, A. Tin, A. P. Elis, J. J. Mann, and V. Arango (2008). Elevated expression of tryptophan hydroxylase-2 mRNA at the neuronal level in the dorsal and median raphe nuclei of depressed suicides. *Mol. Psychiatry* 13, 507–513.

Blier, P. and C. deMontigny (1994). Current advances and trends in the treatment of depression. *Trends Pharmacol. Sci.* 15, 220–226.

Branchek, T. A. and T. P. Blackburn (2000). 5-HT$_6$ receptors as emerging targets for drug discovery. *Annu. Rev. Pharmacol. Toxicol.* 40, 319–334.

Breese, G. R. (1975). Chemical and immunochemical lesions by specific neurotoxic substances and antisera. In *Handbook of Psychopharmacology* (L.L. Iversen, S.D. Iversen and S.H. Snyder. Eds). Plenum Press, New York, vol. 1, 137-190.

Cooper, J. R., F. E. Bloom, and R. H. Roth (2002). *Biochemical Basis of Neuropharmacology*, 8th ed. Oxford University Press, New York.

Gray, J. A. and B. L. Roth (2007). Serotonin systems. In *Handbook of Contemporary Neuropharmacology* (D. R. Sibley, I. Hanin, M. Kuhar, and P. Skolnick, Eds.). Wiley, Hoboken, NJ, pp. 257–297.

Haghighi, F., H. Bach-Mizrachi, Y. Y. Huang, V. Arango, S. Shi, A. J. Dwork, G. Rosoklija, H. T. Sheng, I. Morozova, J. Ju, J. J. Russo, and J. J. Mann (2008). Genetic architecture of the human tryptophan hydroxylase 2 gene: Existence of neural isoforms and relevance for major depression. *Mol. Psychiatry* 13, 813–820.

Heninger, G. R. (1997). Serotonin, sex and psychiatric illness. *Proc. Natl. Acad. Sci. USA* 94, 4823–4824.

Jayanthi, L. D. and S. Ramamoorthy (2005). Regulation of monoamine transporters: Influence of psychostimulants and therapeutic antidepressants. *AAPS J.* 7(3), E728–E738.

Malhotra, A. K., T. Lencz, C. U. Correll, and J. M. Kane (2007). Genomics and the future of pharmacotherapy in psychiatry. *Int. Rev.Psychiatry* 19(5), 523–530.

Murphy, D. L. and K.-P. Lesch (2008). Targeting the murine serotonin transporter: Insights into human neurobiology. *Nature Rev.* 9, 85–96.

Nestler, E. J., S. E. Hyman, and R. C. Malenka (2001). *Molecular Neuropharmacology: A Foundation for Clinical Neuroscience*. McGraw-Hill, New York.

Ricaurte, G. A., J. Yuan, and U. D. McCann (2000). (6)3,4-Methylenediozymethamphetamine ("Ecstasy")-induced serotonin neurotoxicity: Studies in animals. *Neuropsychobiology* 42, 5–10.

Steinbusch, H. W. M. and A. H. Mulder (1984). Serotonin-immunoreactive neurons and their projections in the CNS. In *Handbook of Chemical Neuroanatomy. Classical Transmitters and Transmitter Receptors in the CNS* (A. Björklund, T. Hökfelt, and M. Kuhar, Eds.), Vol. 3, Part II. Elsevier, New York, pp. 68–118.

Steiner, J. A., A. Marin, D. Carneiro, and R. D. Blakley (2008). Going with the flow: Trafficking-dependent and -independent regulation of serotonin transport. *Traffic* 9, 1393–1402

Tzvetkov, M. V., J. Brockmoller, I. Roots, and J. Kirchheiner (2008). Common genetic variations in human brain-specific tryptophan hydroxylase-2 and the response to antidepressant treatment. *Pharmacogenetics Genomics* 18, 495–506.

Watling, K. J. (2006). *The Sigma-RBI Handbook of Receptor Classification and Signal Transduction*, 5th ed. Sigma–Aldrich, St. Louis.

9

Histamine

Since the beginning of this century, when Henry Dale demonstrated that histamine is an endogenous tissue constituent and a potent stimulator of a variety of cells, this substance has been thought to act as a neurotransmitter. However, direct evidence to support this concept accumulated slowly. The challenge posed by histamine to neuropharmacologists has led to a vigorous chase across meadows of enticing hypotheses surrounded by bogs of confusion and dubious methodology. At last, more than 75 years after its isolation from the pituitary by J. J. Abel, the role of histamine in the brain seems to have been resolved by recognizing that this diamine occurs in two types of cells: mast cells (found in some, but not all, mammalian brains) and (more consistently) magnocellular neurons in the posterior hypothalamus.

Most of our previous understanding of the synthesis and degradation of histamine in the brain was based on attempts to simulate in brain tissue data obtained from more or less homogeneous samples of peritoneal mast cells (Fig. 9–1). However, since mast cells were not supposed to be found in healthy brains and since histamine does not cross the blood–brain barrier, it had long been assumed that neurons could also make histamine and therefore that histamine should be considered as a putative neurotransmitter.

In fact, attempts to develop drugs that were histamine antagonists, in the mistaken belief that battlefield shock was compounded by histamine release,

238

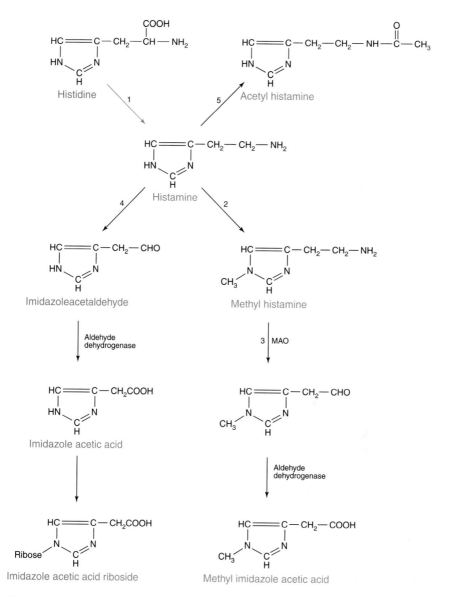

FIGURE 9–1. Metabolism of histamine. (1) Histidine decarboxylase. (2) Histamine methyltransferase. This is the major pathway for inactivation in most mammalian species. (3) Monoamine oxidase. (4) Diamine oxidase (histaminase). (5) Minor pathway of histamine catabolism.

were a key to the subsequent development of antipsychotic drugs. Furthermore, as every hay-fever sufferer knows, most present-day antihistamine drugs clearly produce substantial central nervous system (CNS) actions such as drowsiness and hunger. Finally, in retrospect, the increased content of histamine found in transected degenerating sensory nerve trunks was likely an artifact of mast cell accumulation rather than a peculiar form of neurochemistry. Viewing the other data on CNS histamine through that same retrospectroscope, as they have been illuminated by the innovative experiments of Schwartz and associates, we now have a rather compelling case that histamine qualifies as a putative central neurotransmitter in addition to its role in mast cells.

The major obstacles in elucidating the functions of histamine in the brain had been the absence of a sensitive and specific method to demonstrate putative histaminergic neurons and fiber tracts *in situ*, the lack of suitable methods to measure histamine and its catabolites, and problems in the characterization of histamine receptors in the nervous system. Progress eventually overcame these impediments, and evidence has now accumulated to support the hypothesis that histamine functions as a neurotransmitter in the brain.

HISTAMINE SYNTHESIS AND CATABOLISM

Because histamine penetrates the blood–brain barrier so poorly, brain histamine arises from histamine synthesis *in situ* from histidine. Active transport of histidine by brain slices has been demonstrated, and because histidine loading has been shown to elevate brain histamine, histidine transport could be a controlling factor in brain histamine synthesis.

Two enzymes are capable of decarboxylating histidine *in vitro*: L-AADC (i.e., the DOPA and 5-HTP decarboxylase) and the specific histidine decarboxylase. The pH optimum, affinity for histidine, effects of selective inhibitors, and regional distribution of histamine-synthesizing activity all indicate that it is the specific histidine decarboxylase that is responsible for histamine biosynthesis in the brain (Fig. 9–1). While the instability of histidine decarboxylase and its low activity in adult brain prevented purification of the brain, fetal liver histidine decarboxylase was purified to near homogeneity. Studies of the pH optimum, cofactor (pyridoxal phosphate), requirements, inhibitor sensitivity, and antigenic properties have subsequently demonstrated that the brain and fetal enzymes have similar properties. Indeed, antibodies to liver histidine decarboxylase have been used to map the distribution of this enzyme in the brain by immunohistochemical techniques.

Estimates of the K_m of histidine for brain histidine decarboxylase are much higher than the concentration of histidine in plasma or brain, suggesting that it is not saturated with substrate *in vivo* and consistent with observations that administration of L-histidine will increase brain histamine levels.

There are surprisingly few selective inhibitors of histidine decarboxylase. Most of the effective inhibitors act at the cofactor site, and although they reduce histamine formation, they also inhibit other pyridoxal-requiring enzymes. A selective inhibitor of histidine decarboxylase, α-fluoromethylhistidine, has been identified. This irreversible inhibitor forms a covalent linkage with the serine residue at the active site of the enzyme. It is more selective and potent than other decarboxylase inhibitors and does not inhibit DOPA/5-HTP decarboxylase or other histamine-metabolizing enzymes, such as histamine *N*-methyltransferase and *N*-acetylhistamine deacetylase. Therefore, α-fluoromethylhistidine should prove useful for manipulating histamine actions *in vivo*.

In nonneural tissues, histamine is catabolized by two distinct enzymatic systems in mammals (see Fig. 9–1): (1) oxidation by diamine oxidase to imidazoleacetaldehyde and then to imidazoleacetic acid and (2) methylation by histamine methyltransferase to produce methylhistamine. Mammalian brain lacks the ability to oxidize histamine and nearly quantitatively methylates it. Methylhistamine undergoes oxidative deamination by either diamine oxidase or, in brains that lack diamine oxidase, monoamine oxidase type B. The major route of catabolism of orally ingested histamine is via *N*-acetylation of bacteria in the gastrointestinal tract to form *N*-acetylhistamine.

HISTAMINE-CONTAINING CELLS

There are fluorogenic condensation reactions that can detect histamine in mast cells by cytochemistry, but this method has not been successful in demonstrating histamine-containing nerve fibers or cell bodies because the fluorogenic reagents cross-react with spermidine, whose uniformly high levels overwhelm the underlying histamine-containing cells and fibers. Because the histamine content of mast cells is quite substantial, however, it has been possible to use the cytochemical method to detect mast cells in brain and peripheral nerve. From such studies, Schwartz *et al.* have estimated that the histamine content of brain regions and nerve trunks that show approximately 50 ng histamine/g (i.e., every place except the diencephalon) can be explained on the basis of mast cells. Moreover, the once inexplicable rapid decline of brain histamine in early postnatal development can now also be attributed to the relative decline in the number of mast cells in the brain after its development.

Mast cell histamine shows some interesting differences from what we shall presume is neuronal histamine. In mast cells, histamine levels are high, turnover is relatively slow, and the activity of histidine decarboxylase is relatively low;

moreover, mast cell histamine can be depleted by mast cell-degranulating drugs (48/80 and polymyxin B). In brain, only approximately 50% of the histamine content can be released with these depletors, and for that which remains, the turnover is quite rapid. The activity of histidine decarboxylase is also much greater. Even better separation of the two types of cellular histamine dynamics comes from studies of brain and mast cell homogenates. In the adult brain, a significant portion of histamine is found in the crude mitochondrial fraction that is enriched in nerve endings and released from these particles upon hypo-osmotic shock. In cortical brain regions and in mast cells, most histamine is found in large granules, which sediment with the crude nuclear fraction; this histamine, unlike that in the hypothalamic nerve endings, has the slow half-life characteristic of mast cells.

Despite the encouraging result that histamine may be present in fractions of brain homogenates containing, among other broken cellular elements, nerve endings, it is difficult to exploit that information into a direct documentation of intraneuronal storage. More promising steps in that direction were taken in studies in which specific brain lesions were made. Lesions of the medial fore-brain bundle region produced a loss of forebrain NE and 5-HT along a time course parallel to nerve fiber degeneration in experiments that were done when our understanding of CNS monoaminergic systems was not as far along as it is for histamine today. When such lesions were placed unilaterally and specific histidine decarboxylase activity followed, a 70% decline in forebrain histidine decarboxylase activity was found after 1 week. The decline was not due to the concomitant loss of monoaminergic fibers since lesions made by hypothalamic injections of 6-hydroxydopamine or 5,7-dihydroxytryptamine did not result in histidine decarboxylase loss. The most reasonable explanation is that the lesion interrupted a histamine-containing diencephalic tract; the his-tamine and decarboxylating activity on the ipsilateral cortex was reduced only approximately 40%, suggesting that the pathway may make diffuse contribu-tions to nondiencephalic regions. However, subsequent studies of completely isolated cerebral cortical "islands" showed complete loss of histamine content.

As mentioned previously, antibodies to histidine decarboxylase have also been utilized to map the distribution of this enzyme in rodent brain by immu-nohistochemical techniques. Steinbusch and coworkers have developed an immunohistochemical method for the visualization of histamine in the CNS using an antibody raised against histamine coupled to a carrier protein. Results obtained with this technique are in general agreement with those of studies on the immunohistochemical localization of histidine decarboxylase. The highest density of histamine-positive fibers is found in brain regions known to contain high histamine levels, such as the median eminence and the premammillary regions of the hypothalamus.

Lesion and immunohistochemical studies indicate the presence of a major histamine-containing pathway emanating from neurons in the tuberomammillary nucleus (in the posterior basal hypothalamus) and ascending through the medial forebrain bundle to project ipsilaterally to broad areas of the telencephalon (Fig. 9–2). A descending pathway originating from the hypothalamus and projecting to the brain stem, cerebellum, and spinal cord has also been demonstrated.

In general, brain (neuronal) histamine levels are higher in lower vertebrates with less well-developed cerebral and cerebellar cortices, and mammals have among the lowest amounts. The tuberomammillary (TM) histamine-containing neurons are well innervated by adrenergic, noradrenergic, dopaminergic, and serotonergic neurons, as well as by glutamatergic neurons from the infralimbic, lateral septal, and preoptic areas and intrahypothalamic hypocretin-containing neurons of the perfornical nuclei. TM neurons are also GABA synthesizing; contain adenosine deaminase; and express several neuropeptides, including galanin, proenkephalin, substance P, and brain natriuretic peptide. TM neurons also contain monoamine oxidase B, the major enzyme responsible for deamination of *N*-methylhistamine, a major metabolite of histamine in the CNS. Unraveling the possible roles of such a large number of putative cotransmitter peptides in a single population of magnocellular neurons in the posterior hypothalamus (the TM nucleus) continues to pose an exciting challenge.

The majority of histamine-containing perikarya are composed of a continuous group of magnocellular neurons numbering approximately 2000 in the rat and confined primarily to the tuberal region of the posterior hypothalamus, collectively named the *tuberomammillary nucleus*. A similar organization has also been described in humans, although histamine-containing neurons are more

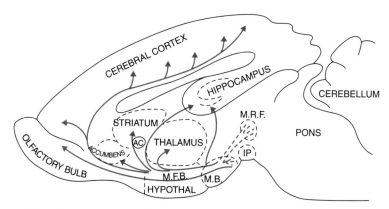

FIGURE 9–2. Schematic illustration of the distribution of histamine-containing neurons in brain. M.R.F., mesencephalic reticular formation; M.B., mammillary bodies; M.F.B., medial forebrain bundle. Modified from Schwartz and Arrang (2002).

abundant (64,000) and occupy a greater portion of the hypothalamus. Like other monoaminergic neurons, the histaminergic system consists of long, highly divergent, mostly unmyelinated, varicose fibers projecting in a diffuse manner to many telencephalic, mesencephalic, and cerebellar structures (Fig. 9–2). Individual neurons appear to project to widely divergent areas but make few typical synaptic contacts.

PHYSIOLOGICAL PROPERTIES OF HISTAMINERGIC NEURONS

Tuberomammillary neurons recorded *in vivo* fire in a regular, but slow, pattern that varies with behavioral state—high during waking and attentive states and slow or silent during slow wave sleep. These patterns support classical clinical descriptions in which patients with posterior hypothalamic lesions were hypersomnolent. TM neurons are also heavily innervated from the GABAergic neurons of the preoptic area, and these neurons are found to fire very rapidly during slow wave sleep, in keeping with the observation that patients with anterior hypothalamic lesions have insomnia. In animals that undergo seasonal hibernation, brain histamine turnover increases, leading to proposals that histamine maintains the hibernation state, perhaps aided by the hypocretin innervation.

The high levels of histamine and the presence of histamine receptors in the hypothalamus, together with the known ability of histamine to alter food and water intake thermoregulation, autonomic activity, and hormone release, indicate a possible role for histamine in these vegetative functions.

Functional assessments of histaminergic neurons have been assessed with two complementary strategies: (1) mice in which histamine synthesis or the histamine receptors have been genetically silenced and (2) human assessments of histamine receptor occupancy with positron emission tomography. In addition to the behavioral state and vegetative functions, these clinical studies have linked histamine functions to epilepsy and pain perception.

HISTAMINE RECEPTORS

Three classes of histamine receptors have been identified in vertebrates and named in the order of their discovery: H_1, H_2, and H_3. Both H_1 and H_2 receptor DNAs were cloned much earlier than the H_3 receptor. They all belong to the G protein-coupled superfamily of receptors with seven transmembrane domains.

H_1 receptors are coupled to inositol phospholipid hydrolysis and involved in a variety of responses, including contraction of smooth muscle, increased capillary permeability mediated by contraction of terminal venules, hormone release, and brain glycogenolysis induced by a rise in the intracellular concentration of free calcium ions. In keeping with the sedating effects of H_1 antagonists, the effects of histamine on neuronal activity are excitatory. H_2 receptors (also generally excitatory in their agonist responses) are positively coupled to adenylyl cyclase via a G_s protein and mediate most of their effects by changes in the intracellular levels of cAMP. The functional responses mediated by H_2 receptors include smooth muscle relaxation, gastric acid secretion, positive chronotropic and inotropic actions on cardiac muscle, and inhibitory effects on the immune system.

Although the presence of H_3 receptors in brain has been appreciated since the mid-1980s, the molecular identity of this receptor had remained elusive. Thus, this receptor had been characterized in the CNS largely on the basis of radioligand binding and pharmacological studies with subtype-specific agents. In general, it was conjectured that the histamine H_3 receptor functions as an autoreceptor coupled to G_i proteins, analogous to dopamine D_2, adrenergic α_2, and serotonergic 5-HT_{1A} autoreceptors. H_3 receptors also appear to function as heteroreceptors regulating the release of other neurotransmitters from their nerve terminals.

Functional studies have provided evidence for presynaptic release modulating H_3 receptors on noradrenergic, serotonergic, dopaminergic, cholinergic, and peptidergic neurons. H_3 receptors are believed to provide a major regulatory mechanism involved in the control of histaminergic activity under physiological conditions. *In vivo* microdialysis studies have demonstrated that administration of selective H_3 receptor agonists reduces histamine release and turnover. Administration of H_3 receptor antagonists, in contrast, enhances histamine turnover and release, suggesting that H_3 autoreceptors are normally under tonic stimulation by endogenous histamine.

The cloning and functional expression of the human H_3 receptor were finally achieved in 1999. With the availability of the cDNA for the H_3 receptor, it will now be possible to develop chemical and biological reagents to address a number of questions concerning the possible role of H_3 receptors in the CNS using molecular biology. The H_3 receptor is negatively coupled to adenylate cyclase, but it can also activate the mitogen-activated protein kinase intracellular response pathway.

The autoradiographic distribution of the three histamine receptors has been mapped in primate brain. H_1 receptors are particularly abundant in the neocortex, whereas H_2 and H_3 receptors, although present in the cerebral cortex, are enriched in caudate and putamen. H_3 receptors are predominant in basal ganglia, with the highest density found in the globus pallidus. Histamine receptors are also found in the hippocampus and cortical areas. Studies on H_3 receptor inverse agonists suggest that the H_3 receptors have a high constitutive activity, and that presynaptically these receptors inhibit the firing of the histamine neurons. The inverse agonists enhance histamine release and have been considered suitable for evaluation in cognitive and in food intake disorders.

A new histamine receptor, H_4, has been reported and characterized, adding a new chapter to the histamine story. This gene encodes a 390–amino acid G_i-coupled receptor with 40% homology to the H_3 receptor and a similar intron–exon structure. The localization of this receptor is quite restricted, and it does not appear to occur in the CNS. Expression appears localized to spleen, thymus, intestine, and immunologically active cells such as neutrophils, eosinophils, and T cells, suggesting a role in the regulation of immune function. If confirmed, this could offer a novel therapeutic potential for histamine receptor ligands in allergic and inflammatory diseases.

H_1 Receptor Agonists and Antagonists

Because of its high affinity and good receptor selectivity, mepyramine remains the agent of choice as a selective H_1 antagonist. A number of H_1 antagonists exist as optical isomers, and in many instances the (+) stereoisomer exhibits higher potency than the (−) stereoisomer. (+)-Chlorpheniramine is such an example. One of the most potent H_1 antagonists is the geometric isomer trans-triprolidine, which has a K_d of 0.1 nM. In humans, a major side effect associated with administration of H_1 antagonists is a high degree of sedation, which has been attributed to the ability of the antagonists to occupy H_1 receptors in the brain. Most of the classic H_1 antihistamines (e.g., diphenhydramine and mepyramine) readily cross the blood–brain barrier and elicit a significant degree of sedation.

A number of new compounds, however, penetrate poorly into the CNS and thus are relatively nonsedating. Terfenadine (Fig. 9–3) is an example of such an agent. Highly selective agonists do not exist for H_1 receptors. 2-Methylhistamine and 2-thiazoylethylamine show some selectivity, but their relative potency at H_1 receptors differs by no more than an order of magnitude from that exhibited at H_2 receptors.

H_2 Receptor Antagonists

Following the successful use of H_2 receptor antagonists such as cimetidine in the treatment of peptic ulcers, a number of these agents have become available. The structures of several H_2 antagonists are illustrated in Figure 9–4. Although a number of more potent agents have been developed, only ranitidine and tiotidine lack antagonist activity on H_3 receptors. These agents have limited access to the CNS. The only selective H_2 receptor antagonist that effectively penetrates into the CNS is zolantidine. This compound has been used extensively in experimental animals but has not been marketed for clinical use. Dimaprit is a fairly selective H_2 agonist that discriminates well between H_2 and H_1 or H_3 receptors. Impromidine is one of the most potent H_2 receptor

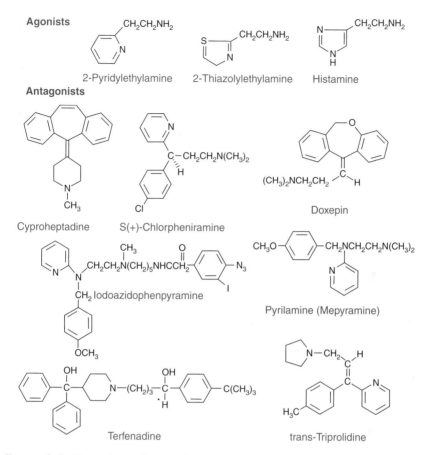

FIGURE 9–3. H_1 agonists and antagonists.

agonists available. Like dimaprit, it has minimal agonist effects on H_1 receptors, but it has more potent H_3 receptor antagonist properties. Amthamine is also a more potent agonist at H_2 receptors than diamaprit and does not affect H_1 receptors. However, this agent exerts weak agonist activity at the H_3 receptor and thus does not exhibit optimal subtype selectivity.

H_3 Receptor Antagonists and Agonists

H_3 receptor antagonists and agonists are illustrated in Figure 9–5. Thioperamide, originally declared to be a potent H_3 receptor antagonist that exhibits good receptor specificity, is now considered to actually be better classified as an inverse receptor agonist, stabilizing the H_3 receptor in an inactive state. Similar effects have been attributed to ciproxifan. Both of these drugs, unlike other H_3 antagonists, cross the blood–brain barrier and have been useful in

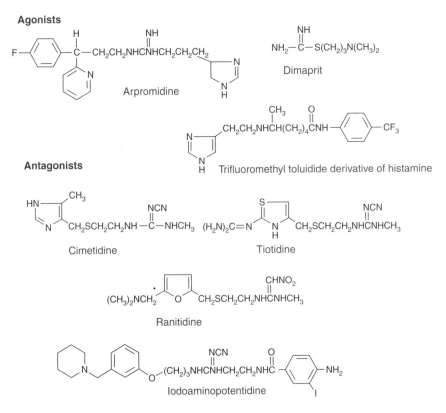

FIGURE 9–4. H$_2$ agonists and antagonists.

evaluating the behavioral role played by H$_3$ receptors in the CNS. A new antagonist, clobenpropit, is the most potent H$_3$ receptor antagonist available for investigating these receptors, but further studies have also characterized its actions as those of an inverse agonist. Nα-Methylhistamine and Nα-Nβ-dimethylhistamine are both potent H$_3$ receptor agonists, but neither shows any marked discrimination between the three histamine receptors. However, substitution of methyl groups in the α or β position of the side chain of the histamine molecule produces agents that exhibit a high degree of selectivity for the H$_3$ receptors. For example, Rα-methylhistamine and Rα,Sβ-dimethylhistamine are 15–20 times more potent than histamine as H$_3$ agonists but possess only approximately 1% of the activity of histamine on H$_1$ and H$_2$ receptors. Imetit is a potent and selective H$_3$ receptor full agonist that is effective both *in vivo* and *in vitro* and 60 times more potent than histamine. Table 9–1 summarizes the pharmacology of histamine receptors and their effector pathways.

In summary, there is compelling evidence that histamine, in addition to its presence in mast cells, exists in neurons, where it probably functions as a

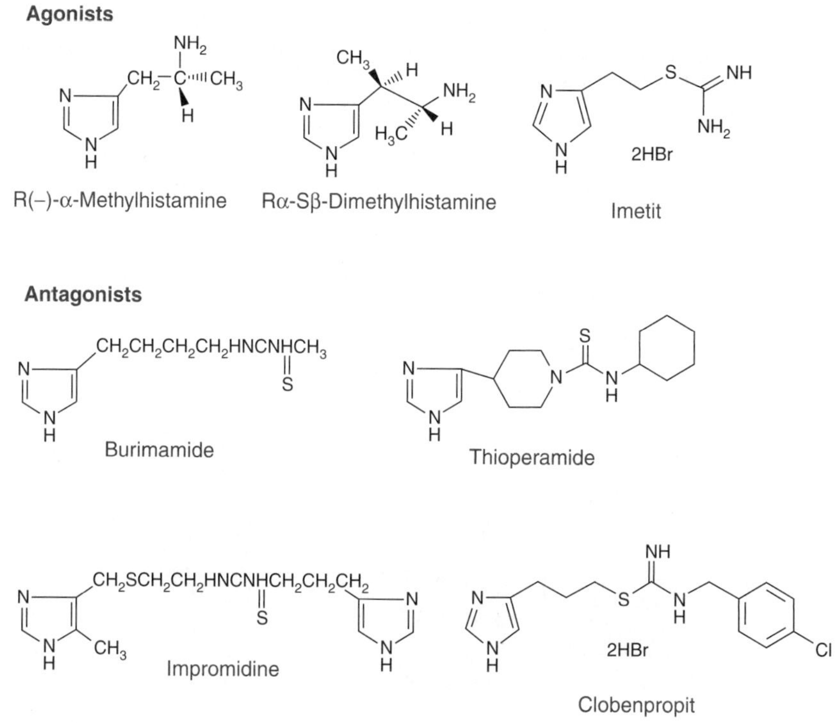

Agonists

R(−)-α-Methylhistamine   Rα-Sβ-Dimethylhistamine

Imetit

Antagonists

Burimamide

Thioperamide

Impromidine

Clobenpropit

FIGURE 9–5. H₃ agonists and antagonists.

TABLE 9–1. Pharmacology of Histamine Receptors

RECEPTOR SUBTYPE	H₁	H₂	H₃
Selective agonists	2-(*m*-Bromophenyl) histamine	Amthamine	(*R*)-α-Methylhistamine[c]
		Impromidine[a] (also an H₃ antagonist)	(*R*)-α(*S*)β-Dimethylhis-tamine[c]
			Imetit[c]
Selective antagonists	Mepyramine[a]	Ranitidine[b]	Thioperamide[c]
	Triprolidine[a]	Tiotidine[b]	Clobenpropit[c]
Effector pathways	↑IP₃/DAG	↑ cAMP	(? G$_{i/o}$)

IP₃/DAG. inositol triphosphate/diacylglycerol: cAMP. cyclic adenosine monophosphate.
[a]See Fig. 9–3.
[b]See Fig. 9–4.
[c]See Fig. 9–5.

neurotransmitter in the CNS. The brain has a similar nonuniform distribution of histamine, a specific histidine decarboxylase, and methylhistamine (the major metabolite of brain histamine). The cerebellum has the lowest levels, whereas the hypothalamus is most enriched. Hypothalamic synaptosomes contain histamine and histidine decarboxylase, suggesting a localization in nerve endings. Depolarization of hypothalamic slices causes a calcium-dependent release of histamine, and tetrodotoxin-sensitive histamine release from neurons has been demonstrated *in vivo*. The turnover of brain histamine is quite rapid, as with other biogenic amine transmitters. The essential elements of the histamine terminal are summarized in Figure 9-6.

Histaminergic Synapse

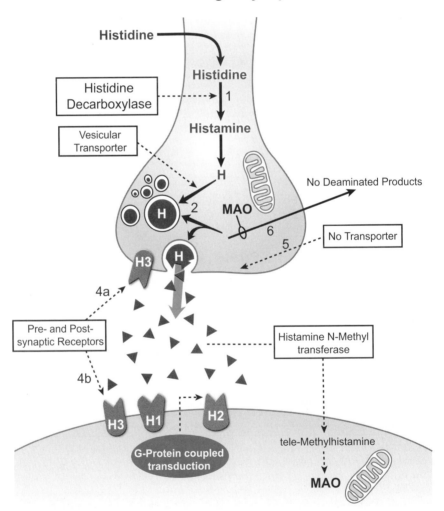

THERAPEUTIC APPLICATIONS OF HISTAMINERGIC DRUGS

The therapeutic role for histaminergic drugs is fairly limited, and the primary pharmacological actions of these agents are often associated with side effects ascribed to other therapeutic agents. For example, several antipsychotic (e.g., clozapine and thioridazine) and antidepressant (e.g., doxepin and amitriptyline) drugs with sedative and weight-gain side effects display potent H_1 antagonist properties. Histamine antagonists have been used therapeutically for only a limited number of conditions. H_1 antagonists such as meclizine are the most commonly used anti-motion sickness drugs. However, it is uncertain whether H_1 blockade is primarily responsible for the effectiveness of these agents. Some H_1 antagonists, notably meclizine and dimenhydrinate, are of benefit in vestibular disturbances such as Meniere's disease. H_1 receptor antagonists are also the ingredients of a number of proprietary remedies sold over-the-counter

←_____

FIGURE 9–4. Schematic model of a central histaminergic neuron indicating possible sites of drug action.

Site 1: *Enzymatic synthesis:* Histidine is taken up into the histamine-containing neuron and converted to histamine by the enzyme histidine decarboxylase. This enzyme can be effectively activated by cyclic AMP activated Protein Kinase A and Ca^{2+}-Calmodulin dependent protein kinase II (CamKII), controlled by H3 autoreceptors, and this activation reversed by protein phosphatase 2A and 1. H3 receptors can be antagonized by clobenpropit and thioperamide.

Site 2: *Storage:* Reserpine and tetrabenazine interfere with the vesicular monoamine transporter uptake-storage mechanism of the amine granules, causing a marked depletion of brain histamine.

Site 3: *Release:* At present, there is no drug available, which selectively blocks the depolarization activated, Ca-dependent release of histamine.

Site 4: *Receptor interaction:* The prototypic agonist of the presynaptic (4A) autoreceptor H3 is R-a-methylhistamine, while the prototypic antagonists are: H1- mepyramine, H2- cimetidine, and H3 thioperamide. Chemical structures for these compounds are shown in Figures 9–2, 9–3 and 9–4 (CBR8, figs 10–12 to 10–14). The H1, H2 and H3 receptors are all G-protein coupled receptors. (4B) H1 signals are transduced through inositol phospholipids hydrolysis, while H2 receptors activate cyclic AMP synthesis. H3 receptors are found on other monoaminergic neurons, cholinergic and peptidergic neurons, and inhibit the release of those transmitters, by negative regulation of cyclic AMP synthesis. A fourth Histamine receptor, H4, exists in non-neural tissues.

Site 5: *Reuptake:* There is no evidence for a histamine transporter that would allow its action to be terminated by reuptake into presynaptic terminals.

Site 6: *Catabolism after release:* While histamine is an excellent substrate for diamine oxidase (DAO), this enzyme has not been shown to exist in brain. Released histamine can be inactivated by histamine-N-methyltransferase (presumed to be post-synaptic), and that substrate can in turn can be catabolized by monoamine oxidase (MAO), yielding imidazole acetic acid; thus histamine catabolism will be diminished by MAO inhibitors.

as sleeping pills for the treatment of insomnia. These preparations are generally ineffective at the recommended dosages, although some sensitive individuals may derive benefit. H_1 antagonists have a well-established and valued place in the symptomatic treatment of hypersensitivity reactions (allergic rhinitis and conjunctivitis). However, their effect is purely palliative, being confined to suppression of the symptoms attributed to the antigen–antibody-induced release of histamine. Despite popular belief, H_1 antagonists are without value in the treatment of the common cold.

Lastly, although not a central nervous system application, the reader should recognize the therapeutic usefulness of the H_2 antagonists in the treatment of gastric and duodenal ulcers. H_2 antagonists are very effective at lowering the basal and nocturnal secretion of gastric acid and that which is stimulated by meals. They both reduce the pain and the consumption of antacids and hasten the healing of ulcers. The incidence of side effects with these H_2 antagonists (cimetidine and ranitidine) is low and can probably be attributed, in part, to the limited function of H_2 receptors in organs other than the stomach and to their poor penetration of the blood–brain barrier.

SELECTED REFERENCES

Arrang, J.-M., S. Morisset, and F. Gbahou (2007). Constitutive activity of the histamine H_3 receptor. *Trends Pharmacol. Sci.* 28, 350–358.

Haas, H. and P. Panula (2003). The role of histamine and the tuberomammillary nucleus in the nervous system. *Nature Rev. Neurosci.* 4, 121–131.

Hill, S. J. (1990). Distribution, properties, and functional characteristics of three classes of histamine receptor. *Pharmacol. Rev.* 42, 45–83.

Honrubia, M. A., M. T. Vilaro, J. M. Palacios, and G. Mengod (2000). Distribution of the histamine H_2 receptor in monkey brain and its mRNA localization in monkey and human brain. *Synapse* 38, 343–354.

Lovenberg, T. W., B. L. Roland, S. J. Wilson, X. Jiang, J. Pyati, A. Huvar, M. R. Jackson, and M. G. Erlander (1999). Cloning and functional expression of the human histamine H_3 receptor. *Mol. Pharmacol.* 55, 1101–1107.

Martinez-Mir, M. I., H. Pollard, J. Moreau, J. M. Arrang, M. Ruat, E. Traiffort, J. C. Schwartz, and J. M. Palacios (1990). Three histamines receptors (H_1, H_2 and H_3) visualized in the brain of human and non-human primates. *Brain Res.* 526, 322–327.

Schwartz, J. C. and J. M. Arrang (2002). Histamine. In *Neuropsychopharmacology: The Fifth Generation of Progress* (K. L. Davis, D. Charney, J. T. Cole, and C. Nemeroff, Eds.). Lippincott Williams & Wilkins, Philadelphia, pp. 179–190.

Staines, W. A. and J. I. Nagy (1991). Neurotransmitter coexistence in the tuberomammillary nucleus. In *Histaminergic Neurons: Morphology and Function* (T. Watanabe and H. Wada, Eds.). CRC Press, Boca Raton, FL, pp. 163–176.

Steinbusch, H. W. M. and A. H. Mulder (1984). Immunohistochemical localization of histamine in neurons and mast cells in brain. In *Handbook of Chemical Neuroanatomy. Classical Transmitters and Transmitter Receptors in the CNS* (A. Björklund, T. Hökfelt, and M. J. Kuhar, Eds.), Vol. 3, part II. Elsevier, New York, pp. 126–140.

Vizuete, M. L., E. Traiffort, M. L. Bouthenet, M. Ruat, E. Souil, J. Tardivel-Lacombe, and J.-C. Schwartz (1997). Detailed mapping of the histamine H_2 receptor and its gene transcripts in guinea-pig brain. *Neuroscience* 80(2), 321–343.

Wouterlood, F. G. and H. W. M. Steinbusch (1991). Afferent and efferent fiber connections of histaminergic neurons in the rat brain: Comparison with dopaminergic, noradrenergic and serotonergic systems. In *Histaminergic Neurons: Morphology and Function* (T. Watanabe and H. Wada, Eds.). CRC Press, Boca Raton, FL, pp. 145–162.

Yanai, K. and M. Tashiro (2007). The physiological and pathophysiological roles of neuronal histamine: An insight from human positron emission tomography studies. *Pharm. Ther.* 113, 1–15.

10

Neuropeptides

Research on neuropeptides has been an active area for more than 30 years, and scientists continue to view this as an area of great future promise. More than 100 small peptides, ranging from 2 to more than 40 residues long, are synthesized and released from neurons in the central and peripheral nervous system. They act potently on specific receptors, often with more than one receptor subtype for each peptide, adding further to the complexity of neuropeptide signaling. The quantities of peptides involved are minute, and the concentrations needed to activate the receptors are commonly sub-nanomolar.

DISCOVERING NEW NEUROPEPTIDES

New neuropeptides used to be discovered by the laborious process of analyzing tissue extracts for molecules possessing some particular biological function. In this way, by processing large amounts of hypothalamic tissue (from hundreds of thousands of animal brains), the various hypothalamic releasing factor peptides were discovered. Similarly, various biologically active gut peptides were extracted from large quantities of gastrointestinal tissue. The techniques of molecular biology have considerably simplified the process nowadays. The neuropeptides are always formed from larger precursor prohormone polypeptides. The cleavage enzymes involved recognize pairs of basic amino acid residues; thus, these cleavage sites can be identified from DNA sequences and new peptides can be predicted. These can then be synthesized and tested for biological activity, and their presence in nervous tissue can be confirmed. The synthetic material can also be used to generate antibodies that can be employed for quantitative measurements (i.e., radioimmunoassay) and to determine the qualitative distribution of the peptide by immunocytochemistry. Once one new neuropeptide has been identified, it becomes a simple matter to search for other potential members of a family of peptides with related amino acid sequences. Another common feature shared by many neuropeptides is that they are protected against enzymic degradation by the presence of a C-terminal amide group (rather than the usual carboxylic acid); tissue extracts can be searched to identify amidated peptides that may reveal novel neuropeptide structures. Recently, cloning of the numerous G protein-coupled receptors from the brain has identified new peptides that can activate the once-orphaned receptors (e.g., orphanin FQ). By refinements of differential display hybridization and searching for region-specific brain peptides by mRNA detection, still other peptides have been identified (cortistatin and hypocretins [also known as orexins]).

WHAT IS DIFFERENT ABOUT PEPTIDES?

Amino acid or monoamine transmitters are formed in nerve terminals from diet-derived amino acids by one or two intracellular enzymatic steps. The active transmitter molecule is then stored in the nerve terminal until release. Neuropeptide synthesis, in contrast, can take place only on ribosomes in the perikaryon or dendrites of a neuron. The synthesized prohormone is then processed by cleavage enzymes and packaged into vesicles in the smooth endoplasmic reticulum and transported from the perikaryon to the nerve terminals for eventual release (see Chapter 4). Peptide-releasing neurons, however, share certain basic properties with all other chemically characterized neurons. The neuropeptides are stored in vesicles in presynaptic nerve terminals, and their release is Ca^{2+}-dependent. Postsynaptically, like the monoamine neurotransmitters, the effects of neuropeptides are mediated by activation of G protein-coupled receptors. The neuropeptides thus act indirectly by regulating ion channel properties through second messengers such as Ca^{2+}, cyclic nucleotides, or inositol triphosphates (see Chapter 4). Furthermore, like the monoamines, peptides identical to those extracted from the nervous system are often made by nonneural secretory cells in endocrine glands and the cells lining hollow viscera such as the intestinal tract (giving rise to the term "gut–brain peptides"). Whether the neuropeptides should be regarded as "neurotransmitters" remains unclear; they act largely as modulators of neural function. In some respects, the actions of neuropeptides resemble those of endocrine peptide hormones. Thus, they may act on targets that are distant from release sites, are of high potency, and have a long time course of effects.

COEXISTENCE OF NEUROPEPTIDES AND NEUROTRANSMITTERS

Traditionally, according to "Dale's law," neurons released only one transmitter. According to this concept (attributed to Henry Dale, one of the pioneer transmitter discoverers), one aspect of a neuron's phenotype—as characteristic as its size, shape, location, circuitry, and synaptic function—was its neurochemical designation as "GABAergic," "cholinergic," "adrenergic," and so on. However, neuroactive peptides started showing up in autonomic neurons, where there was no need for additional transmitters. The presence of coexisting peptides in central as well as peripheral neurons that are already occupied by an amino acid or monoamine or even another neuropeptide is now seen as the norm. Some neurons may contain several different neuropeptides in addition to a conventional neurotransmitter.

Such a revolutionary concept forces us to ask a simple question: If the peptide is not the sole signaling molecule but, rather, a minor, fractional percent of the messenger signaling capacity of the nerve terminal, how do peptides affect signals transmitted by the coexisting amino acid or monoamine? So far, there are few satisfactory answers to this question. However, in the autonomic nervous system some examples of peptide–monoamine interactions have emerged. In the salivary gland, for example, low-frequency stimulation of the parasympathetic nerves releases acetylcholine (ACh), but vasoactive intestinal peptide (VIP) is also released when the cholinergic nerves are stimulated at higher frequency. VIP is a potent vasodilator and augments parasympathetic control of salivation by increasing glandular blood flow, a necessary correlate of secretion. Neuropeptide Y (NPY), found in many sympathetic neurons, is also released at higher frequencies of activation and sensitizes smooth muscle target cells to the accompanying adrenergic signals. Other peptide interactions, although not necessarily between coexisting amino acid or monoamine transmitters, are worth noting. For example, VIP greatly accentuates the cAMP response of cortical neurons to low doses of norepinephrine, and galanin can change the release of ACh in the ventral hippocampus.

One way to recast these players in their proper perspective might be to consider that a peptide usually embellishes what the primary transmitter for a neuronal connection seeks to accomplish. Such an effect may be to strengthen or prolong the primary transmitter's actions, especially when the nerve is called on to fire at higher than normal frequencies.

From the pharmacological perspective, the effects of peptide-directed drugs will depend not only on the location of the receptors and their actions but also on the context of its coexisting signals. Thus, the pharmacology of NPY or neurotensin may be most appropriately understood as a part of the total picture of central noradrenergic pharmacology, given the degree to which these two peptides may participate in that monoaminergic neuron's transmission. Given the relatively modest number of response mechanisms on which peptide messengers may operate through G protein-coupled receptors, a great enrichment of signaling possibilities becomes attainable through the interplay between frequency-dependent and diffusion-dependent release of multiple chemical signaling molecules and response sites.

In terms of the development of drugs active on the nervous system, the past decade has seen breakthroughs in the discovery of nonpeptide drugs that act as potent and selective agonists or antagonists at neuropeptide receptors. Peptides themselves do not make good starting points for drug discovery: The molecules are too large, do not penetrate the blood–brain barrier, and are too easily metabolized. Because they usually lack rigid chemical structures, they do not offer useful pharmacophores for medicinal chemistry. However, progress in identifying novel nonpeptide drugs has been made through the large-scale screening of chemical libraries, often deliberately enriched with chemical groups known to be preferred by G protein-coupled receptors. Once a single chemical lead has been identified, it can be used as a pharmacophore for further computer-based and wet-lab screening. Whereas 20 years ago there were few nonpeptide drugs, these are now commonplace and such compounds are known for most neuropeptide systems. They have provided valuable research tools to probe the physiology and pharmacology of the neuropeptides, although very few clinically useful new medicines have emerged. Hopes for the future remain high, however, and the rest of this chapter reviews some emerging trends in neuropeptide psychopharmacology.

CHOLECYSTOKININ

Among the gut–brain hormones with the longest history is cholecystokinin (CCK). In the periphery, CCK is secreted as a local hormone in the gut in response to food intake, and it regulates gallbladder emptying and pancreatic secretion and intestinal motility. The closely related hormone gastrin regulates acid secretion in the stomach. CCK is an abundant neuropeptide in the central nervous system (CNS), where it exists as the truncated C-terminal octapeptide, with a sulfated tyrosine at position 2 (CCK-8).

CCK coexists with dopamine and neurotensin in the substantia nigra and ventrotegmental area; with VIP, NPY, and GABA in thalamocortical and thalamostriatal connections; and with substance P and 5-HT in medullary neurons. The CCK neurons in spinal cord and brain stem appear to act as an "anti-opioid" system, present in parallel but distinct neuronal pathways from those containing endorphins. CCK reduces the analgesic effects of morphine and related opiates in animal tests.

There are two CCK receptors, CCK-1 and CCK-2 (which is also identical to the "gastrin receptor" in the stomach). The CCK-2 receptor predominates in the CNS of most mammalian species, although this is not true in human spinal cord and brain stem, where CCK-1 is the most common form. The discovery of nonpeptide antagonists of high affinity and potency for both CCK receptors was among the first breakthroughs in the development of neuropeptide pharmacology. The antagonists enhance the analgesic actions of opiates in animal tests, and a pilot scale clinical trial showed that the CCK-1 antagonist devazepide made morphine more effective in treating pain of neuropathic origin. Such drugs could prove valuable adjuncts to opiate therapy in treating intractable pain.

In terms of psychopharmacology, much interest was raised by the discovery that the intravenous administration of small doses of C-terminal fragments of CCK, or the gastrin fragment pentagastrin, reliably induced a psychological state of panic in human subjects. The panic is dose-related and mercifully short-lived. Administration of the CCK-2 antagonist L-365,260 completely blocked this chemically induced panic in volunteers. However, the results of a clinical trial of this drug in patients who suffered spontaneous panic attacks were negative, so it seems unlikely that CCK antagonists will prove useful in the treatment of panic disorders.

CORTICOTROPIN-RELEASING FACTOR

Corticotropin-releasing factor (CRF) is a hypothalamic releasing factor that is released into the blood supply to the anterior pituitary, where it stimulates the release of the hormone corticotrophin (ACTH). This in turn acts on the adrenal gland to stimulate production of glucocorticoids, which are steroid hormones that play a key role in metabolic regulation. The system is self-limiting because excess amounts of glucocorticoids feed back on steroid receptors in the hypothalamus to limit CRF production and release. This is a particularly important system because it mediates the reactions of the so-called hyothalamo–pituitary–adrenal (HPA) axis to stress of various kinds, with increased glucocorticoid production as the end result. Although CRF was discovered in 1981 through the analysis of large quantities of bovine hypothalamic tissue, knowledge of its physiology and pharmacology has continued to accumulate, and it is now regarded as one of the most attractive targets for novel psychopharmaceuticals.

CRF is related to three other neuropeptides, the urocortins, and it acts on two distinct receptors—CRF-1 and CRF-2. The CRF-2 receptor exists in three different splice variants of the same gene—CRF-2α, -β, and -γ. In addition, a soluble CRF-binding protein, derived as a splice variant of CRF-2α, binds CRF with high affinity and may be involved either in modulating the activity of the peptide or in its transport to target sites.

It quickly became clear that CRF was not restricted to the hypothalamus; CRF-containing nerve fibers are widely distributed in extrahypothalamic sites in the brain, notably in cerebral cortex, cerebellum, amygdala, and other limbic forebrain structures and in the monoamine-rich locus ceruleus and raphe nuclei in brain stem. Outside the brain, CRF and urocortins are also widely distributed in male and female reproductive organs, skin, gut, heart, and muscle. In peripheral tissues, the CRF-1 and CRF-2β receptors predominate, whereas brain contains mainly the CRF-1 and CRF-2α receptors.

Both animal and human evidence points to an important role of the CRF system in mediating reactions to stress. Apart from its role in the HPA axis, the extrahypothalamic CRF system, which is not under negative feedback control by glucocorticoids, seems particularly well suited to activate cortical, limbic, autonomic, and central monoamine systems thought to be important in mediating autonomic and behavioral reactions to stress. Administration of CRF intraventricularly in rats leads to physiological and behavioral changes characteristic of stress, including increased heart rate and blood pressure, suppression of exploratory behaviors in an unfamiliar environment, increased grooming, and reduced food intake and sexual activity. In the elevated plus maze test (see Chapter 14), rats spend less time in the open segments and enter these less frequently. At high dose levels, CRF induces seizure activity. The behavioral effects are independent of the HPA axis and can be reproduced by direct injection of CRF into amygdala or other limbic forebrain structures. Animals genetically modified to overexpress the CRF gene display similar signs of stress reactions, whereas knockout mice lacking expression of the CRF-1 receptor show impaired stress responses and decreased anxiety (e.g., spending more time in the light segment of the elevated plus maze). Monkeys or rats exposed to early life stress show elevated concentrations of CRF in hypothalamic and extrahypothalamic sites in adulthood; early life stress is associated with an increased risk of depression in humans.

Clinical findings also suggest a role for CRF in some forms of depression/anxiety disorders. Depressed patients were found to have elevated concentrations of CRF in cerebrospinal fluid, and this was reversed after successful antidepressant treatment. There is also evidence for hyperactivity of the HPA axis in depression.

This evidence has prompted an active search during the past decade for nonpeptide drugs that act as antagonists at the CRF-1 receptor as potential antidepressants/anxiolytics or antistress medicines. Compounds such as CP 154,526, NBI 27914, antalarmin, DMP 696, and NBI 30775, when administered to animals, attenuate CRF-induced behavioral changes, elevations in plasma ACTH levels, or seizure activity.

To date, only one clinical trial has been published—an open-label study of 20 depressed patients treated for 30 days with R121919, a potent water-soluble CRF-1 antagonist with good oral bioavailability. The compound was safe and well tolerated, and at the doses used it did not impair ACTH or cortisol secretion either at baseline or after CRF challenge. Significant reductions in depression and anxiety ratings were observed using both patient and clinician ratings, and these symptoms worsened again at the end of the trial when the drug was withdrawn. Although these are encouraging results, this was a small uncontrolled trial, and the results of larger placebo-controlled trials with this or other CRF-1 antagonists are eagerly awaited.

GALANIN

Galanin is another peptide initially isolated from gut and later found to be present in the CNS. The Swedish "peptide hunters" Viktor Mutt and Katzuhiko Tatemoto searched for C-terminally amidated peptides in extracts of porcine intestines and isolated a 29-amino acid residue amidated peptide. Curiously, the human version of galanin is a 30-amino acid residue peptide lacking the C-terminal amide.

Galanin is widely distributed in both the central and peripheral nervous systems and the endocrine system. It acts on three receptors—GalR1, GalR2, and GalR3. In the CNS, much attention has been paid to the possible function of galanin as a modulator of pain systems in the spinal cord. Galanin is strongly inhibitory, reducing the excitability of target cells or inhibiting presynaptic release of neurotransmitters or other neuropeptides. It is normally present in small amounts in many small-diameter primary sensory fibers, but the expression of the peptide is greatly increased if the nerves are damaged. Galanin is also present in inhibitory GABAergic interneurons in spinal cord dorsal horn, where it may coexist with enkephalins or NPY. When administered directly to spinal cord in normal rats, the effects of galanin are complex, with antinociceptive actions predominant, but some reports also find a hyperalgesic effect. In models of neuropathic pain in which sensory nerve fibers are damaged and galanin is upregulated, spinally administered galanin alleviates the heightened pain sensitivity otherwise seen in such models. Conversely, knockout mice in which galanin expression is blocked show heightened sensitivity to noxious stimuli. These results suggest that a galanin receptor agonist might provide a novel analgesic, and there have been several attempts to develop such a drug. Progress in identifying nonpeptide agonist ligands has been slow, however, the most successful compounds galnon and galmic have micromolar rather than nanomolar affinities. Galnon displays little selectivity for galanin receptor sub-types, whereas galmic has some selectivity for GalR1. Both compounds have been shown to alleviate the increased pain sensitivity seen in animal models of neuropathic and inflammatory pain. Galnon also displayed strong anticonvul-sant properties in rat models, suggesting another possible application for galanin agonist drugs in the treatment of epilepsies.

In the brain, galanin coexists with serotonin in the dorsal raphe nucleus and with norepinephrine in the locus ceruleus—nuclei known to play a key role in the actions of antidepressant drugs (see Chapter 14). When administered into the brain, galanin is a potent inhibitor of serotoninergic transmission, leading to a reduction in serotonin release and a functional blockade of 5-HT$_{1A}$ receptor-mediated responses. Pharmacological and genetic studies suggest a role for galanin in depression-related behavior. Transgenic mice overexpressing galanin display increased immobility in the forced swim test (see Chapter 14), and intra-cerebral administration of galanin increases depression-like behavior—an effect reversed by administration of the peptidic galanin antagonist M35. Impor-tantly, M35 alone produces antidepressant effects, and this has prompted a search for more potent nonpeptide galanin antagonists. Several such antago-nists have been described, with selectivity for the GalR3 receptor subtype. The compounds are capable of crossing the blood–brain barrier and when given systemically show anxiolytic and antidepressant-like activity: enhanced social interaction in rats, reduced guinea pig vocalizations after maternal sep-aration, increased punished drinking behavior in rats, increased swim time in the forced swim test in rats, and decreased immobility time in the tail suspen-sion test in rats (see Chapter 14). These results will encourage increased efforts to identify additional Gal-3 receptor antagonists that might prove to be novel anxiolytic/antidepressant medicines.

NEUROTENSIN

This 13-amino acid peptide is another member of the "gut–brain" family. In the intestine, neurotensin is secreted by mucosal nonneural endocrine cells after food ingestion, and it serves a number of local digestive functions. Its name derives from its ability to lower blood pressure and cause a visible vaso-dilatation in vessels in the rabbit ear. Neurotensin is also found in the CNS as a neuropeptide, with largest amounts in the anterior and basal hypothalamus, the nucleus accumbens and septum, the midbrain dopamine neurons (along with CCK), and selected scattered neurons in the spinal cord and brain stem.

Two G protein-coupled receptors exist, NTS1 and NTS2, and a third less studied receptor, NTS3, has been reported that is not in the G protein-coupled family. Centrally administered neurotensin elicits analgesia, hypothermia, anorexia, accentuation of barbiturate and ethanol sleeping time, and increased release of growth hormone and prolactin. The peptide has been implicated in pain mechanisms, central control of temperature, control of feeding behavior, and in the mechanism of action of antipsychotic drugs. It is the latter possibility that has attracted most research attention.

Neurotensin is present in dopamine-rich areas of brain. In rodents, it coexists with dopamine in midbrain dopaminergic neurons, but this is not the case in human brain. Reduced levels of neurotensin have been reported in postmortem brain samples from schizophrenic patients. The association with dopamine and its behavioral properties has led to the suggestion that it may act as an endogenous neuroleptic. In animals, intracerebral administration of neurotensin leads to behavioral effects similar to those seen after atypical neuroleptics, including blockade of apomorphine-induced yawning, penile erection, and climbing behavior (see Chapter 15). Administration of neuroleptic drugs leads to increased levels of neurotensin in dopamine-rich brain areas, with an interesting differential effect of typical versus atypical drugs. The latter cause elevations in neurotensin only in nucleus accumbens and forebrain, whereas typical neuroleptics lead to increased levels of neurotensin also in basal ganglia regions. This may be a factor in explaining why the atypical drugs are less prone to cause extrapyramidal motor side effects.

Drugs acting as neurotensin receptor (NTR) agonists might represent a novel approach to the development of atypical neuroleptics. To date, the only available NTR agonists are peptide analogues of NT_{8-13} (modified to increase metabolic stability and CNS availability following peripheral administration), for example, NT69L, and PD149163. Similar to atypical neuroleptics, systemic administration of these agonists in animals restores pharmacologically induced (DA agonists, α_1 receptor agonist, dizocilpine, or a 5-HT_{2A} receptor agonist) deficits in prepulse inhibition of the acoustic startle response (see Chapter 15). Systemic NTR agonists also share with neuroleptics the ability to inhibit amphetamine- and phencyclidine-induced hyperlocomotion, as well as preventing haloperidol-induced catalepsy and apomorphine-induced climbing behavior. Given the broad range of other biological activities of neurotensin both in the CNS and in the periphery, it will be a challenge to develop neurotensin-based psychopharmaceuticals that are both effective and safe.

OPIOID PEPTIDES

The discovery of the first opioid peptides, the enkephalins, by John Hughes and colleagues more than 30 years ago sparked a wave of research in this new field of neurobiology. More than 20 opioid peptides (also known as "endorphins") are now known, and they are present in several distinct families. There are four distinct opioid receptors: μ(MOR), δ(DOR), κ(KOR), and ORL$_1$. The opioid peptides are grouped into several different families:

1. The proopiomelanocortin (POMC) peptides are expressed independently in the anterior pituitary, the intermediate lobe of the pituitary, and one main cluster of neurons in the area of the arcuate nucleus of the hypothalamus. The major endorphin agonist produced from POMC is the 31-amino acid C-terminal fragment β-endorphin, the most potent of the natural opioids. In the cortico-tropin-secreting cells of the anterior pituitary, POMC is processed largely to corticotropin and to an inactive form of β-endorphin; in intermediate lobe cells and arcuate neurons, the same precursor is processed to α-MSH and active β-endorphin.

2. The enkephalin pentapeptides Met^5-enkephalin and Leu^5-enkephalin are expressed in wholly separate neuronal systems from the POMC neurons and are much more widely distributed throughout the CNS and peripheral nervous system, including the adrenal medulla and enteric nervous system. The precursor proenkephalin contains multiple copies of the two peptides in almost exactly the 6:1 ratio of Met^5- to Leu^5-enkephalin found in regional brain and gut assays.

3. The prodynorphin peptides consist of C-terminally extended forms of Leu^5-enkephalin arising from a different gene and from a different mRNA that encodes for production of four major peptides: dynorphin A, dynorphin B, and two neoendorphins, α and β. These C-terminally extended peptides act as potent opioid agonists without cleavage down to the enkephalin pentapeptide form, and they are expressed in a separate series of rather generally distributed central and peripheral neurons.

4. Two tetrapeptides, endomorphin-1 and endomorphin-2, are derived from a different prohormone and are also widely distributed in the central and peripheral nervous systems. These peptides display a high affinity and remarkable selectivity for the mu-opioid receptor (MOR), at which they act as partial agonists. MOR is known to be of particular importance in mediating the analgesic and rewarding properties of opiates (see Chapters 18 and 22).

5. The peptide nociceptin (also known as orphanin-Q) is a selective agonist for the ORL$_1$ receptor, at which most of the other opioid peptides are inactive.

6. Certain plant and animal products contain peptides that act as ligands at one or another of the opioid receptors. Thus, for example, the milk protein casein when partially digested gives rise to a series of casomorphins. Other examples include the dermorphins, found in some amphibian skins. Such naturally occurring exogenous opioid peptides are sometimes termed "exorphins."

Although there has been great progress in understanding the cellular actions and the physiology and pharmacology of the opioid peptides, this field of research has been disappointing in that it has not led to the discovery of new medicines. Although some of the opioid peptides are very potent (β-endorphin is more than 1000 times more potent than morphine), they are unable to penetrate into the brain after systemic administration, and most are rapidly degraded metabolically. Indeed, the development of inhibitors of the enzymes responsible for such degradation is seen by some as a possible way of finding novel analgesics. However, pharmaceutical progress in the opioid field has relied on the development of new synthetic opiates that are much more potent analgesics than morphine (e.g., fentanyl) and on the development of new pharmaceutical formulations of morphine and related opiates to provide once-a-day medicines (see Chapter 18).

SUBSTANCE P AND OTHER TACHYKININS

Substance P (SP) is one of the oldest of the neuropeptides. It was discovered in the heroic era of pharmacology, isolated in 1936 by von Euler and Gaddum from extracts of horse intestines. It was not until 1970 that the sequence of this undecapeptide was elucidated by Susan Leeman. SP is a member of a family of related peptides, the tachykinins (so called because they can elicit slow contractions of smooth muscle). The three mammalian neuropeptides are recognized by three receptors—NK-1, NK-2, and NK-3. In recent years, a number of potent nonpeptide receptor antagonists have become available, with selectivity for one or other of these receptors.

Although all three peptides and their receptors are present in mammalian CNS, most research attention has focused on SP and the NK-1 receptor for which it is the preferred agonist. This is largely because SP is present in small sensory nerve fibers projecting into the spinal cord, where SP may play a neurotransmitter or neuromodulator role. Such "C fibers" play an important role in transmitting pain information into the CNS so the idea that SP might act as some form of "pain transmitter" has been extensively studied. The results have been mixed. Many animal experiments have suggested that SP plays a role in pain transmission. Knockout mice, lacking SP or the NK-1 receptor, show blunted responsiveness to painful stimuli. A series of clinical trials of NK-1 antagonists as analgesics, however, proved disappointing, with no benefit seen in trials of inflammatory pain (e.g., arthritis), neuropathic pain (e.g., diabetic neuropathy), or migraine. SP is only one of several different neuropeptides present in sensory nerves, and it coexists with the excitatory amino acid glutamate. Blockade of SP alone is apparently not sufficient to cause analgesia, although SP is upregulated after nerve damage in conditions of neuropathic pain.

The sensory neurons that contain SP also invariably contain a second neuropeptide, calcitonin gene-related peptide (CGRP), and this too has been implicated in pain mechanisms, particularly in migraine, where there is evidence for an increased release of this peptide during migraine attacks. Nonpeptide antagonists of CGRP have yielded positive results in the relief of acute migraine headaches, so such drugs represent another potential approach to novel analgesics.

SP is also present in a number of neural pathways in the brain, especially in the substantia nigra, caudate putamen, amygdala, hypothalamus, and cerebral cortex. Some animal experiments suggest a possible role of SP in mediating stress responses; thus, an increased release of SP is seen in medial amygdala in response to immobilization stress (using indwelling microdialysis cannulae). NK-1 antagonists block the anxiogenic effects of such stress or the anxiogenic effects of microinjections of SP into this brain region. NK-1 antagonists were also reported to have positive effects in a guinea pig model predictive of antidepressant activity (reduced stress calls after maternal separation). There was considerable excitement in 1998 when positive results were reported in the treatment of major depression in a controlled clinical trial with the potent NK-1 antagonist aprepitant, and this was followed by a further positive clinical trial in depression using a second NK-1 antagonist, L-759,274. However, large-scale clinical trials failed to replicate these early results, and it seems unlikely that NK-1 antagonists will find an important role in the treatment of depression/anxiety.

The NK-1 antagonist aprepitant (Emend) is the first of what is hoped to be a new generation of human medicines based on neuropeptide research. It found a clinically useful role in another context—as a novel antiemetic agent used in conjunction with 5-HT$_3$ antagonists in patients undergoing cancer chemotherapy, which tends to cause severe nausea/vomiting. The rationale for this is that SP is present in a majority of the sensory fibers in the vagus nerve, which carry noxious stimuli to the brain stem vomiting center. Blockade of the NK-1 receptors caused a powerful antiemetic effect in animal experiments, and this was followed by successful clinical trials. In the clinic, addition of the NK-1 antagonist to the 5-HT antagonist significantly improves the control of nausea/vomiting, particular in the delayed phase that follows some days after the initial chemotherapy.

Interest in other aspects of tachykinin pharmacology is also developing. Nonpeptide antagonists with selectivity for NK-2 or NK-3 receptors display anxiolytic and antidepressant actions in animal models, and the NK-2 antagonist saredutant (SR48968) is in advanced-stage clinical trials for depression/anxiety. Selective NK-3 antagonists (e.g., talnetant and osanetant) have been proposed as potential antipsychotic agents.

VASOPRESSIN AND OXYTOCIN

These two similar nonapeptideswith internal disulfide bridges are the original mammalian peptide "neurohormones." Both peptides are synthesized in neurons in the hypothalamus that project to the posterior pituitary, from which they are released into the circulation. In addition, oxytocin (OT) and arginine-vasopressin (AVP) neurons innervate various regions of the brain and spinal cord. AVP acts on three related receptors—V_{1a}, V_2, and V_{1b} (sometimes called V3). OT acts on a single OT receptor.

AVP has important roles in the kidney and cardiovascular system, and OT has important roles in the female reproductive system in parturition and lactation. A variety of drugs are under development that target these peripheral actions. In addition, these peptides have an interesting range of centrally mediated behavioral actions. AVP and OT play critical roles in regulating social behaviors, including pair bonding, parental care, and territorial protection. Human brain imaging studies have shown that both maternal love and romantic love activate brain regions that are rich in AVP and OT receptors. Defects in such mechanisms may underlie sexual dysfunction, the social dysfunction in autism, or social phobia. Nonpeptide OT agonists are being explored as possible treatment for such disorders. In the brain, AVP acting at V_{1b} receptors enhances the actions of CRF, both in its pituitary function of releasing ACTH and in extrahypothalamic regions. Nonpeptide antagonists with selectivity for the V_{1b} receptor (e.g., SSR149415) display anxiolytic/antidepressant actions in animal models, particularly those involved with stress. They may represent novel treatments for some forms of depression or anxiety disorders, and one such compound is already in clinical trials.

NEUROPEPTIDES IN APPETITE REGULATION AND OBESITY

The prevalence of obesity is rapidly increasing in developed countries, and it represents a major public health problem. Previous attempts to develop drugs that regulate appetite to control obesity have sometimes ended in disastrous failures (e.g., *d*-amphetamine and *d*-fenfluramine ["fen-phen"]) (see Chapter 21). Despite this, there continues to be strong interest in pharmaceutical solutions, and the neuropeptides offer many potential targets. The control of appetite and body weight is extremely complex and involves numerous central and peripheral mechanisms. The topic cannot be reviewed in detail here, but some of the neuropeptides worth noting are discussed.

Appetite-Stimulating (Orexigenic) Peptides

Neuropeptide Y, a 36-amino acid residue peptide, is one of the most abundant in hypothalamus, particularly in the arcuate nucleus, which is a key feeding control center. NPY is one of the most potent appetite stimulants in animal studies. There are six distinct NPY receptors; of these, five are expressed in the hypothalamus. The Y1 and Y5 subtypes appear most important in mediating the actions of NPY on appetite.

Melanin-concentrating hormone (MCH), a cyclic 19-amino acid neuropeptide, is found in other feeding centers in lateral hypothalamus and zona incerta. It stimulates energy intake in rats and decreases energy expenditure. It acts on two receptors, MCH-1R and MCH-2R. Null mutant MCH or MCH-1R mice are resistant to high-fat diet-induced obesity, whereas mice overexpressing MCH readily become obese when exposed to a high-fat diet. Nonpeptide antagonists of MCH-1R prevent diet-induced obesity and also have anxiolytic and antidepressant effects. They may prove valuable in the treatment of obesity.

Hypocretins (also known as orexins) are a group of closely related neuropeptides. Hypocretin A (33 residues) and hypocretin B (28 residues) are expressed on the same prohormone sequence. There are two closely related receptors, OX_1R and OX_2R. Both peptides and their receptors are present in the hypothalamus, and both peptides stimulate food intake, apparently by delaying normal satiety mechanisms. Nonpeptide antagonists with selectivity for OX_1R (e.g., SB-334867) suppress food intake and advance the onset of satiety. However, orexins are also importantly involved in the control of sleep and wakefulness; null mutant orexin mice develop a form of narcolepsy, with repeated short bouts of sleep. Whether orexin antagonists would be able to avoid such unwanted actions remains unclear.

Appetite-Suppressing (Anorectic) Peptides

Melanocortins are bioactive peptides derived from the precursor POMC. This remarkable prohormone gives rise to ACTH in anterior pituitary, but in hypothalamus it can generate bioactive peptides related to α-MSH that act on the MC4R receptor to inhibit feeding and reduce body weight. MC4R and the related MC3R are unique in that there is an endogenous 132-residue peptide, Agouti-related peptide (AGP), that acts as an antagonist at these receptors. Thus, the balance between melanocortin peptides and AGP may determine at any particular time whether this is an orexigenic or anorectic mechanism. Matters are further complicated by the finding of MC4R receptors on fat cells in the periphery, where they may respond to circulating melanocortins released from the pituitary.

CART (cocaine- and amphetamine-regulated transcript) is an 89-amino acid peptide that was discovered on the basis of its increased expression in rats following repeated administration of cocaine or amphetamine (see Chapter 21). It is localized in various hypothalamic nuclei, where it may coexist with vasopressin or CRF. Intracerebral administration of CART inhibits normal and fast-induced feeding in rats; it also blocks NPY-induced feeding.

Glucagon-like peptides represent another example of how the same peptide prohormone may be processed to give rise to different peptide products in different tissues. In α cells of the pancreas, preproglucagon gives rise to glucagon, a hormone that plays an important role in metabolic control. However, in the brain stem nucleus of the solitary tract, preproglucagon gives rise to various peptides, including the glucagon-like peptides GLP-1 and GLP-2. These play complex roles both in the brain and in the periphery in the control of appetite. In the hypothalamus, GLP-1-containing fibers and the GLP-1 receptor appear to play a key role in the central anorectic actions of GLP-1.

SELECTED REFERENCES

Akil, H., C. Owens, H. Gutstein, L. Taylor, E. Curran, and S. Watson (1998). Endogenous opioids: Overview and current issues. *Drug Alcohol Depend.* 51, 127–140.

Anubhuti, S. A. (2006). Role of neuropeptides in appetite regulation and obesity–A review. *Neuropeptides* 40, 375–401.

Cáceda, R., B. Kinkead, and C. B. Nemeroff (2006). Neurotensin: Role in psychiatric and neurological diseases. *Peptides* 27, 2385–2404.

Hokfelt, T., T. Bartfai, and F. Bloom (2003). Neuropeptides: Opportunities for drug discovery. *Lancet Neurol.* 2, 463–472.

Holzer, P. (Ed.) (2004). Tachykinins. *Handb. Exp. Pharmacol.* 164.

Kehne, J. H. (2007). The CRF-1 receptor: A novel target for the treatment of depression, anxiety, and stress-related disorders. *CNS Neurol. Disord. Drug Targets* 6, 163–182.

Liu, H.-X., and T. Hökfelt (2002). The participation of galanin in pain processing at the spinal level. *Trends Pharmacol. Sci.* 23, 468–474.

Lu, X., L. Sharkey, and T. Bartfai (2007). The brain galanin receptors: Targets for novel antidepressant drugs. *CNS Neurol. Disord. Drug Targets* 6, 183–194.

McCleane, G. (2004). Cholecystokinin antagonists a new way to improve the analgesia from old analgesics? *Curr. Pharmaceutical Design* 10, 303–314.

Navari, R. M. (2004). Role of neurokinin-1 receptor antagonists in chemotherapy-induced emesis: Summary of clinical trials. *Cancer Invest.* 22, 569–576.

11

Purinergic Pharmacology

INTRODUCTION AND HISTORY

Students with prior knowledge of intermediary metabolism will recognize the purine base adenine as the beginning of a triple-threat raw material. As the purine base, adenine is one of the four bases that make up nucleic acids, but its ribonucleoside form, adenosine, and its three nucleotide mono-, di-, and tri- phosphorylated forms (AMP, ADP, and ATP) have probably been much more intensively studied in the energy metabolism of nonneural cells. Their place in textbooks of neuropsychopharmacology was a long time in coming. Although it has been known for more than 80 years that adenosine and ATP can elicit potent pharmacological effects on the cardiovascular system (Drury and Szent-Gyorgy, 1929), studies of their effects on the brain or peripheral nerves by central or systemic injection lagged approximately 20 years. The evidence that endogenous purines regulated the activity of the nervous system was not widely accepted until the 1990s when molecular cloning of the receptors for adenosine and ATP revealed that, like the other transmitters discussed in this book, there was cellular and regional selectivity in their expression sites in the brain, expanding their more general roles in energy metabolism to include additional intercellular signaling functions. Subsequent research on the purinergic systems of the central nervous system has established two main categories of signal transduction: sites where adenosine is the mediator (A receptors; Table 11–1) and sites where ATP (and sometimes UTP) is the mediator, often in conjunction with either a monoamine or a neuropeptide. Subsequent work on the receptors for adenosine as a special kind of intercellular signal, a neuromodulator, but not a classic neurotransmitter, and for ATP as a cotransmitter more firmly established their different physiological roles and the pharmacological roles each system has been found to play in the brain as well as the autonomic nervous system.

ADENOSINE

The seminal work of Rall, Sattin, McIlwain, and others demonstrated that adenosine stimulated the formation of cAMP in brain slices and that methylxanthines such as theophylline and caffeine were competitive pharmacological antagonists of this response. These findings were instrumental in developing much of the interest in adenosine in the mid-1980s. However, unlike other neurotransmitters, adenosine is neither stored in vesicles nor released as a classical neurotransmitter by activity-dependent, Ca^{2+}-mediated release mechanisms. Extracellular levels of adenosine in the brain are not static: Adenosine was found to be released into the extracellular spaces of the brain during hypoxia, ischemia, physical damage, or metabolic stress.

The extracellular concentrations of adenosine clearly vary with some components of neuronal activity, but what is the relationship functionally intended to accomplish? After much debate, a solid hypothesis has been developed that states that whatever the intervening cause, adenosine is released into the extracellular spaces whenever oxygen demand exceeds oxygen supply. The released adenosine increases oxygen supply by its universal ability to dilate vascular beds and decreases oxygen demand by diminishing neuronal activity by decreasing the release of excitatory transmitters and thus neuronal activity. As discussed later, ATP as a coreleased cotransmitter is also released with the activity of some synaptic sites. Biochemically, this ATP can also contribute to the extracellular pool of adenosine through the actions of prevalent 5′-nucleotidases. ATP can also affect adenosine synthesis by the formation of S-adenosylmethionine, a precursor of S-adenosylhomocysteine that can in turn be converted to adenosine by S-adenosylhomocysteine hydrolase.

On the basis of these observations, adenosine is generally considered to be a prototypic modulator—like nitric oxide, prostaglandins, and CO_2—arising from non-synaptic sites of active neurons, yet affecting excitability of adjacent neurons. Evidence also supports the likelihood that glia can also release adenosine. The brain has an especially high concentration of adenosine receptors, and its modulatory actions have been shown to be involved in both normal and

TABLE 11–1. Adenosine Receptors in Brain (Modified from Dunwiddie & Masino, 2001)

ADENOSINE RECEPTOR	G-PROTEIN	TRANSDUCTION MECHANISMS	PHYSIOLOGICAL ACTIONS IN BRAIN	DISTRIBUTION IN BRAIN	RECEPTOR AFFINITY
A1	Gi, Go	Inhibits adenylyl cyclase Activates GIRKs (inward rectifying K-channels Inhibits Ca^{++} channels Activates PLC	Hyperpolarizes neurons Inhibits synaptic transmission (all transmitters) Neuroprotection	Widespread	70 nM
A2A	Gs, G_{olf}	Activates adenylyl cyclase Inhibits Ca^{++} channels Activates channels (?)	Facilitates transmitter release Inhibits transmitter release	Primarily striatum, olfactory tubercle, nucleus accumbens	150 nM
A2B	Gs	Activates adenylyl cyclase Activates PLC	Increases in cAMP in brain slices Modulation of Ca^{++} channel	Widespread	5100 nM
A3	Gi, Gq	Activates PLC Inhibits adenylyl cyclase Increases intracellular Ca^{++}	Uncouples A1 in mGLUR's	Widespread	6500 nM

pathophysiological processes, including regulation of sleep, arousal, neuro-protection, and epilepsy, as well as the brain's responses to ethanol and opi-ates. The pharmacological actions of caffeine and theobromine, which are arguably the most widely used psychoactive drugs throughout the world, are largely attributable to their activity as adenosine receptor antagonists.

Adenosine and adenosine analogues are potent activators of cellular func-tion, altering neuronal activity and affecting behavior as well. Highly specific, high-affinity binding sites for adenosine have also been identified in the cen-tral nervous system, and it is thought that most, if not all, of the physiological actions of adenosine are mediated via the interaction of extracellular adenos-ine with one of these four G protein-coupled receptor sites (see Table 11–1). Since adenosine can be released by most brain cells, including neurons and glia, it is believed that adenosine modulates the activity of the nervous system by acting presynaptically (facilitating or inhibiting transmitter release), post-synaptically, and/or nonsynaptically.

A convincing case has been made for adenosine receptors having a critical function in regulating the activation of multiple nonpurinergic receptors that affect neurotransmitter release and synaptic function. In particular, adenosine receptors regulate N-methyl-D-aspartate and metabotropic glutamate recep-tors, nicotinic cholinergic receptors, and receptors for several neuropeptides such as calcitonin gene-related peptide and vasoactive intestinal polypeptide receptors. Thus, adenosine has been conceptualized to behave as a modulator to fine-tune the actions of other transmitters and neuromodulators.

Perhaps the most comprehensively defined functional role of adenosine is in sleep–wake regulation. McCarley and colleagues built on the early observa-tions of Feldberg that intravenous or intracerebroventricular injections of ade-nosine had sedative, sleep-inducing effects that were antagonized by caffeine and theophylline. Recently, they performed a comprehensive analysis using microdialysis in several different regions of the cat brain to search for sleep–wake-related changes in extracellular adenosine in areas known to register sleep-related electroencephalogram changes. Basal forebrain, cerebral cortex, thalamus, preoptic hypothalamus, dorsal raphe nucleus, and pedunculopon-tine nucleus all showed similar declines in extracellular adenosine during brief periods of spontaneous sleep. However, only in the magnocellular cholinergic portions of the basal forebrain did extracellular adenosine levels rise (by more than 40%) during 6 hours of imposed sleep deprivation. From these and other observations, McCarley and colleagues proposed that adenosine promotes sleepiness by inhibiting the activity of neurons known to promote wakeful-ness, such as these cholinergic basal forebrain neurons. Furthermore, they proposed that adenosine is an endogenous sleep factor mediating the sleepi-ness that follows sleep deprivation. As intriguing as this role in sleep regula-tion has grown for adenosine, in transgenic mice in which the A1 adenosine receptor had been knocked out constitutively, no difference in sleep-wake pattern could be observed between the knock-out mice and non-transgenic litter mate mice. Obviously, some other brain systems can also regulate sleep. The reader should not be surprised.

ATP AS A TRANSMITTER

Gaining acceptance of the concept that ATP should be considered as a neurotransmitter proved to be far more elusive than the saga surrounding adenosine. The hero of this campaign was the physiologist Geoffrey Burnstock, who recognized that sympathetic nerves could still transmit inhibitory junctional potentials to their smooth muscle targets in the presence of potent antagonists of both acetylcholine and norepinephrine. Furthermore, his experiments later demonstrated that these potentials were blocked by tetrodotoxin, a Na channel-blocking, lethal puffer fish toxin that abolishes nerve conduction. The latter observation strongly suggested that intramural nerves were the source of the nonadrenergic, noncholinergic (NANC) transmission. Pursuit of this NANC transmitter eventually satisfied several of the criteria for its identification as ATP:

1. Stimulation of the intramural nerves released ATP.

2. Quinacrine, a fluorescent dye known to bind to high levels of ATP, histochemically reacted with intramural neurons.

3. Close application of ATP to the smooth muscle target mimicked the effects of transmural stimulation.

4. α,β-Methylene ATP, a slowly degradable analogue of ATP, blocked the responses to both ATP and transmural stimulation of the NANC potentials.

Nevertheless, because of the much more prominent role of ATP as an intracellular energy source, its possible role as a transmitter was not readily accepted, even though it later became quite clear that the catecholamine-storing synaptic vesicles were quite rich in ATP, which in part helped stabilize the amines in the vesicles through formation of ternary complexes. The fact that potent extracellular (or ecto-) ATPases were found in most tissues was taken either as a sign of an extracellular role for ATP as a messenger or as a barrier to ATP signaling, depending on one's perspective. However, as with neuropeptides, the concept of ATP being a cotransmitter with either norepinephrine in sympathetic nerves or acetylcholine in parasympathetic nerves has now been generally accepted: The ATP is released rapidly, and this sets the stage for the later, more prolonged responses to the classical autonomic and other central first messengers. Local administration of ATP has been reported to activate the secretion of vasopressin from hypothalamic neurons of the paraventricular nucleus and to activate vasopressor responses when applied to neurons of the ventrolateral medulla, while administration of ATP into the nucleus tractus solitarius of awake rats yields pressor responses and bradycardia dependent in part on exactly where within the nucleus tractus solitarius the injection is made. Much opportunity for further work exists here, especially with regard to determining which P2 receptor types are responsible.

After Burnstock and colleagues set the foundation for ATP as the mediator of NANC junctional transmission in autonomically innervated smooth muscle and glands, the pharmacological exploration accelerated. Although it was originally observed that α,β-methylene ATP is more potent on purine receptors in the vas deferens and arteriolar smooth muscle, other ATP responsive sites have been found, aided by patch clamp recording, on other smooth muscles on which α,β-methylene ATP is relatively ineffective and 2-methlythio ATP is the more potent analogue. In true pharmacological tradition, these receptors were promoted as separate receptor systems and designated as either "P2X" (where α,β-methylene ATP was predominant) or "P2Y" (where 2-methlythio ATP was predominant). During the next few years, the P2 receptor family expanded to several members of the alphabet, but it was quite unclear how large or complex this family might eventually grow to be. Enter receptor cloning.

The receptors for the responses originally labeled P2X were in fact the tip of a small iceberg of ionotropic receptors (receptors that directly regulate ion channel state as open or closed; see Chapter 2). The P2X receptors, of which seven subtypes have been molecularly distinguished, consist of two transmembrane domain subunits in a trimeric or hexameric configuration with a large extracellular loop containing the ATP binding site. In the brain, three of these P2X receptors predominate: $P2X_2$ and $P2X_4$ are homomeric receptors (all subunits the same), whereas the $P2X_4/X_6$ are mixed or heteromeric receptors. An inhibitory cross talk has been reported for the $P2X_2$ receptors and nicotinic and $5-HT_3$ receptors. The distribution of these receptors within the brain is extensive but not ubiquitous, being expressed in cerebral cortex; hippocampus; habenula; substantia nigra pars compacta; the ventromedial, arcuate, supraoptic, and paraventricular hypothalamic nuclei; as well as the vagal complex and nucleus of the solitary tract, cerebellum, and spinal cord (dorsal greater than ventral).

On the other hand, the receptor family represented by the original P2Y receptor (more sensitive to α,β-methylene ATP) turns out to have been a G protein-coupled receptor, and so the later cloned G protein-coupled purine receptors were all placed in the P2Y subfamily. At least 10 different P2Y receptor gene products have been cloned and characterized. These receptors have the molecular configuration typical of G protein-coupled receptors, with seven presumptive transmembrane hydrophobic domains. Several of the P2Y receptors are heavily expressed in brain: $P2Y_1$, $P2Y_6$, and $P2Y_{11-14}$. The $P2Y_1$ receptor is most highly expressed in striatum, nucleus accumbens, putamen and globus pallidus, hippocampus, cerebellum, and many but not all regions of the human cerebral cortex. The $P2Y_1$, $P2Y_{12}$, and $P2Y_{13}$ receptors are currently considered as "ADP preferring" and recognize both nucleotides. Several P2Y receptors also recognize uridine as well as adenine nucleotides. The $P2Y_{14}$ receptor is activated by both adenine and uridine nucleotides, but it is the only member of the P2Y family to respond to nucleotide sugars, UDP glucose and UDP galactose. The $P2Y_1$, $-Y_2$, $-Y_4$, and $-Y_6$ receptors are all linked to activation of phospholipase C, and $P2Y_{12}$ is linked to inhibition of adenylate cyclase.

The molecular events associated with ATP cotransmission are currently a hotbed of activity, with the intent to develop novel ligands with the potency, selectivity, and bioavailability to characterize functions of P2 receptors in the intact animal and thereby better understand their roles in physiology and pathophysiology. Although most attention has been devoted to the short-term actions of the co-released ATP in neurotransmission as a means to enhance the effects of the cotransmitter amine or peptide, it has also been proposed that the ATP message may have longer-term trophic effects that could be pertinent to some sort of neuroprotective effect.

P2Y receptor antagonists have been proposed as potential neuroprotective agents in the brain by modulation of Glu-induced currents at AMPA receptors (see Chapter 5) and by excessive activation of glutamate receptor systems generically implicated in the apoptotic cellular death associated with stroke, epileptic seizures, and neurodegenerative diseases such as Alzheimer's disease, Parkinson's disease, and amyotrophic lateral sclerosis. Endogenous ATP has been claimed to be involved in the regulation of anxiety via stimulation of $P2Y_1$ receptors in the dorsomedial hypothalamus in rats. Currently, none of these therapeutic entities are known to be in the developmental pipeline.

SELECTED REFERENCES

Basheer, R., R. E. Strecker, M. T. Thakkar, and R. W. McCarley (2004). Adenosine and sleep–wake regulation. *Prog. Neurobiol.* 73, 379–396.

Burnstock, G. (2006). Historical review: ATP as a neurotransmitter. *Trends Pharmacol. Sci.* 27, 166–176.

Burnstock, G. (2007). Physiology and pathophysiology of purinergic transmission. *Physiol. Rev.* 87, 659–797.

Burnstock, G. and M. Williams (2000). P2 purinergic receptors: Modulation of cell function and therapeutic potential. *J. Pharmacol. Exp. Ther.* 295, 862–869.

Drury, A.N. and A. Szent-Gyorgyi (1929). The physiological activity of adenine compounds with especial reference to their action upon the mammalian heart. *J. Physiol.* 68, 213–237.

Dunwiddie, T. V. and S. A. Masino (2001). The role and regulation of adenosine in the central nervous system. *Annu. Rev. Neurosci.* 24, 31–55.

Illes, P. and J. A. Ribeiro (2004). Molecular physiology of P2 receptors in the central nervous system. *Eur. J. Pharmacol.* 483, 5–17.

North, R. A. and Barnard, E. A. (1997). Nucleotide receptors. *Curr. Opin. Neurobiol.* 7, 346–357.

Other Interneuronal Signals

The previous chapters were devoted to what we might now consider the "classical" or perhaps "conventional" neurotransmitters. By this, we mean those transmitters that are synthesized within the neuron (cell body or synaptic terminal) that releases them by activity-dependent, Ca^{2+}-dependent mechanisms to act on discrete receptors largely, but not exclusively, on the neuron, smooth muscle, or gland cell opposite the nerve terminal. However, as the wheels of progress have turned, it seems that once again the more we learn about intercellular communication in the nervous system, the more complicated the situation becomes. The purine signals discussed in Chapter 11 provided an appetizer by acting both pre- and postsynaptically, as do many of the other classical transmitters. Nevertheless, through improved methods of substance identification and detection of signal responsiveness, several potent interneuronal signals have been recognized that are not stored in vesicles, or even stored at all, but rather seem to be synthesized and released on demand to act more broadly than the immediate-releasing neuron terminals and to modify the effectiveness of the conventional interneuronal signals.

PROSTAGLANDINS

The prostaglandins are a group of biologically active derivatives of arachidonic acid often referred to as eicosanoids for their basic 20-carbon atom structure.

The two major pathways of eicosanoid metabolism are the cyclooxygenase pathway, which yields the prostaglandins and thromboxanes, and the lipoxygenase pathway, which yields the leukotrienes. A minor pathway termed epoxygenase yields epoxides, which have received scant attention in the central nervous system (CNS). Arachidonic acid is synthesized on demand from dietary linoleic acid by either a G protein-regulated phospholipase A_2 or diglyceride lipase activation (Fig. 12–1), and it yields a very broad array of bioactive metabolites, as shown in Figure 12–2. The three major groups of arachidonic acid-derived metabolites are the prostaglandins, thromboxanes, and leukotrienes.

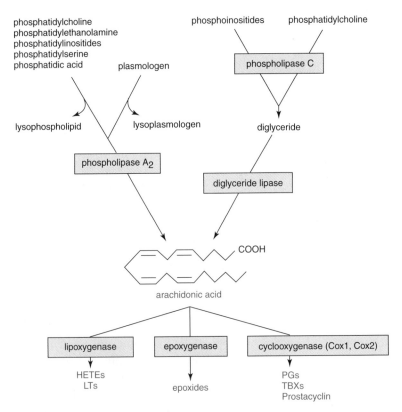

FIGURE 12–1. Pathways for the generation and metabolism of arachidonic acid. Arachidonate can arise directly from phospholipids through the action of phospholipase A_2 or prior action of phospholipase C, followed by the action of diglyceride lipase. Alternatively, the diglyceride may be phosphorylated to phosphatidic acid by the action of diglyceride kinase, and arachidonate can then be released through the action of phospholipase A_2. The released arachidonate may then be metabolized by lipoxygenase, cyclooxygenase, or epoxygenase enzymes to form leukotrienes (LTs), hydroxyeicosatetraenoic acids (HETEs), prostaglandins (PGs), thromboxanes (TBXs), and epoxides. (Modified from Axelrod et al., 1988.)

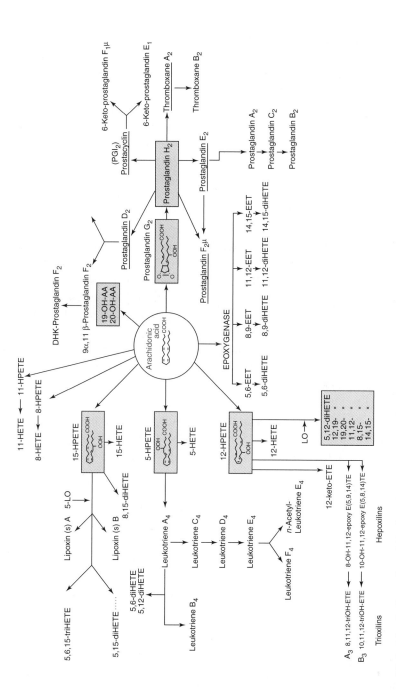

FIGURE 12-2. Metabolism of arachidonic acid (AA) by cyclooxygenase, lipoxygenases (LO), epoxygenase, and corresponding end products (prostanoids). PGI$_2$, prostaglandin I$_2$; HETE, hydroxyeicosatetraenoic acid. (From Schaad et al., 1991.)

Historically, the earliest effect of prostaglandins arose with the recognition in the 1930s that fresh semen could induce contraction of myometrial muscle, and the name arose from the factor's anticipated origin. As chemical detection methods improved in the 1950s, two classes of prostaglandins were recognized—a PGE class that was soluble in ether and a PGF class soluble in phosphate buffer (*fosfat* in Swedish)—and one of their sites of synthesis localized to seminal vesicles. Subsequent work indicated that virtually every organ could manufacture prostaglandins, and several distinct synthetic pathways were recognized. A major advancement occurred when John Vane proposed that aspirin and several other nonsteroidal anti-inflammatory drugs (NSAIDs) worked by inhibiting the prostaglandin-synthesizing enzyme cyclooxygenase. Work in the 1990s revealed that a second cyclooxygenase (COX-2) (and perhaps a third) was also present in the CNS. Since this enzyme was shown to be induced by inflammatory cytokines, it immediately suggested a separate target for relief of inflammatory pain, with the potential for reduced symptoms from the gastrointestinal tract irritation typically evoked by NSAIDs. COX-2 is also induced *in vitro* by the neurotransmitter GLU and inhibited by glucocorticoids. Unfortunately, prolonged use of COX-2 inhibitors has untoward cardiovascular side effects, leading to multiple litigious claims and diverting attention from this once-promising therapeutic modification.

It is well known that the eicosanoids, particularly the prostaglandin series, play an important modulatory role in nervous tissue, but it has been difficult to write a lucid account of specifically how and where they act. This is primarily due to the fact that they are not stored in tissues, nervous or other, but synthesized on demand, particularly in pathophysiological conditions. They act briefly (some with a half-life of seconds) and at extremely low concentrations (10^{-10} M). Although indomethacin is a good inhibitor of cyclooxygenase-1, blocking the conversion of arachidonic acid to prostaglandins, there are few specific inhibitors available to block lipoxygenase and epoxygenase. Thus, although it had been postulated that the E series of prostaglandins modulates noradrenergic release, blocks the convulsant activity of pentylenetetrazol, strychnine, and picrotoxin (possibly by increasing the level of γ-aminobutyric acid [GABA] in the brain), and increases the level of cAMP in cortical and hypothalamic slices, these effects were noted *in vitro* with the addition of substantial amounts of the prostaglandins. There was very little evidence in intact animals to support these neuronal findings. Since we skeptics all hold "*in vivo* veritas" in higher regard, the physiological relevance of the effect was in doubt.

Subsequently, however, direct evidence has established arachidonic acid and lipoxygenases as second messengers. The cascade begins with the binding of a neuroactive agent to its receptor. Then, according to findings from the

Axelrod laboratory, the receptor is coupled to G proteins, which may either activate or inhibit phospholipase A_2, although this has not been conclusively established for all neural tissues. The activated enzyme promotes the release of arachidonic acid, which will then act intracellularly as a second messenger. Arachidonic acid and its metabolites can also leave the cell to act extracellularly as first messengers on neighboring cells. Eicosanoids have been shown to mediate the somatostatin-induced opening of an M channel in hippocampal pyramidal cells and the release of VIP in mouse cerebral cortical slices. At the supracellular level, prostaglandins of the E series have been held to be a mediator of fever and prostaglandins of the D series as regulators of sleep. It is thus becoming clear, despite enormous technological difficulties in assaying eicosanoids, that these agents are major messengers.

Another exciting chapter of the arachidonic acid story has been told separately, namely the endocannabinoids, which are described later in this chapter.

NEUROSTEROIDS

According to their discoverer, Etienne Baulieu, neurosteroids are those steroids that are synthesized in the nervous system either *de novo* from cholesterol or by *in situ* metabolism of blood-borne precursors but are found at levels in the nervous system that are independent of steroid synthesis by adrenals or gonads. Such steroids include at least two previously known steroid precursors, pregnenalone (PREG) and dehydroepiandrosterone (DHEA), that in the nervous system have effects alone or as sulfated esters. In the central and peripheral nervous systems, neurosteroid synthesis has been attributed to oligodendrocytes, astrocytes, and neurons. The peripheral benzodiazepine receptor found on the mitochondrial outer membrane has been suggested to allow cholesterol access to the P450 cleavage enzyme complex on the inner mitochondrial membrane, leading to PREG formation and subsequently to other neurosteroids (Fig. 12–3).

In contrast to the endocrine actions of adrenal steroids on the brain, acting at a distance and at very low concentrations, neurosteroids are thought to act locally as either autocrine (acting on the cells that synthesizes them) or paracrine (acting on cells close to the site of synthesis) signals. In this manner, the ability to activate myelin synthesis in oligodendrocytes may provide a reparative effect in multiple sclerosis. In their sulfated ester forms, both PREG and DHEA have been reported to be potent regulators of $GABA_A$ and NMDA receptor functions, with PREG-S and DHEA-S inhibiting the effects of GABA; however, these effects on the GABA receptor are reduced if the complex contains a δ subunit.

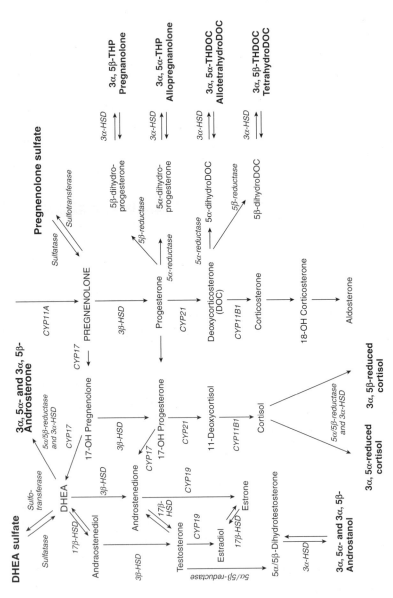

FIGURE 12–3. Biosynthetic pathways from cholesterol to the major neurosteroid end products produced in the central nervous system (Adapted from Morrow, 2007).

In addition, further characterization of the neurosteroids suggests that a small group of pregnenolone-, progesterone-, or tetrahydrodeoxycorticosterone-derived catabolites are the active moieties in the CNS, namely $3\alpha,5\alpha$- and $3\alpha,5\beta$-androsterone, $3\alpha,5\beta$-THP pregnenolone, $3\alpha,5\alpha$-THP allopregnenolone, $3\alpha,5\alpha$-THDOC allotetrahydroDOC, $3\alpha,5\beta$-THDOC tetrahydroDOC, and $3\alpha,5\alpha$- and $3\alpha,5\beta$-androstanol (Morrow, 2007). These are the neurosteroids that are believed to be responsible for the largely GABA-enhancing actions to induce anxiolytic, sedative, and anticonvulsant activity through allosteric modifications at discrete sites on the receptor. Of interest is that systemic doses of ethanol at low to moderate pharmacological levels induce elevation of neurosteroids to levels capable of modifying GABA receptors and contributing to the cellular and behavioral effects of ethanol (see Chapter 18).

NITRIC OXIDE

In 1980, Furchgott and Zawadzki observed that stimulation of vascular endothelium released a factor that relaxed blood vessels. This factor, referred to as the endothelium-derived relaxing factor, was subsequently identified by the Moncada laboratory as nitric oxide (NO). Acting as a second messenger, NO is now known to be involved in an incredible number of systems. Aside from its role in the nervous system, NO is a mediator in the cardiovascular, renal, pulmonary, endocrine, and immune systems, where it is the primary mediator of the bactericidal and tumoricidal actions of macrophages.

NO is synthesized from arginine via the enzyme NO synthase (NOS), a flavin adenine dinucleotide and flavin mononucleotide enzyme, requiring molecular O_2 and with reduced nicotinamide–adenine dinucleotide phosphate as coenzyme and tetrahydrobiopterin as cofactor. The neuronal and endothelial enzyme that is constitutively expressed (cNOS) is activated by Ca^{2+} and calmodulin, whereas the macrophage enzyme that is inducible by cytokines (iNOS) is not. A third form of NOS specifically expressed in neurons (nNOS; also known as NOS-1) is activated by GLU acting at NMDA receptors. nNOS is also a substrate for at least three kinases that are activated by second messengers (see Chapter 4), including cAMP-activated protein kinase A, Ca/calmodulin-dependent protein kinase, and the diacylglycerol activated protein kinase C. After phosphorylation, nNOS activity is reduced. Thus, NO sits within several transductive cascades allowing for precise control of its own modulatory actions.

The synthetic reaction sequence in the brain is shown in Figure 12–4. An unusual feature of this enzyme is that it is a member of the family of cytochrome P450 proteins, which catalyze the hydroxylation of a variety of metabolites as well as drugs.

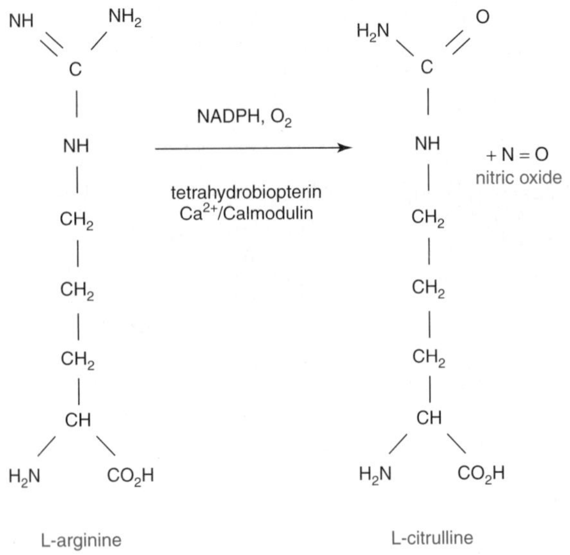

FIGURE 12–4. Synthesis of nitric oxide.

NO synthase is inhibited by a variety of arginine analogs, and this finding has proven to be invaluable in delineating the functions of NO *in vivo*. NO is destroyed by reacting with hemoglobin and other iron-containing compounds. Interestingly, vasodilators such as nitroprusside and nitroglycerin produce NO, and this is considered to be their mechanism of action.

NADPH diaphorase immunoreactivity is co-localized in most, but not all, cells with NOS activity. Detailed analysis of its intracellular location suggests that through its PDZ domain, nNOS is closely, but reversibly, associates with the postsynaptic density protein, PSD95, which in turn also binds the NMDA receptor. Their close association probably accounts for the ability of NMDA receptor occupancy to activate NOS. However, as noted previously, NO is not stored in synaptic vesicles as are most other interneuronal signals but, rather, is released on synthesis for short-range and brief effects on a variety of enzymes and other reactive targets.

The first and primary action of this gaseous molecule is to complex the iron of soluble guanylyl cyclase to stimulate the enzyme and increase the concentration of cGMP. The rise in cGMP will activate cGMP-dependent protein kinases, which catalyze the phosphorylation of substrate proteins, largely unidentified, which then give rise to myriad effects. NO can produce a similar conformational change in the metal centers of other enzymes as well, including cytochrome C oxidase, cytochrome P450, ferritin, and cytosolic aconitase. The latter enzyme can also bind the mRNA for ferritin in cells that are iron depleted, for which it is termed the *iron regulatory protein* (IRP). NMDA transmission mediated by NO enhances this transition to IRP and decreases aconitase activity, perhaps shifting energy reserves to protect neurons during hypoxic periods.

NO also acts to S-nitrosylate cysteine residues on several protein substrates, including ion channels, ion transporters, and several metabolic enzymes. These properties constitute the basis for a growing connection between NO and both protective and toxic effects of NO release, from protein misfolding to mitochondrial toxicity. Most startling from the earliest studies of NO was that it was incriminated as the mediator of a retrograde synaptic signal now termed depolarization-induced suppression of inhibition (DSI), a process character-ized in the cerebellum, hippocampus, and aplysia. In DSI, a chemical signal is released from principal neurons (pyramidal cells in the hippocampus and Pur-kinje neurons in the cerebellum) and transiently inhibits evoked inhibitory postsynaptic currents mediated by GABA release from the terminals of intrin-sic interneurons. The current primary competitive factor for this retrograde signaling is the endocannabinoids.

CARBON MONOXIDE

Another gaseous molecule, carbon monoxide (CO), has garnered attention as a neuromodulating second messenger that also activates guanylyl cyclase. CO is generated via heme oxygenase, the enzyme that in erythrocytes, near the end of their life cycle, catalyzes the conversion of heme to biliverdin, thereby liberating CO. Three heme oxygenases, expressed by separate genes, have been described. Heme oxygenase-1 is inducible and localized mainly in the spleen and liver, with a small (but inducible) concentration in glial cells and in a few neurons. In con-trast, heme oxygenase-2 (HO2) and heme oxygenase-3 are constitutive enzymes and are not inducible. HO2 is found in high concentrations in the brain, particu-larly cerebellum, olfactory bulb, and hippocampus. It is not present in glial cells under normal conditions, but it can be activated by protein kinase C.

As noted previously, CO, like NO, raises the level of cGMP. Whereas the localization of NO synthase does not always correlate with the localization of guanylyl cyclase, the localization of heme oxygenase and guanylyl cyclase is virtually identical and coincides with the presence of cytochrome P450 reductase, a necessary electron donor for heme oxygenase as well as NO syn-thase. The most credible proof for an interneuronal signal mediated by CO is based on the study of enteric neurons of the myenteric plexus, where nNOS and HO2 are co-localized in many neurons. However, mice made deficient in both enzymes by genetic manipulations have virtually no evidence of residually nonadrenergic, noncholinergic transmission of the type attributed to purines in Chapter 11. These mice also show little evidence of cGMP levels and soluble guanylate cyclase activity.

In olfactory neurons, also rich in HO2, HO inhibitors reduce cGMP levels and inhibit the activation of guanyl cyclase in response to odorants. In cultured mammalian olfactory neurons, direct production of CO has been reported. In cultured amphibian olfactory neurons, CO produced by HO mediates olfactory adaptation to odorants by regulating cyclic nucleotide gated channels in a cGMP-dependent manner. Little progress can be expected until better and more selective inhibitors of HO2 are developed.

HYDROGEN SULFIDE

Hydrogen sulfide (H_2S), found in micromolar concentrations in the brain, is a third gaseous signal to which some interneuronal signaling capacity has been attributed. H_2S can be formed by cystathione-β-synthase, and mice in which the gene for this enzyme has been inactivated show no H_2S in their brains. Interestingly, like nNOS, cystathionine-β-synthase is also activated by GLU transmission, and this activity can be further enhanced by Ca^{2+}/calmodulin (Fig. 12–5). Exogenous H_2S added to hippocampal slice preparations in concentrations within the physiological range will facilitate induction of long-term potentiation (LTP) (see Chapter 3) and also raise levels of cAMP. However, mice with cystathione-β-synthase genetically knocked out still retain perfectly good LTP, suggesting more research is required.

ENDOCANNABINOIDS

Just as the discovery of the opiate receptor in brain led to the discovery of the endorphins, the discovery of the cannabinoid receptors prompted a search for and discovery of the naturally occurring ligands (now called *endocannabinoids*). The first was discovered in Israel by Raphael Mechoulam and colleagues, who 30 years earlier had first described THC as the principal active component in cannabis. They succeeded in isolating from pig brain extracts a tiny amount of a fat derivative that was active in the test tube receptor assay and in a smooth muscle bioassay that responded to THC. On chemical analysis, it proved to be a derivative of the fatty acid arachidonic acid, *N*-arachidonyl-ethanolamine, and was named "anandamide" after the Sanskrit word *ananda*, meaning "bliss." Anandamide has essentially all of the pharmacological and behavioral actions of THC in various animal models. Since then, four more endocannabinoids have been described (Fig. 12–6), all of which are derivatives of arachidonic acid and have varying degrees of selectivity for CB-1 or CB-2 receptors. The endocannabinoids are part of a large family of other lipid signaling molecules derived from arachidonic acid that includes the prostaglandins

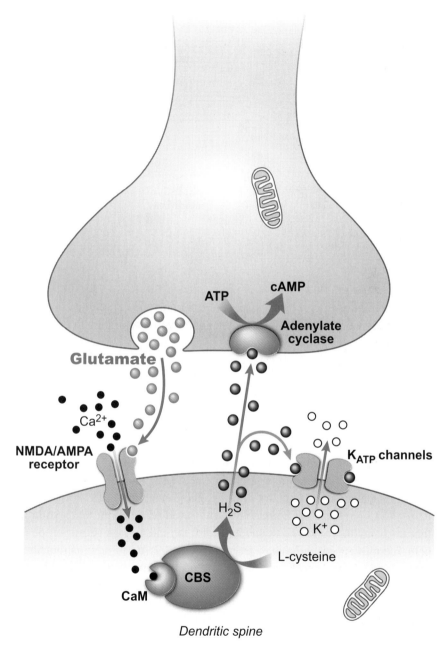

FIGURE 12–5. Hydrogen sulfide synthesis activated by Ca^{2+} entry through GLU channels and the coactivation of cystathionine-β-synthase by Ca/calmodulin; H_2S potentially acts on K^+ channels and presynaptic adenylate cyclase. (From Boehning and Snyder, 2003.)

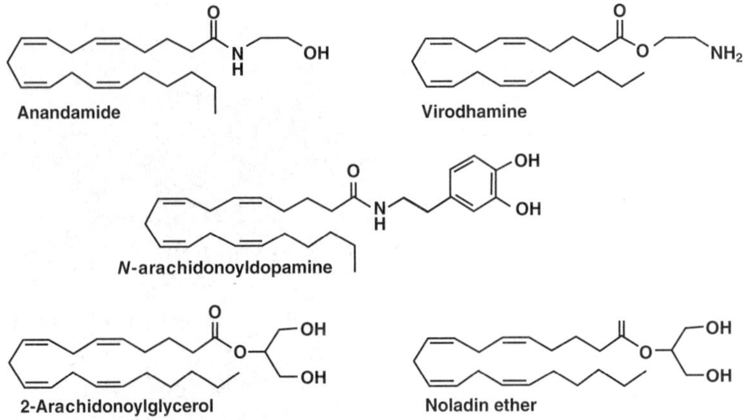

FIGURE 12–6. Endocannabinoids (reprinted with permission from V. Piomelli, 2003, *Nature Neuroscience* 4, 874).

and leukotrienes, important mediators of inflammation. The functions of the natural endocannabinoid control system are only just beginning to emerge.

Biosynthesis and Inactivation of Endocannabinoids

Arachidonic acid is one of the fatty acids commonly found in cell membrane lipids. Anandamide is synthesized by an enzyme known as phospholipase D, but 2-arachidonoylglycerol is synthesized by a different route involving an enzyme known as DAG-lipase. Inhibitors of the biosynthetic enzymes offer an alternative to cannabinoid receptor antagonists in dampening cannabinoid activity, and there has been some progress in discovering such inhibitors. As with the prostaglandins and leukotrienes, the endocannabinoids are not stored in cells awaiting release but, rather, are synthesized on demand. A key stimulus that triggers biosynthesis is a sudden influx of calcium on activation of the cell. The rate of biosynthesis of anandamide and 2-AG in brain is increased, for example, when nerve cells are activated by exposure to the excitatory amino acid L-glutamate. Anandamide release from the living brain can be monitored by microdialysis probes inserted into rat brain.

As with other biological messenger molecules, the endocannabinoids are rapidly inactivated after their formation and release. Both anandamide and 2-AG are broken down by hydrolytic enzymes. An enzyme known as fatty acid amide hydrolase (FAAH) seems likely to play a key role. Immunohistochemical staining of rat brain sections using antibodies against purified FAAH showed that the enzyme was most concentrated in regions containing high densities of CB-1 receptors. More detailed studies suggested that the degrading enzyme might be located particularly in those neurons that were postsynaptic to axon terminals that bore presynaptic CB-1 receptors (see Chapter 24). After their release from cells, a specific transport protein, the endocannabinoid transporter, moves anandamide and other endocannabinoids into cells in which they can be metabolized by FAAH. The rapid inactivation of anandamide accounts for its relatively weak and transient actions when administered *in vivo*.

Physiological Functions of Endocannabinoids

Retrograde signal molecules at synapses

The parallel regional distribution of CB-1 receptors and the enzyme FAAH in brain suggested a complementary relationship between the two at the synaptic level. The existence of a retrograde cannabinoid signaling mechanism has been suggested whereby endogenous cannabinoids released in response to synaptic activation feed back to presynaptic receptors on these axon terminals and are subsequently inactivated by FAAH after their uptake into the postsynaptic compartment. This hypothesis has been supported by neurophysiological findings. A phenomenon known as "depolarization induced suppression of inhibition" (DSI) is a form of fast retrograde signaling from postsynaptic neurons back to the inhibitory cells that innervate them, suppressing inhibitory inputs for 10 seconds or more. In slice preparations of rat hippocampus, DSI induced by depolarizing neurons with minute electrical currents via intracellular microelectrodes was blocked by the CB-1 receptor antagonists AM251 and rimonabant, and it was absent in hippocampal slices prepared from CB-1 receptor knockout mice.

Subsequent research found that retrograde cannabinoid-mediated signaling also applied to DSE (a parallel process involving suppression of excitatory inputs) and to long-term depression, an inhibitory phenomenon lasting several minutes following brief stimulation of neurons in some parts of the brain. These findings suggest that endocannabinoids are involved in the rapid modulation of synaptic transmission in the CNS by a novel retrograde signaling system causing local inhibitory effects on both excitatory and inhibitory neurotransmitter release that persist for tens of seconds or minutes.

Control of energy metabolism and body weight

Endocannabinoids play a complex role in the control of obesity and energy metabolism. It has long been known that cannabis users often experience sudden increases in appetite ("the munchies") (see Chapter 24), and this is probably due to an action of THC on CB-1 receptors in the hypothalamus. CB-1 receptors in fat tissues and in the liver also play an important role in regulating the synthesis of fats from foodstuff. By blocking these peripheral and central CB-1 receptor-mediated mechanisms, the CB-1 receptor antagonist rimonabant may offer an important new treatment for obesity and related metabolic disorders. Rimonabant led to a significant loss of body weight after 1 year (approximately 6 kg) compared to placebo, and this was accompanied by a reduction in biochemical markers of the metabolic syndrome. The compound was approved for medical use in Europe (Accomplia) for obesity linked to cardiovascular risk factors or diabetes, but in the United States approval has been delayed because of concerns about a small but significant incidence of adverse psychiatric side effects, including anxiety, depression, and increased "suicidality."

Regulation of pain sensitivity

Endocannabinoids influence sensitivity to various types of pain. As described in Chapter 24, cannabinoid receptors both in the CNS and in the periphery play a role in modifying pain responsiveness. This situation is complicated in the case of the endocannabinoids because several of these compounds, notably anandamide and NADA, interact not only with cannabinoid receptors but also with another receptor that profoundly influences pain—the vanilloid receptor TRPV-1. This is found in the sensory nerves that carry pain information into the CNS and in some parts of the brain. It is the target for capsaicin, the pungent principle of the Hungarian red pepper. Activation of the TRPV1 protein by capsaicin causes intense pain by activating the pain-sensitive sensory nerves. Paradoxically, anandamide and some other endocannabinoids are also able to activate this mechanism, although not as potently or effectively as capsaicin. Nevertheless, such activation would tend to negate the analgesic effects caused by activation of CB-1 receptors on the same sensory nerves. The physiological significance of this dual action of endocannabinoids is unclear, but it may explain some of the apparently paradoxical effects of the compounds in animal models, in which anandamide can sometimes increase sensitivity to pain rather than cause analgesia. It is possible that the sensitivity of the CB-1 versus TRPV1 targets to endocannabinoids may vary according to the pathological state of the animal.

Endocannabinoids are strongly activated in stressful situations in which pain sensitivity is known to be briefly dulled in some cases (e.g., the wounded soldier or football player does not feel the pain immediately). In an animal model of stress-induced analgesia, much of the effect was blocked by rimonabant, and stress led to rapid accumulations of anandamide and 2-AG in an area of the brain stem (periaqueductal gray) known to play a key role in regulating pain sensitivity.

Cardiovascular control

CB-1 receptors are found in many blood vessels, and cannabinoids relax the smooth muscle of such vessels, causing decreases in blood pressure. However, endocannabinoids do not seem to play an important role in the basal control of blood pressure since treatment of animals or people with rimonabant does not affect blood pressure, and CB-1 receptor knockout mice have normal blood pressure. Endocannabinoid mechanisms may become important in pathological states such as hypertension or in mediating the sudden decreases in blood pressure that occur in conditions of shock—for example, after a sudden loss of blood.

Roles in pleasure and reward mechanisms

People take cannabis because of its pleasurable and rewarding effects. Studies of endocannabinoids and CB-1 receptor knockout mice are beginning to reveal the complex manner in which cannabinoids are involved in pleasure and reward pathways. CB-1 knockout mice display heightened reactions to stress, including increased fear and anxiety behavior when exposed to novel environments or other fearful stimuli. CB-1 knockout mice are less able to forget painful, unpleasant memories. When trained to associate a tone with an electric shock, they are slow to extinguish this memory when tone and shock are no longer paired, suggesting a role for endocannabinoids in the extinction of unpleasant or frightening memories.

Development of a New Endocannabinoid-Based Pharmacology

The discovery and development of drugs that inhibit the inactivation of endocannabinoids via the putative endocannabinoid transporter and/or enzyme FAAH could offer a way to enhance endocannabinoid actions selectively in areas where there was already some activation of the cannabinoid system. Such drugs would be far more selective than externally administered THC or related CB-1 receptor agonists. A number of inhibitors of the endocannabinoid transporter have been reported, but none are completely selective transport inhibitors, all exhibit appreciable activity also as inhibitors of the degradative enzyme FAAH, and some are also capable of activating the vanilloid receptor TRPV-1. An alternative approach has been to develop inhibitors of the degradative enzyme FAAH. FAAH knockout mice have increased levels of anandamide and are very sensitive to anandamide. A number of potent and apparently selective FAAH inhibitors are now available, and their pharmacological properties are promising. In whole animal experiments, these compounds raise pain thresholds and have antianxiety properties but do not cause catalepsy, lowered body temperature, or increased food intake. FAAH inhibitors, however, may not enhance the actions of all the endocannabinoids. The existing compounds do not affect tissue levels of 2-AG, and it may be that a different enzyme, monoacylglycerol lipase, is involved in degrading this endocannabinoid. These early results with inhibitors of uptake or enzymic degradation are encouraging, but it will be some time before they can be translated into new medicines. To be useful, such compounds need to be absorbed when given by mouth, to penetrate readily into the brain and to have a relatively long duration of action. It may take several more years of research to attain these goals.

Reflecting on the myriad mechanisms available to nervous tissue for modulating synaptic transmission, two questions emerge: Could these have evolved simply to open humans' minds to surviving despite whatever the forces of nature challenge us with? and How does all this fine tuning enhance our options for lasting behavioral changes once transient solutions to a new problem have been implemented?

SELECTED REFERENCES

Arancio, O., M. Kiebler, C. J. Lee, V. Lev-Ram, R. Y. Tsien, E. R. Kandel, and R. D. Hawkins (1996). Nitric oxide acts directly in the presynaptic neuron to provide long-term potentiation in cultured hippocampal neurons. *Cell* 87, 1025.

Axelrod, J., R. M. Burch, and C. L. Jelsema (1988). Receptor-mediated activation of phospholipase A$_2$ via GTP-binding proteins: Arachidonic acid and its metabolites as second messengers. *Trends Neurosci.* 11, 117.

Boehning, D. and S. H. Snyder (2003). Novel neural modulators. *Annu. Rev. Neurosci.* 26, 105–131.

Brown, G. C. (2007). Nitric oxide and mitochondria. *Front. Biosci.* 12, 1024–1033.

Calabrese, V., C. Mancuso, M. Calvani, E. Rizzarelli, D. A. Butterfield, and A. M. G. Stella (2007). Nitric oxide in the central nervous system: Neuroprotection versus neurotoxicity. *Nature Rev. Neurosci.* 8, 766–775.

Di Marzo, V., M. Bifulco, and L. De Petrocellis (2004). The endocannabinoid system and its therapeutic exploitation. *Nat. Rev. Drug Discov.* 3, 771–784.

Furchgott, R. F. and J. V. Zawadzki (1980). The obligatory role of endothelial cells in the relaxation of arterial smooth muscle by acetylcholine. *Nature* 288, 373.

Lambert, D. M. and C. J. Fowler (2005). The endocannabinoid system: Drug targets, lead compounds, and potential therapeutic applications. *J. Med. Chem.* 48, 5059–5087.

Moncada, S. and A. Higgs (1993). The L-arginine–nitric oxide pathway. *N. Engl. J. Med.* 329, 2002.

Morrow, A. L. (2007). Recent developments in the significance and therapeutic relevance of neuroactive steroids: Introduction to the special issue. *Pharmacol. Therap.* 116, 1–6.

Muccioli, M., et al. (2006). Fatty acid amide hydrolase inhibitors. *J. Med. Chem.* 49, 417–425.

Nakamura, T. and S. A. Lipton (2007). S-nitrosylation and uncompetitive/fast off-rate (UFO) drug therapy in neurodegenerative disorders of protein misfolding. *Cell Death Differ.* 14, 1305–1314.

Piomelli, D. (1994). Eicosanoids in synaptic transmission. *Crit. Rev. Neurobiol.* 8, 65.

Schaad, N. C., P. J. Magistretti, and M. Schorderet (1991). Prostanoids and their role in cell–cell interactions in the central nervous system. *Neurochem. Int.* 18, 303.

Schuman, E. M. and D. V. Madison (1994). Nitric oxide and synaptic function. *Annu. Rev. Neurosci.* 17, 153.

13

Treatments for Neurological or Psychiatric Disorders: Principles of Central Nervous System Drug Development

The discovery and development of effective medicines for the treatment of a variety of neuropsychiatric disorders is one the great medical achievements of the past 50 years. The great success stories of antidepressants, anxiolytics, and antipsychotics were all developed with limited animal models, no genetic clues, and the involvement of many clever, insightful clinicians. Since then, neuropsychopharmacology research has given us a greatly increased understanding of drug mechanisms and has suggested pointers to future advances.

This chapter briefly reviews the complex processes leading from drug discovery of a potential new central nervous system (CNS) drug to registration and market launch. The six major phases of research and development activity involved can be summarized as follows:

Drug discovery → preclinical → phase I → phase II → phase III → registration

DRUG DISCOVERY

The aim is to discover a potential new CNS drug that is effective in animal models thought to be predictive of clinical efficacy but not necessarily recapitulating the pathophysiology of the human condition. The safety and efficacy of the drug in animals and in human subjects are determined in later stages. Discovering CNS drugs with truly novel molecular mechanisms of therapeutic effectiveness is very difficult and will remain so until greater insight into the mechanisms of the pathophysiology is gained. Many companies have opted for the safer strategy of "me too," making drugs that closely mimic the mechanism of action of existing medicines. Such compounds can offer genuine improvements in secondary factors such as duration of action, improved oral absorption, or reduced unwanted side effects, but they are not quantal leaps forward.

Currently, great hope is placed on the unraveling of the genetic risk factors that predispose people to neurological or psychiatric illness using powerful gene chip and other DNA technology to compare affected and unaffected groups in terms of both haplotypes and patterns of gene expression. This strategy can be complemented by the use of proteomics, searching for alterations in complex patterns of protein expression associated with the disease state. However, although rapid progress is being made in identifying multiple genes that may represent risk factors for disease, it will be a long time before the biological meaning of these findings is fully understood and the knowledge translated into new drug discovery. Perhaps the best example of the success of the genetic approach to date has been in understanding the molecular basis of Alzheimer's disease. In Alzheimer's disease, one of the hallmark signs of pathology at postmortem examination is the "plaques" composed of fragments of a protein of unknown function, named β-amyloid. In some rare cases of familial Alzheimer's disease, mutations in the amyloid precursor protein are thought to lead to abnormal fragments of the protein, releasing potentially neurotoxic fragments that can aggregate into the plaques. This knowledge has helped to unravel the molecular pathology, which in turn has led to the identification of multiple targets (e.g., the enzymes that can cleave the amyloid precursor protein) for new drug discovery, currently the subject of active research and development efforts (see Chapter 16).

Molecular genetic techniques can also be used to create new strains of experimental animals (currently almost always mice). These can represent "knockout" strains in which one can observe the effect of eliminating a putative drug discovery target and perhaps attempt to correct any resulting deficits by treatment with experimental drugs.

Alternatively, strains of mice expressing human mutations identified as causing disease can be created. A prime example is again from Alzheimer's disease research, in which a number of variations of the "Alzheimer mouse" have been developed, which express human mutations in the amyloid precursor protein gene together with alterations in the expression of tau protein or other factors known to be associated with the disease. Such animals come as close as it is possible to an "animal model" of a human disease, and they have proved invaluable in research on this disease. Similar approaches are being used for three other neurodegenerative diseases: Parkinson's, Huntington's, and Lou Gehrig's disease. New methods allow the selective knockout of particular genes in specific organs, such as in brain or even in specific brain regions. A temporary suppression of gene expression can also be achieved by the use of antisense RNA or iRNA methods (see Chapter 2).

After a putative molecular target has been identified, screening of large numbers of chemicals can be initiated to discover potential lead compounds. The molecular target in the CNS is usually a neurotransmitter or neuropeptide receptor, an enzyme, or an ion channel or other cell membrane component. Screening takes many different forms; for example, it may monitor the binding of compounds to the target through displacement of radiolabeled or fluorescent tracers, the activity of enzymes, or the electrical signals generated on occupation of the target by an appropriate ligand. High-throughput screening methods, using laboratory robots, may permit screening of very large numbers of chemicals—as many as 1 million or more is not uncommon. These large numbers of chemicals are generated by combinatorial chemistry, a method that automatically synthesizes a wide range of variants on a particular chemical scaffold, again using robotic techniques. Most pharmaceutical companies have their own "chemical libraries" containing millions of compounds. Such libraries are designed to contain only "druglike" molecules, using the so-called "Lipinski rules," which are named after the chemist who analyzed the common molecular features of the thousands of drugs on the market. These rules restrict molecular weight, chemical reactivity, and lipophilicity.

After a promising chemical lead has been identified, it can be refined by further chemical modifications in a process of "lead optimization," which may yield compounds with improved affinity for the target, greater selectivity, improved water solubility, prolonged duration of action, or better oral absorption properties—factors that are important because most medicines are given by mouth. After this process is complete, the potential new medicine enters a further series of preclinical evaluations prior to testing in human subjects.

PRECLINICAL DEVELOPMENT

General

There are many questions to be answered before the drug candidate can be considered likely to be safe and effective in the intended patient population. We focus on the testing of new compounds in animal behavioral models because this forms a unique and important part of the assessment of novel CNS drugs, whereas other components in preclinical development are common to many other classes of pharmaceuticals.

Chemical stability is needed to ensure adequate shelf life of the product, and metabolic stability and bioavailability also need to be established, the latter by administering the drug to animals by various routes and measuring the resulting plasma levels. The *pharmacokinetic* profile of the drug developed in this way will help to establish whether or not the compound has an adequate duration in the body and to identify major metabolites and whether they have any pharmacological effects on their own. For use in treating chronic CNS disorders, drugs that need to be given only once a day are clearly preferred. For CNS drugs, an added requirement is that they must be capable of penetrating the blood–brain barrier to enter the CNS. There are various methods for assessing this in animals, but initially a simple measurement of drug levels in brain versus plasma will be informative. In clinical studies, the use of imaging methods to establish the ability of the administered test drug to displace a radiolabeled ligand from specific binding sites in brain offers a direct way of establishing CNS penetration.

Establishing the drug's safety in animals is a requirement by regulatory agencies before the testing of a new drug in humans can be allowed. Such safety assessment takes a number of different forms. General safety is established by treating two separate mammalian species with doses up to the maximum safely tolerated dose every day for 6 to 12 months. Biochemical and hematological parameters are monitored in regular blood samples, and at the end of the test period animals are culled and each organ is examined histologically to determine if any damage has occurred. Other *in vitro* and *in vivo* tests will search for *genotoxicity*, assessing the likelihood that the drug induces chromosomal DNA breaks or damage. Other tests in both male and female animals will search for *reproductive toxicity*, changes in fertility or potential damage to the fetus.

Any drug that is intended for chronic human use will also be required to undergo *carcinogenicity* testing, which involves administering a high dose of the drug to two mammalian species every day for 2 years and then examining the effects on tumors or other signs of malignancy.

In vivo pharmacology tests will also establish whether the candidate drug has any unwanted or dangerous effects on peripheral functions, including the cardiovascular, renal, and gastrointestinal systems and the airways. A focus in recent years has been the elimination of effects on the conduction of impulses in the heart, where some drugs can cause prolongation of the so-called "QT interval," potentially increasing the risk of dangerous cardiac arrhythmias.

The Role of Behavioral Testing in Preclinical Evaluation

At its inception, behavioral pharmacology was very much a subdiscipline of pharmacology that emerged as the first widely used drugs for treating psychiatric disorders became available in the 1950s. Since so little was known about the neuropharmacological properties of these drugs prior to the catecholamine revolution, behavioral studies offered an empirical way to characterize and differentiate the major classes of drugs. For many decades, a limited repertoire of behavioral paradigms in rodents provided the means of identifying novel drugs for the treatment of psychiatric disorders. These models remain useful today, but increasingly the challenge has been to understand the psychobiological processes altered in human mental diseases and to devise animal models that place specific demands on the aspects of brain function deemed to be dysfunctional in that disorder. In the early days of psychopharmacology, the term *animal model* often denoted an attempt to reproduce a psychiatric disorder in a laboratory animal. At the other extreme, a more modest goal would be a behavioral response capable of evaluating the efficacy of existing drugs and of detecting similar compounds. This has been termed *pharmacological isomorphism*. Although valuable, this approach is not suitable to detect drugs with novel mechanisms of action. By strict definition, a model is an experimental preparation developed to study a particular condition in the same or different species and involves both an independent variable (i.e., inducing manipulation) and a dependent variable (i.e., the measure(s) used to assess the effects of the manipulation). Hypotheses about the etiology of the disorder ideally inform the choice of manipulation, and the choice of measure(s) is usually based on behavioral abnormalities considered to be core features of the neuropsychiatric disorder being modeled. The variety of manipulations that have proven to be particularly useful pharmacological models are best illustrated in relation to antipsychotics (Chapter 15). Aversive stimuli and stress are used particularly in relation to anxiolytics and antidepressants (Chapter 14). Developmental models, including early lesions or social isolation, and genetic manipulations are also finding an increasingly important place in the behavioral repertoire.

Equally challenging is the choice of measures. Identification of the psychological constructs believed to be affected in the condition would be the ideal way to select measures. Some examples include the impairment of pre-pulse inhibition in schizophrenia, the suppression of responding associated with conflict in anxiety states, and the immobility in the face of unavoidable stress in depressive states. However, many manipulations in widespread use result in profound changes in locomotor behaviors that appear to bear little relevance to a clinical phenotype. An excellent extended review of these points can be found in Geyer and Markou (2002).

The increasingly important field of cognitive neuroscience is identifying neural circuits mediating the building blocks of these complex behaviors. Some, but not all, of these can be modeled in animals. Thus, increasingly, psychopharmacology is turning to studies of normal human volunteers in which the measurement of behavioral responses can be combined with noninvasive brain imaging. This research informs the interpretation of disorders of behavior in terms of neurotransmitters, neural circuits, and the genes critical for their maintenance. As human behavioral paradigms have become available, the process of drug discovery has been transformed. Whereas in the past new drugs were evaluated in psychiatric patients in proof-of-concept clinical trials, increasingly they are evaluated in normal subjects using highly specific tasks of relevance to the psychiatric disorder being targeted by the drug. Promising new drugs can then quickly be moved into clinical trials in psychiatric or neurological patients. However, these are complex and costly studies, and the full range of preclinical evaluation required for new drugs still requires and will continue to require the use of animal tests. The ideal scenario is to have a drug evaluated on equivalent, validated tasks that can be administered to animals, normal volunteers, and patients. One excellent exemplar of this approach is the use of the Cambridge Neuropsychological Test Automated Battery (CANTAB) and its animal parallels to characterize and distinguish cognitive dysfunction in Parkinson's disease (Chapter 17), Alzheimer's disease (Chapter 16), and, recently, psychiatric disorders (Chapter 15). The battery targets a range of higher cognitive functions, notably visual memory, working memory and planning, attention, cognitive flexibility, response control, risk taking, and decision making. A number of the tests have been adapted for use in squirrel and rhesus monkeys using touchscreen technology, and equivalent tasks suitable for work in rodents have also been developed by the CANTAB group.

With respect to preclinical screening, animal and human models of mental illness have always faced the issue of pharmacological validity. Does the laboratory response mirror the clinical drug response? If it does, the model is said to have predictive or empirical validity and will have fulfilled the following criteria according to Carlton: (1) The same range of drugs produce the clinical and experimental responses; (2) the potencies of different drugs should match on clinical and experimental responses; (3) the onset time and the degree of tolerance to the drug should be the same on both responses; and (4) clinical and experimental responses should be antagonized or augmented by the same compounds. An example of the first criterion is well illustrated in Chapter 14, where the use of controlled conflict paradigms provides highly correlated clinical and experimental anxiolytic responses. However, after the first criterion is met, a model still faces the further challenge of differentiating the desired clinical effect from unwanted side effects. Drugs have multiple effects and different combinations of these effects. Carlton suggests the following drug categories: Type 1 drugs both reduce clinical symptoms and have unwanted secondary effects, type 2 drugs have only secondary effects, and type 3 drugs have neither (i.e., they are clinically inert). The ideal laboratory model responds to type 1 drugs and not to the other classes. Some drugs can mimic the secondary effects of clinically efficacious drugs without being efficacious themselves.

This means that the symptom reductions characteristic of some drugs cannot be attributed to these secondary effects; otherwise, all drugs with secondary effects would be efficacious. Antidepressants are excellent examples of type 1 drugs, having secondary anticholinergic effects similar to those of atropine or scopolamine. Antidepressant activity might be ascribed to this secondary effect, but if so, atropine and scopolamine should be clinically effective antidepressants, which they are not. The anticholinergics are therefore type 2 drugs that do not reduce the symptoms of depression and do not show a positive response in validated laboratory models for antidepressants.

The second criterion for a laboratory model is that it should detect the potencies of different drugs in a way that is directly related to the clinical potencies of the same drugs (i.e., laboratory and clinical potencies should match). This is of fundamental importance, and it is critical to undertake wide dose–response investigations in both animals and humans. The correlation of relative potencies is best illustrated graphically, and an excellent example is shown in Fig. 15.2 (Chapter 15), in which the potencies of a wide range of neuroleptic drugs used to control the florid symptoms of schizophrenia correlate highly with their ability to bind to dopamine D2 receptors in an *in vitro* binding study. The third criterion specifies that in both models the temporal onset of the responses should be of the same order and that the development of tolerance to the response (if it occurs with repeated doses) should follow the same pattern. Regarding the temporal onset, there is a striking lack of coherence for antidepressant and antipsychotic drugs, where the experimental response in animals is immediate and the clinical responses require several weeks to emerge. Regarding tolerance, it is notable that when drugs show both symptom reductions and secondary effects, differential tolerance to these effects may be seen. For example, the antipsychotic effects of neuroleptics do not show tolerance, but the acute motor effects do.

How to Evaluate a Novel Psychotropic Drug

In the early days of psychopharmacology, drugs of potential therapeutic value were, after somewhat cursory safety evaluation and extremely basic observations in animals, quickly tested in the relevant psychiatric patients. In a current discovery program, the evaluations of lead compounds proceed within the framework of existing knowledge of the standard classes of drugs in widespread clinical use. For compounds within a particular chemical class, this is quite straightforward if the target is a "me-too" compound with a better separation between type 1 and type 2 effects (i.e., increased efficacy with fewer side effects). It is more challenging when the chemical class is novel and the clinical target does not exactly conform to well-recognized disease phenotypes. For example, in previous decades potential antidepressants were not evaluated for anxiolytic effects and vice versa, whereas a number of newer drugs show both clinical responses. As more refined diagnostic criteria in psychiatry emerged with revision of the *Diagnostic and Statistical Manual of Mental Disorders* diagnostic categories, confidence in the absolute defining characteristics of long-recognized phenotypes waned and novel compounds are now evaluated on a much wider range of experimental models than in the past.

Behavioral Screening Process

The screening process begins with a simple CNS screen, usually tested in mice, designed to detect the effects of drugs on the autonomic and skeletal nervous systems. A range of behavioral and physiological responses are recorded at set times after drug administration. Modifications of a screen originally described by Irwin are most commonly used. One can easily obtain dose–response data, get a good indication of possible side effects, and study time of onset of drug action and its duration. Measures include tremors, ptosis (eyelid droop), temperature, salivation, defecation, hypo- and hyperreflexes, response to pain (tail pinch), motor coordination (rotarod or inclined grid), and catalepsy (abnormal maintenance of distorted posture). These simple screens are also useful for studying drug interactions. Sometimes, drugs have no effect on their own but modify the effect of another drug. For example, antidepressants potentiate the rise in temperature induced by amphetamine, and although they do not increase locomotor activity per se, they reverse the sedation induced by reserpine.

Genetic manipulations, such as knock-outs and transgenic knock-ins in mice, play a central role in attempts to understand how drugs target neurotransmitters in the brain and change behavior. It has therefore been necessary to develop and validate tests originally designed for use in larger animals for different mouse strains.

The second stage of screening consists of studies of simple unconditioned behaviors that commonly involve automated methods of measurement. For example, locomotor activity and exploration in different environments are easily quantified with well-located photocells or computer-assisted video recordings. The "open field" is commonly used to measure exploratory locomotor activity. Animals are placed in an unfamiliar walled space and exploration of the corners or the center of the field, rearing on the walls, and responses to novel or familiar objects placed in the field or to conspecifics can be recorded easily (see Chapter 3). A wide range of other naturalistic behaviors fall into this category of screening.

The third stage of screening consists of more complex conditioned behaviors that assess the response to reinforcement or punishment, the ability to learn and remember, or the ability to attend to and manipulate information in more complex tasks. As we have seen, schedules of reinforcement or punishment play a dominant role in the first of these enabling measurements of the stable performance of acquired responses over repeated testing sessions. In the latter areas, in addition to discrete trial procedures (mazes and shock-avoidance boxes), computer-controlled cognitive tasks (of which the CANTAB is an example) are increasingly playing an important role and are of particular value in developing equivalent tasks for rats, monkeys, and humans. In the final screening stage, the aim is to move beyond empirical validity based on the pharmacological criteria discussed previously to the use of models with face and construct validity.

These are the behavioral tasks in animals and humans targeted specifically at the neuropsychiatric disorder or disorders for which the drug is being developed. Most recent developments rely on mimicking only specific signs or symptoms associated with the psychopathological conditions, rather than attempting to model the entire syndrome. For example, drugs for treating memory impairment in Alzheimer's disease are usefully evaluated using the Morris water maze (see Chapter 16), but ultimately a task that puts pressure on the ability to hold and manipulate information in recent memory (episodic and working memory) would be deemed of most relevance (e.g., the working memory and planning components of CANTAB). Similarly, although impairment of discriminated active shock avoidance associated with maintenance of shock escape has traditionally been a cornerstone for the evaluation of potential antipsychotic drugs, the antagonism of dopamine-mediated amphetamine-induced locomotor activity or motor stereotypy would now be regarded as tests of more pharmacological relevance for this class of psychotropic drug. It is in this final phase of preclinical screening that some of the most innovative developments in behavioral pharmacology are occurring, with the goal being the reconciliation of laboratory and clinical empirical validity using behavioral measures.

At the heart of this process lies the difficult distinction between face and empirical validity: A model of the clinical phenomenon is not the same as a model of the clinical drug response. It may be fortuitous that the most commonly used empirical animal models of anxiety also have face validity—the suppression of behavior encourages us to believe that the animal is feeling anxious. On the other hand, discriminated shock avoidance, which has been critical in the search for antipsychotics, has empirical validity but no claim to face validity. The ideal model would be useful for both the clinical phenomenon and the clinical drug response. Currently, models of anxiety come closest to this ideal, but for depressive conditions the task remains a challenge, despite some progress. In the field of psychosis, there are few psychological models, and research continues to be heavily dependent on pharmacological models. Additional examples of disease-specific models are discussed later.

CLINICAL TRIALS

Provided that the potential new drug has passed all of the hurdles outlined previously, it can enter the even more complex stage of clinical trials. All of the data obtained in the preclinical stages of pharmacology, safety assessment, and drug metabolism/pharmacokinetic studies will have been in accord with the strict guidelines in the Good Laboratory Practice manual, and the purity of the drug samples used will have been ensured by compliance with Good Manufacturing Practice. Now the clinical tests will also have to meet the standards laid down in Good Clinical Practice guidelines (all the "good practice" manuals are published by the Organisation for Economic Co-operation and Development [www.oecd.org]) and the ethical standards set out by the World Medical Association in the Declaration of Helsinki (www.wma.net/e/policy).

Before starting any clinical trial, permission must be obtained from the relevant regulatory agency—the Food and Drug Administration (FDA) in the United States or its counterparts in other countries. The agency will want to scrutinize the entire package of preclinical data to determine that it meets the required standards and justifies exposure of human subjects to the drug. Before entering the more advanced stages of clinical trial development, the company will have had discussions with the FDA to agree on how large a study is needed and what outcome measures need to be fulfilled to possibly obtain registration of the new drug.

Phase I

The first trials of a new drug in human subjects will aim to determine that it is safe and well tolerated and also whether it causes adverse effects. Such trials are almost always performed in healthy young male volunteers. Initially, the drug will be administered in single doses, starting with very small doses and gradually increasing the dose. If dose-dependent adverse effects are seen, this may establish the *maximum tolerated dose*. Single-dose studies will be followed by further trials in volunteers using repeat doses and lasting for several days. At the same time, measurements of the drug and its metabolites in blood and urine will help to establish the human *bioavailabilty, pharmacokinetics*, and *drug metabolism*, which will not always mirror the parameters measured in experimental animals. The data obtained from phase I trials will help to determine the appropriate dose regimen to be used in subsequent clinical trials and will alert investigators to potential adverse side effects.

A variant on traditional phase I trial design is the use of "microdosing," in which minute doses of the test drug, sometimes radioactively labeled, are administered to volunteers to obtain an initial profile of bioavailability, pharmacokinetics, and drug metabolism. Because the dose used is very small, there is less concern of toxicity and only minimal animal safety data may be needed.

Phase II

Provided that the results obtained in phase I trials show the compound to be safe and well tolerated, and to have acceptable bioavailability and duration, the first clinical trials in the intended patient population can begin. These are relatively small-scale trials with perhaps only 100 subjects. There are several objectives: to establish that the compound is safe to use in the patients as opposed to the healthy volunteers used up to now, to obtain at least preliminary evidence that the compound is effective (i.e., it has beneficial effects on the chosen outcome measures), and to obtain further pharmacokinetic data to guide the choice of the optimal clinical doses. Phase II trials are sometimes subdivided into phase IIa, which has these aims, and a subsequent phase IIb, which will also be in the intended patient population but use the precise formulation of the drug intended for use in the larger phase III trial to follow and in subsequent marketing and also hone in on the final clinical dose range to be tested.

All of the clinical trials involving patients will be controlled to avoid any bias in either patient or doctor. Some patients will receive no active test drug but instead will take placebo pills or capsules that are identical in appearance to those containing active drug. Patients will be randomly assigned to drug or placebo groups, and the code will be held by someone independent of the clinical investigators and broken only when the trial is complete. Different groups of patients may be assigned to placebo or drug, or there may be a "crossover" design, in which patients are treated on two or more different occasions with either test drug or placebo. In either case, in assessing the outcome it will be necessary to demonstrate a statistically significant benefit in those patients receiving active drug versus those receiving placebo. This is a major issue for drugs used in neuropsychiatric disorders, in which a significant benefit is often observed in response to placebo treatment. The placebo effect may be so large that it renders the result with test drug not statistically significant. Even in trials of new pain-relieving medicines, a substantial placebo effect may be seen. However, there may be ethical concerns about giving a very ill patient a placebo rather than an older drug of modest effectiveness.

Phase III

The final stage of clinical development will involve administering the test drug to a much larger number of patients, sometimes several thousand. This will involve multiple medical centers and require sophisticated coordination and data collection. The size of the trial and the exact outcome measures to be used will have been agreed upon beforehand with the FDA or other regulatory body and given the status of a "pivotal trial." If positive outcomes can be obtained in two such pivotal trials, it may be possible to apply for registration of the compound as a new medicine. By their nature, phase III trials are very expensive and usually take a long time to complete and analyze. Even when positive results are obtained in phase II trials, it is not uncommon for phase III trials to fail to yield the expected benefits. In this case, the company has the choice of performing a new and costly phase III trial or abandoning the compound at this stage.

REGISTRATION

Upon satisfactory completion of at least two pivotal phase III trials, the company may apply to the regulatory agency for registration of the compound as a new prescription medicine. This takes place through the formal submission of a New Drug Application (NDA), which contains all of the relevant preclinical and clinical data on the compound. This is a huge data package, and it is now submitted in digital electronic form.

The FDA or other agency will often take 1 year or more to evaluate the contents of the NDA and will usually have a list of questions to be answered by the company or ask for further clinical trials. If successful, official registration will be followed by marketing of the new medicine, implementing a plan carefully constructed beforehand by the company.

In some countries, a further economic analysis may be applied to assess the value of the new medicine to the health service in relation to its cost (i.e., *pharmacoeconomics*). In countries in which the government reimburses the costs of prescription medicines, such analysis may determine whether or not the new medicine will be reimbursable.

In all countries, a *postmarketing surveillance* system will encourage individual doctors to report any unusual or serious adverse side effects seen after treatment with the new medicine. Despite the fact that large numbers of patients are exposed in phase III trials, some very rare side effects may go undetected until the compound enters the market. An adverse event occurring with a frequency of 1:2000 requires exposure of 6000 patients before its occurrence can be guaranteed with 95% certainty. Some serious adverse effects may also be observed only after prolonged periods of treatment, which again cannot be emulated in clinical trials.

The overall process of developing a new CNS medicine is complex and lengthy. It is not uncommon for it to take 10 years or more from laboratory idea to marketed product—a process costing millions of dollars. There are many risks and pitfalls along the way—less than 1 in 10 of the development candidate compounds that make it through the preclinical stages will eventually succeed in gaining registration.

The medical and social burden of CNS disorders is immense and rapidly growing as our population ages, partly because effective pharmaceutical treatments for cardiovascular disease and cancer are available. The psychopharmaceuticals needed to treat neuropsychiatric disorders are usually chronic medications so they need to be safe and effective. There remains an urgent need to continue pharmaceutical innovation in this field.

SELECTED REFERENCES

Bansal, A. T. and M. R. Barnes (2008). Genomics in drug discovery: The best things come to those who wait. *Curr. Opin. Drug Discov. Dev.* 11, 303–311.

Carlton, P. L. (1983). *A Primer of Behavioral Pharmacology*. Freeman, New York.

Geyer, M. and A. Markou (2002). The role of preclinical models in the development of psychotropic drugs. In *Neuropsychopharmacology: The Fifth Generation of Progress* (K. Davis, D. Charney, J. Coyle, and C. Nemeroff, Eds.). Lippincott Williams & Wilkins, Philadelphia, pp. 446–455.

Leeson, P. D. and B. Springthorpe (2007). The influence of drug-like concepts on decision-making in medicinal chemistry. *Nat. Rev. Drug Discov.* 6, 881–890.

Lipinski, C. A. (2000). Drug-like properties and the causes of poor solubility and poor permeability. *J. Pharmacol. Toxicol. Methods* 44, 235–249.

Warne, P. (2003). *How Drugs Are Developed: An Introduction to Pharmaceutical R&D*, SRIP Reports No. BS 1238. PJB Publications, Richmond, UK.

14

Antidepressants and Anxiolytics

THE DISORDERS

Depression and anxiety are among the most common psychiatric disorders. Worldwide sales of antidepressant drugs of more than $20 billion make this one of the most important classes of central nervous system medicines. Although some may think of depression as a form of moral deficiency from which individuals could get better if they just "pulled themselves up by the bootstraps," the reality is that it is an illness, not a choice, and it represents a major cause of disability, preventing sufferers from work and pleasure. It is also a syndrome of different symptoms, only one of which is depressed mood. The diagnostic criteria suggested by the *Diagnostic and Statistical Manual of Mental Disorders*, fourth edition (*DSM-IV*; Table 14–1), make this clear and readily distinguish major depression from normal reactions to life events such as bereavement.

Major depression affects as many as 5% of the population, and the percentage may be even higher because it is commonly underdiagnosed. At the other extreme, mania affects approximately 1% of the population and is associated with persistently elevated mood, decreased sleep, inflated self-esteem, and hyperactivity. Classically, mania and depression are "poles apart," hence the term *unipolar depression* for those suffering only depression and the term *bipolar disorder* for those suffering cycles from mania to depression.

TABLE 14–1. *DSM -IV* Diagnostic Criteria for a Major Depressive Episode

A. Five (or more) of the following symptoms have been present during the same 2-week period and represent a change from previous functioning; at least one of the symptoms is either (1) depressed mood or (2) loss of interest or pleasure. *Note*: Do not include symptoms that are clearly due to a general medical condition or mood-incongruent delusions or hallucinations.

   1. Depressed mood most of the day, nearly every day, as indicated by either subjective report (e.g., feels sad or empty) or observation made by others (e.g., appears tearful). *Note*: In children or adolescents, can be irritable mood.
   2. Markedly diminished interest of pleasure in all, or almost all, activities most of the day, nearly every day (as indicated by either subjective account or observation made by others).
   3. Significant weight loss when not dieting or weight gain (e.g., a change of more than 5% of body weight in a month), or decrease or increase in appetite nearly every day. *Note*: In children consider failure to make expected weight gains.
   4. Insomnia or hypersomnia nearly every day.
   5. Psychomotor agitation or retardation nearly every day (observable by others, not merely subjective feelings of restlessness or being slowed down).
   6. Fatigue or loss of energy nearly every day.
   7. Feelings of worthlessness or excessive or inappropriate guilt (which may be delusional) nearly every day (not merely self-reproach or guilt about being sick).
   8. Diminished ability to think or concentrate, or indecisiveness, nearly every day (either by subjective account or as observed by others).
   9. Recurrent thoughts of death (not just fear of dying), recurrent suicidal ideation without a specific plan, or a suicide attempt or a specific plan for committing suicide.

B. The symptoms do not meet criteria for a mixed episode (i.e., bipolar illness).

C. The symptoms cause clinically significant distress or impairment in social, occupational, or other important areas of functioning.

D. The symptoms are not due to the physiological effects of a substance (e.g., a drug of abuse, a medication, or other treatment) or a general medical condition (e.g., hyperthyroidism).

E. The symptoms are not better accounted for by bereavement (i.e., after the loss of a loved one); the symptoms persist for longer than 2 months or are characterized by marked functional impairment, morbid preoccupation with worthlessness, suicidal ideation, psychotic symptoms, or psychomotor retardation.

Source: Reprinted with permission from the *Diagnostic and Statistical Manual of Mental Disorders,* Text Revision, Fourth Edition (Copyright 2000), American Psychiatric Association.

Bipolar disorder or "manic depressive disorder" is treated with both antidepressants and neuroleptics.

Untreated episodes of depression may last 6–24 months before recovery, but patients will usually suffer recurrent episodes. Regarding the effects of treatment with antidepressant drugs, five terms beginning with the letter "R" can be used to describe the improvement or worsening seen: response, remission, recovery, relapse, and recurrence. The term *response* generally means that a depressed patient has experienced at least a 50% reduction in symptoms as assessed on a standard psychiatric rating scale such as the Hamilton Depression Rating Scale. This generally corresponds to a global clinical rating of the patient as much improved or very much improved. *Remission*, on the other hand, is the term used when essentially all the symptoms go away, not just 50% of them. The patient is not just better, but well. If this lasts for 6–12 months, then this is considered to be *recovery*. However, if the patient worsens before remission has turned into recovery, then this is described as a *relapse*. If a patient worsens some time after recovery, this is described as a *recurrence*.

Anxiety disorders are also common and occur in many different forms. Anxiety can be thought of as a normal emotion experienced in circumstances of threat, as part of the "fight-or-flight" reaction, for example. However, nowadays the presence of anxiety is more often maladaptive and constitutes a psychiatric disorder. The largest group of sufferers can be diagnosed in the category of *generalized anxiety disorder* (GAD; Table 14–2). GAD often

TABLE 14–2. *DSM-IV* Diagnostic Criteria for Generalized Anxiety Disorder

A. Excessive anxiety and worry (apprehensive expectation), occurring more days than not for at least 6 months, about a number of events or activities (such as work or school performance).

B. Difficulty in controlling the worry.

C. Anxiety and worry associated with three or more of the following six symptoms, with at least some symptoms present for more days than not for the past 6 months. (*Note*: Only one item required for children).
   1. Restless or feeling keyed up or on edge
   2. Easily fatigued
   3. Difficulty in concentrating or mind going blank
   4. Irritability
   5. Muscle tension
   6. Sleep disturbance (difficulty falling asleep or staying asleep, or restless and unsatisfying sleep)

D. The focus of the anxiety and worry is not confined to features of an Axis I disorder. For example, the anxiety or worry is not about having a panic attack (as in panic disorder); being embarrassed in public (as in social phobia); being contaminated (as in obsessive–compulsive disorder); gaining weight (as in anorexia nervosa); or having a serious illness (as in hypochondriasis); and the anxiety and worry do not occur exclusively during posttraumatic stress disorder.

E. The anxiety, worry, or physical symptoms cause clinically significant distress or impairment in social, occupational, or other important areas of functioning.

F. The disturbance is not due to the direct physiological effects of a substance (e.g., a drug of abuse or a medication), or to a general medical condition (e.g., hyperthyroidism) and does not occur exclusively during a mood disorder, a psychotic disorder, or a pervasive developmental disorder.

Source: Reprinted with permission from the *Diagnostic and Statistical Manual of Mental Disorders*, Text Revision, Fourth Edition (Copyright 2000), American Psychiatric Association.

overlaps with depression, and it may emerge as the predominant feature in depressed patients who show only an incomplete response to treatment with antidepressants. However, GAD is only one of a spectrum of other anxiety disorders. These include *obsessive–compulsive disorder*, characterized by obsessions and/or compulsions that are intrusive and inappropriate and cause marked anxiety and distress. The obsessions take many forms, as do compulsions, for repeated cleaning/washing, counting, ordering/arranging, and many others. Another group of anxiety disorders includes a number of phobias (e.g., agoraphobia and social phobia); posttraumatic stress syndrome, in which a specific event can trigger a panic attack; and, at the extreme, panic disorder, in which panic attacks occur spontaneously. Anxiety states are also commonly associated with insomnia, a condition commonly treated with hypnotics to aid sleep. All of these conditions can be alleviated in part by various medicines, and these will form the basis of the review in this chapter.

ANTIDEPRESSANT DRUGS

Most antidepressants act by enhancing the neurotransmission of serotonin (5-hydroxytryptamine; 5-HT), norepinephrine (NE), or both (Table 14–3 and Fig. 14–1). They do so by blocking the reuptake (transport) of neurotransmitter, by blocking the metabolism of neurotransmitter (i.e., monoamine oxidase inhibitors; MAOIs), or by direct action on neurotransmitter receptors that

TABLE 14–3. Antidepressant Drugs Currently on the Market

GENERIC NAME	PROPRIETARY NAME, UNITED STATES	PROPRIETARY NAME, EUROPE	MECHANISM OF ACTION[a]	DAILY DOSE RANGE (MG)
Amitriptyline	Elavil	Lentizol	TCA–NE/5-HT	50–200
Amoxapine	Asendin	Asendis	TCA–NE/5-HT	100–250
Bupropion	Wellbutrin	Wellbutrin	Other	300–450
Citalopram	Celexa	Cipramil	SSRI	20–60
Clomipramine	Anafranil	Anafranil	TCA–NE/5-HT	30–150
Desipramine	Norpamin		TCA–NE prefer	100–300
Desvenlafaxine	Pristiq		Mixed NE/5-HT	50–100
Dothiepin		Prothiade	TCA–NE/5-HT	75–150
Doxepine	Sinequan	Sinequan	TCA–NE/5-HT	10–100

(Continued)

TABLE 14–3. Antidepressant Drugs Currently on the Market (*Continued*)

GENERIC NAME	PROPRIETARY NAME, UNITED STATES	PROPRIETARY NAME, EUROPE	MECHANISM OF ACTION[a]	DAILY DOSE RANGE (MG)
Duloxetine	Cymbalta	Ariclaim	Mixed NE/ 5-HT	60–80
Escitalopram	Lexapro	Cipralex	SSRI	10–20
Fluoxetine	Prozac	Prozac	SSRI	20–60
Fluvoxamine	Luvox	Faverin	SSRI	100–200
Imipramine	Tofranil	Tofranil	TCA–NE/5-HT	50–200
Lofepramine		Gamanil	TCA–NE prefer	140–210
Maprotiline	Ludiomil	Ludiomil	NE selective	25–75
Mianserin		Tolvon	Serotonergic	10–30
Mirtazapine	Remeron	Zispin	Other	15–45
Moclobemide		Manerix	MAO reversible	300–600
Nefazodone	Serzone	Dutonin	Serotonergic	100–400
Nortriptyline	Aventyl	Allegron	TCA–NE prefer	75–150
Paroxetine	Paxil	Seroxat	SSRI	20–60
Phenelzine	Nardil	Nardil	MAOI	30–45
Protriptyline	Vivactil		TCA–NE prefer	15–60
Reboxetine	Edronax	Edronax	NE selective	8–12
Sertraline	Zoloft	Lustral	SSRI	50–200
Venlafaxine	Effexor	Effexor	Mixed NE/5-HT	75–225

[a] Mechanism of action: TCA–NE/5-HT, tricyclic drug active on both NE and 5-HT uptake; TCA–NE prefer, tricyclic drug with preferential affinity for NE transporter; SSRI, serotonin selective reuptake inhibitor; NE selective, drug with selective affinity for NE transporter; mixed NE/5-HT, newer nontricyclic drug with mixed action on NE and 5-HT uptake; seritonergic, drug with action on 5-HT/ NE receptors; MAOI, irreversible monoamine oxidase inhibitor; MAO reversible, reversible MAO inhibitor.

regulate monoamine release. Agents that block neurotransmitter reuptake can be further divided into those that are nonselective (e.g., tricyclic antidepressants with mixed action), serotonin selective reuptake inhibitors (SSRIs), and norepinephrine selective reuptake inhibitors (NSRIs). Nomenclature has become a bit unwieldy in that the newer nonselective agents are referred to as

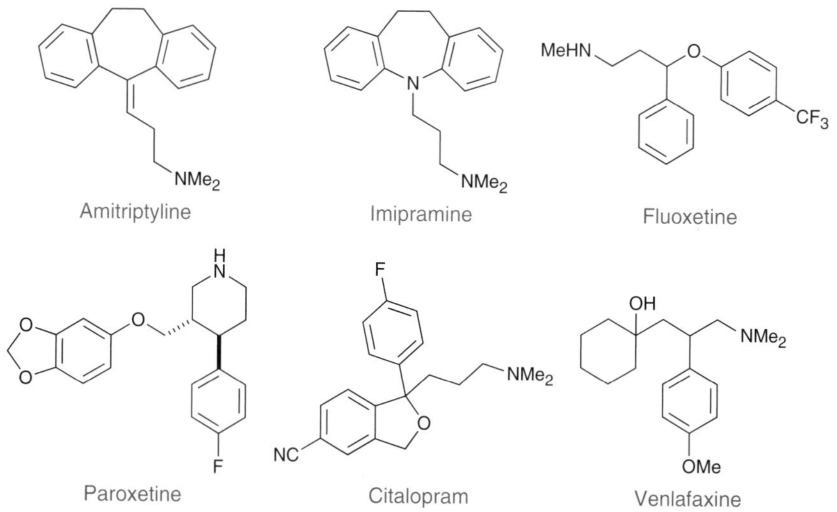

FIGURE 14–1. Commonly used antidepressants.

serotonin and norepinephrine selective reuptake inhibitors (SNRIs) to distinguish them from the earlier generation of nonselective tricyclic antidepressants.

All antidepressants are administered orally, usually on a once-a-day dosing regime. A typical course of treatment lasts 3 months. Clinical trials invariably employ self-reporting of symptoms using standardized questionnaires. The tool most often used is the 17- or 21-item Hamilton Rating Scale for Depression (HAM-D). A positive response to drug treatment is usually defined as a decrease of at least 50% in the baseline HAM-D score.

There are several puzzling features of antidepressant drug action. The first is that regardless of which drug is used, one third or more of those treated fail to show any significant response. All drugs seem effective in approximately 60–70% of those treated, but placebo response rates range from 30% to 50% (Fig. 14–2). Thus, the true efficacy of antidepressant drugs may only be seen in less than 50% of those treated. The high placebo response occurs partly because some patients show a spontaneous remission from their depression during the 6–8 weeks of the drug trial and partly because of the genuine power of the placebo effect, which is particularly noticeable in the treatment of psychiatric illnesses. The magnitude of the placebo effect is exceptionally large in trials of antidepressants, often at least as great as that attributable to the antidepressant drug. In practice, this means that it may be impossible to obtain a statistically significant difference between drug-treated and placebo groups in clinical trials. An analysis of 74 phase III clinical trials for 12 antidepressants submitted to the Food and Drug Administration (FDA) between 1987 and 2004 revealed that only half of these trials succeeded in demonstrating a statistically significant benefit from drug treatment. The placebo effect is variable; for example, it is

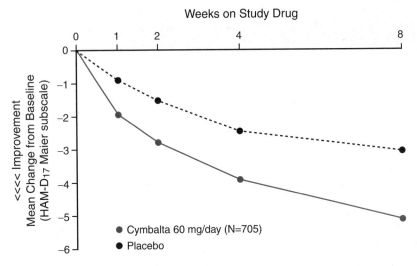

FIGURE 14–2. Typical antidepressant clinical trial data.

Improvements in a subset of the Hamilton Depression score measuring the core emotional symptoms of depression in depressed patients receiving placebo (n = 488) or duloxetine (Cymbalta®) 60 mg/day (n = 706). Pooled results from 4 studies. As early as one week patients in the drug-treated group showed significantly more improvement than those receiving placebo; nevertheless, there was a significant placebo effect. (*www.insidecymbalta.com*)

larger in patients with milder depression than in those with more severe forms of the illness. For this reason, clinical trials that include such patients are less likely to demonstrate any significant benefit from drug treatment.

The various classes of antidepressant drugs exhibit few differences in their clinical efficacy; the advantages of the newer mixed NE/5-HT compounds are related to their improved side effect profiles rather than to a more powerful antidepressant action. This may be surprising at first, but selective NE uptake inhibitors have a similar overall efficacy to selective 5-HT uptake inhibitors, so presumably both mechanisms influence some common downstream mechanism.

A second unexplained feature of antidepressant drug action is that the maximum clinical benefit is not seen until treatment has been continued for several weeks. Although a significant improvement in HAM-D scores can sometimes be detected after 2 weeks of treatment, it takes 4–6 weeks to obtain the maximum response (Fig. 14–2). The fact that all drugs, regardless of their mechanism of action, require a period of several weeks before they become fully effective suggests that they modify gene expression in the brain and that the resulting altered biochemical state takes a long time to become stabilized. Many theories have been proposed, including alterations in the expression of α- and β-adrenergic receptors, changes in transcription factors and/or neurotrophic

TABLE 14–4. Additional Indications for SSRI and Mixed NE/5-HT Antidepressants

Bulimia nervosa

Panic disorder

Obsessive–compulsive disorder

Generalized anxiety disorder

Social anxiety disorder

Posttraumatic stress syndrome

---

factors, and even alterations in the rate at which new neurons are generated in the hippocampus or other parts of the brain. Treatment of animals with antidepressant drugs or electroconvulsive shock accelerates the process of neurogenesis, whereas exposure to stress or corticosteroids has the opposite effect.

However, controlled trials have shown that the glutamate NMDA receptor antagonist ketamine causes an almost instant and persistent antidepressant action, indicating that it may be possible to discover antidepressants that act far more rapidly than the existing medicines. This finding also suggests that it is glutamatergic pharmacology that may offer the way forward in the future.

Depression is often associated with anxiety or other forms of psychiatric disorder, and the SSRIs and the newer mixed NE/5-HT uptake inhibitors in particular have come to be used increasingly in a variety of conditions other than major depression. Table 14–4 summarizes the uses for which SSRIs have been formally approved, based on the finding of significant beneficial effects in controlled clinical trials. In addition, agents in this class have shown usefulness in controlled trials for premenstrual dysphoria, borderline personality disorder, obesity, smoking cessation, and alcoholism.

ADVERSE SIDE EFFECTS

MAOIs

The first-generation MAOIs irreversibly inhibit the enzyme in the brain and liver, leaving patients vulnerable to adverse cardiovascular effects caused by absorption of such dietary vasoactive amines as tyramine into the general circulation—the so-called "wine and cheese" syndrome. The syndrome can include severe headache and hypertension, and it may lead to cerebral hemorrhage and death.

The second-generation MAOI moclobemide selectively targets one form of the enzyme, monoamine oxidase A, leaving monoamine oxidase B in the liver active and capable of detoxifying tyramine and other dietary vasoactive amines.

Moclobemide is also a reversible inhibitor of the enzyme, so its effects are not cumulative. It represents a real advance in terms of its safety profile over the earlier MAOIs, but the class as a whole remains largely out of favor. Another MAOI, selegeline (Deprenyl), is a selective inhibitor of MAO-B. It is also used in treating major depression, and a once-a-day transdermal patch formulation (Emsam) is approved by the FDA for this indication.

Tricyclic Antidepressants

The older antidepressant drugs in this class exhibit a variety of adverse side effects, most of which are related to their secondary pharmacological actions on targets other than the monoamine transporters. Whereas some of these side effects are uncomfortable but not serious, others are life threatening, and the tricyclic antidepressants (TCAs) have only a narrow therapeutic index. Serious toxicity can occur at doses that are only two to six times therapeutic. TCA overdose was among the most common causes of drug-related deaths in the United States in the early 1980s. The most serious effects of the older drugs are due to direct quinidine-like actions on the heart, interfering with normal conduction and causing prolongation of the QRS or QT interval. Death is most commonly due to cardiac arrhythmia and arrest. Other toxic effects include respiratory depression, delirium, seizures, shock, and coma.

In therapeutic doses, the TCAs also cause a variety of less serious unwanted side effects, including cholinergic side effects such as dry mouth and urinary retention, and also histamine H_1 receptor and α adrenoceptor-related sedation. Orthostatic hypotension is another side effect related to α_1-adrenergic blockade, possibly causing syncope and falls in the elderly. Another unwanted feature of the older drugs is their tendency to cause significant weight gain, which may reduce patient compliance with the drug treatment regime. Sexual dysfunction may also be associated with tricyclic use; however, these effects are much more common in patients treated with the newer SSRIs.

SSRIs

Since their introduction in the mid-1980s, SSRIs have become the most widely used of all antidepressants. This is largely due to their improved safety and tolerability in clinical use. Although the SSRIs are no more efficacious or rapid in onset of action than the tricyclics, they lack most of the serious toxicity and adverse side effects associated with the first-generation drugs. The relative absence of cardiac toxicity makes the SSRIs relatively safe in overdose. The relative safety of the SSRIs has led to their being prescribed more freely than the earlier antidepressants and their use in a number of indications in addition to the treatment of major depression (see Table 14–4).

A common side effect in the acute use of SSRIs is nausea, which clinical trial data indicate affects approximately 20% of patients taking fluoxetine, fluvoxamine, paroxetine, and citalopram. All SSRIs also tend to cause sexual dysfunction, including loss of libido, erectile dysfunction, and delayed or absent orgasm. Both men and women are affected, and the incidence of these side effects is quite high, occurring in as many as 50–70% of patients taking SSRIs and 30–40% of all those on antidepressant medication of any kind.

A debate has raged for several years over the alleged association between the use of SSRIs and the occurrence of suicidal thoughts and suicide. However, meta-analysis of the available clinical data has failed to show any such association. Nevertheless, manufacturers of SSRIs are required to include a warning in patient information leaflets about the possibility of suicidal thoughts when patients begin taking the products, particularly when used by children or adolescents.

SSRIs are metabolized by cytochrome P450 enzymes in the liver. Most SSRIs inhibit CYP2D6, fluvoxamine inhibits CYP1A2, and fluoxetine inhibits CYP3A4. Consequently, these drugs may interfere with the metabolism of a number of other agents. Given concurrently with TCAs, they may cause serious adverse effects. SSRIs should never be given with MAOIs because a fatal "serotonin syndrome" has been reported with fluoxetine in this combination.

Bupropion is a weak inhibitor of dopamine (DA) reuptake that has not been widely used outside the United States as an antidepressant. However, it has received a new worldwide lease on life as an effective means of treatment for tobacco smoking cessation (see Chapter 26). It has few sedative, cholinergic, hypotensive, or cardiotoxic properties. However, there are some adverse side effects related to the ability of this drug to enhance dopaminergic function, including insomnia, agitation, nausea, weight loss, and, sometimes, psychosis.

Venlafaxine is an inhibitor of serotonin and norepinephrine uptake, but unlike the TCAs, it has little affinity for muscarinic, histamine, or α-adrenergic receptors. Consequently, it does not exhibit the cholinergic, sedative, or hypotensive side effects seen with the earlier compounds. Nevertheless, the side effect profile includes headache, dry mouth, sedation, and constipation in up to 15% of patients. At high doses, close monitoring of blood pressure is needed because the drug tends to cause hypertension. Venlafaxine appears to have little cardiac toxicity and seems to be safe in overdose.

Trazodone is a weak inhibitor of serotonin uptake and is an antagonist at 5-HT and α_1-adrenergic receptors. These properties appear to be related to the side effects of sedation and hypotension (leading to dizziness) seen with the drug and common at high doses. Trazodone lacks cardiac toxicity and appears safe in overdose.

Nefazodone is chemically related to trazodone but acts in a different manner, largely through inhibition of serotonin uptake and antagonism at

5-HT_{2A} receptors. Adverse effects are mild and infrequent. It is considered safe to use in epilepsy, and there appears to be no overdose risk.

Reboxetine is a selective NE uptake inhibitor that lacks affinity for most of the monoamine receptors. Thus, it does not exhibit the typical side effect profile of the tricyclics. There is no evidence of cardiotoxicity, and sexual dysfunction seems to be rare. In contrast to some of the earlier tricyclics that are sedative, reboxetine is nonsedating and can cause insomnia.

BEHAVIORAL PHARMACOLOGY OF ANTIDEPRESSANT DRUGS

The first clinically efficacious antidepressants came into use at approximately the same time as the neuroleptics. Using the behavioral technology of the time, it was impossible to differentiate these two classes of very different psychotropic drugs. Both imipramine and chlorpromazine were reported to depress locomotor activity and depress operant responding maintained by FR or FI schedules for food reinforcement. In the squirrel monkey, responding for food or shock escape results in equated baseline behavior, and both are reduced by imipramine and chlorpromazine.

However, as more tricyclics and MAOIs came into clinical use and a range of animal models were developed, the antidepressants were demonstrated to have a specific behavioral profile and distinctions between antidepressants emerged. For example, the tricyclics did not enhance intracranial self-stimulation (ICSS) but could potentiate the stimulant effect of amphetamine on reward function. By contrast, MAOIs increased ICSS but, unlike tricyclics, reversed tetrabenazine-induced depression of shock avoidance behavior in the rat.

Animal Models for Evaluating Antidepressant Drugs

Considerable progress has been made in developing models with predictive validity (correspondence between drug actions in the model and in the clinic), face validity (phenomenological similarities between the model and the disorder), and construct validity (a sound theoretical framework) (see Chapter 3). There are more than 20 paradigms of varying value for the evaluation of antidepressants. As we shall see, despite progress, challenges remain. First, although a wide range of these models respond to acute drug treatment, the experience in the clinic is that depressive symptoms take weeks, not days, to respond to drug treatment, at least when used in normally accepted doses. Second, most of these models are thought to reflect pharmacological manipulation of NE, 5-HT, or combinations of both, with or without some effect on DA. The drug discovery process is therefore circular: The existing pharmacological models are capable only of detecting more compounds of the same class. How would antidepressants acting through entirely novel pharmacological substrates be recognized?

More than 30 years ago, McKinney and Bunney articulated the minimum requirements for an animal model of depression as follows:

1. The model is "reasonably analogous" to the human disorder in its manifestations or symptomatology (i.e., it has a degree of validity).

2. There is a behavioral change that can be monitored objectively.

3. The behavioral changes observed should be reversed by the same treatment modalities that are effective in humans. The Carlton criteria described in Chapter 13 underpin the demonstration of this pharmacological isomorphism.

4. The model should be reproducible between investigators.

The phenotype in major depressive disorder is complex in expression and almost certainly in etiology. Therefore, the aim has been to model one or another simple endophenotypic feature (i.e., one clear-cut behavioral output) rather than attempt to model the complex disorder.

Pharmacological Models

The tricyclics and the MAOIs were discovered in the early days of the catecholamine era as drugs able to enhance the availability of NE and 5-HT at the synapse. Catecholamine dysfunction was soon regarded as the biological determinant of depression, and the earliest animal models invoked the reversal of the behavioral effects of catecholamine depletion. Reserpine, a drug that depletes NE, 5-HT, and DA, induces sedation in humans, and reserpine-induced sedation in animals was soon widely used as a first-line screen for antidepressants. Tetrabenazine has similar pharmacological and behavioral effects. Clinically significant antidepressant agents almost universally antagonize this effect of reserpine and other autonomic effects of the drug, including ptosis, miosis, hypersecretion of tears and saliva, and hypothermia. However, some of the newer antidepressants are not consistently active in this model. It has been noted that although reversal of reserpine-induced sedation indicates antidepressant action, drug-induced states of hyperactivity in animals do not. Amphetamine, for example, produces reliable stimulation of motor activity but is not an effective antidepressant. However, the nonselective depletion of transmitters meant that the reserpine model was not useful for detecting drugs acting more selectively on NE or 5-HT pathways or for drugs with novel combinations of action on these transmitters or novel putative antidepressants acting on neither catecholamine nor indoleamine sites. Indeed, early tests based on NE-mediated behaviors did not detect SSRIs. This is equally true of other behavioral endpoints involving nonselective manipulation of catecholamines and 5-HT. These include the potentiation of the behavioral effects of amphetamine, muricide (mouse killing by rats), and stimulation of low rates of operant responding maintained by DRL schedules of reinforcement.

There is thus a continuing need to identify the contributions of NE, 5-HT, and DA to the different endpoints in these pharmacological models in order to maximize their value in detecting selective drugs for treating different aspects of major depressive disorder.

Behavioral Models

The diagnosis of major depression in *DSM-IV* places special emphasis on two core symptoms—depressed mood and anhedonia—and it is generally accepted that stress models in animals produce similar behavioral endpoints. The most important of these are described in more detail, but more complete reviews can be found in Cryan, Markou, and Lucki (2002) and in Willner (1991).

The existing behavioral models have been grouped as stress models, separation models, and miscellaneous and linked to six major depressive symptoms: reduced activity, increased activity, decreased motivation and persistence, impulsivity, decreased social contact, and anhedonia. By far the most significant models relate to stress, resulting as they do in reduced activity, decreased motivation/persistence, and anhedonia. Some appear to model the reduced activity and lack of motivation and persistence, whereas others change the response to rewarding stimuli.

Learned helplessness is an animal model with strong construct validity demonstrating reduced activity, reduced motivation and persistence, and anhedonia. Seligman, in now classic studies in dogs, explored the response to unavoidable and repeated electric shocks in situations in which escape or avoidance was impossible. Conditioned immobility resulted, and animals became unable to cope in new learning situations. This has been likened to reactive depression in humans. The escape deficits seen in rats respond to a wide range of antidepressants, but the behavioral effects are short-lived and can therefore demonstrate only the acute effects of drugs. By contrast, a modification, the *chronic mild stress* paradigm in rats, results in prolonged behavioral changes in sucrose consumption, an effect reversed by chronic treatment with antidepressants with either NE or 5-HT selectivity including the SSRI fluoxetine and the nonselective NE/5-HT uptake inhibitor imipramine.

The *forced swim test* (FST) was developed by Porsolt and is currently the most widely used test for assessing antidepressant activity preclinically and is deemed to result in reduced motivation and persistence. Rats are placed in a cylinder filled with water and have no means of escape. Initially, they show escape-orientated movements, before adopting an immobile posture. The latency to assume this posture is recorded. If replaced 24 hours later, they quickly reassume this immobile posture, interpreted as a failure in persistence to escape or development of passive behavior that essentially relieves the animal of the need to cope with the stressful situation. If treated with antidepressants acutely between the two exposures, escape-directed behaviors persist longer and the rodents are protected against ulcers induced by the stress of water immersion. In mice, only a single exposure is required to generate stable immobility. A wide range of typical antidepressants and MAOIs reduce immobility. However, SSRIs cannot be detected with this form of the model. Some modifications have been made to increase the sensitivity of this test (Lucki, 1998). The depth of the water was increased from 15 to 30 cm and the response measured using time sampling of predominant behaviors over 5-second intervals. Three behaviors are measured: (1) climbing behavior (known as thrashing), defined as upward-directed movements of the forepaws along the side of the cylinder; (2) swimming behavior—crossing quadrants of the cylinder; and (3) immobility—head above the water.

Under these testing conditions, less immobility is observed. Antidepressants targeted on NE increase climbing behavior, whereas 5-HT-related compounds, notably SSRIs, are now active and although they decrease immobility, they increase swimming behavior. Drugs act acutely in the original FST to reverse immobility, whereas in the modified procedure antidepressants are inactive when given acutely but active when administered chronically. This is considered to further validate this model since several weeks of drug treatment are required clinically to achieve mood elevation.

Tail suspension is another model that induces behavioral despair. The immobile behavior assumed by rodents on this task responds to both typical and atypical antidepressants that are not active in other tasks. Unfortunately, a number of other drugs devoid of antidepressant activity also test positive on this task, including GABA agonists, Ca^{2+} antagonists, and atypical antipsychotics.

Models of Anhedonia

Chronic Mild Stress

Since its introduction in 1987, the chronic mild stress (CMS) paradigm has been widely investigated for its validity as a model of anhedonia in rodents. Unlike earlier paradigms in which intense aversive stimuli were employed, in CMS rodents are exposed in the home cage to a variety of different microstressors, scheduled in a relatively unpredictable sequence over a period of several weeks. The consequent almost continuous exposure to periods of water deprivation, small temperature reductions, or changes of cage mates result in a reduction of the intake of a sucrose solution when this highly rewarding stimulus is freely available. Saccharin solution intake is also reduced, and these effects can be measured by free intake or preference in a two-bottle test.

All of these behavioral changes are reversed by chronic but not acute treatment with all classes of clinically effective antidepressant drugs, but not by drugs known to be ineffective as antidepressants. This paradigm has been extensively studied for its reliability; it avoids the use of intense aversive stimuli that are ethically unacceptable; and the effects have been shown to be independent of changes in body weight. Interestingly, CMS increases the duration of immobility in the FST in both rats and mice, suggesting that immobility in FST and CMS-induced anhedonia involve similar brain mechanisms.

Drug Withdrawal

On withdrawal from most drugs of abuse, a behavioral syndrome referred to as the "crash" occurs. This is characterized by unpleasant psychological and somatic symptoms. In the case of psychostimulants, the state shows a remarkable resemblance to the symptoms of major depressive disorder in humans (see *DSM-IV* criteria in Table 14–1) and has been developed in rodents as a model of depression that is proving valuable for screening antidepressant compounds. Pharmacologically, psychostimulants increase synaptic availability of DA, NE, and 5-HT, but after withdrawal reversal of this neurochemical tone induces an emotional state opposite to the initial euphoria and enhanced mood associated with drug intake. This has been conceptualized within a theoretical framework by Koob and others, and it has been described as the *opponent-process theory of motivation.* Withdrawal is associated with anhedonia, lethargy, and anxiety, but unlike major depressive disorder, the effect is transient (days, not months). Nevertheless, these rodent models have face and construct validity for many of the symptoms of major depressive disorder, including changes in levels of sleeping and eating activity and cognition. Depressed mood is difficult to measure in animals, but there is experimental evidence of a dysphoric state during psychostimulant withdrawal. For example, conditioned place aversion develops to an environment associated with cocaine withdrawal, and in a drug discrimination paradigm rats chose the lever associated with haloperidol injection (known to be an aversive drug cue) during amphetamine withdrawal.

Anhedonia can be assessed objectively and reliably in rodents with paradigms designed to quantify the salience of rewarding stimuli, including natural rewards. However, the use of ICSS is the most powerful and sensitive method for measuring changes in the value of reinforcement (see also Chapter 20). This involves quantifying the amount or frequency of current required to maintain responding for brain stimulation. During withdrawal from psychostimulants, rats require a higher intensity of electrical current to sustain brain stimulation. Tricyclics, SSRIs, and MAOIs are active in this model. Interestingly, combining fluoxetine with a 5-HT$_{1A}$ antagonist enhances its effect.

Other Animal Models

Brief mention should be made of the olfactory bulbectomy model of depression. Bilateral removal of the olfactory bulbs in rats results in a complex constellation of behavioral, neurochemical, and neuroendocrine effects, some of which are also seen in major depressive disorder. The rationale for this model is obscure; however, some of the behavioral changes, particularly hyperactivity in stressful situations, are reliably changed by chronic, rather than acute, antidepressant treatment.

Social separation, particularly during development, enjoyed a prominent position in early attempts to model depression in animals. The classic studies of Harlow and colleagues on the adverse behavioral consequences of isolating newborn rhesus monkeys from their mothers resonated with Bowlby's studies of the impaired behavioral development of children separated from their mothers for long periods of time (so-called anaclitic depression). Early adverse experiences of this kind result in reduced social contact and activity, but it is not clear that these changes are indicative of depressed mood or anhedonia. However, in animal models these social behaviors are not reliably normalized with antidepressants, although daily desipramine has been reported to significantly reduce distress and self-directed behavior and reinstate play in young maternally deprived monkeys.

Finally, genetic models are assuming importance in the test batteries for antidepressants. There are marked strain differences in the ability of rodents to withstand or respond to stressors of various kinds, including differences in behavioral and neuroendocrine endpoints. Also, the use of genetically altered mice provides models to demonstrate the involvement of different classes of NE, 5-HT, and DA receptors and catecholamine-specific enzymes (e.g., MAO) in the response to antidepressants.

MOOD STABILIZERS

Lithium, usually administered as lithium carbonate, remains first-line therapy for the treatment of the mood swings associated with bipolar disorder. Although the discovery of its effectiveness in these disorders is one of the major achievements of psychopharmacology in the past 50 years, the mechanism of action remains unclear. Among the suggested mechanisms are inhibition of the enzyme inositol monophosphatase, importantly involved in the metabolism and synthesis of inositol phosphate second messengers; inhibition of the enzyme glycogen synthase kinase-β, an enzyme thought to be important in regulating gene expression; and modulating G protein function.

Chronic treatment with lithium not only treats acute episodes of mania and hypomania but also helps to prevent recurrence of these mood swings.

However, it is effective in only 40–50% of patients, and many patients are unable to tolerate it because of the numerous adverse side effects. These include gastrointestinal symptoms such as dyspepsia, nausea, vomiting, and diarrhea, as well as weight gain, hair loss, acne, tremor, sedation, impaired cognition, and incoordination. There are also long-term adverse effects on the thyroid and kidney. There is a narrow therapeutic window, and for this reason patients require monitoring of plasma lithium levels at regular intervals.

Alternative treatments that have been shown to be effective include the use of certain anticonvulsant drugs, particularly sodium valproate and carbamazepine, although benefits have also been claimed for lamotrigine, gabapentin, and topiramate. A pharmaceutical formulation of valproate called Depakote, which reduces gastrointestinal side effects, is approved for the acute treatment of bipolar disorder and is widely used in long-term treatment. However, it can have a number of adverse effects, including hair loss, weight gain, and sedation.

Classical neuroleptics such as chlorpromazine and haloperidol have long been used to treat the agitation and psychosis associated with the manic phase of bipolar disorders. Atypical neuroleptics, particularly olanzapine, risperidone, and quetiapine, have been increasingly used as long-term therapy, although whether the chronic use of such drugs is beneficial remains unclear.

ANXIOLYTICS AND HYPNOTICS

For many years, the treatment of anxiety disorders was dominated by one class of drugs, the benzodiazepines (Fig. 14–3). The discovery of the tranquilizing effects of chlordiazepoxide (Librium) and diazepam (Valium) was another of the great leaps forward in psychopharmacology in the past 50 years. These drugs were safe in overdose and rapidly replaced meprobamate or the barbiturates that had previously been used as anxiolytics but that could be lethal in overdose.

Both the barbiturates and the benzodiazepines bind to specific sites on the $GABA_A$ receptor and enhance the actions of the inhibitory neurotransmitter GABA (see Chapter 5). For many years, the benzodiazepines were among the most widely used of all psychotropic medicines. Companies developed a wide range of different compounds that differed mainly in their pharmacokinetic properties rather than in any more fundamental way (Table 14–5).

In addition to their effectiveness in treating anxiety, benzodiazepines have other useful actions as anticonvulsants for the treatment of epilepsy, particularly in managing acute seizures (see Chapter 19); as muscle relaxants; and as sedatives, anesthetics, and hypnotics. However, some of these actions may also be considered adverse effects in the long-term treatment of anxiety. Muscle relaxant effects, for example, can lead to ataxia and may make it dangerous to drive a car or use complex machinery. By far the most serious adverse effect

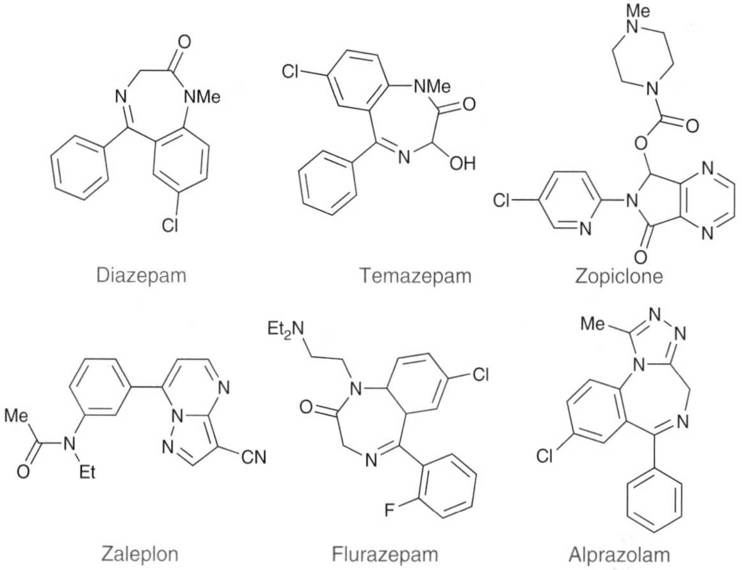

FIGURE 14–3. Commonly used anxiolytics/hypnotics.

TABLE 14–5. Benzodiazepine Tranquilizers and Hypnotics

Alprazolam (Xanax)

Brotizolam (Lendormin)

Chlordiazepoxide (Librium)

Clobazam (Frisium)

Clonazepam (Klonopin)

Clorazepate (Tranxene)

Diazepam (Valium)

Flunitrazepam (Rohypnol)

Loprazolam (Dormonoct)

Lorazepam (Ativan)

Lormetazolam (Noctamid)

Midazolam (Versed)

Mitrazepam (Remeron)

Oxazepam (Serax)

Prazepam (Centrex)

Temazepam (Restoril)

Triazolam (Halcion)

of long-term treatment with benzodiazepines is the risk of dependence. This was only recognized after these drugs had been widely used for many years. This was partly because of the gradual evolution of concepts of addiction and dependence during the latter part of the 20th century (see Chapter 20) and partly because of the absence of evidence from animal studies that chronic use could lead to dependence. This changed dramatically with the discovery of flumazenil, a drug that acts as an antagonist at the benzodiazepine receptor on the $GABA_A$ complex. When animals that have been treated chronically with benzodiazepines are challenged with flumazenil, they display an obvious behavioral withdrawal syndrome, not unlike that seen in opiate withdrawal (see Chapter 20). At the same time, careful clinical analysis revealed that benzodiazepine dependence was not uncommon in patients treated with these drugs for any prolonged period, making it difficult for them to stop taking the drugs because of a craving for the drugs and the unpleasant psychological withdrawal symptoms. For this reason, the long-term use of benzodiazepines in the treatment of anxiety is no longer common, although they may be used for the short-term stabilization of symptoms.

Pharmacologists recognize a spectrum of drug actions on the benzodiazepine receptor, from the full agonists used as medicines to partial agonists and antagonists (e.g., flumazenil) and inverse agonists that act to depress $GABA_A$ receptor function. Some inverse agonist β-carbolines, when tested in human volunteers, proved capable of precipitating unpleasant acute panic attacks associated with fear and a sense of impending death. Although many attempts have been made to develop partial agonist benzodiazepines that might retain anxiolytic effects while lacking sedative or ataxic effects, none of these have been successful.

The benzodiazepines and tricyclic antidepressants were popular in an era when psychiatry viewed depression and anxiety as two entirely distinct illnesses. Nowadays, the two conditions are seen to have very significant overlaps. This is reflected in the fact that the drugs most commonly used to treat anxiety disorders and the related phobias are the newer antidepressants, including some of the SSRIs and the mixed NE/5-HT compounds. Venlafaxine was the first drug to be formally approved by the FDA for the treatment of both major depression and generalized anxiety disorder. It is currently a best seller in the United States, with sales approaching $4 billion annually. The related antidepressant drug duloxetine and the SSRI escitalopram are also approved for the treatment of generalized anxiety disorder. Surprisingly, some atypical neuroleptics (see Chapter 15) also appear to be effective in treating generalized anxiety disorder, and quetiapine, risperidone, and aripiprazole may be used for this indication.

By far the most common use of benzodiazepines is in treating insomnia. Insomnia is associated with a range of different sleep disorders, including those associated with a psychiatric disorder (e.g., depression and anxiety); a painful medical condition; restless legs syndrome; or jet lag. A number of different benzodiazepines, and nonbenzodiazepine compounds (which nevertheless act as partial allosteric modulators at the benzodiazepine receptor; see Chapter 5), are available. To induce sleep at night without causing residual sedation during the next day, drugs have been designed that are rapidly metabolized and thus have short half-lives (Table 14–6).

There are several problems associated with using these drugs for the treatment of insomnia. If the dose used is too high, there may be carryover effects of sedation and interference with memory or other cognitive function on the morning after. Longer-term difficulties are associated with the development of tolerance in many patients so that the medicines stop working after a week or so. To avoid this, it is recommended that patients not take the medicine every night. However, if patients persist in taking the medicines for long periods of time, they may suffer withdrawal symptoms upon stopping them, including "rebound insomnia."

An alternative to hypnotics acting on the $GABA_A$ receptor is the natural hormone melatonin, secreted by the pineal gland and involved in natural circadian sleep rhythms. A sustained-released formulation of melatonin (Circadin) is available in Europe as a treatment for primary insomnia in patients aged 55 years or older.

TABLE 14–6. Sedative/Hypnotic Agents

Benzodiazepines

    Triazolam (Halcion)

    Temazepam (Restoril)

    Estazolam (ProSom)

    Flurazepam (Dalmane)

    Quazepam (Dormalin)

Novel nonbenzodiazepines (PAMs)

    Eszopiclone (Lunesta)

    Zaleplon (Sonata)

    Zolpidem (Ambien)

    Zopiclone (Imovane)

PAMs, partial allosteric modulators (see Chapter 5).

BEHAVIORAL PHARMACOLOGY OF ANXIOLYTIC DRUGS

Compared with the efforts to characterize antidepressant drugs, the operant conditioning techniques of the 1960s proved highly satisfactory in the case of the anxiolytics. At the time, the terms *major* (neuroleptics) and *minor* (anxiolytics) *tranquilizers* were much in vogue. Neuroleptics were active in discriminated and nondiscriminated shock avoidance, whereas anxiolytics were active only in the latter. Subsequent work established that the neuroleptics were manipulating the relationship between the warning signal and the shock, not the effect of the shock per se. By contrast, anxiolytics manipulate the response to the shock, probably through fear mechanisms. This important distinction weakened the significance of the terms major and minor tranquilizers, which suggested a continuum of action in one dimension.

The barbiturates in small doses were used extensively for their anxiolytic properties in the 1950s, before the safer drug, meprobamate, was introduced only to be superseded rapidly by the discovery and clinical adoption of the benzodiazepines. Barbiturates and meprobamate at nonsedative doses were demonstrated to have a rate-increasing effect on behavior controlled by schedules of positive reinforcement. Low rates of responding on DRL schedules were markedly increased and showed rate dependency. However, the use of animal models involving conditioned fear (Estes–Skinner procedure) and conflict were soon adopted as being of special validity in the evaluation of anxiolytics. Classically conditioned emotional responses (CERs) have been widely studied.In the basic paradigm, the unconditioned stimulus (foot shock) is paired with a conditioned stimulus (light), and conditioned freezing is eventually elicited by the presentation of the light in the absence of shock. This procedure has been modified in the potentiated startle paradigm. Rats are first trained to associate a stimulus (e.g., a light) with the onset of foot shock. Subsequently, this conditioned "fear" stimulus is presented with an unexpected loud noise. The elicited startle reflex is greater (i.e., potentiated) compared to the natural response to that noise. This task has been very useful in defining the neural circuits mediating classically conditioned fear responses and is now finding a role in screening for novel anxiolytic drugs. In a further modification of the paradigm that avoids the need for memory of the conditioning experience, acoustic startle is tested in very bright conditions (900 lux) or in the dark. The bright light acts as an unconditioned aversive stimulus. The startle response is greater in the bright condition, and this light-enhanced startle response is decreased by chlordiazepoxide and the 5-HT_{1A} receptor agonist flesinoxan, but the SSRI fluvoxamine is inactive. The Estes–Skinner procedure (see Chapter 3) is another form of CER in which a conditioned stimulus signals adventitious punishment at a later time, and again through Pavlovian conditioning, operant conditioning in the presence of that signal is suppressed.

Conditioned suppression under strong discriminative control can yield baselines that are sensitive to anxiolytic drugs. In a classic study, Kelleher and Morse (1964) trained pigeons on a multiple schedule during which the pecking key was alternately illuminated by orange or white light. In the presence of the orange light, an FR30 schedule for food reinforcement operated until 5 reinforcements had been earned (150 responses). The light then switched to white. The same FR30 for food remained in operation but the first 10 responses in each FR30 run were followed by a 35-ms mild shock to electrodes implanted around the pubic bone. High rates of responding in the orange periods were followed by almost total suppression of responding during the white periods. Pentobarbital released responding during the white periods to almost the same level as responding for food during the orange light periods. When the white light condition was subsequently on throughout the session, total suppression was seen that was released by the barbiturate to levels that would have been expected under food reinforcement (Fig. 14–4).

It is generally accepted that paradigms involving immediate punishment (i.e., consequent on the animal's behavior) yield more reliable results with anxiolytic drugs than those involving adventitious punishment. The discovery of the benzodiazepines prompted the introduction of a wider range of behavioral tasks in animals to measure and distinguish the sedative, hypnotic, anticonvulsant, and anxiolytic properties of this class of drug. The unique effect of these compounds is on behavior suppressed by punishment (see Chapter 3). Meprobamate increased the number of shocks a rat would tolerate in a conflict situation, even when intense shocks were used. The effects of barbiturates were elegantly demonstrated in pigeons using a multiple VI food/VI punishment schedule, in which the drug simultaneously stimulated reinforced responding on the VI for food and released punished responding on the alternate segments of the schedule. However, the effects on punished behavior cannot be ascribed to general stimulation since amphetamine, despite its rate-dependent stimulation of a range of unconditioned and conditioned behaviors, does not release punished responding. On the contrary, amphetamine further increases the suppression associated with punishment.

The Geller–Seifter procedure involving immediate punishment has become the most widely used and reliable model for evaluating benzodiazepines and other anxiolytic drugs. In a classic study, a rat was first trained on a VI-2 minute schedule for liquid reinforcement and then shifted to a VI-2 minute/CRF schedule. The change from VI to CRF was signaled by a tone. The rat experienced 15 minutes on the VI, followed by 3 minutes on the CRF. However, during the 3-minute periods, every response yielded reinforcement accompanied by foot shock of a sufficient strength to virtually suppress all responding during that sector of the schedule (see Fig. 3–5). Initial studies with pentobarbital showed that the drug increased the response rate during the "conflict segment" by 350%.

A

Non-Punished and Punished

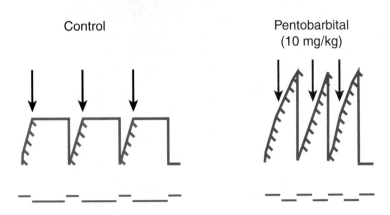

Control

Pentobarbital
(10 mg/kg)

B

Punished Only

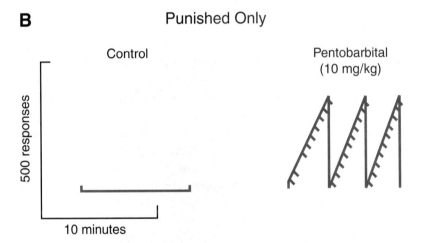

Control

Pentobarbital
(10 mg/kg)

500 responses

10 minutes

FIGURE 14–4. Pentobarbital increases responding in the conditioned suppression test in pigeons.
(A) Upward displacements of the bottom record indicate non-punished segments, with an FR30 schedule of reinforcement accompanied by an orange light. During punished segments (indicated by downward displacement of bottom record), an FR30 schedule was accompanied by a white light. In this part of the multiple schedule the first 10 responses in each 30 response section produced a brief (35 ms) 6-mA electric shock. Pecking was suppressed during these punishment segments in controls. With pentobarbital treatment, pecking responses occurred during both punished and non-punished segments. The termination of each punishment component is indicated by the resetting the recording pen. (B) The punishment procedure in the presence of a white light was in effect throughout each session. The control condition shows no responding, while after pentobarbital treatment pecking was continuous during the session. (Modified from Kelleher and Morse, 1964.)

Oxazepam had a similar effect, and benzodiazepines are now routinely evaluated on this paradigm, which has become the gold standard in the field.

The water lick suppression task is similar in principle but has the advantage of requiring little training since it utilizes an unconditioned behavior. Thirsty rats readily lick the tip of a small metal spout for water when it is inserted into the cage for 3 minutes. After every 20th lick, the rat receives a mild shock (0.4 mA, 0.5 seconds in duration) to the mouth. A marked suppression of licking is observed, and the minimally effective dose of an anxiolytic drug is defined as the average dose producing significant increase in licking rate during the test.

The drug discrimination paradigm has also been of great value in the search for new benzodiazepine drugs, allowing an assessment of their potency relative to known compounds, and in testing hypotheses about the neurochemical basis of their anxiolytic action. Rats are trained to press one of a pair of levers placed side by side for food rewards. Drug days and saline days alternate (see Figure 20–2). On the former, at an appropriate time after drug administration, rats are rewarded for pressing the right lever. Presses on the left lever are unrewarded. On saline days, the opposite is the case and presses on the left lever are rewarded. On a drug day, the rat's score is the percentage of responses made on the drug lever up to the first reinforcement. On a drug day, a well-trained rat might make 2 responses on the saline lever and 10 on the drug lever, with the final one being rewarded with highly palatable milk mixture. The rat's score would be 10/12 or 83.3%. On a saline day, the distribution might be 10 responses on saline to 3 on drug, yielding a score of 77%. Reliable discrimination would be indicated by a score of approximately 91% for 3 consecutive days. Having reached this level of accuracy, the threshold dose of drug required to yield at least 75% accuracy needs to be determined. This provides a baseline against which to test a new compound. If the animal responds to the drug lever, the interoceptive cue is recognized as being similar to the trained compound; 80% consistency on the drug lever is generally considered to represent generalization, and the dose at which this occurs gives an indication of the potency of the novel compound relative to the training drug. A less potent compound will require a higher dose than the training drug to achieve this response level. This methodology is invaluable for establishing similarities or differences between drug classes, their relative potencies, and the potencies of antagonists. It also played a significant role in the discovery of inverse agonists at the benzodiazepine receptor—compounds with anxiogenic as opposed to anxiolytic properties (see Chapter 20).

Aversive stimuli induce fear and stress correlated with a range of endocrine responses, including release from the adrenal gland of corticosterone, epinephrine, and NE. Anxiolytic drugs block stress-induced steroid release and the similar effects induced by anxiogenic drugs. The animal models involving stress and conflict most commonly involve highly aversive stimuli, such as electric shock. The paradigms involve extensive training, although once established, animals can be used for extended periods on the multiple schedules described previously, permitting dose–response data to be collected from individual animals in a balanced order design. However, efforts have been made to develop less time-consuming animal models, avoiding highly aversive stimuli or the need to manipulate motivation by food or water deprivation. The trend is to use simple biologically prepared responses (i.e., unconditioned responses). However, there are disadvantages to such an approach: (1) Many factors that are difficult to control influence such behaviors; (2) animals can only be used on one test occasion since experience would modify the baseline; (3) consequently, large groups of animals need to be used to obtain reliable dose–response data with a compound; (4) there is frequently a lack of reliability between experimenters and labs; and (5) drug effects on motor performance can compromise the interpretation of the drug effects. Despite these problems, a number of such tests for evaluating anxiolytics are in widespread use. They all depend to some extent on the conflict between an innate tendency to perform a response and the aversive consequences of doing so in a particular environment.

The elevated plus maze (EPM) is probably the most widely used of such tests. The apparatus is a simple cross-shaped maze raised approximately 50 cm above the floor. It has four arms—two opposite open arms and two opposite walled arms with no roof. The distribution of behavior is determined by the rodent's aversion to heights and open spaces. The rat or mouse is placed in the center of the maze, and the number of entries and time spent in the open as opposed to the closed arms are recorded. Saline-treated controls exhibit a preference for the closed arms and show fear-related responses (freezing and defecation) and raised plasma corticosterone when in the open arms. Anxiolytic drugs induce selective increases in open arm activity and anxiogenic drugs (caffeine and β-carbolines) reduce normal levels of activity in the open arms. The EPM is thought to model generalized anxiety (Fig. 14–5).

The light–dark crossing box (sometimes called black–white) is similar in principle. Rodents experience an arena of two interconnected compartments, one brightly lit and the other dark and enclosed. The number of crossings between the boxes and the overall motor activity in the boxes are recorded. Normally, the dark side is preferred. Anxiolytics enhance activity in the bright box, resulting in dose-related increases in activity on both sides and increased numbers of crossings, with their potencies in this task matching clinical experience with the drugs. In evenly lit open-field situations, anxiolytics do not increase general motor activity, suggesting that in the brightly lit box normal activity levels are suppressed by the associated fear.

Novelty-induced hypophagia is another useful test in rodents. Typically, mice are presented with highly palatable condensed milk for several days

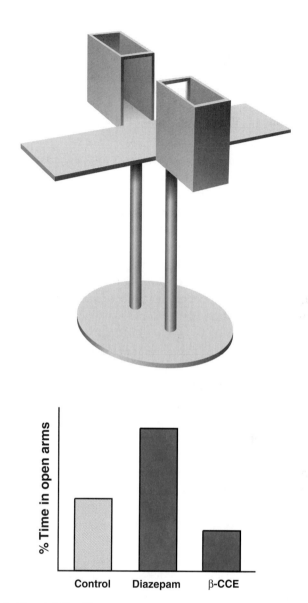

FIGURE 14–5. Elevated Plus Maze.

The apparatus is raised above a table, and consists of two arms that intersect to form a plus sign. The sides of one arm are enclosed with sides; the other arm is open. A rat is placed at the intersection, and the amount of time it spends in the open versus closed arms and the number of entries into the arms is measured. Rodents normally prefer the closed arm, suggesting that they find the open brightly lit arm fearful or anxiety-provoking. Anxiolytic drugs, such as diazepam (illustrated), significantly increase the amount of time animals spend in the open arms, whereas in contrast β-carboline (an inverse agonist at the benzodiazepine receptor, known to be anxiogenic in man) reduces the amount of time animals spend in the open arms. (Modified from Nestler et al. 2001.)

before being given a test day drinking in their home cage under dim light conditions. The following day, they are placed in new clean cages with no bedding and under bright lighting (1200 lux)—a highly aversive environment. Milk is available, and the latency to drink and the amount drunk compared with that in the familiar home cage situation are recorded. The aversive environment increases latency and reduces consumption. Anxiolytic drugs reduce this suppression of milk intake.

A more dynamic conflict between approach and withdrawal is seen in the defensive burying paradigm, which has been used to demonstrate anxiolytic drug effects but also to predict the propensity of rats to consume alcohol. Defensive burying is a species-specific defense reaction. Rats are habituated to a cage with deep bedding litter for 30 minutes over 4 days. On day 5, a probe protrudes into the cage that when touched delivers a 5-mA shock. The behavior of the rat is recorded for 10 minutes after the first contact with the probe. The latency to bury the probe with bedding, the number of burying bouts separated by a minimum of 30 seconds of nonburying, vertical activity, grooming, freezing, and immobility are recorded. Anxiety can also be induced in social situations. Levels of social interaction between male rats in a brightly lit arena are increased after anxiolytic treatment, although this test is less reliable. The ultrasonic vocalizations emitted by rat or guinea pig pups when isolated from their mother are another social response modified by anxiolytics. These responses can be measured during the first 2 weeks of life, and benzodiazepines reduce the intensity of these calls without reducing overall activity.

However, the effects of anxiolytic drugs on unconditioned behaviors can be compromised by the dose-related tendency of these drugs to either increase or decrease spontaneous motor behaviors. Care must therefore be taken in interpreting drug effects in these models. This is particularly the case for behavior in the open field, which could be considered the simplest anxiolytic task in the behavioral repertoire (see Chapters 3 and 13). Rats placed in a large (40×40 cm) open arena experience approach/avoidance conflict as the urge to explore conflicts with the fear of open space. Manipulating the overhead lighting can influence this balance. A number of behavioral measures can be made either by observation or with automation: (1) entries into the center of the field, (2) time spent in the center, (3) distance traveled in the center divided by the total distance, and (4) total distance traveled (i.e., overall motor activity). As one might expect from the results of other tests, anxiolytics increase behavior in the center, presumably because of fear reduction. However, so do drugs that activate the mesolimbic DA pathway, including amphetamine, and substance P or enkephalin injected into the ventral tegmental area. These effects are not ascribed to fear reduction.

As with research on depression, genetic studies are playing an increasingly significant role in the search for more selective benzodiazepines and other novel anxiolytic compounds. This is well illustrated in a study that used behavioral tasks to investigate the role of $GABA_A$ receptor subtypes in the sedative as opposed to the anxiolytic effects of benzodiazepines. Mice with an α_2 subunit point mutation (H101R) lacked anxiolytic responses to diazepam assessed in the light–dark box and the EPM. By contrast, an α_3 subunit mutation (H126R) had no such effect. Neither mutant lost the ability to show the sedative, motor, and anticonvulsant effects of diazepam, as measured with locomotor activity, rotarod, and PTZ-induced seizures.

DRUGS WITH BOTH ANTIDEPRESSANT AND ANXIOLYTIC PROPERTIES

There is a growing convergence of opinion that major depressive disorder and anxiety states overlap in their phenotypic expression and share a number of overlapping neuropharmacological (NE, 5-HT, and DA) and neuroanatomical brain circuits. This view is supported by the *DSM-IV* diagnostic criteria. We now view these disorders as overlapping clusters of symptoms, each with their own clinical continuum.

Several interesting experimental approaches are emerging in an effort to differentiate the effects of anxiolytics and antidepressants. These include new behavioral models for teasing apart different dimensions of anxiety states and major depressive disorders. This involves finding the most behaviorally sensitive preparations and identifying, with gene manipulation, the contribution of different neurotransmitter receptors in the expression of these behavioral phenotypes. For example, in a new theoretical construct of anxiety-related defensive behavior it has been proposed that two processes are involved: avoidance and escape. Inhibitory avoidance has been equated with generalized anxiety, and escape has been equated with panic disorder. A modified form of the EPM has been used to quantify these two behavioral dimensions in one test situation. The elevated T-maze consists of three arms: One enclosed by 40-cm high walls is set perpendicular to two opposed open arms. The whole apparatus is elevated 50 cm above the floor. After acclimatization to the lab, the rat is placed in one of the open arms that has been isolated from the rest of the maze. Twenty-four hours later, the rat is placed at the distal end of the enclosed arm facing the intersection of the arms. The time taken to leave this arm is recorded, and this trial is repeated a second time. The rat is then placed at the end of the open arm and the latency to leave this arm is recorded over three trials. Anxiolytic drugs have been shown to reduce avoidance while leaving escape behavior unchanged. By contrast, escape was impaired by chronic imipramine, chlorimipramine, and the SSRIs fluoxetine and paroxetine. These results correlate with clinical experience that generalized anxiety is ameliorated by anxiolytic drugs, whereas panic disorders respond to SSRIs. Escitalopram, the S-enantiomer of racemic citalopram, is an example of a drug already in clinical use for anxiety, panic, and social phobia as well as for depressive disorders. The drug is more potent, faster acting, and has fewer side effects than the original racemic drug. It has been evaluated in the elevated T-maze and compared with imipramine. On chronic administration, both drugs had anxiolytic and antipanic effects.

The increasing interest in drugs with activity on multiple receptors poses a particular challenge to behavioral pharmacology. This is very clearly illustrated in the efforts to discover atypical anxiolytics and antidepressants with improved clinical profiles and to determine the role of particular neurotransmitter receptors in these drug effects. In this endeavor, genetically modified mice are playing an increasingly important role. For example, mice with global disruption of 5-HT_{2A} receptor signaling capacity were evaluated in the open field, dark–light box, EPM, and novelty suppressed feeding. Since in humans anxiety and depression often coexist and 5-HT signaling has been implicated in the etiology of both disorders, the mice were also studied using the forced swim test and the tail suspension test. The mice were found to have reduced inhibition in conflict paradigms, but fear-conditioned and depression-related behaviors were not affected.

Animal models sensitive to chronic but not acute antidepressant treatment are particularly valuable. The BALB/c strain of mouse shows high levels of anxiety and is sensitive to the effects of chronic fluoxetine in the forced swim test (using the Lucki modification), the open field, and the novelty-induced hypophagia test. The mice thus exhibit a pattern of behavioral effects consistent with the fact that SSRIs have profound mood-altering effects in both depressed and anxious patients.

SELECTED REFERENCES

Banasr, M. and R. S. Duman (2007). Regulation of neurogenesis and gliogenesis by stress and antidepressant treatment. *CNS Neurol. Disord. Drug Targets* 6, 311–320.

Barr, A. M., A. Markou, and A. G. Phillips (2002). A "crash" course on psychostimulant withdrawal as a model of depression. *Trends Pharmacol. Sci.* 23, 475–482.

Cryan, J. F., A. Markou, and I. Lucki (2002). Assessing antidepressant activity in rodents: Recent developments and future needs. *Trends Pharmacol. Sci.* 23, 238–245.

Davis, M., W. A. Falls, S. Campeau, and M. Kim (1993). Fear potentiated startle. I: A neural and pharmacological analysis. *Behav. Brain Res.* 58, 175–198.

Geller, I. and J. Seifter (1980). The effects of meprobamate, barbiturates, d-amphetamine and promazine on experimentally induced conflict. *Psychopharmacologia* 1, 482–492.

Graeff, F. G., et al. (1998). The elevated T-maze, an experimental model of anxiety. *Neurosci. Biobehav. Rev.* 23, 237–246.

Kelleher, R. T. and W. H. Morse (1964). Escape behavior and punished behavior. *Fed. Proc.* 23, 808–817.

Koob, G. F., et al. (1997). Opponent process model of psychostimulant addiction. *Pharmacol. Biochem. Behav.* 57, 513–521.

Lucki, I. (1998). The spectrum of behaviors influenced by serotonin. *Biol. Psychiatry* 44, 151–162.

Maeng, S. and C. A. Zarate Jr. (2007). The role of glutamate in mood disorders: Results from the ketamine in major depression study and the presumed cellular mechanism underlying its antidepressant effects. *Curr. Psychiatry Rep.* 9, 467–474.

McKinney, W. T. Jr. and W. E. Bunney (1969). Animal models of depression. I: Review of evidence: Implications for research. *Arch. Gen. Psychiatry* 21, 240–248.

Nestler, E. J., S. E. Hyman, and R. C. Malenka (2001). In *Molecular Neuropharmacology.* McGraw Hill, New York.

Neubauer, D. N. (2007). The evolution and development of insomnia pharmacotherapies. *J. Clin. Sleep Med.* 3(5 Suppl.), S11–S15.

Newberg, A. R., L. A. Catapano, C. A. Zarate, and H. K. Manji (2008). Neurobiology of bipolar disorder. *Expert Rev. Neurother.* 8, 93–110.

Papakostas, G. I., M. E. Thase, M. Fava, J. C. Nelson, and R. C. Shelton (2007) Are antidepressant drugs that combine serotonergic and noradrenergic mechanisms of action more effective than the selective serotonin reuptake inhibitors in treating major depressive disorder? A meta-analysis of studies of newer agents. *Biol. Psychiatry* 62, 1217–1227.

Perlis, R. H. (2007). Treatment of bipolar disorder: The evolving role of atypical antipsychotics. *Am. J. Manag. Care* 13(7 Suppl.), S178–S188.

Porsolt, R. D., A. Lenegre, and R. A. McArthur (1991). Pharmacological models of depression. In *Animal Models in Psychopharmacology* (B. Olivier, J. Slangen, and J. Mos, Eds.). Birkhauser-Verlag, Berlin.

Turner, E. H., et al. (2008). Selective publication of antidepressant trials and its influence on apparent efficacy. *N. Engl. J. Med.* 358, 252–260.

Willner, P. (1991). Animal models as simulations of depression. *Trends Pharmacol. Sci.* 12, 131–136.

Antipsychotics

THE DISORDERS

The discovery of the unique ability of chlorpromazine to treat the bizarre thought disorders, delusions, and hallucinations that accompany schizophrenia was one of the great advances in psychopharmacology in the 20th century. It was a serendipitous discovery that relied on the astute clinical observations of the French physicians involved. Chlorpromazine was synthesized as a potential antihistamine, and it was the surgeon Henri Laborit who first observed its unique calming effect in a human subject. However, it was Pierre Deniker and his assistant Jean Delay who first successfully tested the drug in schizophrenic patients, with results reported in 1952. Many believe that the discovery of chlorpromazine was as important to psychiatry as the discovery of penicillin was to the rest of medicine. Chlorpromazine was widely adopted for the treatment of schizophrenia in Europe and the United States, and it revolutionized the management of the disorder. Schizophrenic patients need no longer be locked up in custodial mental hospitals but are largely treated in the community. Many other antipsychotic drugs evolved from chlorpromazine, with a range of improvements in dosage, formulations, and modifications to their pharmacological profile to minimize adverse side effects and to broaden the scope of symptom coverage. Early studies of these drugs in animal models showed that they tended to cause suppression of activity and indifference to external stimuli—a condition known as neurolepsis—so the drugs are often referred to as "neuroleptics."

Psychosis comprises a syndrome of different symptoms, which present in a large variety of different combinations. At a minimum, these include bizarre thought disorders, hallucinations, and delusions, and these are often accompanied by disorganized speech and behavior. Although schizophrenia is the classical psychotic disorder, a number of other conditions include psychosis as a key symptom. These include substance-induced psychosis (e.g., induced by excessive doses of amphetamine, phencyclidine, or cannabis), schizophreniform disorder, schizoaffective disorder, and psychotic disorders associated with a medical condition. In addition, psychosis often occurs in other psychiatric disorders, including mania, major depression, cognitive disorders, and Alzheimer's disease. Antipsychotic drugs are increasingly used in the treatment of bipolar illness and major depression. They are also used in the treatment of psychosis associated with Alzheimer's disease, although this is not yet a formally approved indication, and carries a "black box" warning in the USA because of an increased risk of mortality.

Schizophrenia is the classical psychotic illness. It has a worldwide incidence of approximately 1%, and its onset occurs most commonly in men in their mid-twenties and in women in their late twenties. It tends to be a lifetime disorder, with periods of remission and exacerbation. Schizophrenia presents in many different forms. However, there are agreed upon diagnostic criteria, which are summarized in Table 15–1.

Although not part of the formal diagnostic criteria, many authors have found it useful to subdivide the symptoms of schizophrenia into five categories: positive symptoms, negative symptoms, cognitive symptoms, aggressive/hostile symptoms, and depressive/anxious symptoms. These are useful distinctions, particularly because these groups of symptoms vary in their responsiveness to treatment with conventional antipsychotic drugs. The British psychiatrist Tim Crow was the first to describe the overlapping syndromes of positive and negative symptoms, which are summarized in Table 15–2.

The importance of this distinction is that whereas the positive symptoms of the disorder generally respond well to antipsychotic drug treatment, the negative symptoms respond less well, if at all, and may be made worse by treatment with conventional antipsychotics. Similarly, the often severe cognitive impairments associated with schizophrenia are largely drug resistant, and this has prompted a search in recent years for new medicines to treat these symptoms, which include disorganized thinking; slow thinking; poor concentration; poor memory; difficulty understanding; difficulty expressing thoughts; and difficulty integrating thoughts, feelings, and behavior. This has reinforced the view that impaired cognition should be considered as an important symptom

TABLE 15–1. Diagnostic Criteria for Schizophrenia

A. *Characteristic symptoms:* Two (or more) of the following, each present for a significant portion of time during a 1-month period (or less if successfully treated):

1. Delusions
2. Hallucinations
3. Disorganized speech (e.g., frequent derailment or incoherence)
4. Grossly disorganized or catatonic behavior
5. Negative symptoms (i.e., affective flattening, alogia, or avolition)

Note: Only one Criterion A symptom is required if delusions are bizarre or hallucinations consist of a voice keeping up a running commentary on the person's behavior or thoughts, or two or more voices conversing with each other.

B. *Social/occupational dysfunction:* For a significant portion of the time since the onset of the disturbance, one or more major areas of functioning such as work, interpersonal relations, or self-care are markedly below the level achieved prior to the onset (or when the onset is in childhood or adolescence, failure to achieve expected level of interpersonal, academic, or occupational achievement).

C. *Duration:* Continuous signs of the disturbance persist for at least 6 months. This 6-month period must include at least 1 month of symptoms (or less if successfully treated) that meet Criterion A (i.e., active-phase symptoms) and may include periods of prodromal or residual symptoms. During these prodromal or residual periods, the signs of the disturbance may be manifested by only negative symptoms or two or more symptoms listed in Criterion A present in an attenuated form (e.g., odd beliefs and unusual perceptual experiences).

D. *Schizoaffective and mood disorder exclusion:* Schizoaffective disorder and mood disorder with psychotic features have been ruled out because either (1) no major depressive, manic, or mixed episodes have occurred concurrently with the active-phase symptoms; or (2) if mood episodes have occurred during active-phase symptoms, their total duration has been brief relative to the duration of the active and residual periods.

E. *Substance/general medical condition exclusion:* The disturbance is not due to the direct physiological effects of a substance (e.g., a drug of abuse or a medication) or a general medical condition.

F. *Relationship to a pervasive developmental disorder:* If there is a history of autistic disorder or another pervasive developmental disorder, the additional diagnosis of schizophrenia is made only if prominent delusions or hallucinations are also present for at least a month (or less if successfully treated).

Source: Reprinted with permission from the *Diagnostic and Statistical Manual of Mental Disorders,* Text Revision, Fourth Edition (Copyright 2000), American Psychiatric Association.

cluster alongside the hallucinations/delusions and negative symptom cluster. In the United States, the National Institute of Mental Health and the Food and Drug Administration have launched a major initiative to encourage the discovery of such medicines (the MATRICS program [www.matrics.ucla.edu]). Many believe that the cognitive impairments that schizophrenic patients suffer

TABLE 15–2. Positive and Negative Symptoms of Schizophrenia

Positive symptoms

Delusions are firmly held erroneous beliefs due to distortions or exaggerations of reasoning and/or misinterpretations of perceptions or experiences. Delusions of being followed or watched are common, as are beliefs that comments, radio or TV programs, etc. are directing special messages directly to him or her.

Hallucinations are distortions or exaggerations of perception in any of the senses, although auditory hallucinations ("hearing voices" within, distinct from one's own thoughts) are the most common, followed by visual hallucinations.

Disorganized speech/thinking, also described as "thought disorder" or "loosening of associations," is a key aspect of schizophrenia. Disorganized thinking is usually assessed primarily based on the person's speech. Therefore, tangential, loosely associated, or incoherent speech severe enough to substantially impair effective communication is used as an indicator of thought disorder by the *DSM-IV.*

Grossly disorganized behavior includes difficulty in goal-directed behavior (leading to difficulties in activities in daily living), unpredictable agitation or silliness, social disinhibition, or behaviors that are bizarre to onlookers. Their purposelessness distinguishes them from unusual behavior prompted by delusional beliefs.

Catatonic behaviors are characterized by a marked decrease in reaction to the immediate surrounding environment, sometimes taking the form of motionless and apparent unawareness, rigid or bizarre postures, or aimless excess motor activity.

Negative symptoms

Affective flattening is the reduction in the range and intensity of emotional expression, including facial expression, voice tone, eye contact, and body language.

Alogia, or poverty of speech, is the lessening of speech fluency and productivity, thought to reflect slowing or blocked thoughts, and often manifested as short, empty replies to questions.

Avolition is the reduction, difficulty, or inability to initiate and persist in goal-directed behavior; it is often mistaken for apparent disinterest. (Examples of avolition include no longer interested in going out and meeting with friends, no longer interested in activities that the person used to show enthusiasm for, no longer interested in much of anything, and sitting in the house for many hours a day doing nothing.)

are the most intractable and debilitating, and they represent one of the major impediments to patients' full integration into work and society. There is increasing evidence of dysfunction in the prefrontal cortex underlying the cognitive impairments. Schizophrenia has many clinical presentations, and it is likely to involve a number of distinct states, varying in severity and chronicity. Each may be associated with distinct brain pathology and neurotransmitter dysfunction involving a spectrum of genes, which together account for no more than 50% of the risk.

In broad terms, individuals fail to understand the external world or how to react appropriately to it and thus lose touch with reality and the people around them.

ANTIPSYCHOTIC DRUGS

A list of the commonly available antipsychotic drugs is given in Table 15–3 (see also Fig. 15–1).

Along with the antidepressants (see Chapter 14), these are among the most widely used of all psychopharmaceuticals, with sales in excess of $10 billion annually. The drugs come from a variety of different chemical classes. Many are phenothiazines, such as chlorpromazine; several of the others are thioxanthenes (e.g., flupentixol), butryophenones (e.g., haloperidol), or substituted benzamides (sulpiride). Whereas the dose of chlorpromazine can be as high as 1 g per day, some of the second-generation drugs are up to 1000 times more potent, with daily doses of only a few milligrams. Although the antipsychotics are usually administered orally, some have been formulated as depot injectables or other sustained-release formulations. The depot products can be injected intramuscularly to provide a constant supply of active drug for prolonged periods, sometimes up to several weeks. These are valuable in the outpatient treatment of schizophrenic patients to improve drug compliance.

Mode of Action

All of the antipsychotic drugs have a common mechanism of action: They antagonize the effects of dopamine at the dopamine D_2 receptor in brain. The elucidation of this mechanism was another major achievement of basic research in neuropsychopharmacology. Although it was increasingly clear in the 1960s that blockade of dopamine was a key action of these drugs, it was not until biochemical methods became available to assess drug actions on individual dopamine receptor subtypes that the relationship of clinical effects and potency to the dopamine D_2 receptor became clear. The relationship depicted graphically in Figure 15–2 became one of the most widely quoted of all basic research findings in this field.

By using positron emission tomography imaging methods, it is possible to measure the ability of antipsychotic drugs to displace a D_2 receptor radioligand in human brain. The results of such experiments have shown that when tested in their normal clinical dose range (established empirically by trial and error), most of the antipsychotic drugs occupy 70–80% of the available D_2 sites. Doses that give higher degrees of D_2 occupancy are liable to cause unacceptably severe adverse side effects, particularly extrapyramidal motor effects.

TABLE 15–3. Available Antipsychotic Drugs

GENERIC NAME	TRADE NAME
Typical neuroleptics	
Acetophenazine	Tindal
Amisulpride	Solian
Chlorpromazine	Thorazine, Largactil
Chlorprothixene	Taractan
Flupentixol	Fluanxol
Fluphenazine	Prolixin, Permitil
Fluspirilene	Imap, Redeptin
Haloperidol	Haldol
Loxapine	Loxitane
Mesoridazine	Serentil
Molindone	Moban, Lidone
Perphenazine	Trilafon
Pimozide	Orap
Piperacetazine	Quide
Prochlorperazine	Compazine
Thioridazine	Mellaril
Thiothixene	Navane
Trifluoperazine	Stelazine
Trifluopromazine	Vesprin
Atypical neuroleptics	
Clozapine	Clozaril
Olanzapine	Zyprexa
Quetiapine	Seroquel
Paliperidone[a]	Invega
Risperidone	Risperdal, Consta
Ziprasidone	Geodon
Zotepine[b]	Nipolept, Lodopin
Other	
Aripiprazole	Abilify

[a] Paliperidone is an active metabolite of risperidone with a similar pharmacological profile; it is a once-a-day sustained-release formulation.
[b] Zotepine is available only in Germany and Japan.

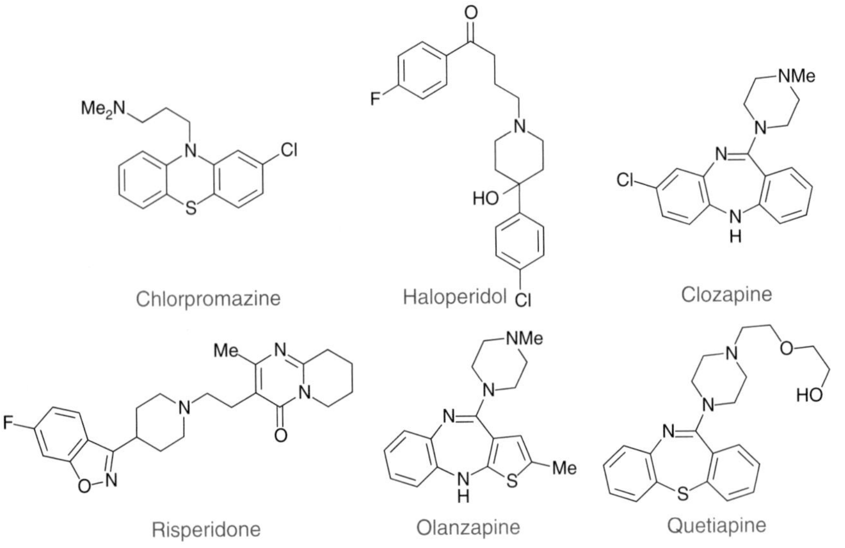

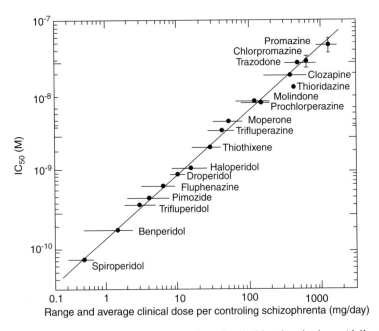

FIGURE 15–1. Commonly used antipsychotics.

FIGURE 15–2. Correlation of clinical potencies of antischizophrenic drugs (daily dose) with *in vitro* affinities for dopamine D_2 receptors in a test tube radioligand binding assay. (From Iversen, 2008.)

Although D_2 receptor occupancy is achieved acutely after a single test dose of drug, the clinical effects of the antipsychotic drugs, like those of antidepressants, do not reach their maximum until after 3 or 4 weeks of continuous drug treatment, although careful longitudinal studies show that reductions in psychosis ratings start within the first few days of treatment. Hundreds of double-blind, placebo-controlled clinical trials have shown the overall clinical benefits of these drugs versus placebo in terms of a reduction in various rating scales of psychotic symptoms. As with other psychotropic drugs, there are also significant placebo effects. In terms of clinical effectiveness, there are few, if any, significant differences among the many drugs available. However, in recent years the emphasis has been on "atypical neuroleptics," which have some advantages over the conventional antipsychotics.

It is interesting to speculate how blockade of the synaptic actions of dopamine in brain can lead to complex pharmacological effects, such as a reduction in delusions or hallucinations. The psychiatrist Shitij Kapur suggested that this may be explained in terms of our improved understanding of the functional role of dopamine in the brain, not only in relation to "reward" and "punishment" mechanisms but also in terms of "motivational salience"—the process whereby an animal comes to link reward-associated stimuli with goal-directed behavior. The dopamine system is thus involved in determining the "salience" of ongoing events to the animal. It is hypothesized that in schizophrenia this system is dysregulated so that patients are exposed to an excessive activation of this system and may thus attribute salience inappropriately to everyday life events. In order to rationalize their exaggerated reactions to such events, patients may construct complex delusions that they come firmly to believe. By interrupting this dopaminergic dysfunction, the antipsychotic drugs may act to neutralize the apparent causes of such delusions.

Atypical Neuroleptics

Currently, the market for antipsychotics is dominated by a series of these drugs, of which the first was clozapine, followed by olanzapine, paliperidone, quetiapine, risperidone, ziprasidone, and zotepine. These are defined by virtue of their ability to produce an effective suppression of psychotic symptoms at doses that fail to elicit significant extrapyramidal motor side effects. There is also some evidence that these drugs have beneficial effects in treating the negative symptoms and cognitive deficits that are unresponsive to conventional antipsychotics, although the evidence for this conclusion remains somewhat equivocal. Clozapine, the archetypal atypical neuroleptic, has the clearest benefits on negative symptoms and cognition, but its pharmacology is very complex, with multiple actions on monoamine receptors in brain. Clozapine is also unusual in causing a much lower occupancy of dopamine D_2 receptors in human brain at clinically effective doses (only 30–40%). With new brain imaging methods using the sensitive dopamine D_2 receptor radiotracer [^{18}F]fallypride, it has been possible to measure drug occupancy of D_2 receptors outside the striatum. Whereas the atypical drugs clozapine and quetiapine occupied only 35–45% of dopamine D_2 sites in human putamen, occupancy was 50–60% of D_2 sites in temporal cortex. Some attribute these differences to the relatively low affinity that atypical neuroleptics have for dopamine D_2 receptors, making them less able to compete with the high levels of endogenous dopamine in striatum. Although the mechanism of action of clozapine and the other atypical drugs is not conclusively established, a widely held hypothesis is that the atypical drugs owe their unique pharmacology to a combination of their ability to act as antagonists at both dopamine D_2 receptors and serotonin 5-HT_{2A} receptors. There is some rationale for this combination if one considers the way in which serotonin interacts with dopamine in the various dopamine pathways in brain. In the nigrostriatal pathway, serotonin exerts a powerful negative influence on dopamine release, acting both on dopamine cell bodies in substantia nigra and presynaptically on dopaminergic terminals in striatum—in both cases involving 5-HT_{2A} receptors. Blockade of these receptors will tend to encourage dopamine release in striatum and alleviate the consequences of dopamine D_2 receptor blockade. For similar reasons, 5-HT_{2A} receptor blockade will tend to increase dopamine release in mesocortical dopamine pathways, which tends to ameliorate the effects of dopamine D_2 blockade in worsening negative symptoms. At the level of the hypothalamic–pituitary dopamine pathway, 5-HT_{2A} receptor blockade will again tend to negate the effects of dopamine D_2 blockade in causing increased prolactin secretion because the serotonin receptors are needed for this response. Finally, in the mesolimbic dopamine pathways, 5-HT_{2A} receptor blockade does not weaken the desired blockade of dopamine via D_2 receptors, thought to be fundamental to the antipsychotic effects, because the interaction between serotonin and dopamine is weaker in this brain region. These differences can be demonstrated by direct measurements of the effects of the atypical drugs on dopamine release in different brain regions: Whereas release is increased in prefrontal cortex, there is no such effect in nucleus accumbens. At clinically effective doses, all of the atypical neuroleptics occupy 70–80% of 5-HT_{2A} receptors in brain and a lower proportion of dopamine D_2 sites in striatum.

Adverse Side Effects

Many adverse side effects are associated with the use of antipsychotic drugs. These can be classified as those related to dopamine receptor blockade and those related to secondary pharmacological properties, often unique to individual compounds. Chlorpromazine, along with several of the other classical phenothiazines, has potent effects as an antagonist at cholinergic, histamine, and other monoamine receptors in brain. Interaction with these sites can cause adverse peripheral cholinergic side effects or, in the case of blockade of histamine H_1 receptors, may lead to excessive sedation. Interaction with H_1 histamine receptors also seems to be a common property of antipsychotic drugs that lead to weight gain. Although this is seen even with chlorpromazine, it is most marked in the atypical neuroleptics clozapine and olanzapine, where weight gain can be sufficiently serious to increase the risk of new-onset diabetes. Other serious side effects include prolongation of the QTc interval in the heart, with the risk of sudden death, seen particularly with ziprasidone and thioridazine. Clozapine can cause a serious blood disorder, agranulocytosis, in 1% or 2% of those taking the drug; thus, patients on clozapine need careful monitoring of blood samples at regular intervals, which limits the usefulness of this otherwise highly effective compound.

The side effects related to blockade of dopamine D_2 receptors other than the desired effects in the mesolimbic pathways are predictable. Blockade of dopamine function in the hypothalamic–pituitary pathway, where dopamine normally acts as an inhibitor of prolactin release in the anterior pituitary, leads to increased secretion of prolactin, which can cause breast enlargement in men or galactorrhea. Blockade of dopamine in the striatum mimics the condition seen in Parkinson's disease and leads to characteristic extrapyramidal motor symptoms, including rigidity and paucity of voluntary movement. After chronic drug use, these symptoms may develop into a hyperkinetic movement disorder known as tardive dyskinesia, characterized by constant chewing, tongue protrusion, and facial grimacing, along with jerky body movements. Blockade of dopamine function in the mesocortical pathway is thought to underlie the worsening of negative and cognitive symptoms caused by many antipsychotics.

BEHAVIORAL ACTIONS OF NEUROLEPTICS

In the absence of animal models of schizophrenia with convincing validity, pharmacologists sought behavioral parameters that could be used to characterize and differentiate antipsychotic drugs from other psychoactive agents. The term *neuroleptic* refers to the depressant actions initially observed with the phenothiazines. These effects are demonstrated in reductions in a range of unconditioned behavior—for example, exploratory locomotor activity in photocells or open field. At higher doses, the first-generation neuroleptics induced catalepsy (sustained and abnormal posture). However, their antipsychotic property cannot be ascribed to this effect since drugs such as barbiturates, which are potent depressants, do not relieve the symptoms of schizophrenia.

Neuroleptics also block conditioned behavior maintained by positive and negative reinforcement. Indeed, in one of the earliest accounts of the pharmacology of chlorpromazine, Courvoisier described impairment on a signaled active avoidance task in which a rat climbed a pole when a tone sounded in order to avoid an electric shock to the feet. Despite the failure of avoidance, neuroleptic-treated animals still escaped to the pole when the shock was presented. It might be assumed that this is due to general sedation, but if the delay between the warning signal and shock is lengthened, avoidance is still impaired. Furthermore, neuroleptics also impair passive avoidance where an active step-down response indicates failure, suggesting that sedation per se is not an adequate explanation of these deficits. Rather, antipsychotics produce an indifference to environmental stimuli without significant sedation. Conditioned shock avoidance has been a cornerstone in drug discovery programs searching for novel antipsychotics. Neuroleptics depress unconditioned behaviors and food-reinforced and shock avoidance responses in a dose-dependent manner. Particularly striking was the demonstration in squirrel monkeys that multiple schedules (FI/FR) for food reinforcement or for removal of electric shock produced identical patterns of responding and were equally depressed by chlorpromazine (see Fig. 3–4). Neuroleptics also depress behaviors maintained by access to sexual behavior, intracranial self-stimulation, and access to drugs of addiction. Motivational variables and the nature of the reinforcement are thus irrelevant determinants of the effect of neuroleptics; rather, they manipulate the relationship between the environment and the animal.

Typical Neuroleptics: Phenothiazines and Butyrophenomes

Once the dopamine-blocking properties of the various classes of neuroleptics had been discovered, behavioral pharmacologists soon capitalized on the properties of the forebrain dopamine pathways to provide behavioral assays. This fruitful period of research resulted in a range of pharmacological models with robust behavioral endpoints. Initially, the behavioral effects of the stimulant drug amphetamine were studied. Amphetamine releases dopamine, which results in profound changes in unconditioned motor behaviors (see Chapter 3). For example, after low doses of amphetamine (approximately 1.5 mg/kg in rats), marked increases in locomotor activity can readily be measured in rats habituated to photocell cages. Exploratory behaviors such as rearing and climbing also increase. At higher doses (approximately 5 mg/kg), rats no longer run around but remain largely in one place, repeating elements of motor behavior. In rats, this stereotypy escalates through sniffing, licking, and head movements to gnawing. Simple observational rating scales can be used to measure the intensity of the behavior. Stereotypy is usually studied in rodents but is observed in other species including humans. Amphetamine addicts may repeat highly complex motor routines, including mechanical clock maintenance, housecleaning, and sorting behavior, a phenomenon sometimes described as "punding." Neuroleptics block, in a dose-dependent manner, amphetamine and apomorphine-induced locomotor and stereotyped behavior, with their relative potencies correlated with their ability to block dopamine D_2 receptors. We now know that the locomotor response is dependent on the mesolimbic dopamine pathway and stereotypy on the nigrostriatal system (see Chapter 21).

A classic paper published by Janssen in 1965 described a simple behavioral screen in rodents for predicting neuroleptic activity. It included (1) drug-induced catalepsy and ptosis (drooping eyelid), (2) antagonism of amphetamine-induced stereotypy, (3) drug effect on shock avoidance in jumping box, (4) antagonism of apomorphine-induced stereotypy, (5) alterations of food intake, (6) open field activity (rearing and ambulation), (7) drug effects on mortality caused by epinephrine or norepinephrine injection, (8) antagonism of tryptamine-induced limb convulsions, and (9) resistance to rotational trauma. Forty antipsychotic drugs available at that time (mainly phenothiazines and butyrophenones) were tested, their ED_{50}s calculated, and these values plotted as "activity spectra." The two classes of typical neuroleptics were clearly distinguishable.

Atypical Neuroleptics

Clinical experience soon identified tardive dyskinesia as a major side effect of the typical neuroleptics. From animal studies it became clear that compounds that had profound and generalized depressant effects on behavior blocked dopamine D_2 receptors in both mesolimbic and striatal dopamine systems. Consequently, they induced catalepsy, impairment of conditioned avoidance behavior, and blockade of amphetamine-induced motor behavior (both locomotion and stereotypy) at very similar doses. The mantra soon emerged that neuroleptics with a reduced risk for tardive dyskinesia should, in animal tests, block amphetamine- or apomorphine-induced locomotion at much lower doses than those required to block stereotypy or induce catalepsy. This is referred to as the extrapyramidal side effects (EPS) separation (Fig. 15–3). The goal has been to discover drugs acting selectively on the mesolimbic system. Although this degree of selectivity has not been achieved, a number of atypical neuroleptics have improved EPS separation.

However, as neuropharmacological research on the forebrain systems implicated in schizophrenia progressed, other hypotheses about how to achieve novel antipsychotic drugs with efficacy in controlling the three different symptom clusters in the disease have emerged. As we have seen, these atypical neuroleptics are not selective dopamine antagonists but interact with a range of neurotransmitter receptors. The behavioral screens currently in use reflect

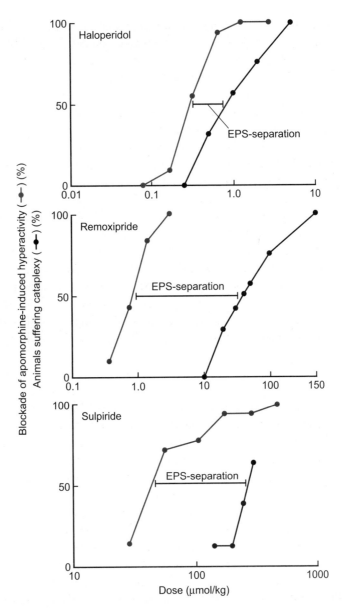

FIGURE 15–3. EPS separation neuroleptic drugs. Dose–response curves for haloperidol, remoxipride, and sulpiride in blocking apomorphine-induced hyperactivity (predictive of clinical antipsychotic efficacy) and in inducing catalepsy (predictive of clinical EPS) in rats. The horizontal line on each graph indicates the degree of EPS separation. Drugs were injected intraperitoneally 60 minutes prior to apomorphine. The atypical neuroleptic remoxipride is no longer used. (Modified from Gerlach, 1991.)

this broad neuropharmacological profile. Compounds continue to be evaluated on screens akin to Jannsen's with particular attention to the EPS separation, but other drug-induced motor behaviors have come into routine use in assessing the ability of atypical compounds to interact with nondopaminergic receptors, particularly $5HT_{2A}$ and glutamate receptors. Interest in these other transmitter systems has been driven by two findings. First was the discovery that a common property of many atypical neuroleptics is antagonism of $5HT_{2A}$ receptors. The selective $5HT_{2A}$ agonist DOI induces a head twitch response in rodents that is blocked by these atypical compounds and is now routinely used to evaluate this particular aspect of their pharmacology. Second was the realization that the well-known fact that ketamine, MK-801 (dizocilpine), and phencyclidine (PCP) induce an acute schizophrenic-like psychosis in humans could be indicating something important about the disease. It had become apparent that all of these compounds were noncompetitive antagonists at the NMDA receptor, suggesting that glutamate was involved in the pathophysiology of schizophrenia. Noncompetitive NMDA antagonists produce characteristic stimulation of motor behaviors in rodents, and these were rapidly adopted into standard screens for atypical neuroleptics. These effects are blocked by typical and atypical compounds, as are the responses to amphetamine and apomorphine.

The neuropharmacological and neuroanatomical basis of the interaction between dopamine, $5HT_{2A}$, and glutamate receptors at cortical and subcortical sites is attracting interest because of the possibility that, particularly at the cortical level, such interaction may provide a target for treatment of the cognitive and negative symptoms of psychosis. The behavioral evaluation of novel agonists acting at the mGLU2/mGLU3 receptors represents a breakthrough and has elicited considerable excitement and research. In rats, LY379268 and LY354740 suppress the release of glutamate and behavioral disruptions induced by PCP via a presynaptic mechanism that may also involve $5\text{-}HT_{2A}$ receptors. The drugs have no effect on glutamate levels and do not effect PCP-induced DA release. LY354740 reduced PCP-induced locomotor activity and attenuated the impairment of working memory assessed in a T-maze, indicating potential pro-cognitive effects. No impairment of general motor behavior was observed, and although amphetamine-induced locomotor activity was blocked, stereotypy was not, suggesting a reduced risk of tardive dyskinesia. Compounds of this class are likely to be valuable in treating a range of central nervous system disorders involving excessive glutamate release, including not only schizophrenia but also anxiety, seizures, drug withdrawal, and neurodegeneration.

Thus, although dopamine overactivity continues to figure prominently in theories of schizophrenia, glutamatergic overactivity associated with frontal hypofrontality is now commonly discussed in this context. These ideas have been developed by Krystal et al. (2003) in a model in which an interaction between dopamine and glutamate is proposed to be critical in the emergence of delusions. In particular, it is suggested that experimentally induced ketamine psychosis in humans provides a powerful method for studying the changes in cognitive processes that lead to the experience of delusions.

PCP abuse in humans produces a schizophrenia-like psychosis, including social withdrawal and affective blunting as well as hallucinations, formal thought disorder, paranoia, and delusions. Cognitive dysfunction, a prominent symptom of schizophrenia, is also seen. The PCP-induced cognitive impairment resembles that seen in schizophrenia or that following frontal lobe lesions or substantial depletion of dopamine from the dorsolateral prefrontal cortex (DLFC). The symptoms include increased perseveration and abnormalities in working memory, behavioral inhibition, attention, and planning. Chronic treatment of monkeys with PCP for 14 days reduces basal and evoked dopamine utilization in DLFC and results in a severe impairment on an "object retrieval with detour" task. Detour ability is an important component of problem solving and skilled action involving changing relationships between the self and objects through movement. Monkeys were trained to retrieve a reward from a transparent box fixed to a tray and attached to the side of the home cage. The box had one side open, which could be directed to the front, left, or right from the monkey's perspective. When the open side was directed to the left or right, the monkey had to inhibit a strong instinctive response to reach directly to the visible reward. Success was scored if the monkey obtained the reward in one reach without touching the closed transparent face of the box. The success rate was significantly reduced in monkeys chronically treated with PCP, which also showed high levels of reaches to the closed transparent front of the box and perseverative errors to a closed side that had previously been open. These impairments persisted when PCP treatment was terminated, indicating that they were not due to a direct effect of the drug; the deficits could be ameliorated with clozapine. Chronic PCP treatment in rats (2 mg/kg for 7 days) also induces a significant deficit in memory performance on the novel object recognition task (NOR). Rats have a strong propensity to respond to novel objects, but to do so they must remember the familiar object. In the NOR test, rats are exposed to two identical objects for 3 minutes. After a 1-minute delay in the home cage, they are returned to the cleaned box with a copy of the familiar object together with a novel object. Time spent exploring the two objects is recorded. This is an ethologically relevant and simple test that is included in the NIMH MATRICS initiative as relevant for studying visual learning and memory deficits in schizophrenia and for screening potential novel antipsychotic drugs. The PCP-induced impairment on this task in rats was significantly attenuated by clozapine and risperidone but not by haloperidol.

The development of validated models of other aspects of cognition relevant to schizophrenia would be of great value to this field of research and to drug discovery. Some progress has been made. Interest has focused on the abnormal processing of sensory information in schizophrenia. Earlier theories proposed that sensory overload caused by deficits in early information processing was a central feature of the disorder, citing deficits in the habituation (simple learning) of the startle response to tactile or auditory stimuli. A related process, prepulse inhibition (PPI), has been more extensively studied in human volunteers, patients, and animals by Geyer and colleagues. PPI is a phenomenon in which a reflexive auditory startle reaction elicited by an intense pulse stimulus is attenuated by presenting a weak prepulse stimulus shortly before the pulse. It is commonly considered a form of sensorimotor gating. Schizophrenics and schizotypic individuals show deficits in PPI and in its associated P50 electrophysiological correlate. PPI is impaired in schizophrenic patients, and it is reported to be restored by typical and atypical antipsychotics. PPI and its response to drugs have also been studied extensively in normal volunteers, but the results have not been as useful or consistent as those obtained in rats. PPI is now considered a valuable model since there are very few validated tests of cognitive function relevant to schizophrenia. PCP and ketamine disrupt PPI, as do apomorphine, amphetamine, and cocaine, through a dopamine D_2 mechanism. Whereas the apomorphine PPI model does not distinguish typical and atypical antipsychotics, the NMDA model does so. The compounds clozapine, olanzapine, and quetiapine, which lack antipsychotic activity in some standard behavioral assays (e.g., blockade of apomorphine- and amphetamine-induced stereotypy), are active in the apomorphine PPI model. The NMDA antagonist disruption, however, is not reversed by dopamine D_1 or D_2 antagonists but is reversed by the same group of atypical neuroleptics. It is therefore useful to include both these pharmacological PPI models in an antipsychotic test battery for identifying novel typical or atypical antipsychotics.

There are limited clinical and animal data to support pro-cognitive effects of atypical antipsychotics. Indeed, typical drugs clearly impair aspects of cognition in normal volunteers, monkeys, and rats. Further investigation of the novel mGlu2/3 agonists is warranted, and promising results have been reported with novel 5-HT_6 antagonists, demonstrating their ability to enhance memory in the Morris swim test and improve acquisition of autoshaping. Both of these effects have been difficult to replicate.

The quest for other models of schizophrenia continues. Since there is a growing consensus that schizophrenia is a developmental disorder with a number of predisposing risk factors, developmental models are of interest. Neonatal excitotoxic lesions of the ventral hippocampus in rats result in a range of behavioral disorders in adulthood and in the response to drugs. These include increased spontaneous activity, disruption of PPI, impaired working memory, and hypersensitivity to stress. In relation to drug responses, the lesions result in potentiation of apomorphine-induced stereotypies and of NMDA antagonist-induced locomotion. It is obvious why this abnormal behavioral phenotype is considered to be of relevance to schizophrenia, although the model has not been exploited in the evaluation of antipsychotics. A more promising approach involves isolation rearing of rats, a developmental experience that also results in PPI deficits. This may be, like the apomorphine-induced effect on PPI, sensitive but not specific in its ability to identify atypical antipsychotics.

Little progress has been made in modeling the negative symptoms in schizophrenia. Chronic high-dose amphetamine treatment of rats living in a large and interesting arena has been reported to result in a lack of behavior, particularly social contact and abnormal withdrawal to isolated sleeping areas. Similar phencyclidine studies have been reported in monkeys and rats. These effects are not blocked by haloperidol or chlorpromazine, but clozapine and quetiapine are active in monkeys showing social isolation induced by amphetamine. Thus, the treatment of the cognitive deficits and negative symptoms of schizophrenia remains a major challenge to psychopharmacology.

FUTURE DEVELOPMENTS

Research on schizophrenia and antipsychotic drugs is an active area, and there are considerable reasons to be optimistic about future developments. Several new drug mechanisms are under active development. One involves the use of dopamine D_2 receptor partial agonists as a more subtle means of regulating dopaminergic synaptic function. One such drug, aripiprazole, is already available for the treatment of schizophrenia. The advantage of a partial agonist is that in conditions in which there is dopamine underactivity the drug can partially stimulate the dopamine D_2 receptors, but when there is excessive dopamine release the partial agonist will partly block its effects. The difficulty in developing such drugs, however, is determining what level of partial agonism/antagonism is most effective. A compound with too much dopamine agonist action is liable to be an amphetamine-like psychostimulant.

Another promising line of research involves glutamate pharmacology. The "glutamate hypothesis" of schizophrenia is based on considerable basic research and animal behavioral data suggesting that an insufficiency of glutamate may underlie the symptoms of psychosis. This is based partly on the dramatic psychotomimetic effects of drugs such as ketamine and phencyclidine, which act as antagonists at the NMDA subtype of glutamate receptors in brain. In human volunteers, these drugs cause a paranoid psychosis, resembling in many respects that seen in schizophrenia. The difficulty in glutamate pharmacology is to avoid interfering or unbalancing the ubiquitous actions of this amino acid, the universal excitatory neurotransmitter in brain. However, this appears to be possible by targeting the G protein-coupled metabotropic glutamate receptors, whose function is modulatory (see Chapter 5). A novel series of drugs that act as highly selective agonists or allosteric activators at mGlu2/3 receptors (a subclass of these receptors) are active in animal behavioral models that respond to conventional antipsychotic drugs, and a pilot clinical trial with one of the drugs in schizophrenic patients yielded significant positive antipsychotic effects with no extrapyramidal side effects, hyperprolactinemia, or weight gain. It seems likely that this breakthrough in nondopaminergic mechanisms will lead to increased activity to develop improved drugs of this kind in the future.

A number of novel drugs are being evaluated as adjuncts to neuroleptics in an attempt to alleviate the cognitive impairments associated with schizophrenia. These include selective antagonists acting at 5-HT$_6$ or histamine H$_3$ receptors (see Chapters 8 and 9) that have shown promise as cognition enhancers in animal studies, donepezil and other cholinesterase inhibitors, and drugs that possess agonist actions at muscarinic M$_1$ receptors.

The other great promise for the future is to unravel the genetic risk factors that undoubtedly exist for schizophrenia. First-degree relatives of schizophrenic patients have a 10-fold increased risk of developing the disorder. Genetic research in this field is still in its infancy, but some risk factor genes have been identified and replicated in several different studies throughout the world. Genes involved in neurodevelopment, such as *neuroregulin* and *dysbindin*, are strong contenders. Although there are likely to be many discoveries in this field, it will require many years to understand the underlying biology and at least as long to use this new knowledge to develop safe and effective new treatments for schizophrenia.

SELECTED REFERENCES

Agid, O., P. Seeman, and S. Kapur (2006). The "delayed onset" of antipsychotic action—An idea whose time has come and gone. *J. Psychiatry Neurosci.* 31, 93–100.

Corlett, P. R., G. D. Honey, and P. C. Fletcher (2007). From prediction error to psychosis: Ketamine as a pharmacological model of delusions. *Psychopharmacology* 21, 238–252.

Creese, I., D. R. Burt, and S. H. Snyder (1976). Dopamine receptors and average clinical doses. *Science* 194, 546.

Di Pietro, N. C. and J. K. Seamans (2007). Dopamine and serotonin interactions in the prefrontal cortex: Insights on antipsychotic drugs and their mechanism of action. *Pharmacopsychiatry* 40(Suppl. 1), S27–S33.

Gerlach J.(1991) New antipsychotics: classification, efficacy, and adverse effects. *Schizophr Bull.* 17, 289–309.

Geyer, M. A., K. Krebs-Thomson, D. L. Braff, and N. R. Swerdlow (2001). Pharmacological studies of pre-pulse inhibition models of sensorimotor gating deficits in schizophrenia: A decade in review. *Psychopharmacology* 156, 117–154.

Geyer, M. and B. Moghaddam (2002). Animal models relevant to schizophrenia disorders. In *Neuropsychopharmacology: The Fifth Generation of Progress* (K. Davis, D. Charney,

J. Coyle, and C. Nemeroff, Eds.). Lippincott Williams & Wilkins, Philadelphia, pp. 689–701.

Gray, J. A. and B. L. Roth (2007). The pipeline and future of drug development in schizophrenia. *Mol. Psychiatry* 12, 904–922.

Iversen, L. L. (2008). *Speed, Ecstasy, Ritalin: The Science of Amphetamines*. Oxford University Press, Oxford.

Iversen, S. D. and L. L. Iversen (2007). Dopamine; 50 years in perspective. *Trends Neurosci.* 30, 188–193.

Janssen, P. A. J., C. J. E. Niemegeers, and K. H. L. Schellekens (1965). Is it possible to predict the clinical effects of neuroleptic drugs (major tranquillizers) from animal data? Part I: "Neuroleptic activity spectra" for rats. *Arzneim-Forsch.* 15, 104–117.

Jentsch, J. D., et al. (1997). Enduring cognitive deficits and cortical dopamine dysfunction in monkeys after long-term administration of phencyclidine. *Science* 277, 953–955.

Kapur, S., R. Mizrahi, and M. Li (2005). From dopamine to salience to psychosis—Linking biology, pharmacology and phenomenology of psychosis. *Schizophr. Res.* 79, 59–68.

Krystal, J. H., et al. (2003). NMDA receptor antagonist effects, cortical glutamatergic function, and schizophrenia: Toward a paradigm shift in medication development. *Psychopharmacology* 169, 215–233.

Meltzer, H. Y. (2004). What's atypical about atypical neuroleptics? *Curr. Opin. Pharmacol.* 4, 53–57.

Pani, L., L. Pira, and G. Marchese (2007). Antipsychotic efficacy: Relationship to optimal D_2-receptor occupancy. *Eur. Psychiatry* 22, 267–275.

Seeman, P. (2006). Targeting the dopamine D_2 receptor in schizophrenia. *Expert Opin. Ther. Targets* 10, 515–531.

Stone, J. M., P. D. Morrison, and L. S. Pilowsky (2007). Glutamate and dopamine dysregulation in schizophrenia—A synthesis and selective review. *J. Psychopharmacol.* 21, 440–452.

Sullivan, P. F. (2008). Schizophrenia genetics: The search for a hard lead. *Curr. Opin. Psychiatry* 21, 157–160.

Wood, M. and C. Reavill (2007). Aripiprazole acts as a selective dopamine D_2 receptor partial agonist. *Expert Opin. Investig. Drugs* 16, 771–775.

16

Cognitive Disorders

There are many interacting processes involved in cognitive behavior, including attention, different forms of memory, planning and executive function, flexibility, and response control. Equally, there are many different paradigms in the experimental psychology literature for measuring these functions in both animals and humans, and some of these were mentioned in Chapters 3 and 13. Since various aspects of cognitive behavior are impaired in a number of different clinical conditions, a wide range of cognitive models now play a central role in the drug discovery process to find drugs intended to restore cognitive function toward normal in these disorders (Fig. 16–1). Impairment of aspects of cognition is the dominant behavioral symptom in attention deficit hyperactivity disorder (ADHD) and Alzheimer's disease, and the behavioral evaluation of drugs targeted for these disorders is discussed in detail. The behavioral pharmacology of the frontal lobes is also reviewed since the working memory component of executive function is known to have specific pharmacological properties and should therefore be amenable to modulation by specific drugs. Whether drugs can enhance normal cognitive function is also considered.

In a number of central nervous system disorders other than ADHD and Alzheimer's disease, cognitive deficits are at least part of the clinical picture, and it should be recognized that the development of drugs to alleviate these

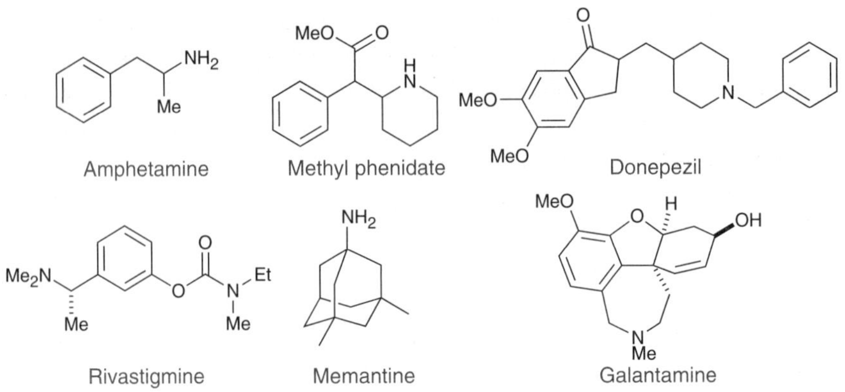

FIGURE 16–1. Commonly used cognition enhancers.

symptoms is an equally important challenge for drug discovery. These include aspects of cognitive dysfunction in advanced Parkinson's disease, schizophrenia (as discussed in Chapter 15), obsessive–compulsive disorder, posttraumatic stress disorder, depression of the elderly, and drug addiction.

THE DISORDERS

ADHD and Alzheimer's disease are the most common forms of cognitive disorder, and they are reviewed in detail in this chapter. In addition, there are many other rarer clinical forms of cognitive dysfunction, which are discussed briefly here.

AIDS dementia complex (ADC; also known as HIV dementia, HIV encephalopathy, and HIV-associated dementia) is a neurological disorder associated with HIV infection and AIDS. It is becoming less common as the use of highly active antiretroviral therapy has become more widely used and effective. The essential features of ADC are disabling cognitive impairment accompanied by motor dysfunction, speech problems, and behavioral change.

Dementia with Lewy bodies (DLB) is the second most frequent cause of hospitalization for dementia in the elderly after Alzheimer's disease. Approximately 60–75% of diagnosed dementias are of the Alzheimer's and mixed (Alzheimer's and vascular dementia) type, whereas 10–15% are DLB, characterized by the development of abnormal proteinaceous (α-synuclein) cytoplasmic inclusions, called Lewy bodies, throughout the brain. These inclusions have similar structural features as "classical" Lewy bodies seen subcortically in Parkinson's disease (see Chapter 17). When Lewy body inclusions are found in the cortex, they often co-occur with Alzheimer's disease pathology found primarily in the hippocampus.

Frontotemporal dementia is a clinical syndrome caused by degeneration of the frontal lobe of the brain and may extend back to the temporal lobe. It is one of three syndromes caused by neurodegeneration. Symptoms can be classified (roughly) into two groups, which underlie the functions of the frontal lobe: behavioral symptoms (and/or personality change) and symptoms related to problems with executive function (inability to organize a coherent future plan).

Multi-infarct dementia, also known as vascular dementia, is another common form of dementia in the elderly. The term refers to a group of syndromes caused by different mechanisms, all resulting in vascular lesions in the brain. Mixed Alzheimer's and vascular dementia is common.

Pick's disease is a rare frontotemporal neurodegenerative disease. It is the cause of approximately 0.4–2% of all dementia and affects women more than men. This disorder causes progressive destruction of nerve cells in the brain and causes tau protein to accumulate into the "Pick bodies" that are a defining characteristic of the disease.

ADHD

ADHD is a neurobehavioral developmental disorder affecting approximately 3–5% of the world's population younger than the age of 19 years. It typically presents during childhood and is characterized by a persistent pattern of inattention and/or hyperactivity, as well as forgetfulness, poor impulse control or impulsivity, and distractibility. ADHD is most commonly diagnosed in children, and during the past decade it has been increasingly diagnosed in adults. Approximately 60% of children diagnosed with ADHD retain the condition as adults. Methods of treatment usually involve some combination of medications, behavior modifications, lifestyle changes, and counseling.

ADHD has attracted an enormous amount of attention in recent years, not least because of the controversy surrounding the use of psychostimulant drugs in its treatment. A Google search for "ADHD" yields more than 30 million items. Some have argued that there is no real medical disorder, merely "naughty children," but there is little doubt that ADHD does exist. According to the *Diagnostic and Statistical Manual of Mental Disorders*, fourth edition (*DSM-IV*), three patterns of behavior indicate ADHD:

1. *Hyperactivity*. Hyperactive children always seem to be "on the go" or constantly in motion. They dash around touching or playing with whatever is in sight, or they talk incessantly. Sitting still at dinner or during a school lesson or story can be a difficult task. They squirm and fidget in their seats or roam around the room. They may wiggle their feet, touch everything, or noisily tap

their pencil. Hyperactive teenagers or adults may feel internally restless. They often report needing to stay busy and may try to do several things at once.

2. *Impulsivity.* Impulsive children seem unable to curb their immediate reactions or think before they act. They will often blurt out inappropriate comments, display their emotions without restraint, and act without regard for the later consequences of their conduct. Their impulsivity may make it difficult for them to wait for things they want or to take their turn in games. They may grab a toy from another child or hit when they are upset. Even as teenagers or adults, they may impulsively choose to do things that have an immediate but small payoff rather than engage in activities that may take more effort yet provide much greater but delayed rewards.

3. *Inattention.* Children who are inattentive have a difficult time keeping their minds on any one thing and may get bored with a task after only a few minutes. If they are doing something they really enjoy, they have no trouble paying attention. However, focusing deliberate, conscious attention to organizing and completing a task or learning something new is difficult. Homework is particularly difficult for these children. They will forget to write down an assignment or leave it at school. They will forget to bring a book home or bring the wrong one. The homework, if finally finished, is full of errors and erasures. Homework is often accompanied by frustration for both parent and child.

Children with ADHD may show all three types of behavior, or one or another behavior may predominate. Thus, there are three subtypes of ADHD recognized by professionals: the predominantly hyperactive–impulsive type (that does not show significant inattention); the predominantly inattentive type (that does not show significant hyperactive–impulsive behavior), sometimes called ADD (an outdated term for this disorder); and the combined type (that displays both inattentive and hyperactive–impulsive symptoms).

Because everyone shows some of these behaviors at times, the diagnosis requires that such behavior be demonstrated persistently to a degree that is inappropriate for the person's age. The diagnostic guidelines also contain specific requirements for determining when the symptoms indicate ADHD. The behaviors must appear early in life, before age 7 years, and continue for at least 6 months. Most important, the behaviors must create a real handicap in at least two areas of a person's life, such as in the classroom, on the playground, at home, in the community, or in social settings. Therefore, someone who shows some symptoms but whose schoolwork or friendships are not impaired by these behaviors would not be diagnosed with ADHD. Nor would a child who seems overly active on the playground but functions well elsewhere receive an ADHD diagnosis.

An Inherited Disease?

A number of family studies have shown that ADHD runs in families: Parents exhibiting symptoms of adult ADHD have a 1 in 4 risk of having a child with ADHD. Studies of identical twins have shown a concordance rate of 0.8 (i.e., if one twin develops ADHD, the other has an 80% chance of also developing the disorder). More detailed genetic analysis has suggested that ADHD may be caused by several interacting genes rather than a single gene. ADHD thus fits into the common genetic models of psychiatric illnesses, which have a complex multigene basis. Consistent evidence for association exists for four genes in ADHD: the dopamine D_4 and D_5 receptors and the dopamine and serotonin transporters. It is notable that three of the genes for which evidence of association is strongest are associated with dopamine function in the brain, suggesting the possibility that ADHD is associated with abnormalities in dopamine systems. However, one fifth of all cases of ADHD are estimated to be caused by trauma or toxic exposure.

Drug Treatment of ADHD

Methylphenidate

The most common drug used to treat ADHD is methylphenidate (MP; Ritalin). The compound exists in several isomeric forms; it is the racemic mixture of the *D* and *L*-isomers of *threo*-methylphendiate that is used medically. MP bears an obvious structural resemblance to *D*-amphetamine (see Fig. 16–1), and it is also similar in its pharmacology. MP is a potent inhibitor of dopamine and norepinephrine uptake in monoamine neurons by virtue of its affinity for the catecholamine transporters. However, unlike *D*-amphetamine, MP has little affinity for the serotonin transporter, and it is less effective than *D*-amphetamine in displacing catecholamines from their vesicular storage sites. In rats, MP elicits behavioral changes similar to those seen after *D*-amphetamine, with increased locomotor activity followed by repetitive stereotyped behavior after large doses of MP. In terms of both behavioral stimulation and its ability to promote catecholamine release in the brain, MP is approximately 10 times less potent than *D*-amphetamine.

Brain imaging techniques have shown that clinically used doses of orally administered MP cause more than 50% occupancy of the dopamine transporter sites in brain, comparable to the effect of the powerful psychostimulant drug cocaine, which also acts as an inhibitor of dopamine uptake in brain (see Chapter 21). Unlike cocaine, however, orally administered MP does not cause marked euphoria and is unlikely to lead to dependence. This is thought to be because the effect of orally administered MP on the dopamine transporter is slow in onset, whereas that of inhaled or insufflated cocaine is very rapid (see Figure 21–2).

This seems to be an example of the phenomenon that the rate at which drugs enter the brain and bind to their targets plays a crucial part in their reinforcing and addictive properties (see Chapter 20). MP is more likely to cause dependence if the powdered tablets are insufflated or injected; however, new dosage forms make this more difficult. Because of MP's short duration of action, the drug needs to be taken more than once a day, creating difficulties for schools to manage drug dosing and providing opportunities for inappropriate use of drug supplies. This problem has been partly overcome by the development of slow-release formulations of MP (Concerta and Metadate) that extend the duration of action to 7 or 8 hours, making drug administration during the school day unnecessary; these formulations are also impossible to crush or to dissolve for injection. A further development has been the marketing of D-MP as a separate single isomer form of the drug (Focalin and Attenade). The D-isomer seems to account for essentially all of the activity of DL-MP. Another pharmaceutical advance is the development of a skin patch formulation for delivering MP (Daytrana). Another approach uses a prodrug form of MP chemically linked to the amino acid L-lysine. The compound, lisdexamfetamine (Vyvanse), is pharmacologically inert and can only release MP when digested in the gut, thus precluding administration by any other route; this again reduces the risk of misuse.

Adderall

Adderall has become popular in recent years and accounts for nearly one fourth of U.S. sales of prescription medicines for ADHD. This drug is a complex mixture of different salt forms of amphetamine, such as D- and L-amphetamine sulfates, D- and L-amphetamine aspartate, and D-amphetamine saccharate, with a ratio of D- to L-amphetamine of 3:1. There seems to be little rationale for this mixture. Clinical trials comparing D- and L-amphetamine in treating hyperactive children have shown that L-amphetamine is effective, although as expected, less so than the pharmacologically more potent D-isomer. Adderall has an action that lasts for 6 or 7 hours, and this has been extended further by the preparation of a slow-release formulation (Adderall-XR). Comparisons of Adderall with MP have shown the two drugs to be of similar efficacy, although the longer duration of action of Adderall compared with standard-release MP is an advantage.

In addition to Adderall, D-amphetamine (Dexedrine) is also marketed for the treatment of ADHD.

Atemoxetine

This is a selective norepinephrine (NE) uptake inhibitor. It is the first non-stimulant, nonscheduled drug approved for the treatment of ADHD, although antidepressants such as bupropion, desipramine, and imipramine have long been viewed as alternatives to amphetamine or MP. It is not entirely clear that atemoxetine is as effective as MP or amphetamine in treating ADHD symptoms.

Modafinil

This stimulant drug, of unknown mechanism, was developed initially for the treatment of narcolepsy, but large-scale clinical trials have shown that it is also effective in treating the cognitive symptoms of ADHD. However, the Food and Drug Administration (FDA) has failed to approve modafinil for use in this indication because of rare adverse dermatological effects.

What Are the Effects of Amphetamines in Children and Adults with ADHD?

The approval of psychostimulant drugs as prescription medicines for the treatment of children with ADHD depended on concrete evidence that they were effective and safe. A variety of different rating scales have been devised to assess the effects of these drugs on ADHD symptoms. Commonly used rating scales include the Conners Teachers Scale and Conners Parents Scale, which are backed up by large databases of information on the effectiveness of these drugs, often from the first day of treatment, in normal and ADHD children of various ages. These and other similar rating scales use the diagnostic criteria for ADHD and ADD defined by the *DSM-IV* to provide numerical scores. Today, approval of a new medicine for ADHD relies on positive data from a variety of outcome measures involving teachers, parents, and physicians, including some form of global clinical assessment measure of improvement.

How can one explain the apparently paradoxical effects of psychostimulants in calming children with ADHD and improving their cognitive function? One hypothesis invokes the theory of rate dependency for CNS drug actions (see Chapter 3). Rate dependency refers to the observation that low baseline rates of response are increased by a drug, whereas higher rates are found to increase to a lesser extent or to decrease as a result of drug treatment. Response rate is thus an inverse function of baseline rate, as described in the following model:

$$\log (D/C) = (a - b) \log (C)$$

where D is response rate on drug, C is baseline response rate, and a and b are constants.

Many studies on a wide range of species have documented rate-dependent effects of amphetamine on fixed interval and fixed ratio schedules of reinforcement. Such effects have been shown for amphetamine doses as low as 0.1 mg/kg, with doses between 0.3 and 1.0 mg/kg found to produce decreases in high base rate responding. Thus, it appears that decreases in motor activity can be produced by amphetamines at doses lower than those that generate stereotypy and associated reduction in locomotor activity.

It has been suggested that the decrease in spontaneous motor activity seen in children with ADHD after treatment with stimulant drugs is attributable to rate-dependent effects. An analysis of raw data from several drug studies of ADHD children and data from a National Institute of Mental Health study of drug effects on normal children, normal adults, and children with ADHD yielded a good fit with the rate-dependency equation. The greatest reductions in activity were found for the most active ADHD children, whereas increases in activity were found for some normal adults within the group who started from low baselines of activity.

How Safe Are Ritalin and Adderall?

Both Ritalin and Adderall are remarkably safe drugs when used in the correct oral dosage regimes as recommended. However, as with any medicines, there are adverse side effects, some serious and others less so. The most serious adverse side effects are associated with the sympathomimetic actions of these drugs. Amphetamines and amphetamine-like drugs act on the peripheral sympathetic nervous system to promote NE release. This can cause an increase in heart rate and blood pressure, which in most healthy young people is of little consequence. However, there have been reports of serious adverse events associated with the cardiovascular system and even some deaths. This led to the temporary suspension of Adderall XR in Canada in 2005, and the FDA now requires manufacturers to include warnings of possible adverse cardiovascular and psychiatric side effects for all drugs used to treat ADHD, including atomoxetine. These risks are increased when children being treated with psychostimulants indulge in strenuous exercise or sports activities, which by themselves activate the cardiovascular system.

Behavioral side effects sometimes occur that are reminiscent of the stereotyped repetitive patterns of behavior seen in laboratory animals after high doses of amphetamine (see Chapter 21). These include abnormal movements, perseverative/compulsive behaviors, lip smacking, lip licking, and stereotyped behavior (e.g., picking at fingernails/finger tips, rubbing eyes or face, head jerking, and eye blinking). Children treated with Ritalin or Adderall may suffer loss of appetite and sleep disturbances. Loss of appetite may be so severe that growth is significantly impeded, but both of these side effects are usually controllable by adjusting the dose and by ensuring that the first dose of the day is given after breakfast rather than before. There is no evidence for long-term growth impairment. Instances of abuse and dependence liability with Ritalin or Adderall are rare, but this is largely because they are administered orally and build up slowly in the brain. There is little doubt that both methylphenidate and amphetamine can cause euphoria and are likely to have abuse potential if administered intravenously or by other fast-absorption routes.

A concern that has often been voiced by critics of Ritalin is that exposing children to powerful psychotropic drugs will make them more likely to abuse drugs later in life. Along with the comparison of Ritalin to cocaine, this concept has become embedded in the popular media as proved. However, the evidence from longitudinal studies of the subsequent drug history of children treated with Ritalin has actually led to precisely the opposite conclusion. A meta-analysis analyzed data from six published studies, involving a total of 674 children treated with Ritalin or related drugs and 360 unmedicated subjects, and concluded that childhood use of Ritalin was protective against adult alcohol or drug misuse. Children treated with psychostimulants were nearly six times less likely to use alcohol or illegal drugs in adolescence, and the protective effect persisted into adulthood, although it was reduced to an odds ratio of 1.5.

Animal and Human Models of Relevance to ADHD

Impulsivity is the most prominent clinical feature in ADHD underpinning profound deficits in attentional behavior. A number of animal models have been developed, and experimental studies with these led to the conclusion that impulsivity is not a unitary phenomenon. It almost certainly involves several overlapping neuropharmacological and neuroanatomical systems. Therefore, no one animal model is likely to replicate the full range of deficits found in ADHD, and the optimal drug treatments of the different forms of impulsivity are likely to require drugs that target several receptors. The 5-choice serial reaction time task (5-CSRTT), originally developed to study visuospatial attention in rats, has proved useful for understanding impulsivity. This is an automated discrete trial procedure in which the rat faces an array of five apertures, each fitted with a light and a food dispenser. Trial by trial, one of the apertures is briefly illuminated and the rat is required to make a nose poke to trigger a reward. The apertures are illuminated randomly, so the rat cannot know the location of the next stimulus and needs to attend to the spatial array of apertures. With training, rats learn to inhibit making responses before the light comes on. The number of responses before the onset of visual stimuli is used as the measure of impulsivity. Delayed aversion is another widely used task. Rats are faced with two response options in a food reward situation: immediate but small rewards or larger delayed rewards. Rats and humans who have a high level of impulsivity are generally more delay aversive and prefer immediate small rewards. A third paradigm, the stop-signal reaction time task (SSRT), is also proving useful. It measures the time taken to inhibit an already initiated motor response. On this task, rats initiate a trial by a nose poke to a central food well, after which the left lever and light are presented. A left lever press results in the appearance of the right lever and light and the disappearance of the left lever. The right lever is available for only a short time, and a quick reaction to the right lever is required to secure reward. Methylphenidate, amphetamine, and modafinil increase premature responding on both 5-CSRTT and SSRT in rats and normal volunteers. These effects are dependent on baseline levels of behavior, and this accounts for the fact that impulsivity is reduced by these drugs in ADHD. The selective NE reuptake inhibitor atamoxetine improved performance on all three of these models of impulsivity.

Lesions to the frontostriatal pathways, particularly to different sectors of the dopaminergic system and to the frontal cortex, impair impulsivity on these two tasks in different ways, strengthening the view that impulsivity has a number of dissociable dimensions. This is also true of the effects of drugs on these paradigms.

ALZHEIMER'S DISEASE

The first case described by Louis Alzheimer in Munich in 1907 was a woman in her fifties. On examination of the brain postmortem, Alzheimer was the first to observe the characteristic senile plaques and neurofibrillary silver-staining tangles that characterize the neuropathology of this disease. This was the first time that any psychiatric disorder had been linked directly to organic brain damage. For many years, Alzheimer's disease (AD) was considered to be a "presenile dementia" affecting people younger than the age of 65 years, but it is now known that AD is the most common cause of dementia no matter the age of the patients, and it accounts for approximately two thirds of all cases.

Dementia is the term used to describe the progressive decline in cognitive function due to damage or disease in the brain beyond what might be expected from normal aging. Although dementia is far more common in the geriatric population, it may occur in any stage of adulthood. Affected areas in cognition may be memory, attention, language, and problem solving. Higher mental functions are affected first in the process. Especially in the later stages of the condition, affected persons may be disoriented in time (not knowing what day of the week, day of the month, month, or even what year it is), in place (not knowing where they are), and in person (not knowing who they are). The most common form of dementia in the elderly is AD, which is characterized by a series of underlying neuropathological changes.

AD is progressive, resulting in impairment in cognitive function and, ultimately, loss of vital functions. Death occurs on average 8–10 years from disease onset. The clinical symptoms associated with the disease include memory loss, language disorders, visuospatial impairment, and behavioral disturbances.

AD may present with a variety of symptoms, but difficulties with memory are common to all. For a diagnosis of probable AD, the criteria adapted from the National Institute of Neurological and Communicative Disorders and the Stroke and Alzheimer's Disease and Related Disorders Association (NINCDS–ADRDA) include the following:

- Dementia established by examination and objective testing (characterized by the *DSM-IV* as a syndrome of multiple cognitive deficits, which include memory impairment and at least one of the following: aphasia, apraxia, agnosia, or disturbance in executive functioning. Social or occupational function is also impaired.)
- Deficits in two or more cognitive areas
- Progressive worsening of memory and other cognitive functions
- No disturbance in consciousness
- Onset between ages 40 and 90 years

The absence of systemic disorders or other brain diseases, which could account for the deficits in memory and cognition, should also be established.

Although a definitive diagnosis rests on confirmation of the characteristic neuropathology postmortem, careful application of NINCDS–ADRDA criteria provides approximately 90% accuracy of diagnosis of AD.

Neurobiology of Alzheimer's Disease

Knowledge of the underlying molecular pathology of AD has advanced dramatically in the past two decades. In postmortem brain, the neuropathology consists of numerous senile plaques, deposited particularly in the temporal cortex and hippocampus, together with the presence of silver-staining fibrillary tangles in dead or dying neurons and an accompanying loss of neurons from these brain regions. The senile plaques consist largely of an aggregated insoluble protein known as β-amyloid, and the neurofibrillary tangles represent an aggregated form of the cytoskeletal protein tau in a hyperphosphorylated state. β-Amyloid is a 40- to 42-amino acid residue self-aggregating protein derived from a larger cell membrane protein, amyloid precursor protein (APP), by two cleavage enzymes, the β- and γ-secretases (Fig. 16–2). APP can also be a substrate for a third enzyme, α-secretase, which cleaves within the β-amyloid sequence, thus preventing β-amyloid formation. These different processing pathways occur normally in brain and in many peripheral tissues. In AD, the pathways of APP processing favor increased formation of β-amyloid, and this leads to an accumulation of this protein in brain. β-Amyloid aggregates initially as soluble oligomers and later in an aggregated

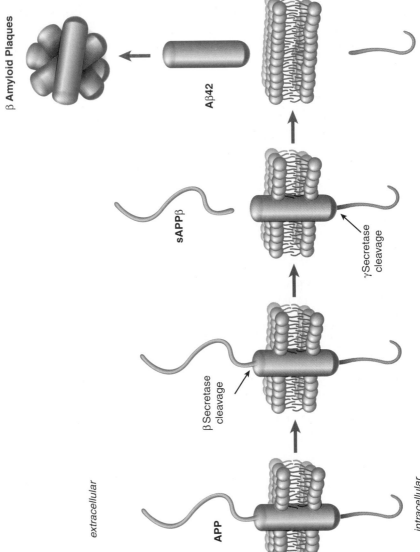

β Amyloid Plaques

Aβ42

sAPPβ

γSecretase cleavage

βSecretase cleavage

extracellular

APP

intracellular

form in senile plaques. It is this process that is thought to underlie the death of neurons, perhaps because β-amyloid provokes a local inflammatory reaction in those areas of brain affected. It is probable that β-amyloid accumulation leads in turn to the formation of tau-containing fibrillary tangles, but the nature of such a link is not clear. Mutations in the tau protein underlie frontotemporal dementia in some rare familial cases.

The β-amyloid hypothesis was greatly strengthened by the discovery of mutations found in rare familial cases of the disease, involving various different genes. Point mutations in the APP protein at or near the β-secretase cleavage points were the first to be discovered, and these promote increased β-amyloid formation, as do mutations in the presenilins, which are proteins that form part of the γ-secretase enzyme complex. In each case, the mutations tend to favor the formation of β-amyloid (1–42), which is particularly prone to self-aggregate. Mutations in the sortilin-related receptor 1 gene are also found in familial AD and again appear to act by shifting APP processing toward the β-secretase pathway.

Drug Treatment of Alzheimer's Disease

Currently available drug treatments for AD alleviate the symptoms rather than their underlying causes. A number of older drugs are still used in the United States and Europe.

Co-dergocrine (Hydergine), a combination of four different dihydroderivatives of ergotoxine, has been available since 1949. Although little used nowadays, most reviews are in agreement that the drug can improve activities of daily living and self-care but has no specific antidementia effect. The mild stimulant effect of the drug may elevate mood. It is approved as an adjunct in the management of mild to moderate cases of AD in the United Kingdom and for treatment of idiopathic decline in mental capacity in the United States.

FIGURE 16–2. The Beta-amyloid hypothesis of AD.
Beta-amyloid (Aβ), a 4 kDa protein, originates from the proteolytic cleavage of amyloid precursor protein (APP) by two proteases, β-secretase and γ-secretase. Cleavage by β-secretase at the amino terminus of APP results in a soluble β-APP and a 12 kDa membrane-bound carboxyl terminal fragment (CTF). The latter in turn becomes the substrate for γ-secretase to yield a soluble Aβ peptide (1–40), or the slightly longer, insoluble peptide amyloid β protein fragment Aβ (1–42). APP can also be cleaved by a third enzyme, α-secretase, leading to the production of soluble α-APP peptide and a 10 kDa CTF. Aβ (1-42) constitutes the major component of the nonfibrillar extracellular plaques that precede the development of the dense, fibrillar neuritic plaques characteristic of AD. (www.sigmaal-drich.com)

Nootropic agents, the "racetam" group of agents, include the pyrrolidinone derivatives piracetam, oxiracetam, aniracetam, nefiracetam, and levetiracetam. They have long been designated as cognitive enhancers or "nootropics." They have been employed for a number of cognitive disorders, including dementia, postconcussion syndrome, and dyslexia. However, their mechanism of action remains unclear, and the efficacy of these compounds is under debate. Despite this, some of these compounds continue to be used in Europe.

Naftidrofuryl (Praxilene) is thought to act by stimulating cerebral metabolism of cerebral blood flow. Some studies report benefits, although there are no clear signs of cognitive improvement. This is unlikely to gain approval under the strict criteria currently used.

The most important of the newer medicines are the acetylcholinesterase inhibitors (AChEI) (see Chapter 6). Their use in AD is based on the finding of severe damage in AD brain to the cholinergic neurons in a projection from the subcortical nucleus basalis to various regions of cerebral cortex and hippocampus. This ascending system is of key importance in cognitive function, particular in the laying down of new memories. In analyses of AD postmortem brain, it was found that the extent of the damage to cortical cholinergic nerves (measured by reductions in the biosynthetic enzyme choline acetyl transferase; see Chapter 6) correlated well with the density of senile plaques, a measure of AD disease progression. The first AChEI to be approved was tacrine (Cognex); it was the first to demonstrate that such drugs could improve cognitive function in AD patients, effectively setting the clock back 6–12 months. However, the drug is little used today because its short half-life requires frequent dosing, and there is a risk of liver damage. In 1997, donepezil (Aricept) was approved for treatment of AD based on positive effects in patients with mild to moderate dementia. The drug has a very long half-life (70–80 hours), allowing a gradual buildup of dose and maximal inhibition of the enzyme without causing too severe side effects, although like all AChEI gastrointestinal symptoms (including nausea, vomiting, and diarrhea), sweating and bradycardia can be dose limiting. Significant improvements are seen in primary cognitive function endpoints and in global clinical improvement, and these are maintained in long-term treatments of several years' duration. Overall, it appears that approximately 40% of AD patients benefit from treatment with donepezil.

A similar pattern of positive response is seen with the other available AChEIs rivastigmine (Exelon), which requires twice-daily dosing, and galantamine (Reminyl). The latter drug in addition to AChEI acts as an allosteric positive modulator of nicotinic receptors in brain, which may improve its cognitive enhancing effects, although this remains to be proved.]

The cholinesterase inhibitors represent an important advance in AD therapy, but a meta-analysis of the clinical data suggested that, at best, they yield minimal improvements lasting for 6 months or less (Kaduszkiewicz et al., 2005).

The only other recently approved drug for AD is memantine (Ebixa and Namenda) (see Fig. 16.1), which is believed to act by virtue of its weak gluta-mate NMDA receptor-blocking properties, perhaps protecting neurons against damage from excess glutamate release in AD. Whatever its mechanism, clini-cal trials have shown significant benefits in cognition and other symptoms. Surprisingly, these are seen in the most advanced cases of AD rather than in mild to moderate stages of the disease; memantine is the only drug approved for the treatment of advanced AD. Combination of memantine with acetylcho-linesterase inhibitors enhances its effectiveness.

Future Treatment for Alzheimer's Disease

The new insights into the molecular basis of AD have prompted an intense international research effort aimed at developing new medicines that may interfere with AD pathology at one or another stage in the hope that such treat-ments might slow down or block the progression of the disease. Although no such medicines are yet available, there are encouraging signs that this may eventually provide radical new treatments for AD. The most advanced clinical trials include the following compounds:

1. The γ-secretase inhibitor flurbiprofen (Flurizan): Positive phase II clinical trial data for flurbiprofen have been reported, but a phase III clinical trial failed to demonstrate any significant positive outcomes. Several other γ-secretase inhibitors remain in development (e.g., LY7450139).

2. A monoclonal antibody directed against β-amyloid: Bapineuzumab, designed to bind and remove β-amyloid, yielded positive phase II clinical trial data, but only in patients lacking the apolipoprotein E4 allele (ApoE4) (known to predispose to early onset AD).

3. The antidiabetic drug rosiglitazone yielded positive results in a phase II clini-cal trial, but again this was only if ApoE4 gene carriers were excluded.

4. The antihistamine drug Dimebon has been in use for AD in Russia since 1983. Results of a Phase III clinical trial in AD reported positive efficacy in all 5 outcome measures at 6 and 12 months.

In earlier stages of development are several inhibitors of the enzyme β-secretase and a variety of nonsteroidal anti-inflammatory drugs, some of which modulate β-amyloid synthesis. Treatments that target the underlying disease process are likely to be most effective if given to patients at the earliest stages of AD. The problem is that by the time clinical signs of memory loss and dementia become apparent, substantial cortical damage may already have occurred. New methods for the early diagnosis of AD are urgently needed. Progress is being made, for example, in devising radiotracers that bind to β-amyloid that can be used in brain imaging studies to measure the amount of β-amyloid accumulated in brain long before clinical signs become apparent.

Transgenic Animal Models of Alzheimer's Disease

AD is a rare example of how knowledge of the human disease has prompted the development of animal models that genuinely reflect some of the key aspects of the pathology underlying the human disorder. Small laboratory animals such as mice and rats do not normally develop β-amyloid-containing deposits or neurofibrillary tangles as they age. However, by genetic engineering it has been possible to develop several strains of so-called "Alzheimer mice." These express, for example, the point mutations in APP discovered in human familial cases of AD. As predicted, such mice synthesize abnormally large amounts of β-amyloid in their brains, initially as soluble oligomers and later (6–12 months) as insoluble deposits of aggregated protein. This is accompanied by cognitive deficits in various tests of learning and memory as the animals age, and the excessive formation of β-amyloid is accompanied by tau pathology in some models. A number of different mice expressing several of the human mutations are available. Although these mice show β-amyloid deposition, and sometimes excess tau accumulation, none have the other characteristic pathological feature of neurofibrillary tangles. However, by developing strains of mice that express both an APP mutation and a tau mutation, it has been possible to generate animals that show the typical cortical plaque and tangle pathology.

These experimental animals have proved very valuable in assessing new treatments for AD. For example, the use of antibodies against β-amyloid as a means of removing excessive amounts of the protein was first tested in such mice. Initially, the animals were vaccinated with β-amyloid. This generated an immune response with a number of antibodies that bound and removed β-amyloid. This proved remarkably successful in removing β-amyloid deposits from brain and this was accompanied by an amelioration of the cognitive deficits. Unfortunately, a clinical trial of the β-amyloid vaccine in AD patients had to be terminated because some patients developed a serious inflammatory reaction in the brain by antibodies that triggered a T cell response. A safer way of using immunotherapy may be to use monoclonal antibodies directed against β-amyloid, and one such product (bapineuzumab) is in advanced stages of clinical trials. The Alzheimer mouse also permits a detailed study of the molecular processes underlying brain damage following β-amyloid deposition, and these animals have formed the basis of a large international research effort.

ANIMAL AND HUMAN MODELS OF COGNITIVE FUNCTIONS

Until recently, the only drugs used for cognitive enhancement were a small group of so-called nootropics, which, although widely prescribed for dementias, have few reproducible effects in specific tests of memory in animals or humans. As new generations of cognitive enhancers are discovered, their efficacy will be judged by their effects on tests of aspects of cognitive dysfunction specific to a particular disease. Since the neurochemical and neuroanatomical circuits underpinning these functions are highly interrelated, it is not surprising that there are common aspects of cognitive dysfunction in clinical conditions that may in other respects be very different. For this reason, as new compounds are discovered, they will be explored for effects on a variety of cognitive functions and for a variety of clinical disorders. The range of models in this area of research is very wide, but here we focus on tasks for evaluating attention, long-term declarative memory, and working memory.

Of particular value for the future are tasks that can be developed in parallel for use in both animals and humans. The Cambridge Neuropsychological Test Automated Battery (CANTAB) test battery in humans, with its animal counterparts, is an excellent example of this approach. The subsets of tests are based on a number of learning and memory paradigms drawn from well-established neuropsychological test batteries, such as word-pair association learning from the Wechsler Memory Scale (Table 16–1). However, CANTAB also draws in a novel way on animal paradigms from the realm of learning theory. With the exception of long-term memory for verbal information, it has proved possible to design a variety of parallel tasks for rats, monkeys, and humans. The use of operant discrete trial procedures has the advantage of avoiding tester bias, as does the use of touch screen technology in humans and nonhuman primates.

Animal Models of Long-Term Memory

In AD, declarative memory for specific facts and events is severely impaired and is usually the first clear clinical symptom to emerge. It has been known for approximately 50 years that this aspect of long-term memory is dependent on the medial temporal lobe. Patients with bilateral damage to this area, which includes the hippocampus and overlying cortex, have profound anterograde amnesia. In AD, the progressive degenerative changes associated with plaque and neurofibrillary tangle deposition are first seen in the transitional region between the cortex and the hippocampus and spread rapidly in the temporal lobe. This explains the prominence of deficits in declarative memory. Psychologists have long studied different aspects of learning and memory in animals. The memory for a particular event (sometimes termed episodic memory)

TABLE 16–1. CANTAB Test Battery

TEST	DESCRIPTION	KEY MEASURES
Visual memory		
DMS	A four-choice test of simultaneous and delayed matching to sample of abstract patterns that share color or pattern with the distractors.	Percent correct Decision latency
PAL	A test of learning and memory. The ability to form visuospatial associations and the number of reminder presentations required to learn all the associations are assessed.	First trial memory score (sum of patterns correctly located on first presentation) Total errors Total trials to success Errors at the six-box level
PRM	A two-choice test of abstract visual pattern recognition memory (immediate and after a delay).	Percentage correct Response latency (ms)
SRM	A two-choice test of recognition for location of a white box on the computer screen.	Percent correct Response latency (ms)
Working memory and planning		
SWM	A test of spatial working memory and strategy performance to find individually hidden "blue tokens" without returning to a box where one has previously been found.	Strategy score Total between errors (returning to a box where a token has been found) Total within errors (returning to a box that has already been inspected)
SSP	A test of spatial memory span to recall the order in which a series of boxes were highlighted.	Span length Total errors
SOC	A spatial planning test involving planning a sequence of moves to achieve a goal arrangement and physically moving the balls by touching them on the VDU. The problems increase in difficulty by requiring more moves.	Problems solved in minimum moves Mean moves to success Initial planning time Subsequent movement time
OTS	A spatial planning test involving planning a sequence of moves to achieve a goal arrangement of colored balls without moving the balls. The problems increase in difficulty by requiring more moves.	Mean attempts Latency (ms)

TABLE 16–1. CANTAB Test Battery *(Continued)*

TEST	DESCRIPTION	KEY MEASURES
Attention		
RVP	A test of sustained attention to detect infrequent three-digit sequences from among serially presented digits.	Mean Latency A' (measure of ability to detect sequences) B' (measure of the tendency to respond regardless of whether target is present)
RTI	A "release and touch" test of speeded response to appearance of a visual stimulus. There are simple (single location) and five-choice (five possible locations) conditions.	Mean response time Mean movement time For single and five-location conditions
Cognitive flexibility, response control, risk taking, and decision making		
IED	Discrimination learning, testing the ability to selectively attend to and set-shift between shape, color, or number stimulus dimensions.	Total errors Total extradimensional shift errors Stages reached
SST	Ability to inhibit prepotent responses. Choice reaction time.	Stop signal reaction time (a measure of response inhibition) Median "go" reaction time Errors (incorrect discrimination responses on "go" trials)
AGN	Reaction time to stimuli of positive and negative affective valence.	Happy RT Sad RT Commission errors when the response valence changes on successive blocks of trials
CGT	A test of decision making. Patients decide whether a randomly hidden token is more likely to be in a red or blue box (the ratio of which varies within a display of 10 boxes). They then place bets (in ascending and descending order) on their choice being correct.	Probability of choosing the most likely outcome (red or blue—depends on the ratio) Percentage of available points bet (ascend and descend conditions) Initial deliberation time to "red" or "blue"

(Continued)

TABLE 16–1. CANTAB Test Battery (Continued)

TEST	DESCRIPTION	KEY MEASURES
IST	A test of predecisional reflection as measured by information sampling rates in revealing the color of cells in a 5 × 5 matrix and deciding on the majority color. Low memory demands.	Average number of boxes opened (a measure of reflection) Errors (wrong color choice)

DMS, Delayed Matching to Sample; PAL, Paired Associates Learning; PRM, Pattern Recognition Memory; SRM, Spatial Recognition Memory; SWM, Spatial Working Memory; SSP, Spatial Span; SOC, Stockings of Cambridge; OTS, One Touch Stockings of Cambridge; RVP, Rapid Visual Information Processing; RTI, Reaction Time; IED, Intra-Extra Dimensional Set Shifting; SST, Stop Signal Task; AGN, Affective go/no-go; CGT, Cambridge Gambling Task; IST, Information Sampling Task.
SOURCE: www.cantab.com.

depends on a sequence of processes—in basic terms, the acquisition or encoding of the information, the storage or consolidation of that information, and its subsequent retrieval. Dysfunction of any one of these component processes results in a loss of memory. Considerable effort has been made throughout the years to design animal and human tests of declarative memory capable of distinguishing the effects of brain damage or pharmacological manipulations on these component processes. It is beyond the scope of this discussion to review the evidence that a wide range of neurotransmitters contribute to learning and long-term memory. Among the most significant are well-established roles for the circuits mediated by the neurotransmitters ACh and 5-HT, but more recently there is increasing evidence that aspects of glutamate transmission also play a critical role in different stages of memory processing. Drugs with specific effects on these transmitter functions would be predicted to either impair or enhance aspects of normal long-term memory or be used to improve memory in neuropsychiatric diseases, particularly in AD and other dementias.

It is difficult to demonstrate improved memory if normal performance is at a high level. Therefore, the principle is to have a task that challenges normal performance to a level that can be improved by the drug. This can be done by putting pressure on the encoding process but is normally achieved by increasing the delay between acquisition and retrieval. Delay-related decrements in performance can be demonstrated with all long-term memory tasks. In rats, one-trial memory tasks have been used most frequently, but the interpretation of results from such tests depends critically on the design of the experiment, as depicted in Figure 16–3. Passive avoidance and contextual fear conditioning are examples involving electric shock. With these paradigms, it is important to ensure that the effects of a drug are on memory and not on changes in motor behavior.

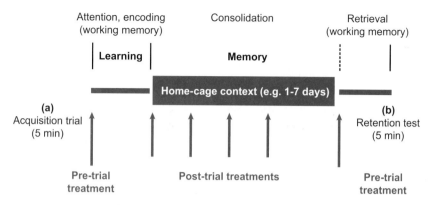

FIGURE 16–3. Pharmacological analysis of stages of memory processing. Depicted are two trials of any standard learning paradigm: (**a**) acquisition training and (**b**) retention testing. Pharmacological interventions before acquisition can potentially affect a range of sensory, perceptual, attentional, motivational and motor performance factors, in addition to learning and memory processes. A lack of effect on retention indicates a specific effect on learning or memory-related processes such as encoding or memory consolidation. A lack of effect in initial training in acquisition accompanied by an effect on retention usually indicates an effect on memory consolidation or retrieval. The time-limited nature of consolidation means that post-trial treatments soon after the first trial will affect memory consolidation, indicated by performance in the retention test, typically 1 – 7 days later. Working memory is an active process of memory that is usually engaged soon after perceptual processing to encode memory traces into passive storage. However, memories that are activated by memory cues also place retrieval memory traces into an active form in working memory for the guidance of behavior. (Modified from Robbins and Murphy, 2006.)

Some novel rodent tasks have been introduced that do not involve memory for aversive events. For example, one-trial place memory is tested in an arena with a 7×7 grid of circular holes covered by lids that can be removed to insert sand wells. A trial consists of an encoding and retrieval phase. In the encoding phase, the rat must search for a food reward buried in a sand well in a trial-specific place. All other possible sand well locations are closed and covered by sawdust. The rats dig in the sand to find a food reward and are then removed from the arena. In the retrieval phase, beginning after a delay during which the rat is returned to its home cage, food is buried in the sand well in the same place as in the encoding phase and sand wells without food are now open in four novel places. To find food efficiently, the rat must use one-trial place memory according to a win-stay rule. Start positions for the encoding and retrieval phases on each trial vary among the four start boxes on the four walls of the arena. Therefore, the task cannot be solved by habit but puts pressure on place memory guided by prominent visual cues provided around the arena (allocentric place memory). Memory is robust on this task, lasting for at least

6 hours, and it has been shown that hippocampal NMDA receptors are required for encoding but not retrieval, whereas AMPA receptors are involved in retrieval.

Using the same apparatus, a rat equivalent of paired-associate learning has been developed. Paired-associate learning typically consists of a study phase of pairs of items (e.g., word pairs) followed by a test of cued recall. Rats enter the arena from a start box and are trained to dig in a single uncovered sand well at a particular location to find a flavored food pellet and during a second sample trial to dig at another location for a different flavored pellet. The recall cue is a pellet of one of these two flavors that the rat eats while confined to a different start box. After this 30-second recollection interval, the rat is released back into the arena and faced with the same two uncovered sand wells. If the cue was the same as the first flavor experienced, digging at the first location is rewarded, whereas digging at the other location is rewarded if the cue was the same as the second flavor. Rats thus learn a unique association between an event and a place (i.e., what and where). On this task, blockade of hippocampal NMDA function was found to impair memory encoding but not retrieval, whereas AMPA blockade impaired both encoding and recall. The emerging pattern of pharmacological results on a variety of these long-term memory tasks suggests that in this area of pharmacology, novel cognitive-enhancing drugs are likely to be discovered.

It remains the case that the most commonly used rat models capitalize on their remarkable ability to learn about and remember spatial events. These include the Morris water maze and the 8-arm maze, both of which were described in Chapter 3 and are widely used for pharmacological and lesion studies. These are not strictly one-trial tasks but can be used to study the effects of drugs on acquisition or delay-dependent retrieval, again depending on when the treatment is given. A form of the Morris water maze is now widely used to evaluate spatial reference memory in mice genetically modified in different ways to model the progressive neuropathological changes in AD or the expression of different levels of neurotransmitter receptors implicated in different aspects of memory. Performance on these spatial memory tasks again depends critically on NMDA-mediated processes in the hippocampus.

However, the long-term memory of objects as opposed to spatial events depends critically on the perirhinal cortex. The episodic memory for objects proved more difficult to measure in animals but was eventually achieved in monkeys using a delayed nonmatching-to-sample task, tested in the Wisconsin Test Apparatus using a three-well test board. Monkeys can be trained to inspect a list of common junk objects presented one by one covering a rewarded food well. After a delay, the same list of objects is re-presented one at a time, but now with a pair of familiar objects being presented with a novel object. A reward can be found under the novel object. The familiar objects are presented in the same order in which they were already seen. Monkeys can remember long lists of objects so that delays of many minutes separate the first and second presentation of a particular object. Using this nonmatching-to-sample paradigm, long-term object memory was convincingly demonstrated for the first time and shown to be disrupted by medial temporal lesions. The perirhinal cortex has proved to be the critical part of this lesion with regard to object memory. The task can now be tested more easily using visual graphics presented with touch screen computer technology. It has been demonstrated that physostigmine enhances performance on this task and that NMDA receptors are also critical for this form of memory. In monkeys trained to remember a list of 20 graphics for 10 minutes, systemic treatment with D-cyloserine, a partial agonist at the glycine modulatory site on the NMDA receptor, significantly improved performance and reversed an impairment induced with the NMDA antagonist dizocilpine (MK-801).

A rat one-trial object recognition task has been described. Each trial consists of two phases. In the sample phase, two identical objects are placed in a Y-shaped apparatus, one at the end of each exploration arm. The rat is released into the exploration area and allowed to explore the objects for 25 seconds. It is then removed from the apparatus for a delay period before being returned to the apparatus, in which one copy of the sample (familiar) object is in one arm and a new object is in the other. The rat explores the objects for 2 minutes and a discrimination ratio is calculated (the proportion of total exploration time spent exploring the novel object). The retention delay between sample and choice phases can be varied. Blockade of AMPA and NMDA receptors in perirhinal cortex disrupts different aspects of encoding, consolidation, and retrieval of object memory.

However, animal models of long-term memory have proved to be of most value to the drug discovery process in the field of cholinergic pharmacology. The cholinergic deficiency hypothesis of AD focused attention on the study of drugs able to enhance brain cholinergic function. It has proved difficult to demonstrate reliable enhancement of normal levels of memory with cholinomimetics, not least because of the adverse peripheral effects of these compounds. The paradigm most widely adopted involves the use of the cholinergic antagonist scopolamine to disrupt memory. The putative cognitive enhancer is then evaluated for its ability to reverse this disruption. The effects of cholinesterase inhibitors, including those currently in clinical use, were demonstrated to have efficacy in this way. In principle, any of the animal models discussed previously lend themselves to this use and, indeed, have been used. However, discrete trial operant tasks are particularly useful for drug evaluation since well-trained animals can be used over extended periods of time to obtain dose–response data on novel compounds. This is not impossible with one-trial tests, but it is more difficult because large matched groups of animals are required.

Delayed matching to sample of spatial position has been widely used for the evaluation of cholinomimetics. In rats, it is not clear that the impairment induced by scopolamine is primarily on memory since the impairment is not delay dependent. In monkeys, a touch screen task has been used. A trial starts when a white square appears at one of nine positions on the screen. The animal presses the square, it disappears immediately, and after a delay all nine identical white squares appear at all the possible locations on the screen. The monkey is required to touch the square occupying the same spatial position as the acquisition stimulus in order to obtain a reward. Training continues with intermingled blocks of trials with delays increasing from 2 to 20 seconds. Scopolamine produces a delay-dependent impairment on this task that is reversed in a dose-dependent manner by physostigmine (Fig. 16–4) and other cholinesterase inhibitors in clinical use and by muscarinic agonists. Although the cholinergic hypothesis provided the first clinically approved drugs for the treatment of AD, cholinergic deficits are no longer believed to be the primary cause of memory loss in AD.

In humans, the episodic memory impairments in AD can be evaluated with a wide range of classical neuropsychological tests. The memory components of CANTAB are particularly valuable both to characterize the mnemonic deficits in AD and to compare their pattern of impairments with that seen in other degenerative diseases involving forebrain pathophysiology, such as Parkinson's disease (PD), or in psychiatric conditions (e.g., depression in the elderly). Equally important is the fact that these tasks closely model animal tests of long-term and working memory. The components used for a comparison of AD and PD were (1) pattern recognition (Pattern Recognition Memory), (2) spatial recognition (Spatial Recognition Memory), (3) matching to sample (Delayed Matching to Sample), and (4) visuospatial associative learning (Paired Associates Learning). The details of these tasks can be found in Sahakian et al. (1988). The AD patients tested were early in the course of the disease and were classified as stage 1 on the Clinical Dementia Rating Scale. They were significantly impaired in both spatial and visual pattern recognition memory, and they exhibited a delay-dependent deficit in delayed matching to sample, whereas simultaneous matching was unimpaired. They were also severely impaired on the visuospatial associative learning task, as would be expected from frequently reported deficits on paired associate word learning. This latter task is also able to detect a subgroup of patients diagnosed as suffering from questionable dementia, who fail this task and have been shown to go on to develop global cognitive decline. Such a marker of future AD will be invaluable when drugs become available that will halt or slow the degenerative processes in dementias. Concerns have been raised about the appropriateness of testing such drugs in well-advanced AD, but with no reliable method of

PHYSOSTIGMINE

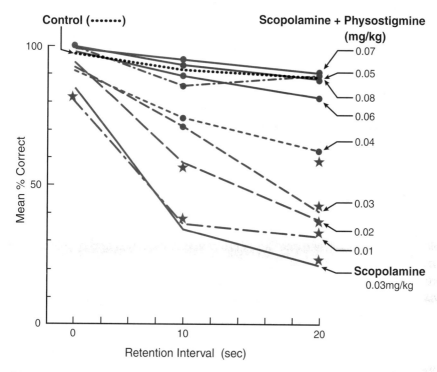

FIGURE 16–4 Reversal of scopolamine-induced spatial memory impairment in rhesus monkeys by the acetylcholinesterase inhibitor physostigmine.

Physostigmine was co-administered with scopolamine (0.03 mg/kg intramuscularly) 30 minutes prior to behavioral testing (n = 4-6 at each dose).* = P < 0.05 when compared to undrugged control; • = P < 0.05 when compared to scopolamine treatment alone. (Modified from Rupniak et al., 1989.)

detecting the disease before memory deficits become obvious, there has been no alternative.

Working Memory and the Prefrontal Cortex

Working memory depends on accessing information, holding and manipulating it on line, and using it to guide behavior. It is short term compared with some of the forms of long-term reference memory discussed previously. The spatial matching tasks mentioned previously are therefore sometimes described as short-term or working forms of memory. Since working memory deficits are seen in AD, these ACh-dependent tasks remain useful for evaluating cognitive enhancers of this pharmacological class.

However, the classical working memory tasks in the literature were described more than 50 years ago in monkeys and are known to depend critically on the integrity of the dorsolateral frontal cortex (DLFC). In monkeys, bilateral surgical removal of this sector of DLFC severely impairs performance on the delayed response and delayed alternation tasks. So too do 6-OHDA lesions targeted to the sulcus principalis of DLFC that severely depletes the mesocortical dopaminergic input to pyramidal neurons. Goldman-Rakic and colleagues extended these earlier studies to demonstrate that, unlike the situation in the striatum, dopamine D_1 receptors dominate in DLFC and that their selective pharmacological manipulation changes working memory performance and the neurophysiological correlates of that behavior. These studies used an occulomotor task of working memory. Monkeys fixate a target in the center of a screen and, while fixated, a brief visual stimulus is presented at one of six positions in the peripheral visual field. After a delay, the fixation stimulus goes off and this is the signal for the monkey to make a saccadic eye movement to the location where the target had been seconds before. This secures a fruit juice reward directly into the mouth. Because the position of the target varies randomly from trial to trial, the monkey has to continually update its memory of the target position. This is a well-controlled task compared with the delayed response or delayed alternation tasks tested in the Wisconsin General Test Apparatus (see Chapter 3). Using this task, it has been demonstrated that local intracerebral injections of the selective D_1 antagonists SCH23390 and SCH39166 increase errors and increase the latency of the response. The deficit is delay dependent and pharmacologically specific since the dopamine D_2 antagonist raclopride had no effect on performance. Subsequently, these studies were extended by combining iontophoretic analysis of dopamine receptors with single-cell recording during behavior. It was found that dopamine D_1 antagonists can selectively potentiate prefrontal neurons that subserve this form of working memory. At first sight, this was an unexpected result since it had already been shown that dopamine D_1 antagonists impair performance. However, from it has emerged one of the most significant findings for cognitive pharmacology—the so-called *inverted U-shaped function* (Fig. 16–5). Simply stated, optimal behavioral performance demands the appropriate degree of activation of receptors. Too little or too much dopamine D_1 receptor activation results in less than optimal working memory. Dopamine D_1 antagonists push dopamine D_1 receptor activation to the left and reduce performance. On the other hand, if dopamine D_1 receptor activation is already high and beyond the optimal level, D_1 antagonists can bring the receptor activation back into the normal range for optimal working memory performance. The nature of the inverted U relation constrains the degree to which cognition can be enhanced by activating dopaminergic mechanisms.

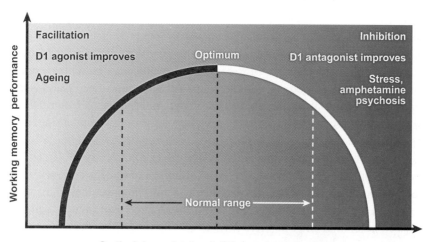

Cortical dopamine levels/D1 receptor activation

FIGURE 16–5. Inverted 'U' shaped function for the role of dopamine D_1 receptor in pre-frontal mechanisms for working memory.
When either prefrontal dopamine levels or D_1 activity are below the optimal range, as may occur with ageing, or above the optimal range, as may occur with stress or amphetamine-induced psychosis, working memory performance is impaired. In such instances dopamine D_1 agonists or antagonists, respectively, may restore performance to the optimal range. (Modified from Desimone, 1995.)

It has been suggested that working memory is heavily dependent on access-ing appropriate information, a process heavily dependent on attention, and that the classical delayed response task does not challenge. A task has been developed for the rat that allows simultaneous assessment of attention to a spatial visual stimulus and memory for that stimulus. In the 5-CSRTT para-digm, the rat is required to nose poke in the food magazine to trigger a light in one of the five apertures. A response to that aperture within 5 seconds triggers a delay during which the rat is required to nose poke in the food magazine until two apertures light up simultaneously (the original target plus one dis-tracter). A response to the original target is rewarded with two food pellets in the magazine. This task puts pressure on attention by varying the duration of the target and on memory by increasing the delay between the sample stimu-lus and the choice. The selective dopamine D_1 agonist SKF 81297 infused into prefrontal cortex modulates the attentional and memory components of per-formance but at a given dose may improve attentional accuracy and disrupt or facilitate working memory in a delay-dependent manner, providing one of the clearest demonstrations of the significance of the inverted U-shaped relation-ship in understanding the effects of drugs on cognition.

Working memory impairments are seen in PD, and MPTP-treated monkeys are impaired on delayed response and delayed alternation tasks and on a barrier detour task that involves working memory because the animal must guide the direction of its hand movements by a representation of the goal rather than by direct visualization of the stimulus. Working memory deficits are also a prominent feature of the cognitive dysfunction in schizophrenia, and it has been proposed that the interaction between dopamine D_1 and glutamate receptors on the dendritic spines of pyramidal neurons in the DLPC (Fig. 16–6) may represent an important target for drugs to treat cognitive deficits associated with psychosis.

The DLFC and other sectors of the frontal cortex also receive 5-HT and NE input, and there is much interest in the neurotransmitter interactions with different classes of cortical neurons and interneurons. Pharmacological manipulations of these transmitter systems also result in cognitive changes, and this offers a number of other possible ways to enhance cognition. Indeed, components of cognition may well depend on a number of interacting neurotransmitters, each operating on the inverted U-shaped relationship. It is therefore difficult to predict the profile of a drug likely to be of benefit for a particular cognitive deficiency. There is substantial evidence that NE in the prefrontal cortex also contributes to working memory performance. A number of variables influence working memory performance, including stress levels and age. Both influence performance of monkeys on the delayed response task, and

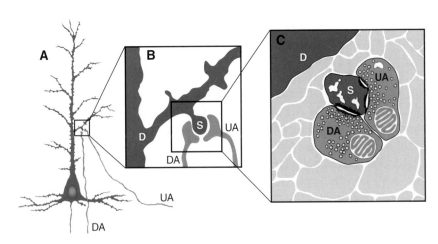

FIGURE 16–6. Synaptic arrangements of dopamine input to the cortex.
A) Dopamine (DA) afferents labeled with a specific antibody terminate on the dendritic spine of a pyramidal cell in the prefrontal cortex, together with an unidentified axon (UA); B) Enlargement of synapse illustrated in A showing apposition of the DA input and a presumed excitatory input that makes an asymmetrical synapse on the same dendritic (D) spine (S); C) Diagram of synaptic arrangement illustrated in B; the DA terminal (darkened by antibody staining) forms a symmetrical synapse; the unidentified axon forms an asymmetrical synapse with the postsynaptic membrane. (With permission from Goldman-Rakic, 1992.)

these decrements in performance can be alleviated with α_2-adrenergic receptor agonists. Clonidine has been extensively investigated in normal volunteers, aged monkeys, and rat models and shown to enhance working memory when high levels of attention are required. Much research interest has therefore focused on patients with ADHD. Guanfacine, a selective α_{2A}-adrenergic receptor agonist, has a superior cognitive enhancing profile with fewer side effects, demonstrating the importance of this receptor subtype. α_1-Adrenergic receptor agonists, in contrast, impair performance, and activation of these receptors is thought to be associated with high stress levels. β-Adrenergic receptor activation with clenbuterol has also been shown to improve working memory modestly in aging monkeys, but it is also known to enhance performance in inhibitory avoidance tasks. β-Adrenergic blockers such as propranolol are being investigated in posttraumatic stress disorder for their ability to block emotional memories, but it is possible that selective β_1 antagonists may be more clinically effective.

COGNITION ENHANCERS: "SMART DRUGS"?

There is great interest in the possibility that so-called "smart drugs" can enhance normal human cognitive performance. A Google search yields almost half a million entries. This class of psychoactive substance includes drugs with the potential to enhance cognitive performance not only in patients with neurological or cognitive disorders but also in normal, healthy people. *Cognition* refers to the internal brain processes that underlie mental activity, such as attention, perception, learning, memory, language, planning, and decision making. Cognitive performance depends on a number of important factors, such as arousal (i.e., level of wakefulness) and motivation. Thus, in theory, a cognition "enhancer" may produce its effects indirectly by acting on arousal or motivation, and this is probably how psychostimulants act to influence cognitive performance.

A major impetus for the emergence of cognition enhancers has been the interest shown by the pharmaceutical industry in the treatment of dementia (including AD, Pick's disease, and Lewy body dementia, as well as the dementia associated with PD) and, recently, stroke, schizophrenia, and ADHD. Although some drugs for the treatment of cognitive disorders are potentially suitable for use by healthy individuals, many are ineffective or potentially unsafe. There are no programs in the pharmaceutical industry to develop cognition enhancers for the healthy population, and there is no regulatory or legal framework in place to approve such drugs for human use. However, it is likely that some cognitive enhancing drugs, including those developed to treat specific clinical conditions, may be suitable for healthy subjects. It is clear that claims spread by word of mouth, the media, and the Internet have led to considerable "off-label" use. Cognition enhancers and "smart drugs" are widely advertised and sold on the Internet, often with exaggerated claims for their efficacy.

Caffeine

Caffeine is the most widely consumed psychoactive drug in the world, with approximately 90% of the population (including children) in the United States regularly consuming caffeine-containing soft drinks, coffee, or tea. Caffeine is a legally available cognition enhancing drug, although its effects are mild. In animals, caffeine has similar properties to classical psychostimulants such as cocaine or amphetamines. It stimulates motor behavior and improves performance on repetitive cognitive tasks. In drug discrimination tests, caffeine partly cross-generalizes to amphetamine in animals trained to recognize the amphetamine cue. There is little doubt that caffeine is mildly rewarding, and many habitual users develop dependence on the drug. If switched to caffeine-free products, they develop a withdrawal syndrome that may include headache, fatigue, decreased energy, depressed mood, difficulty concentrating, and irritability. These unpleasant effects are thought to play a role in maintaining human habitual caffeine consumption.

Caffeine acts as a relatively nonselective antagonist at adenosine receptors (see Chapter 11). Its psychostimulant actions are due to its ability to indirectly stimulate dopaminergic systems in the brain. In animals, the motor stimulant effects, which underlie the ability of caffeine to act as a discriminative cue, are blocked by dopamine depletion or dopamine antagonists. Like other psychostimulants, caffeine causes an increase in dopamine release in the nucleus accumbens. At the synaptic level, the mechanism of action is unusual because the actions of caffeine seem to depend on its activation of adenosine A_1 and A_{2A} receptors present as heterodimers with dopamine D_1 and D_2 receptors, respectively, in dopamine-rich areas of brain. Activation of the adenosine receptor in these heterodimers renders dopamine less effective in activating the D_1 or D_2 receptor. One hypothesis about the mode of action of caffeine is that by blocking the effects of adenosine, normally present as a "brake" on dopamine receptor function, the drug mildly stimulates dopaminergic function.

Nutraceuticals and Vitamins

Many food extracts claimed to have a medicinal benefit on human health are currently available, and many are said by various sources to improve cognition. Such supplements are usually well tolerated with no known abuse potential, and they are regulated in the United States by the FDA and in the United Kingdom under the Food Safety Act 1990. They include vitamins E, B_6, B_{12}, folate, thiamine, lecithin, neurosteroids such as dehydroepiandrosterone, and ginkgo biloba. A group of antioxidants claimed to promote mitochondrial function and to enhance cognition includes α-lipoic acid, acetyl-L-carnitine, and coenzyme Q. The latter compound was found to be partially protective against the neurotoxin MPTP in a primate model, and it has been proposed as a treatment for PD and Huntington's disease (see Chapter 17).

For most of these supplements, there is insufficient evidence to assess efficacy, either because the trials were too small or too few in number or included only poor measures of effectiveness. Studies in healthy individuals have produced some suggestive effects, such as associations between vitamin B_6 and memory, but these findings remain inconclusive.

Cholinergic Drugs

Several existing cognitive enhancers are based on the concept of enhancing neural transmission through the cholinergic system, known to be important in the cerebral cortex in cognitive functions such as attention. Whether or not enhancing cholinergic function can yield "smart drugs," it is fairly clear that antagonists of cerebral cholinergic function can be regarded as "dumb drugs." For example, the muscarinic receptor antagonist scopolamine causes well-documented impairments in learning and memory in human volunteers.

Cholinesterase Inhibitors

As described previously, cholinesterase inhibitors are important in the treatment of AD. Cholinesterase inhibitors have been found to induce cognitive improvements in laboratory tests in healthy volunteers, although effects on different types of cognition can vary between individuals. One study showed that donepezil enhanced the performance of healthy middle-aged pilots after flight simulator training. Clearly, such drugs have some potential to be considered "smart drugs," although they cause a variety of unpleasant and potentially hazardous adverse side effects.

Nicotine and Related Compounds

Nicotine has long been known to be effective in promoting attention, and it appears to also have beneficial effects on learning and memory (see Chapter 26). Nicotine has been shown to improve performance in laboratory tests of sustained attention in young adults and elderly volunteers who are already smokers (see Chapter 26). The synthetic drug varenicline (Chantix), introduced for cessation of tobacco smoking, targets a particular nicotinic receptor subtype in brain. Other drugs that target nicotinic receptors are in development as potential cognitive enhancers for treating the cognitive deficit in schizophrenia.

Psychomotor Stimulant Drugs

Psychomotor stimulant drugs such as a D-amphetamine (Dexedrine and Adderall) and methylphenidate (Ritalin) are most widely known for their use in treating ADHD. However, such drugs are also known to exert some mild beneficial effects on cognition in normal adults, especially under conditions of fatigue. Effects on vigilance, verbal learning, and long-term memory are often relatively small, but the ability of these drugs to permit subjects to continue cognitively demanding tasks for long periods of time is real. This feature probably accounts for the popularity of these drugs with students studying for examinations or in preparing lengthy essays. Small percentage increments in performance can result in the difference between an A grade and lower grades.

However, the effects of these drugs cannot simply be ascribed to their prevention of drowsiness. Stimulant drugs may enhance the efficiency of cortical processes by enhancing the signal-to-noise ratio. This enhancement may be brought about through actions on the dopaminergic and noradrenergic systems that innervate the cerebral cortex. Animal studies have demonstrated that both dopaminergic and noradrenergic systems are implicated in mediating functions such as working memory in "higher" brain regions, including the prefrontal cortex. Such actions of psychostimulant drugs appear to be at least partially distinct from their effects on subcortical brain regions implicated in mediating their "rewarding" or "reinforcing" effects.

Related drugs such as L-DOPA can also effect improvements in healthy subjects in forms of learning that are guided by rewarding feedback.

Atypical Stimulants: The Unusual Case of Modafinil

Modafinil (Provigil) is licensed for the treatment of excessive daytime sleepiness associated with narcolepsy and disorders of breathing during sleep (sleep apnea). The drug is also approved for the treatment of sleep disorders resulting from shift work. Studies have shown that non-sleep-deprived volunteers may also benefit in certain domains of cognitive function. Tests on young adults have shown improvements in verbal working memory, visual recognition, planning performance, and executive inhibitory control (stop signal reaction time). However, improvements were not seen in other tests of learning and memory, suggesting that the beneficial effects of modafinil may be limited to particular brain systems. Volunteers treated with modafinil are able to sustain long periods (24–48 hours) without sleep, without obvious adverse effects. The beneficial effects of modafinil, together with its lack of obvious toxic effects or apparent abuse liability, appear to have led to considerable off-label use of this compound. In addition, it is used by the U.S. military as an alternative to D-amphetamine in maintaining wakefulness in air crews involved in prolonged flight missions.

A major question concerning modafinil relates to its mechanism of action, which is unclear. Early suggestions that it acts on the noradrenergic and dopaminergic systems were later replaced by claims of actions on the orexin neuropeptide system, known to be importantly involved in the control of sleep–wake cycles. Understanding the mode of action of modafinil will be important for the future development of further cognitive enhancing drugs.

Cerebral Vasodilators and Nootropics

Cerebral vasodilators are agents that act to widen blood vessels in the brain, increasing blood flow. Vasodilators such as naftidrofuryl have been proposed to enhance cognition in disorders such as vascular or multi-infarct dementia, but there are few controlled clinical trials. Several other agents, including phosphodiesterase inhibitors and calcium channel blockers (e.g., nimodipine), may also affect cerebral metabolism and blood flow. These agents may also have a role as cognition enhancers. A review of the clinical data on the calcium channel blocker nimodipine suggested benefits for cognition in dementia but not in overall functioning. Inhibition of phosphodiesterase by such agents as rolipram and papaverine can lead to increases in cellular signaling by molecules such as cyclic AMP, which has been implicated in cellular processes underlying memory. However, there are few data to indicate any therapeutic potential of these drugs.

Hydergine

The mixture of ergot derivatives called hydergine is available for use in elderly patients with mild to moderate dementia, and it has positive effects on mood if not on cognition per se.

SELECTED REFERENCES

Azron, N. H. and W. C. Holtz (1966). Punishment. In *Operant Behavior: Areas of Research and Application* (W. K. Honig, Ed.). Appleton, New York, pp. 300–447.

Ballon, J. S. and D. Feifel (2006). A systematic review of modafinil: Potential clinical uses and mechanisms of action. *J. Clin. Psychiatry* 67, 554–566.

Bobb, A. J., F. X. Castellanos, A. M. Addington, and J. L. Rapoport (2005). Molecular genetic studies of attention deficit hyperactivity disorder 1991–2004. *Am. J. Med. Genet. B Neuropsychiatr. Genet.* 132, 109–125.

Clark, C. M., C. Davatzikos, A. Borthakur, A. Newberg, S. Leight, V. M. Lee, and J. Q. Trojanowski (2008). Biomarkers for early detection of Alzheimer pathology. *Neurosignals* 16, 11–18.

Desimone, R. (1995) Is dopamine a missing link? *Nature* 376, 549–550.

Ferré, S. (2008). An update on the mechanism of the psychostimulant effects of caffeine. *J. Neurochem.* 105, 1067–1079.

Ferster, C. B. (1966). Animal behavior and mental illness. *Psychol. Rev.* 16, 345–356.

Goldman-Rakic, P. S. (1992). Dopamine-mediated mechanisms of the prefrontal cortex. *Semin. Neurosci.* 4, 149–159.

Imbimbo, B. P. (2008). Therapeutic potential of gamma-secretase inhibitors and modulators. *Curr. Topics Med. Chem.* 8, 54–61.

Kaduszkiewicz, H., T. Zimmermann, H. P. Beck-Bornholdt, and H. van den Bussche (2005). Cholinesterase inhibitors for patients with Alzheimer's disease: Systematic review of randomised clinical trials. *BMJ.* 331, 321–327.

Leonard, B. L., D. McCartan, J. White, and D. J. King (2004). Methylphenidate: A review of its neuropharmacological, neuropsychological and adverse clinical effects. *Hum. Psychopharm.* 19, 151–180.

Lichtlen, P. and H. Mohajeri (2008). Antibody-based approaches in Alzheimer's research: Safety, pharmacokinetics, metabolism and analytical tools. *J. Neurochem.* 104, 859–874.

Liu, J. (2008). The effects and mechanisms of mitochondrial nutrient α-lipoic acid on improving age-associated mitochondrial and cognitive dysfunction: An overview. *Neurochem. Res.* 33, 194–203.

Mehta, M. A. and W. J. Riedel (2006). Dopaminergic enhancement of cognitive function. *Curr. Pharm. Des.* 12, 2487–2500.

Robbins, T. W. and E. R. Murphy (2006). Behavioural pharmacology: 40+ years of progress, with a focus on glutamate receptors and cognition. *Trends Pharmacol. Sci.* 27, 141–145.

Rupniak, N. M., M. J. Steventon, M. J. Field, C. A. Jennings, and S. D. Iversen, (1989) Comparison of the effects of four cholinomimetic agents on cognition in primates following disruption by scopolamine or by lists of objects. *Psychopharmacology (Berl).* 99, 189-95

Sahakian, B. J., R. G. Morris, J. L. Evenden, et al. (1988). A comparative study of visuospatial memory and learning in Alzheimer-type dementia and Parkinson's disease. *Brain* 111, 695–718.

Sarter, M. (2006). Preclinical research into cognition enhancers. *Trends Pharmacol. Sci.* 27, 602–608.

Seow, D. and S. Gauthier (2007). Pharmacotherapy of Alzheimer disease. *Can. J. Psychiatry* 52, 620–629.

Serretti, A., P. Olgiati, and D. De Ronchi (2007). Genetics of Alzheimer's disease. A rapidly evolving field. *J. Alzheimers Dis.* 12, 73–92.

Swainson, R., J. R. Hodges, C. J. Galton, et al. (2001). Early detection and differential diagnosis of Alzheimer's disease and depression with neuropsychological tasks. *Dement. Geriatr. Cogn. Disord.* 12, 265–280.

Zhang, Y. W. and H. Xu (2007). Molecular and cellular mechanisms for Alzheimer's disease: Understanding APP metabolism. *Curr. Mol. Med.* 7, 687–696.

17

Movement Disorders

Movement disorders are neurological conditions that affect the speed, fluency, quality, and ease of movement. Abnormal fluency or speed of movement (*dyskinesia*) may involve excessive or involuntary movement (*hyperkinesia*) or slowed or absent voluntary movement (*hypokinesia*). Movement disorders include the following conditions:

- Ataxia (lack of coordination, often producing jerky movements)
- Dystonia (causes involuntary movement and prolonged muscle contraction)
- Huntington's disease (also called chronic progressive chorea)
- Multiple system atrophies (e.g., Shy–Drager syndrome)
- Myoclonus (rapid, brief, irregular movement)
- Parkinson's disease
- Progressive supranuclear palsy (rare disorder that affects purposeful movement)
- Restless leg syndrome (RSD) and periodic limb movement disorder (PLMD)
- Tics (involuntary muscle contractions)
- Tourette's syndrome
- Tremor (e.g., essential tremor and resting tremor)

- Wilson's disease (inherited disorder that causes neurological and psychiatric symptoms and liver disease)

PARKINSON'S DISEASE

This is by far the most common of the movement disorders, affecting 1% of people older than age 65 years and 2% of those older than 80 years. It is the second most common neurodegenerative disorder after Alzheimer's disease (see Chapter 16). Consequently, Parkinson's disease (PD) is the focus of a major portion of the research in the movement disorder field. The pathological hallmark of PD is the Lewy body, an accumulation of filamentous material derived from cytoskeletal components and aggregates of the protein α-synuclein. Lewy bodies are found in the pigmented monoamine neurons in brain stem, and their accumulation is associated with the progressive degenerative loss of dopamine and norepinephrine (NE) neurons. The gradual loss of the nigrostriatal dopamine (DA) neurons leads to the classical extrapyramidal motor symptoms of bradykinesia, tremor, and rigidity that characterize the disease. There is a remarkable degree of redundancy within the nigrostriatal system in that up to 80% of the DA neurons may be lost before clinical symptoms begin to appear. Apart from the movement dysfunction, which varies considerably from one patient to another, there are numerous other symptoms, including autonomic dysfunction, cognitive impairments, and sleep disturbance.

The etiology of PD remains obscure. An epidemic of PD of viral origin followed an epidemic of encephalitis in the early 20th century, but recent research has focused on the discovery of genetic risk factors. Valuable clues have come from the study of rare cases of familial disease. These have revealed a number of mutations in risk factor genes, including α-synuclein (a major protein in Lewy bodies), in which single mutations, duplications, and triplications have been found; the *parkin* and *UCHL1* genes, associated with the ubiquitin–proteasome system thought to be involved in promoting α-synuclein aggregation; *DJ1* and *PINK* genes involved in mitochondrial metabolism; and the *LRRK2* gene, in which a number of mutations and variants occur. As with all such breakthroughs in human genetic research, it will take time to translate these findings into practical new treatments, but their future promise is exciting.

DYSTONIAS

Common forms include *spasmodic torticollis*, which affects muscles of the head, face, and neck, and *blepharospasm*, which causes involuntary closing of the eyelids.

TOURETTE'S SYNDROME

Tourette's syndrome has a prevalence of 1% and is characterized by multiple motor and vocal tics, including involuntary movements and vocal noises. The symptoms start in childhood, often between 5 and 7 years, and are usually worst at approximately 11 years and often improve into adulthood. The syndrome may include involuntary swearing and compulsion to say or do socially unacceptable things, including echophenomena (irritating repetition of words or phrases said by themselves or others). The disorder has a strong genetic component, but other possible risk factors include birth injury, streptococcal autoimmunity, and psychosocial stress. The behavioral phenotype is heterogeneous. Only approximately 10% of patients present with tics alone. The remainder have additional comorbidities, most commonly obsessive–compulsive disorder (OCD) and attention deficit hyperactivity disorder (ADHD).

HUNTINGTON'S DISEASE

This is an inherited autosomal dominant disease caused by a mutation in the gene encoding the protein Huntington. There are approximately 30,000 patients in the United States. Although the mutation was identified almost 20 years ago, the molecular pathology remains obscure. The disease is characterized by progressive physical and mental deterioration, including characteristic "choreiform" convulsive body movements. Physical symptoms include the following:

- Development of tics (involuntary movement) in the fingers, feet, face, or trunk
- Increased clumsiness
- Loss of coordination and balance
- Slurred speech
- Jaw clenching or teeth grinding
- Difficulty swallowing or eating
- Continual muscular contractions
- Stumbling or falling

These are accompanied by mental symptoms, including forgetfulness and memory decline, poor judgment, and difficulty making decisions or answering questions. They are also accompanied by emotional changes, including hostility/irritability and disinterest in life (lack of pleasure or joy). Patients may also exhibit psychosis, including delusions, hallucinations, inappropriate behavior (e.g., unprovoked aggression), and paranoia.

ESSENTIAL TREMOR

This is a neurological disorder characterized by shaking of hands (and sometimes other parts of the body including the head), evoked by intentional movements. It is the most common type of tremor and probably the most commonly observed movement disorder. Half of the cases are due to gene mutation and transmitted dominantly. There are two main loci: ETM1 and ETM2. The rest are idiopathic. Essential tremor generally presents as a rhythmic tremor (4–12 Hz) that is present only when the affected muscle is exerting effort (in other words, it is not present at rest). Any sort of physical or mental stress will tend to make the tremor worse, often creating the false impression that the tremor is of psychosomatic origin. It is typical for the tremor to worsen in "performance" situations, such as when writing a check at a checkout stand.

TREATMENTS

General

A wide variety of drugs are used in the treatment of movement disorders. Table 17–1 summarizes some of the most important, and it is clear that there is considerable overlap in the treatment of different disorders. The muscle relaxant actions of benzodiazepines, for example, are used to treat a variety of conditions.

A remarkable treatment for a variety of dystonias and other movement disorders is botulinum toxin (Botox, Dysport, or Myobloc). This is a protein toxin synthesized by the bacterium *Clostridium botulinum* and is one of the most deadly poisons known. In 19th-century Germany, it was known as the "sausage poison" because outbreaks of botulism were often associated with poorly prepared meat products. The toxin selectively blocks neuromuscular transmission by interfering with the release mechanism for acetylcholine; it kills by paralyzing the respiratory muscles. Medically, it is used in minute doses, injected locally into a particular muscle area. At the cholinergic nerve terminal, botulinum toxin-A binds to one of the key proteins involved in acetylcholine release, called SNAP-25, and degrades it. This irreversibly inactivates the cholinergic terminal, and recovery occurs only when a fresh supply of the SNAP-25 protein is delivered by the slow process of axonal flow. This means that the actions of a single minute dose of the toxin can persist for

TABLE 17–1. Drugs Used to Treat Movement Disorders

PARKINSON'S DISEASE	HUNTINGTON'S DISEASE	TOURETTE'S SYNDROME	DYSTONIAS	RESTLESS LEGS SYNDROME	ESSENTIAL TREMOR
L-DOPA			L-DOPA	L-DOPA	
DA agonists			DA agonists	DA agonists	
	Neuroleptics	Neuroleptics (pimozide)[a]	Neuroleptics		
Anticholinergic			Anticholinergic		
	Benzodiazepine		Benzodiazepine		Benzodiazepine
	SSRIs	SSRIs	Baclofen		
	Lithium				
		Clonidine	Botulinum toxin		Botulinum toxin
					Propranolol
	Tetrabenazine				Primidone

SSRIs, selective serotonin reuptake inhibitors.

[a] Pimozide is approved by the FDA for this indication.

weeks or months. The medical use of botulinum toxin has proved very successful, and the product is approved by the Food and Drug Administration (FDA) for the treatment of blepharospasm, cervical dystonia, and excessive underarm sweating (also controlled by a cholinergic mechanism). However, botulinum toxin is used for the treatment of a wide range of other movement disorders. In recent years, there has also been a rapidly growing use of the toxin for cosmetic purposes—for example, to smooth out facial wrinkles. A cosmetic version (Botox Cosmetic) has received FDA approval.

Parkinson's Disease

The understanding that the symptoms of PD are largely caused by a loss of dopaminergic neurons from brain led to the use of the DA precursor L-DOPA, the first rational development of drug treatment for a central nervous system condition (Table 17–2). This has been of enormous benefit to millions of sufferers of this disabling disease. L-DOPA therapy has been improved by the combination of L-DOPA with carbidopa or benserazide, compounds that inhibit the metabolism of L-DOPA in the liver by the enzyme DOPA decarboxylase, thus making more drug available to enter the brain. The metabolism of L-DOPA by the enzyme catechol-O-methyl transferase (COMT) can be blocked by the use of the COMT inhibitors entacapone or tolcapone. One product, Stalevo, combines L-DOPA with both carbidopa and entacapone. A problem in using L-DOPA, however, is that the duration of action is relatively short and patients may thus suffer swings in the efficacy of symptoms control with "off" periods. To smooth out such fluctuations, sustained-release formulations of L-DOPA have been developed, and for treatment-resistant patients a constant intraduodenal infusion of a viscous gel containing L-DOPA can be used.

Another way of making L-DOPA treatment more effective is to use drugs that act directly as DA receptor agonists. The constant injection of the agonist apomorphine is a very effective way of controlling symptoms, but the complexity and expense of this limits its use. Other DA agonists given orally, or by transdermal patch (rotigotine [Neupro]), are widely used. Some can be used as monotherapy in the treatment of early stage PD, and bromocriptine and ropinirole have been shown to be as effective as L-DOPA in such patients. In later stages of the disease, DA agonists are frequently used as add-ons to L-DOPA in order to have a "levodopa sparing" effect and to reduce the fluctuations between on and off periods. There seems to be little difference in the efficacy of the various DA agonists, and they all target both dopamine D_2 and D_3 receptors (Table 17–3).

Another class of drugs used to treat PD is the monoamine oxidase B inhibitors rasagiline and selegiline. The precise mechanism of action of these is not

TABLE 17–2. Drugs Used in the Treatment of Parkinson's Disease

DRUG	TRADE NAME
L-DOPA	
L-DOPA + carbidopa	Sinemet
L-DOPA + benserazide	Madopar
L-DOPA + carbidopa + entacapone	Stalevo
Dopamine agonists	
Apomorphine (parenteral)	Uprima
Bromocriptine	Parlodel
Cabergoline	Dostinex, Cabase
Pramipexole	Mirapex
Ropinirole	Requip
Rotigatine	Neupro[a]
COMT inhibitors	
Entacapone	Comtan
Tolcapone	Tasmar
Monoamine oxidase B inhibitors	
Rasagiline	Azilect
Selegiline	Eldepryl
Anticholinergics	
Benztropine	Cogentin
Orphenadrine	Norflex
Trihexyphenidyl	Artane
Amantadine	Symmetril

[a] Not available in the United States.

clear, but they may inhibit the inactivation of DA in the central nervous system. A metabolite of selegeline also possesses mild amphetamine-like stimulant properties. Some physicians favor the use of selegiline as monotherapy in early stage patients. It is available in a fast-absorbed oral disintegrating tablet formulation (Zelapar) and also as a once-a-day transdermal patch (Emsam). The newly introduced rasagiline has the advantage of being a once-a-day oral medicine. Some long-term studies with selegeline suggest that the compound may exert a neuroprotective effect, slowing the course of the disease. However, other studies have failed to confirm this finding.

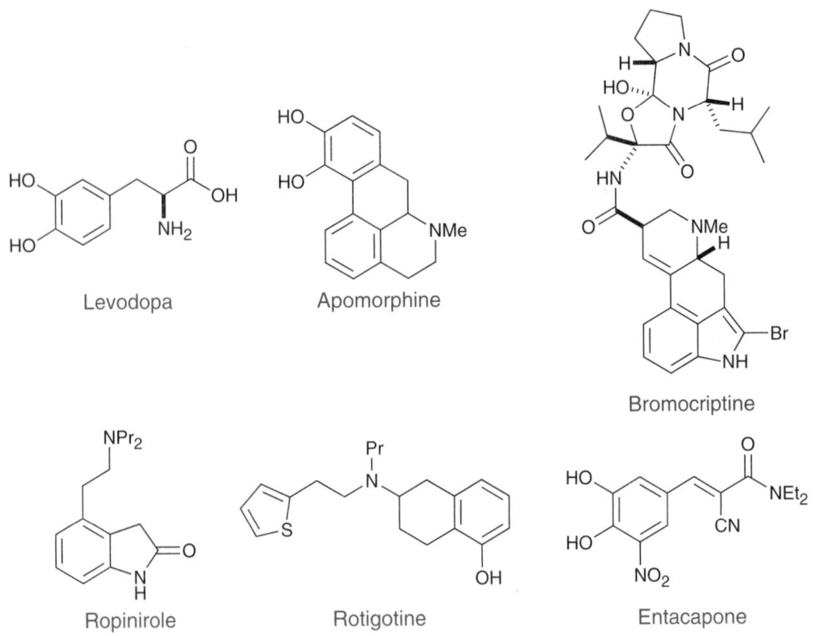

FIGURE 17–1. Drugs used in Parkinson's Disease.

It should be emphasized that PD also involves damage to other nondopaminergic neurons, including those that employ NE or acetylcholine, and there are a variety of nonmotor symptoms that do not respond to L-DOPA or dopaminergic agonists (e.g., emotional disturbance, sleep disorders, and gastrointestinal and urinary dysfunction) (see Rothstein and Olanow, 2008).

Amantadine, originally developed as an antiviral agent, is rarely used in treating PD, but it may be helpful in treating L-DOPA-induced dyskinesias in advanced stage patients. The mechanism of action is unclear.

TABLE 17–3. Dopamine Agonist Receptor Profiles

AGONIST	ERGOT DERIVATIVE?	DOPAMINE D_1	DOPAMINE D_2	DOPAMINE D_3
Bromocriptine	Yes	–	++	++
Cabergoline	Yes	++	++++	?
Primipixole	No	–	+++	++++
Ropinirole	No	0	+++	++++
Rotigotine	No	++	+++	++++

Other medicines include anticholinergic drugs such as trihexyphenidyl and orphenadrine, which were widely used in the pre-DOPA era but are only rarely used today. These drugs may, however, be helpful in controlling acute dystonic reactions. Their use is associated with troublesome side effects, including cognitive impairments and frank confusional state. The antitremor effects of these drugs may still occasionally be useful.

A potentially important new class of nondopaminergic drugs are adenosine antagonists that target the adenosine A_{2A} class of receptors. These receptors are expressed in highdensity in basal ganglia, where they may form heteromeric functional complexes with dopamine D_2 receptors. Drugs that act as antagonists at adenosine A_{2A} sites are effective in animal models of PD, and one such compound, istradefylline, is in advanced stages of clinical development. This would be the first time that a heteromeric receptor complex has been targeted.

Animal Models of Parkinson's Disease

The symptoms of PD largely reflect the profound depletion of forebrain dopaminergic neurons, and this has guided the development of animal models. Pharmacological treatments (e.g., reserpine and α-methyl-p-tyrosine) that deplete brain catecholamine stores result in a loss of motor behaviors. These syndromes can be temporarily reversed by L-DOPA. Lesion models have proved more useful. The discovery of the selective catecholamine neurotoxin 6-hydroxydopamine (6-OHDA) led to a breakthrough in experimental studies of forebrain DA pathways. 6-OHDA can be injected locally into regions containing catecholamine cell bodies or into terminal areas that they innervate. The toxin can also be injected intracerebroventricularly, resulting in a depletion of both NE and DA. Selective DA depletion can be achieved by pretreating with desipramine, which blocks the uptake of the 6-OHDA into NE neurons. However, it is difficult to achieve controlled lesions to the DA pathways with this toxin. Lesions need to result in greater than 80% depletion of striatal DA in order to observe reliable motor deficits. Lower levels of depletion are rapidly compensated for by increases in activity of the remaining DA neurons. At depletion levels greater that 90%, DA receptor upregulation is observed in the striatum, again enhancing the remaining function. However, despite these problems, 6-OHDA lesions have been widely studied.

Soon after the distribution of the DA neurons and their ascending projections was described in the rat brain, Ungerstedt used unilateral injections of the selective neurotoxin 6-OHDA into the substantia nigra to lesion the nigrostriatal pathway on one side of the rat brain. These rats had motor deficiencies contralateral to the lesion side, and they showed rotational behavior when treated with indirect or direct DA agonists. Whereas amphetamine induces turning ipsilateral to the side of the lesion, the agonist apomorphine induces contralateral rotation because it acts preferentially on the sensitized DA receptors on the lesioned side. This model, using a "rotometer" apparatus (Fig. 17–1), has proved valuable in assessing novel D_2 receptor agonists of potential value in treating PD.

Bilateral 6-OHDA lesions to the substantia nigra (SN) have also been studied, using local SN infusion or intracerebroventricular injection. The bilateral depletion of striatal DA results in profound deficits in motor behaviors including bradykinesia that are somewhat alleviated by L-DOPA. Indeed, careful observation of these animals reveals a wide variety of the clinical features seen in PD. However, the bilateral 6-OHDA lesion also severely impairs feeding and drinking behavior, and the rats require a level of husbandry that limits its usefulness as an experimental model. Current research focuses on the unilateral 6-OHDA lesion model in both rats and monkeys, in which a hemiparkinsonian syndrome is described. In the rat, use of the rotometer model has overshadowed the wide range of contralateral motor and sensorimotor deficits that can be observed in rodents and serve as valid models of PD. These are proving valuable for evaluating not only drugs but also neuronal grafts.

Another major breakthrough in PD research came with the fortuitous discovery of the neurotoxin 1-methyl-4-phenyl-1,2,3,6-tetrahydropyridine (MPTP). This story is one of the most fascinating in modern pharmacology. In 1976, an amateur chemist in Maryland was attempting to synthesize 1-methyl-4-phenyl-4-propionoxypiperidine (MPPP), an analog of the analgesic meperidine, with known psychotropic properties. He injected himself with the drug intravenously and after some doses developed the clinical symptoms of PD, which were successfully treated with L-DOPA. Chemical analysis of the drug revealed the presence of MPTP, which produced short-lasting motor effects when injected into rats. The case was published and nothing more thought of it until a few years later in 1982, when a group of young heroin addicts in northern California also experienced a rapid-onset PD syndrome. Chemical analysis of the contaminated drug they were abusing revealed the presence of MPTP. Langston, a neurologist, recognized the link between these cases and the earlier report. It eventually emerged that the illicit drug manufacture in both cases had taken a shortcut in the chemical synthesis process and produced, by mistake, not MPPP but MPTP. The systemic injection of MPTP into experimental animals of various species results in a specific parkinsonian syndrome associated with severe damage to the nigrostriatal DA system. The drug is converted by monoamine oxidase-B to 1-methyl-4-phenylpyridinium (MPP+), which is concentrated by the DA transporter in DA neurons, where it acts as a mitochondrial toxin. Rats are relatively insensitive to MPTP, but this is not the case in monkeys, in which daily intravenous dosing with MPTP for

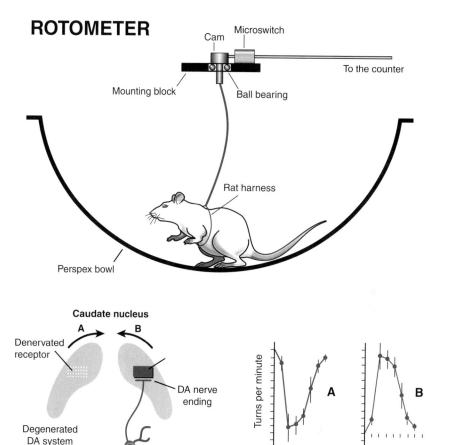

FIGURE 17–2. The rotometer. (Left) Schematic drawing of the rotometer, a half-spherical bowl in which movements of the rat are transferred by a steel wire to a microswitch mounted above. The animals were prepared previously by unilateral injection of the DA neurotoxin 6-OHDA in the striatum to cause a unilateral DA depletion. (Top) When stimulation of the sensitized DA receptor on the denervated side occurs, animals turn away from the lesion (A). If stimulation takes place only on the innervated side, animals turn toward the lesion (B). (Bottom right) Rotational behavior in response to apomorphine (direct acting agonist) (A) and amphetamine (indirect DA stimulant) (B). Negative values are obtained when the denervated side predominates, and positive values are obtained for the innervated side. (Iversen and Iversen, with permission from Ungerstedt, 1971.)

5–8 days results in a severe parkinsonian syndrome with a full range of clinical motor symptoms. The primate model has become a gold standard in the behavioral repertoire for evaluating novel drugs for treating PD.

Animal Models of Cognitive Dysfunction in Parkinson's Disease

The MPTP model in the monkey has been suggested to mimic both the pathophysiological and the behavioral sequelae of human idiopathic PD. However, in addition to profound motor impairments, PD also results in neuropsychological deficits reminiscent of frontal lobe dysfunction and distinct from the dementia often seen later in this progressive disease. The object retrieval/detour task described in Chapter 15 and used to characterize PCP-induced cognitive deficits in monkeys has also been used to investigate the behavioral impairments in MPTP-treated monkeys, in which damage to the ascending DA systems involves striatal and cortical DA depletion. This task is able to assess speed of directed actions and also the cognitive flexibility required to retrieve food when direct reaching is precluded by a transparent barrier. Systemic treatment of monkeys with MPTP (0.3–0.4 mg/kg over 5 days) results in severe debilitating autonomic and motor impairments in some animals but leaves others with no gross behavioral symptoms. The baseline level of the DA metabolite homovanillic acid measured in this latter group of animals at various times after treatment was found to be reduced by 65% at 1 year. These monkeys were tested on the object retrieval detour task 8–12 months following MPTP treatment and found to show (1) impairment on the acquisition of the task, (2) motor deficits (number of reaches and time to initiate them), and (3) cognitive deficits (reaches into the barrier, perseverative responses, and awkward reaches). In this study, the task was modified to increase the motor difficulty by placing the reward in less accessible areas of the transparent box and changing the direction of the open side after one or more trials (which encourages perseveration).

Cognitive deficits have also been reported in PD on tasks such as the Wisconsin Card Sorting Task (WCST) that demand flexibility and the ability to change strategy in the face of changing circumstances. Subjects are given a pack of 60 cards on which are printed one to four symbols (triangle, star, cross, or circle) in one of four colors (red, green, yellow, or blue). No two are the same. Subjects are instructed to place the cards one by one under four sample cards. After each card is placed, the tester says "correct" or "incorrect," and from this feedback the subject must work out the correct sorting strategy—that is, by color, shape, or number. Once the subject adopts the required sorting strategy and 10 correct placements have been made, the rule is changed and the subject must find the next required sorting strategy. The normal order used is color followed by form and then number, repeating until all the cards have been sorted. Performance is measured by how many correct sorting strategies are achieved with the pack of cards. In humans, frontal lobe lesions also impair performance. Tasks of this kind are often described as set shifting and are usually automated with graphics and touch screen technology. The Intra-Extra Dimensional Set Shifting task (IED) of the Cambridge Neuropsychological Test Automated Battery (CANTAB) is one such task. Humans and monkeys are able to attend selectively to one dimension of a compound stimulus that is reliably correlated with reinforcement and shift easily to novel stimuli constructed from new exemplars of the original stimulus dimension. (intradimensional shift [IDS]). If, however, the relevant dimension is switched to the previously irrelevant dimension, the task becomes much more difficult (extradimensional shift [EDS]).The WCST requires a form of EDS and therefore it was predicted and found that patients with PD are impaired on EDS but not IDS.

Adverse Effects of L-DOPA and Dopamine Agonists

The adverse effects of L-DOPA and the DA agonists are similar. Both can cause nausea and vomiting, and drug-induced orthostatic hypotension is common (patients may faint on rising from their bed or chair). The drugs ameliorate the motor symptoms of PD but can also cause dyskinesias, with uncontrolled movements of head or trunk. As the disease progresses, L-DOPA and the agonists become less effective, leading to increases in the doses used. This may lead to disturbed sleep, nightmares, psychotic thought disturbance, and confusion. These symptoms can be so severe as to be dose limiting, and they are sometimes treated with an atypical neuroleptic (e.g., quetiapine), although pharmacologically this is paradoxical. In advanced stages of PD, patients may suffer from a form of dementia, and this may be treated with an acetylcholinesterase inhibitor (e.g., rivastigmine). Ergot derivatives (bromocriptine and cabergoline) may cause pleuropulmonary fibrosis in a small percentage of patients, but this can become severe and life-threatening. One ergot dopamine agonist, pergolide, was withdrawn because of this risk. A bizarre side effect has been observed in some PD patients treated with pramipexole or ropinirole who developed compulsive gambling behavior, despite never having previously displayed such behavior. Fortunately, this is a rare side effect, seen in less than 1% of treated patients.

Animal Models of L-DOPA-Induced Dyskinesia

L-DOPA-induced dyskinesia (abnormal involuntary movements) is one of the most debilitating side effects seen in parkinsonian patients treated with L-DOPA. These movements are generally choreiform. Initial attempts to develop an animal model used 6-OHDA to lesion the nigrostriatal pathways. 6-OHDA lesioned rats treated chronically with L-DOPA exhibit abnormal movements. In the unilateral lesioned preparation, the drug induces clear involuntary movements in the forelimb, trunk, and orofacial musculature contralateral to the lesion. These movements are described as deformed fragments of motor programs that interrupt normal behavioral activities; they do not resemble the stereotyped behaviors induced by DA agonists. Drugs with reported anti-dyskinetic efficacy in PD, including amantadine, clozapine, and α_2-adrenergic receptor antagonists, reduce the severity of these involuntary movements. The validity of this rat model has been questioned with claims that the abnormal movements are merely compensatory to the marked body turning and rotation induced by the lesion. However, the two lesion-induced syndromes can be dissociated. Of more widespread use is the unilateral intracarotid infusion of the toxin MPTP in monkeys, which results in a contralateral hemiparkinso-nian syndrome. When treated chronically with L-DOPA, abnormal involun-tary movements, particularly involving the forelimb and the orofacial musculature, emerge on the body side contralateral to the lesion. These are strikingly similar to those seen in L-DOPA-treated PD patients.

Tourette's Syndrome

The treatment of Tourette's syndrome has remained the same for many years. Polypharmacy typifies the clinical drug treatment but is different for the two clinical clusters—that is, predominantly tics or tics together with OCD/ADHD. Multiple complex tics are treated with typical neuroleptics with potent dopamine D_2 receptor-blocking activity. In the United States, pimozide and haloperidol are FDA approved for this indication. The parallels with schizo-phrenia are striking both in terms of the brain systems thought to be involved in the disorder and in terms of the challenges of discovering better drug treat-ments. The use of neuroleptics is associated with sedation, weight gain, acute dystonic reactions, and tardive dyskinesia. There is optimism that atypical antipsychotics, such as risperidone, may offer a treatment with fewer side effects, but their improved efficacy in the treatment of Tourette's syndrome remains unproven. It is not clear why typical neuroleptics are effective in this condition. There is no consistent evidence of DA overactivity, but modest increases in DA receptors and in the DA transporter have been reported. As with schizophrenia, novel compounds with activity at receptors other than or in addition to dopamine D_2 are seen to be the hope for the future. These include 5-HT_{2A}, GABA, and glutamate. In patients with tics plus behavioral disorders, the first-line treatment remains the α_2-adrenergic receptor agonists clonidine and guanfacine. α_2-Adrenergic receptors control the terminal release of NE in the forebrain and the firing of NE neurons in the locus ceruleus.

There are currently no specific animal models of Tourette's syndrome. Novel compounds identified using models in the antipsychotic test battery will no doubt be explored for possible use in the treatment of complex multiple tics.

Huntington's Disease

Treatment focuses on reducing symptoms and preventing complications. A wide variety of medicines are used to help control emotional and movement symptoms, including the following:

- Antipsychotics to control hallucinations, delusions, and violent outbursts (haloperidol, chlorpromazine, and olanzapine)
- Antidepressants to treat depression and/or obsessive–compulsive behavior (fluoxetine, sertraline, and nortriptyline)
- Benzodiazepines or propranolol as muscle relaxants
- Mood stabilizers to control mania or bipolar disorder (lithium, valproate, and carbamazepine)
- Botulinum toxin (dystonia and jaw clenching)
- Tetrabenazine (tremors)

Essential Tremor

Drug treatment may include benzodiazepines, beta blockers, and antiepileptic drugs; botulinum toxin may be injected into the affected muscles. The two medicines that are prescribed most commonly for control of essential tremor symptoms are the anticonvulsant primidone (Mysoline) and the beta blocker propranolol (Inderal).

SELECTED REFERENCES

Cenci, M. A., I. Q. Whishaw, and T. Schallert (2002). Animal models of neurological deficits: How relevant is the rat? *Nature Rev. Neurosci.* 3, 574–579.

Dawson, T. M., A. S. Mandir, and M. K. Lee (2002). Animal models of PD: Pieces of the same puzzle? *Neuron* 35, 219–222.

Downes, J. J., A. C. Roberts, B. J. Sahakian, et al. (1989) Impaired extra-dimensional shift performance in medicated and unmedicated Parkinson's disease: evidence for a specific attentional dysfunction.*Neuropsychologia.* 27, 1329-43.

Fernandez, H. H. and J. J. Chen (2007). Monoamine oxidase-B inhibition in the treatment of Parkinson's disease. *Pharmacotherapy* 27, 174S–185S.

Fuxe, K., D. Marcellino, S. Genedani, and L. Agnati (2007). Adenosine A(2A) receptors, dopamine D(2) receptors and their interactions in Parkinson's disease. *Mov. Disord.* 22, 1990–2017.

Iversen, L. L. and S. D. Iversen (1981). *Behavioral Pharmacology*, 2nd ed. Oxford University Press, New York.

Jankovic, J. (2008). Parkinson's disease and movement disorders: Moving forward. *Lancet Neurol.* 7, 9–11.

Kenney, C., S. H. Kuo, and J. Jimenez-Shahed (2008). Tourette's syndrome. *Am. Fam. Physician* 77, 651–658.

Kostrzewa, R. M. and J. Segura-Aguilar (2007). Botulinum neurotoxin: Evolution from poison to research tool. *Neurotox. Res.* 12, 275–290.

Robertson, M. M. (2000). Tourette syndrome, associated conditions and the complexities of treatment. *Brain* 123, 425–462.

Rothstein, T. L. and C. W. Olanow (2008). The neglected side of Parkinson's disease. *Am. Sci.* 96, 218–225.

Schapira, A. H. (2007). Future directions in the treatment of Parkinson's disease. *Mov. Disord.* 22(Suppl. 17), S385–S391.

See, S. and R. Ginzburg (2008). Skeletal muscle relaxants. *Pharmacotherapy* 28, 207–213.

Stacy, M. and A. Galbreath (2008). Optimizing long-term therapy for Parkinson disease: Levodopa, dopamine agonists, and treatment-associated dyskinesia. *Clin. Neuropharmacol.* 31, 51–56.

Taylor, J. R., J. D. Elsworth, R. H. Roth, J. R. Sladek, Jr., and D. E. Redmond, Jr. (1990). Cognitive and motor deficits in the acquisition of an object retrieval/detour task in MPTP-treated monkey. *Brain* 113, 617–637.

Ungerstedt, U. (1971). Striatal dopamine release after amphetamine or nerve degeneration revealed by rotational behaviour. *Acta Physiol. Scand. Suppl.* 367, 49–68.

18

Pain

Clinically, there are many different varieties of pain, and it is associated with many different disorders. This chapter reviews the major categories of analgesic drugs used to treat some of the most common of these conditions and some of the preclinical animal models used to assess these drugs

PRECLINICAL MODELS FOR ASSESSING ANALGESIC DRUGS

A number of simple animal tests are available for assessing analgesic drugs. The simplest tests use unconditioned behaviors to measure the effects of drugs in acute pain models. In the tail flick test, a beam of light is focused on a small segment of the rat's tail. The initial low intensity of the light beam is increased incrementally until the normal pain threshold is reached and the tail is reflexively flicked out of the beam. Analgesic drugs increase the latency to respond to that level of pain. The hot plate test is an equally reliable test using thermal heat. A metal plate at the base of a cylinder is maintained at a temperature between 55 and 70°C. When placed on the hot plate, the rat is observed and the latency to kick the back legs and attempt to escape from the cylinder is recorded (Fig. 18–1).

The flinch jump procedure uses electric shock to a grid floor. At low intensities, the shock induces a flinch response and no general agitation; as the shock

A. Tail-flick test

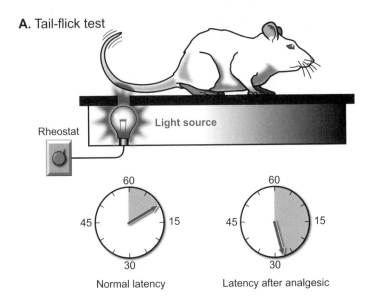

Rheostat

Light source

60
45   15
30

Normal latency

60
45   15
30

Latency after analgesic

B. Hot plate test

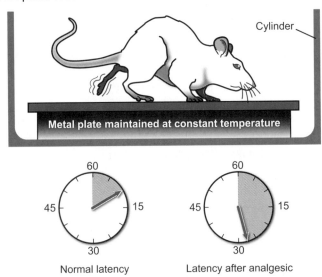

Cylinder

Metal plate maintained at constant temperature

60
45   15
30

Normal latency

60
45   15
30

Latency after analgesic

FIGURE 18–1. Acute tests of analgesia.
(A) The tail-flick test measures the response to a painful thermal stimulus by measuring the time between the onset of the radiant heat beam and reflex removal of the tail. (B) The hot plate test measures the latency to kicking with the hind paws or attempting to escape when a rat is placed on a metal plate maintained at constant temperature (55-70°F). (Modified from Hamilton and Timmons, 1990.)

intensity increases, the rat removes three or more paws from the grid, a so-called jump response often accompanied by emotional responses including vocalization. It has been suggested that this task differentiates perception of pain from the emotional arousal it induces. Clinically, pain is commonly chronic, as in cancer or peripheral neuropathy. The search for effective analgesics to treat such conditions moves beyond the simple acute test to models involving the neuropathological correlates of specific diseases. For example, in the study of inflammatory pain, models of rheumatoid arthritis are used in which an antigen (e.g., yeast or carrageen) is injected into a leg joint or paw—the "carrageen paw test." This sets up a slowly developing painful inflammation, and the animal will become increasingly unwilling to place that limb on the cage floor. The ability of analgesics to modify this behavior can then be assessed. Another inflammatory pain model, the formalin skin test, involves the intradermal injection of formalin, which causes an immediate chemically induced pain reaction, followed by a delayed period of developing inflammatory pain. Animal models of neuropathic pain often involve partial section or crush of the rat sciatic nerve (Chung or Bennett models). This leads to the gradual development of neuropathic pain in the affected limb, and the animal becomes reluctant to place the limb on the cage floor, allodynia may develop with light touch becoming a painful stimulus, and the animal will nurse the affected paw. All these behaviors can be modified by the drugs known to be effective in treating clinical conditions of neuropathic pain (gabapentin, carbamazepine, ω-conotoxin, and intrathecal morphine).

TREATMENT OF SEVERE PAIN WITH OPIATES

Morphine and related opiate analgesics are among the most effective drugs for the treatment of severe pain. The neurobiology of the opiate systems in brain and the family of naturally occurring morphine-like peptides, the endorphins, are described in Chapters 10 and 22. The analgesic action of these drugs is due to their ability to activate the mu-opiate receptor in spinal cord, brain stem, and forebrain pathways involved in the transmission of painful stimuli from the peripheral sensory system into the CNS. At each of the synaptic relay stations along these pathways there is a high density of opiate receptors and endorphins. The conclusion that activating the mu-opiate receptor, rather than the kappa or delta subtypes, is key to opiate analgesia is fairly clear. It stems from experiments on knockout strains of mice lacking expression of one or the other opiate receptor. Mice that lack expression of the mu-opiate receptor show no analgesic response to morphine or other opiates.

Patients with pain who are given morphine in therapeutic doses report that the pain is less intense, or entirely gone; they often report an accompanying drowsiness, and some patients report euphoria. Because the chronic use of opiates can lead to dependence, physicians are reluctant to prescribe opiates for the treatment of chronic severe pain. This is particularly true in the United States, where the use of opiate analgesics tends to be restricted mainly to the treatment of pain in terminally ill cancer patients. Opiate prescribing practice varies considerably from country to country. In Europe, for example, the number of scripts written for opiate analgesics in Denmark is approximately five times higher per capita than the European average.

Opiate Analgesics

Morphine, the natural alkaloid produced by the opium poppy, is still widely used, but when given orally it has a short duration and must be readministered every 3 or 4 hours. The availability of increasingly sophisticated sustained-release formulations, however, has permitted the use of morphine as a once or twice a day medicine. In addition, many synthetic drugs are available that act on the same opiate mechanism (Table 18–1).

Fentanyl and its analogues, sufentanil, alfentanil, and remifentanil, are more than 100 times more potent than morphine. Because of their powerful analgesic effects, these drugs are given intravenously as anesthetics for short surgical procedures. Fentanyl is also available for pain relief, in the form of a transdermal skin patch (Matrifen, Duragesic) that provides sustained drug exposure for up to 24 hours or as a "lollipop" (Actiq) that can be used for urgent pain relief in

TABLE 18–1. Opiate Analgesics

DRUG	TRADE NAME	EQUIVALENT ANALGESIC DOSE
Morphine		30 mg (3–4 hours)
Codeine		130 mg (3–4 hours)
Diamorphine	Diagesil	2.5 mg s.c.
Fentanyl	Actiq, Duragesic	<1 mg (oral lollipop or skin patch)
Hydromorphone	Dilaudid	7.5 mg (3–4 hours)
Hydrocodone	Lorcet, Lortab	30 mg (3–4 hours)
Levorphanol	Levo-Dromoran	4 mg (6–8 hours)
Meperidine	Demerol	300 mg (2–3 hours)
Methadone	Dolophine	20 mg (6–8 hours)
Oxycodone	Roxicodone, Oxycontin	30 mg (3–4 hours)
Pethidine	Demerol	100 mg (4–6 hours)
Propoxyphene	Darvon	130 mg
Tramadol	Ultram	100 mg

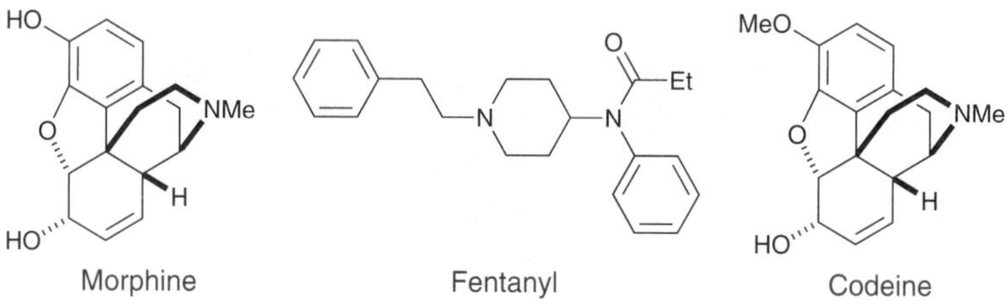

FIGURE 18–2. Some commonly used opiate analgesics.

cancer patients. Unfortunately, the fentanyl products are susceptible to diversion for nonmedical uses. Diamorphine (otherwise known as heroin; see Chapter 22) is an acetylated derivative of morphine that crosses the blood–brain barrier more readily. When given intravenously, it can provide rapid pain relief. Although used in Europe for terminally ill cancer patients, it is not available in the United States.

Oxycodone is a synthetic opiate that gained some notoriety in the United States. A sustained-release formulation called OxyContin provided effective sustained pain relief and came to be widely prescribed in physician's offices. Unfortunately, a substantial part of the medical supply was diverted to recreational use, creating an epidemic of opiate dependence (see Chapter 22).

Codeine, at the other end of the spectrum of potency, is an O-methylated derivative of morphine that is not directly active on the mu-opiate receptor. However, it is partially metabolized to morphine when taken orally. This provides a weak analgesic effect that is not adequate for treating severe pain conditions but is useful in many other contexts. Codeine and its congener, tramadol, are often formulated together with aspirin as a mild over-the-counter analgesic remedy. Another weakly active opiate, propoxyphene, has a similar profile to codeine.

The choice of an opiate analgesic for pain relief involves a number of factors, including potency, pharmacokinetics, duration of action, and available routes of administration. Intravenous injection avoids the substantial metabolism of active drug in the liver, and it can provide more rapid pain relief. Injection devices that permit "patient-controlled analgesia" are commonly used, with careful controls to avoid overdose. Administration into the epidural or intrathecal space provides a more direct access to key target sites in the spinal cord, and suitable formulations exist for morphine and various synthetic opiates; this too can be via a patient-controlled device (e.g. Pethidine in chidbirth). Other routes include rectal suppositories and the oral transmucosal route (e.g., fentanyl lollipop [Actiq]).

Adverse Side Effects

Morphine and related opiates depress respiration, and this effect is discernible at therapeutic dose levels. Death from morphine overdose is almost always due to respiratory arrest, but this occurs very rarely with standard therapeutic doses. However, the effects on respiration may be potentiated by the combination of opiates with other sedative or anesthetic drugs. Nausea and vomiting are common unpleasant side effects, seen most often when treatment is initiated. Opiates also cause peripheral vasodilatation, so patients may suffer orthostatic hypotension and fainting. A combination of opiate actions in the gastrointestinal tract commonly leads to constipation, which can become severe. The chronic use of these drugs often requires the parallel administration of stool softeners and laxatives. Another approach is to administer a mu-opioid receptor antagonist that has been chemically modified so that it can act peripherally but cannot cross the blood–brain barrier. One such compound, methylnaltrexone, has been approved. Side effects of opiates include dizziness, mental confusion, and drowsiness.

ASPIRIN, ACETAMINOPHEN, AND RELATED ANALGESICS

Aspirin and acetaminophen (paracetamol, Tylenol) are by far the most widely used of all pain remedies. They are effective for the treatment of mild pain, particularly of muscular origin, or mild headache. Aspirin acts in part on the brain to inhibit cyclooxygenase enzymes responsible for prostaglandin synthesis, and it also has this action as a classical anti-inflammatory agent in various conditions in which tissue inflammation is present. The precise mode of action of acetaminophen remains obscure, but it appears to act exclusively on a similar mechanism in the CNS. Both of these drugs have proved to be remarkably safe and well tolerated, although the chronic use of aspirin and related anti-inflammatory drugs can lead to gastric and intestinal irritation and lesions, and acetaminophen can cause life-threatening liver damage if used in excess.

A large number of aspirin-like drugs have been developed as anti-inflammatory/analgesic agents and are widely used in the treatment of painful conditions such a rheumatoid arthritis (Table 18–2). Several compounds are much more potent than aspirin, but unfortunately the more potent drugs are also more likely to cause gastric irritation/lesions.

With the exception of celecoxib, all of these compounds share a common mechanism of action with aspirin—namely inhibition of cyclooxygenase enzymes COX-1 and COX-2. These exist in several different forms. COX-1 is present in normal undamaged tissues including the stomach and intestine. Inhibition of this enzyme is thought to mediate the adverse gastric irritant effects of the nonsteroidal anti-inflammatory drugs (NSAIDs). A second enzyme, COX-2, is expressed only in damaged or inflamed tissue, and it is the therapeutic target for the NSAIDs, both peripherally and possibly also in spinal cord

TABLE 18–2. Commonly Used Nonsteroidal
Anti-inflammatory Drugs in the United States

Aspirin

Celecoxib (Celebrex)

Diclofenac (Voltaren)

Diflunisal (Dolobid)

Etodolac (Lodine)

Ibuprofen (Motrin)

Indomethacin (Indocin)

Ketoprofen (Orudis)

Ketorolac (Toradol)

Nabumetone (Relafen)

Naproxen (Aleve, Naprosyn)

Oxaprozin (Daypro)

Piroxicam (Feldene)

Salsalate (Amigesic)

Sulindac (Clinoril)

Tolmetin (Tolectin)

---

and brain. (However, a third enzyme, COX-3, has been proposed as the CNS target for these drugs and for acetaminophen.) A new generation of highly selective COX-2 inhibitors was developed, and these drugs were initially hailed as a significant advance in the treatment of painful inflammatory disorders, with a reduced risk of gastric irritation or damage. However, it became apparent that the long-term use of such drugs carried a small but significant increased risk of heart attacks or stroke; consequently, most of the initial COX-2 drugs have been withdrawn from the market. The one that is still available, celecoxib (Celebrex), is widely prescribed, although the FDA has issued a warning about its possible cardiovascular risks and is closely monitoring the clinical experience with this compound.

TREATMENT OF NEUROPATHIC PAIN

Chronic pain can result from lesions to peripheral sensory nerves or to CNS pathways. These occur in a variety of different conditions (Table 18–3).

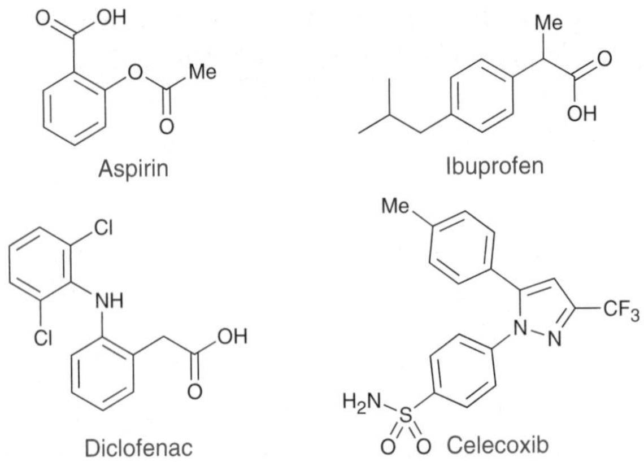

FIGURE 18–3. Commonly used aspirin-like analgesics

Neuropathic pain is always perceived in the sensory field normally innervated by the damaged nerve. After limb amputation, for example, the damaged sensory nerve fibers will sometimes generate neuropathic pain, which the patient perceives in the "phantom limb." Painful neuropathies may lead to continuous spontaneous pain and/or stimulus-evoked pain. In extreme cases, pain may be evoked by light mechanical stimuli that would normally be innocuous—a condition known as *allodynia*. This can be highly disabling to the unfortunate sufferers. Not all patients who suffer nerve damage will experience neuropathic pain; it is estimated that 5% of those who suffer traumatic nerve injuries

TABLE 18–3. Conditions in which Neuropathic Pain May Occur

PERIPHERAL	CENTRAL
Traumatic nerve injury	Stroke
Nerve compression/entrapment	Multiple sclerosis
Polyneuropathy	Spinal cord injury
Diabetic neuropathy	Syringomyelia
Plexus injury	Epilepsy
Root compression	Space-occupying lesions
Herpes zoster/postherpetic neuralgia	
Trigeminal neuralgia	
Cancer chemotherapy or radiation induced	
AIDS neuropathy	

will experience pain, 8% of patients with stroke will experience pain, and 28% of those with multiple sclerosis will experience pain.

Neuropathic pain is difficult to treat; less than half of patients with this type of pain will obtain substantial pain relief from any of the currently available drug treatments. In the vast majority of cases, conventional analgesics are ineffective, and opiate analgesics are of limited effectiveness. There is debate about the use of opiates for treating chronic nonmalignant pain, so physicians restrict their use in treating chronic neuropathic pain conditions.

A number of drugs are used to treat neuropathic pain, but not all patients will respond to drug treatment. Commonly used drugs include a number of antidepressants, including selective serotonin reuptake inhibitors (SSRIs); some antiepileptic drugs (believed to act by blocking neural sodium channels); some local anesthetics; and a variety of others (Table 18–4). The antiepileptic gabapentin and its closely related congener pregabalin, which block a neural calcium channel mechanism, have found particular favor in recent years. An unusual product is the 25-amino acid peptide omega-conotoxin MVIIA (ziconotide), a naturally occurring marine product marketed as Prialt. This acts as a potent antagonist at presynaptic N-type calcium channels. Because the peptide cannot penetrate into the CNS, it is administered by intrathecal injection into the spinal cord and has proved effective in treating severe neuropathic pain of spinal cord origin.

There is considerable research activity aimed at developing improved medicines to treat neuropathic pain. Several different approaches are being assessed. Among these are the search for agonists of the sensory nerve neuropeptide galanin (see Chapter 10); the GABA transporter inhibitor tiagabine; the cannabis sublingual spray Sativex; memantine and other antagonists acting at the glutamate NMDA receptor; botulinum toxin; and nonpeptide drugs acting on the N-type calcium channel.

TABLE 18–4. Drugs Used to Treat Neuropathic Pain

Antidepressants (amitriptyline, maprotiline, imipramine, SSRIs)

Antiepileptics (gabapentin, pregabalin, carbamazepine, clonazepam, lamotrigine, topiramate, phenytoin)

Local anesthetics

Baclofen

Ketamine

Guanethidine

Opiates (dextrorphan, methadone, fentanyl, tramadol)

Omega-conotoxin MVIIA (ziconitide, Prialt)

TREATMENT OF MIGRAINE HEADACHE

Migraine headache is a common and disabling pain condition. It is more common in women than in men, and it affects mainly those in the 30- to 49-year-old age group. The pain is due to a local inflammation of the meninges covering the brain that is thought to be caused by a burst of nerve impulses originating from the brain and traveling down the sensory fibers of the trigeminal sensory nerve that innervates the meninges. At the sensory nerve endings, the nerve impulses release a mixture of sensory neuropeptides, including substance P and calcitonin gene-related peptide (CGRP), which cause a local vasodilatation and "neurogenic inflammation" that becomes painful. Drugs used to treat migraine are listed in Table 18–5. The traditional pharmacological treatment for migraine was ergotamine or dihydroergotamine, which act on serotonin receptors on blood vessels to cause vasoconstriction, which neutralizes the vasodilatation underlying the migraine. However, ergotamines are not selective for the arteries in the brain, and their repeated use can cause severe vasoconstriction in the periphery, leading to possible damage to extremities deprived of adequate blood flow. A breakthrough occurred with the discovery of sumitriptan, a compound that is a selective agonist at the 5-HT–1B/1D receptor subtypes, which effectively relieves inflammation in the meningeal

TABLE 18–5. Drugs Used to Treat Migraine Headache

Triptans	Preventative
Almotriptan (Axert)	Propranolol
Eletriptan (Relpax)	Verapamil
Frovatriptan (Frova)	Amitriptyline
Naratriptan (Amerge)	Nortriptyline
Sumatriptan (Imitrex)	Gabapentin
Rizatriptan (Maxalt)	Pregabalin
Zolmitriptan (Zomig)	Valproic acid (Depakote)
	Topiramate (Topamax)
Other	Diphenhydramine (Benadryl)
Ergotamine	Cyproheptadine (Periactin)
Dihydroergotamine	
Prochlorperazine	
Promethazine	
Acetaminophen/codeine	

membranes without causing peripheral vasoconstriction. Sumatriptan was the first medicine that could stop a migraine headache after it had already started. It was followed by a series of related triptans with a similar mechanism of action but improved pharmacokinetics (e.g., faster absorption and onset of action and also longer duration); some can be administered by nasal spray (naratriptan), whereas others are absorbed by the orobuccal route (rizatriptan) (Table 18–5).

Several other drugs are commonly used as prophylactics to reduce the frequency of occurrence of further migraine attacks. These include amitriptyline, sodium valproate, topiramate, and propranolol. Novel treatments of migraine may include antagonists of the neuropeptide CGRP, which have shown promise in clinical trials (see Chapter 10).

SELECTED REFERENCES

Botting, R. M. (2006). Inhibitors of cyclooxygenases: Mechanisms, selectivity and uses. *J. Physiol. Pharmacol.* 57(Suppl. 5), 113–124.

Doods, H., K. Arndt, K. Rudolf, and S. Just (2007). CGRP antagonists: Unravelling the role of CGRP in migraine. *Trends Pharmacol. Sci.* 28, 580–587.

Dworkin, R. H., A. B. O'Connor, M. Backonja, et al. (2007). Pharmacologic management of neuropathic pain: Evidence-based recommendations. *Pain* 132, 237–251.

Guindon, J., J. S. Walczak, and P. Beaulieu (2007). Recent advances in the pharmacological management of pain. *Drugs* 67, 2121–2133.

Hargreaves, R. (2007). New migraine and pain research. *Headache* 47(Suppl. 1), S26–S43.

Miljanich, G. P. (2004). Ziconotide: Neuronal calcium channel blocker for treating severe chronic pain. *Curr. Med. Chem.* 11, 3029–3040.

Riley, J., E. Eisenberg, G. Müller-Schwefe, et al. (2008). Oxycodone: A review of its use in the management of pain. *Curr. Med. Res. Opin.* 24, 175–192.

Singh, P. and A. Mittal (2008). Current status of COX-2 inhibitors. *Mini Rev. Med. Chem.* 8, 73–90.

Waldhoer, M., S. E. Bartlett, and J. L. Whistler (2004). Opioid receptors. *Annu. Rev. Biochem.* 73, 953–990.

19

Epilepsy

THE DISORDERS

Epilepsy is one of the most common of the serious neurological disorders. The prevalence of active epilepsy is approximately 5–10 per 1000 people. Seizure types are organized first according to whether the source of the seizure within the brain is localized (*partial* or *focal* onset seizures) or distributed (*generalized* seizures). Partial seizures are further divided based on the extent to which consciousness is affected. If it is unaffected, then it is a *simple partial* seizure; otherwise, it is a *complex partial* (*psychomotor*) seizure. Generalized seizures are divided according to the effect on the body, but all involve loss of consciousness. These include *absence* (*petit mal*), *myoclonic, clonic, tonic, tonic–clonic* (*grand mal*), and *atonic* seizures.

There are many different epilepsy syndromes, each presenting with its own unique combination of seizure type, typical age of onset, EEG findings, treatment, and prognosis. A number of syndromes affect children, including *infantile spasms* (*West syndrome*), *childhood absence epilepsy*, *benign focal epilepsies of childhood*, and *juvenile myoclonic epilepsy*. The most common epilepsy of adults is *temporal lobe epilepsy*.

416

ANIMAL MODELS

There are many sophisticated animal models, each designed to simulate one of the many forms of human epilepsy. A detailed review is not possible here, but many models involve the use of a number of different convulsant agents administered systemically, focally, or topically. These include the GABA antagonists pentylenetetrazol, bicuculline, and picrotoxin; the glutamate agonist kainic acid; and the cholinergic agonist pilocarpine. *Kindling*, a phenomenon whereby repetitive, focal application of initially subconvulsive electrical stimulation ultimately results in intense partial and generalized convulsive seizures, continues to be an informative model, particularly for temporal lobe epilepsy. Although it is not routinely observed, the validity of this model as an epilepsy model is strengthened from the observation that different species of kindled animals can develop spontaneous recurrent seizures, reinforcing the idea that brain networks become permanently hyperexcitable after repeated partial seizures. To date, all animal species examined are susceptible to kindling, including frogs, reptiles, rats, mice, rabbits, dogs, cats, rhesus monkeys, and baboons. The kindling model emphasizes the importance of a better understanding of the factors underlying the development of epilepsy so that prophylactic treatments can be targeted at prevention rather than symptomatic relief. A range of genetic strains of rats and mice that are prone to seizures have also proved valuable in assessing novel antiepileptic drugs.

DRUG TREATMENT

A variety of antiepileptic drugs are available (Table 19–1) and are often used in combination, with the goal of balancing the inhibitory and excitatory synaptic activity to suit the individual patient. Too much inhibition means loss of the ability to function, whereas too little inhibition risks seizure onset. The drug treatment of seizures started in 1850 with the introduction of bromides, followed in 1910 by phenobarbital, which became the drug of choice for many years. A number of other barbiturates were developed, including primidone. In 1940, phenytoin was found to be an effective drug for the treatment of epilepsy, and since then it has become a major first-line antiepileptic drug in the treatment of partial and secondarily generalized seizures. During the second half of the 20th century, carbamazepine was introduced for partial seizures, ethosuximide became the first-choice drug for the treatment of absence seizures, and valproate became the drug of choice in primary generalized epilepsies. These anticonvulsants were the mainstays of seizure treatment until the 1990s, when several newer antiepileptic drugs with good efficacy, fewer toxic effects, and better tolerability were developed, including topiramate, vigabatrin, tiagabine, and oxcarbazine.

TABLE 19–1. Commonly Available Antiepileptic Drugs

DRUG	TRADE NAME
Carbamazepine	Tegretol
Chlormethiazole	Heminevrin*
Clobazepam	Frisium*
Clonazepam	Rivotril
Diazepam	Valium, Stesolid
Diazemuls	Valclair
Ethosuximide	Zarontin, Emeside
Fosphenytoin	Pro-Epanutin
Gabapentin	Neurontin
Lamotrigine	Lamictal
Levetiracetam	Keppra
Methylphenobarbitone	Prominal
Oxcarbazine	Trileptal
Phenobarbitone	
Phenytoin	Dilantin, Epanutin
Piracetam	Nootropil
Primidone	Mysoline
Sodium valproate	Epilim
Tiagabine	Gabitril
Topiramate	Topamax
Valproic acid	Depakene, Convulex
Vigabatrin	Sabril
Zonisamide	Zonegren

* Not available in the United States.

SODIUM CHANNEL BLOCKERS

Sodium channel blockade is the most common and well-characterized mechanism of currently available antiepileptics. Drugs that target neuronal sodium channels prevent the return of the channels to the active state by stabilizing the inactive form. In doing so, repetitive firing of the neurons is prevented. The presynaptic and postsynaptic blockade of sodium channels of the axons causes stabilization of the neuronal membranes, blocks and prevents posttetanic

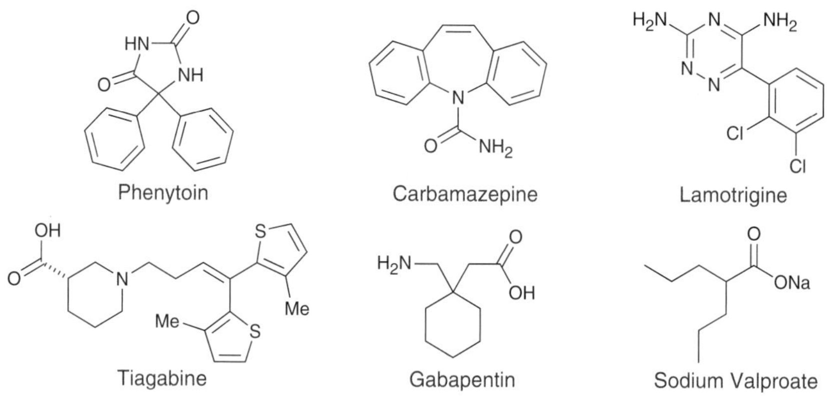

FIGURE 19–1. Commonly used antiepileptic drugs.

potentiation, limits the development of maximal seizure activity, and reduces the spread of seizures. Drugs with this mechanism include carbamazepine, phenytoin, lamotrigine, and zonisamide.

Carbamazepine

Carbamazepine is a major first-line drug for the control of partial seizures and generalized tonic–clonic seizures. Adverse effects include dizziness, nausea, ataxia, and blurred vision. It is metabolized by liver cytochrome P450 and chronic use may lead to induction of CYP3A4, which in turn can cause troublesome drug-interaction effects. However, carbamazepine is still one of the most widely used antiepileptics. The extended-release preparations, Tegretol XR and Carbatrol, are better tolerated than the immediate-release preparations. Oxcarbazine is an analogue of carbamazepine with a similar action but a more benign adverse effect profile; it is also less likely to lead to liver enzyme induction.

Phenytoin

Since its introduction in 1938, phenytoin has been a major first-line antiepileptic in the treatment of partial and secondary generalized seizures. It blocks movement of ions through the sodium channels during propagation of the action potential and therefore blocks and prevents posttetanic potentiation, limits development of maximal seizure activity, and reduces the spread of seizures. It also has secondary effects on calcium channels and calmodulin. However, the adverse effect profile (e.g., gingival hyperplasia and coarsening of facial features in women) and slow absorption make its use less desirable in some patients. An injectable prodrug, fosphenytoin, gives rise to effective plasma levels more rapidly and is used in the acute treatment of seizures (*status epilepticus*).

Lamotrigine

Lamotrigine is chemically unrelated to any of the other antiepileptics. Its major mechanism of action is blocking voltage-dependent sodium channel conductance. It has been found to inhibit depolarization of the glutamatergic presynaptic membrane, thus inhibiting release of glutamate. Lamotrigine is a very effective and well-tolerated drug with relatively few adverse CNS effects. Therefore, it is one of the preferred choices in treating elderly patients or patients who are pregnant.

Zonisamide

Zonisamide acts to reduce neuronal repetitive firing by blocking sodium channels and preventing neurotransmitter release. It also exerts influence on T-type calcium channels and prevents influx of calcium; it may also exhibit neuroprotective effects through free radical scavenging. Zonisamide has a long half-life and can be used once daily without significant fluctuation of blood levels. In addition, it does not have the cosmetic and pharmacokinetic problems of phenytoin. Its mechanism of action, inhibiting thalamic T calcium currents, may make it effective in the treatment of absence epilepsy and juvenile myoclonic epilepsy.

GABA AGONISTS

Another group of antiepileptic drugs act by enhancing the actions of the inhibitory neurotransmitter GABA, the main "off" signal in neural circuits. The drugs act by stimulating the benzodiazepine receptor on the $GABA_A$ receptor complex to enhance the synaptic effects of GABA (see Chapter 5) or by blocking the inactivation of GABA by reuptake or metabolism.

Benzodiazepines

Clonazepam is used specifically to treat myoclonus, but it is also used widely in children because of its relatively benign side effect profile. Clobazepam is less sedative in animal tests, but both benzodiazepines exhibit sedation as a primary adverse side effect, along with possible dizziness and ataxia. Because of their anxiolytic effects (see Chapter 14), they may be useful in treating epileptic patients with concomitant anxiety disorders.

Barbiturates

These act like the benzodiazepines on the $GABA_A$ receptor to enhance the synaptic effects of GABA. Phenobarbitone was one of the most widely used antiepileptic drugs during the 20th century. Primidone acts as a prodrug that is converted to phenobarbitone. Both are highly effective anticonvulsants, but they have many drawbacks. Barbiturates tend to produce intense sedation, which may be accompanied by other CNS effects, including psychomotor slowing, poor concentration, depression, irritability, ataxia, and decreased libido; at high doses they can be lethal. These drugs also strongly induce liver cytochrome P450 enzymes, which in turn can lead to problems of drug interactions. For these reasons, they are rarely used for the chronic treatment of epilepsy, although they remain valuable in controlling status epilepticus.

Inhibitors of GABA Uptake or Metabolism

Tiagabine was the first GABA uptake inhibitor to be introduced as an antiepileptic. It blocks the GAT-1 neuronal GABA transporter, which is important in the inactivation of synaptically released GABA. Use of tiagabine is limited to adjunctive therapy in refractory partial epilepsy. It should not be used in absence epilepsy or in partial epilepsies with generalized spike wave because it can worsen seizure control or cause status epilepticus. The most troublesome side effects are dizziness, asthenia, nervousness, tremor, depressed mood, and emotional lability.

Vigabatrin is a close structural analogue of GABA that binds irreversibly to the active site of the GABA degrading enzyme GABA transaminase. *In vivo* studies in human and animal subjects have shown that vigabatrin significantly increases extracellular GABA concentrations in the brain. It is partially effective in patients with refractory partial seizures, but it is less effective against primarily generalized tonic–clonic seizures and may worsen myoclonic seizures or generalized absence seizures. Vigabatrin is very effective in the treatment of infantile spasms; therefore, it is the drug of choice for this indication in many countries. Unfortunately, because of this drug's toxicity (CNS and visual), its use is restricted. It has not been approved by the FDA because of its adverse visual effects.

Other Antiepileptic Drugs

Gabapentin was developed to have a structure similar to that of GABA; however, it has little or no action on the GABA receptor. It binds with the $\alpha_2\delta$ subunit of neuronal calcium channels in the cerebral neocortex, hippocampus, and spinal cord. This mechanism of action may be important for its efficacy both in epilepsy and in the control of neuropathic pain (see Chapter 18). It is relatively well tolerated, although it does have some adverse effects, particularly in high doses, but these are usually relatively minor. Gabapentin is more commonly used to treat pain rather than epilepsy.

Valproate is the drug of choice for primary generalized epilepsies, and it is also approved for the treatment of partial seizures. The mechanism of action is uncertain. It enhances GABA function, but this effect is observed only at high concentrations. It also produces selective modulation of voltage-gated sodium currents during sustained, rapid, repetitive neuronal firing. Adverse effects include nausea, vomiting (mainly during initiation of therapy and improved by administration of enteric-coated preparations), tremor, sedation, confusion or irritability, and weight gain. Although valproate is a very potent antiepileptic drug, due to its adverse effect profile, it is being replaced by newer drugs. The extended-release preparation may decrease dose-related adverse effects and be better tolerated.

Topiramate is a very potent anticonvulsant. It has multiple mechanisms of action: It exerts an inhibitory effect on sodium conductance, decreasing the duration of spontaneous bursts and the frequency of generated action potentials; enhances GABA by unknown mechanisms; inhibits the AMPA subtype glutamate receptor; and is a weak inhibitor of carbonic anhydrase. It is unclear which of these is most important. Comparisons of topiramate with other new antiepileptics have shown greater effects from topiramate than from any of the other drugs compared to placebo. It has also been effective in drug-resistant generalized epilepsies as adjunctive therapy. The most common adverse effects of topiramate include ataxia, impairment of concentration, confusion, dizziness, fatigue, paresthesia in the extremities, somnolence, disturbance of memory, depression, agitation, and slowness of speech; however, these are seen mainly with higher doses.

Levetiracetam is a piracetam derivative. It is a unique antiepileptic drug because it is ineffective in classic animal seizure models that screen potential compounds for antiseizure efficacy such as maximal electroshock and pentylenetetrazol in rats and mice. During preclinical evaluations, however, it was found to be effective in several models of seizures, including tonic and clonic audiogenic seizures in mice, tonic seizures in the maximum electroshock seizure test in mice, and tonic seizures induced in rodents by chemoconvulsants. The mechanism of action is unknown, but a brain-specific stereoselective binding site for the drug has been identified. Levetiracetam is a potent antiepileptic with a significant effect in generalized epilepsies. It was approved by the FDA in 2007 for primary generalized tonic–clonic seizures in adults and children age 6 years or older.

SELECTED REFERENCES

Ben-Menachem, E. (2008). Strategy for utilization of new antiepileptic drugs. *Curr. Opin. Neurol.* 21, 167–172.

Bertram, E. (2007). The relevance of kindling for human epilepsy. *Epilepsia* 48(Suppl. 2), 65–74.

Falip, M., A. Gil-Nagel, C. Viteri Torres, and J. Gómez-Alonso (2007). Diagnostic problems in the initial assessment of epilepsy. *Neurologist* 6(Suppl. 1), S2–S10.

Helbig, I., I. E. Scheffer, J. C. Mulley, and S. F. Berkovic (2008). Navigating the channels and beyond: Unravelling the genetics of the epilepsies. *Lancet Neurol.* 7, 231–245.

Karceski, S. C. (2007). Seizure medications and their side effects. *Neurology* 69, E27–E29.

Löscher, W. (2002). Animal models of epilepsy for the development of antiepileptogenic and disease-modifying drugs. A comparison of the pharmacology of kindling and post-status epilepticus models of temporal lobe epilepsy. *Epilepsy Res.* 50, 105–123.

Sarkisian, M. R. (2001). Overview of the current animal models for human seizures and epileptic disorders. *Epilepsy Behav.* 2, 201–216.

20

Recreational Psychoactive Drugs

Humans seem to have an irresistible urge to alter their state of consciousness, and the use of psychoactive drugs is one popular means of achieving this. Alcohol and intoxicant drugs derived from plants have been used for many thousands of years, supplemented more recently by man-made synthetic compounds. Understanding how such drugs act on the brain, and how their use can turn into abuse and addiction, is an important part of neuropsychopharmacology, which is why we review this subject in detail. This section of the book covers psychoactive drugs used for nonmedical reasons, so the legal substances alcohol and nicotine are included along with the illicit narcotics. Individual chapters cover each of the major recreational drugs.

Although the misuse of psychoactive drugs can damage or even kill the user, and may cause grave damage to society, there are also positive aspects to the recreational use of psychoactive drugs. The moderate use of alcohol or other intoxicants gives much pleasure to the users, who find the effects relaxing, helping to counteract the stresses and worries of everyday life. One could argue that the moderate use of alcohol may be equivalent to using benzodiazepines or other prescription antianxiety agents, and this may not be too fanciful since both act on similar brain mechanisms (see Chapters 14 and 25). The use of recreational drugs can also act as an important "social lubricant" making it easier to make social contacts and friendships. The drug Ecstasy is a particular example of this phenomenon, creating a strong feeling of empathy with those around, even though they may be complete strangers. Others argue that the psychedelic drugs can offer metaphysical insights into the user's psyche.

However, users of recreational psychoactive drugs also risk adverse effects and possible damage to society. The repeated use of such drugs can cause temporary or longer term damage to neural or psychological function. In many cases, use becomes uncontrolled and leads to addiction, an irresistible compulsion to continue taking the drug even in the face of obvious evidence of harm. Addicts may indulge in criminal activities to obtain continuing supplies of the drug. Damage is caused to society by this criminal behavior, by the added burden of health costs associated with accidents or violence that occur during the intoxicated state or associated with the treatment of addiction, and by the adverse effects on the family and the local community. For such reasons, the availability of psychoactive drugs has been strictly regulated. A number are considered so dangerous that they are illegal, and those caught in possession of these drugs or supplying them to other users are subject to severe criminal penalties. Even the legal drugs, alcohol and nicotine, are strictly regulated. They cannot be purchased by minors, and their sales are subject to high rates of tax by governments. In Europe, since 2007, the smoking of tobacco has been prohibited in any public place, and similar regulations have been enacted in several states in the United States.

Despite the criminal penalties associated with the use of illicit psychoactive drugs, they continue to be widely used throughout the world, and the continuing expansion in their use in developed countries is considered one of the most serious of all social problems. The United Nations (UN) *World Drug Report* gives an annual review of global patterns of drug use (Table 20–1). Approximately 200 million people admit to using illicit drugs, with the great majority using cannabis. The production and sale of illicit psychoactive drugs is big business worth many billions of dollars. The UN estimated that approximately 423,000 metric tons of herbal cannabis are produced annually, along with 40 metric tons of amphetamines, 700 metric tons of cocaine, and 100 metric tons of opiates. The cultivation of coca for cocaine production dominates the economy of some Latin American countries, and the cultivation of the opium poppy in Afghanistan accounts for 90% of the world's production of opium, the raw ingredient for the manufacture of heroin. Ironically, U.S. and European users

TABLE 20–1. Global Data on Illicit Drug Use—2005–2006 (Millions of Users)

ANY ILLICIT DRUG	CANNABIS	AMPHETAMINES	OPIATES	COCAINE	ECSTASY
200	159	25	15.6	14.3	8.6

Data from UN *World Drug Report* (2007).

TABLE 20–2. Illicit Drug Use by 12th-Grade Students in the United States—2007 (% Ever Used)

ANY ILLICIT DRUG	CANNABIS	AMPHETAMINES	PSYCHEDELIC	COCAINE	ECSTASY
50	42	11	10	8	6

Data from NIDA "Monitoring the Future" (2007).

of heroin help to fund the terrorist organizations in Afghanistan that benefit from opium production.

In the United States, the National Institute on Drug Abuse (NIDA) publishes an annual report on drug use by U.S. schoolchildren, a project called "Monitoring the Future." The latest data from their 2007 report (Table 20–2) show that the use of illicit psychoactive drugs is common, even among 12th graders, with approximately 50% admitting to ever having used one or another of these drugs. Again, cannabis is by far the most commonly used substance.

THE REGULATION OF ILLICIT PSYCHOACTIVE DRUGS AND MEASURES OF HARM

Different countries have sought to control the availability of psychoactive drugs by legislation that makes it a criminal offense to supply or possess such substances. Penalties vary from country to country and, in the United States, from state to state. However, possession of even modest amounts of these drugs can often carry a substantial prison sentence or fine. Countries have tried to classify the dangers posed by psychoactive drugs according to how harmful they are, with the most harmful carrying the most severe criminal penalties. In addition to this classification, psychoactive drugs—including those used in treating neuropsychiatric illnesses—are also scheduled according to their medical importance and possible harmfulness. Schedule 1 is the most severe, restricted to drugs that are considered harmful but have no recognized medical use. Despite claims for genuine medical applications, cannabis continues to be regarded as a Schedule 1 drug in both Europe and the United States. At the other extreme, Schedule 4 drugs have recognized clinical indications but still require careful recording and storage to limit their diversion to nonmedical use. Many have been critical of the current classification system used in both Europe and the United States, which is largely based on historical accident rather than on scientific evidence of the degree of harm posed by individual drugs.

In a freedom-loving society in which the liberal tradition of John Stuart Mill guides a good deal of law reform (i.e., that no conduct should be criminalized unless it is harmful to others), it is crucially important to be clear about the harms that using drugs can cause. In considering how the harmfulness of psychoactive drugs might be measured, there are many factors to consider, some of which are summarized in Table 20–3.

In considering individual psychoactive drugs, the following questions might be asked:

Lethality—How common is death through overdose? Different drugs have varying safety margins—that is, the ratio between the intoxication dose and the lethal dose. This ratio is less than 10 for heroin and more than 1000 for cannabis.

Long-term effects on health—Are there serious adverse health effects associated with long-term use? Injected drugs carry a high risk of infection with such viruses as HIV or hepatitis B and/or C. Smoking tobacco products carries a severe risk of lung cancer and many other forms of cancer.

Impaired brain function—Does use of the drug impair the user's ability to undertake demanding cognitive or motor tasks? Many intoxicants produce such impairments, making it dangerous to drive after drinking alcohol, for example.

TABLE 20–3. Major Health and Social Harms of Illicit Recreational Drug Use

HARM	MAIN DRUGS
Overdose and other drug-related deaths	Heroin (especially if administered by injection), other opiates, cocaine, MDMA and amphetamines
Infections by blood-borne viruses: HIV, hepatitis B, hepatitis C; bacterial infections: endocarditis, tuberculosis	Injecting drug use
Dependence syndrome	Opiates/heroin, cocaine, amphetamines, cannabis
Psychosis	Amphetamines, cannabis
Respiratory disorders/cancer	Smoking drugs: cannabis, crack, heroin
Adverse effects on fetal and child development	Opiates/heroin, crack, cannabis
Road traffic accidents and other injuries	All
Adverse impact on school and work performance	Cannabis and all drugs
Family adversity, deprivation, and intergenerational substance misuse	Early onset of cannabis use or use of other substances, including heroin, cocaine
Crime	Heroin and crack

TABLE 20–4. Relative Dependence Risks of Psychoactive Drugs

DRUG	CAPTURE RATIO (%)
Tobacco	33
Heroin	23
Cocaine	17
Alcohol	15

Data from the U.S. Comorbidity Study.

There is also evidence that repeated drug use may cause persistent cognitive deficits; the evidence is clear for alcohol but less so for cannabis.

Dependence liability—How likely is the user to become an addict, whose life becomes dependent on a continuing supply of the drug? Different drugs vary in their dependence liability. The U.S. Comorbidity Study measured what was termed a "capture ratio"—that is, the percentage of people who had ever used the substance who were likely to become addicted. The results were startling (Table 20–4).

Harms to the family and community—In addition to harm to the individual user, we need also to ask how much harm drug use does to the family or community. This occurs in a variety of forms. The intoxicated user may lose inhibitions and become aggressive. A considerable amount of domestic violence and public disorder can be attributed to the excessive use of alcohol, for example. Intoxicated users are also more likely to have accidents, which incur medical costs. Addicts may also be driven to crime to fund their habit; a considerable proportion of domestic burglary is committed for this reason.

It is not our intention to attempt to rank the recreational psychoactive drugs in terms of their harmfulness. Almost everyone would agree that the top of the list of harm would be occupied by heroin and cocaine, which together probably account for the most harm to users and to society among the illicit drugs. However, the legal substances alcohol and nicotine also have massive social and medical costs, partly because they are widely used.

ANIMAL BEHAVIORAL MODELS FOR STUDYING ADDICTIVE DRUGS

Behavioral Tasks For Evaluating the Acute Reinforcing Properties of Addictive Drugs

Addictive drugs, like natural reinforcers, sustain responding on schedule controlled and discrete trial procedures. *Drug self-administration* is tested in an operant chamber designed so that appropriate lever pressing results in the delivery of the drug bolus to the jugular vein via an implanted cannula (Fig. 20–1). Oral administration of these drugs is less widely studied, except in the case of alcohol, where intragastric cannulae or inhalation chambers are used.

A wide range of drugs can be shown to act as reinforcers in rats and monkeys, with their relative reinforcement potential and patterns of drug taking closely resembling those seen in humans. In addition, drugs such as neuroleptics or hallucinogens which are not self-administered in animals appear to lack reinforcing properties, or may be aversive., The acute presentation of rewarding drugs sustains rates and patterns of responding on different schedules of reinforcement that are indistinguishable from those controlled by natural reinforcers. Similarly, through classical conditioning, stimuli paired with drug infusion acquire conditioned reinforcing properties that can be useful in establishing second-order schedules in which completion of an individual component of

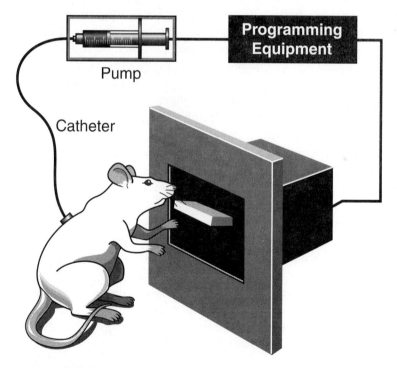

FIGURE 20–1. Self-administration apparatus. Rats implanted with intravenous catheters are trained to self-administer drugs by pressing a lever. They are generally trained on an FR-1 or FR-5 fixed ratio (FR) schedule. With FR-1, each lever press delivers a metered amount of drug, and with FR-5 drug is delivered on every fifth lever press. Rats learn to regulate the amount of drug administered so that if the dose is reduced below that used for training, they will increase the number of intravenous infusions and vice versa. (After Caine et al., 1993.)

the schedule produces the terminal event (drug infusion) according to another overall schedule. Typically, a brief visual stimulus is presented after the nth response of each FR component schedule and then together with the drug infusion after the first FR completed at the end of a fixed interval (15 minutes). The visual stimulus acquires conditioned or secondary reinforcing properties and sustains responding throughout the fixed interval, and thus the acute effects of the drug infusion on responding are minimized. Initially developed in monkeys, second-order schedules are now widely used in rodent research and considered excellent models of human drug-seeking behavior, where drug taking is preceded by a series of behaviors (e.g., procurement and preparation). Putative medicines for controlling drug-seeking behavior, such as dopamine D_3 receptor partial agonists or antagonists, have been shown to attenuate the cue-controlled seeking of cocaine without influencing the acute reinforcing effect of the drug. Multiple schedules can also be used where self-administration of drug can be one component and a nondrug natural reinforcer the other. Progressive ratio schedules of drug administration are valuable for determining the relative reinforcement strength of different reinforcers, including drugs.

By the process of classical conditioning, the interoceptive stimuli associated with a drug can be readily conditioned to environmental stimuli. Based on this principle, the *conditioned place preference task* is a technically simple nonoperant procedure for demonstrating the reinforcing efficacy of drugs. The apparatus consists of a two-chambered box (Figure 20–2). The two sides are highly discriminable. During daily conditioning trials, animals are injected either with drug or with vehicle and confined (e.g., for 30 minutes) to either one or the other distinct chamber. The animal thus has the opportunity to associate two discriminable internal states with two distinct environments. After conditioning, a drug-free test trial is given, in which animals have free access to both chambers. A rewarding drug results in the animal spending markedly more time in the chamber in which the drug was experienced, whereas drugs inducing aversive interoceptive stimuli result in animals avoiding the chamber in which they have experienced such a drug (Fig. 20–2).

The interoceptive cues induced by the drug can also act as discriminative stimuli. The *drug discrimination* paradigm described in Chapter 3 is based on this principle. It is used to compare the subjective pleasant or aversive experiences induced by related groups of drugs and continues to be useful in drug discovery programs. The choice of lever that follows administration of an unknown test compound provides valuable information about the similarity of that drug's interoceptive cue properties to those of the training drug. With this task, the relative potencies of related compounds can be readily assessed (Fig. 20–3), and drugs capable of antagonizing the reinforcing effect of addictive drugs can be identified. The test also gives an indication of whether or not a novel chemical entity is likely to be abused.

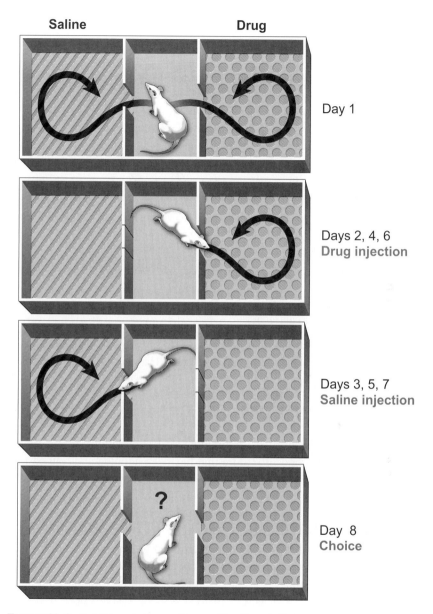

Saline   **Drug**

Day 1

Days 2, 4, 6
Drug injection

Days 3, 5, 7
Saline injection

Day 8
Choice

FIGURE 20–2. Conditioned place preference. The diagram illustrates the place conditioning procedure in the rat. Animals are placed in the middle of a three-compartment cage from which they can enter either of two other compartments, each with distinct features. After familiarization with the environments on Day 1, on Days 2, 4, and 6 the animals are kept in one of the two environments and treated with test drug; on Days 3, 5, and 7 they are kept in the other environment without drug treatment. On Day 8, they are given a choice between the two environments. The time spent in the drug- versus nondrug-associated environment gives an index of the reinforcing value of the test drug (or, alternatively, its aversive properties). (Modified from Swerdlow et al., 1989.)

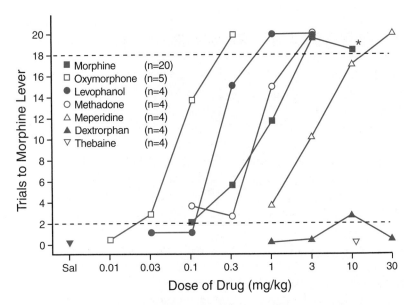

FIGURE 20–3. Drug Discrimination.
A range of opiate analgesics and the inactive analogs dextrorphan and thebaine were tested in animals trained to discriminate between an intravenous infusion of morphine or saline. The ordinate is the maximum number of trials (out of 20) that were completed on the morphine-appropriate lever. Most of the drugs tested showed complete cross-generalization to morphine, and the test offers a useful way of comparing their *in vivo* potencies. *(Modified from Shannon, H.E. and Holtzman, S.G., 1976)*

Intracranial self-stimulation (or brain reward stimulation) is one of the most important behavioral procedure that has been adopted and refined in a number of different ways to study the neural basis of reward and the changes in reward associated with drugs of addiction. It provides a sensitive measure of the effects of addictive drugs on brain reward systems.

In 1954, Olds and Milner reported the now classic experiment in which they demonstrated that rats could be conditioned to press a lever delivering brief (250-ms), direct electrical stimulation to the medial forebrain bundle, the major pathway connecting the ventral midbrain with the forebrain. Intracranial self-stimulation (ICSS), as it came to be known, sustains operant behavior, as do natural reinforcers. We now know that the electrode placements in the medial forebrain bundle activate components not only of forebrain dopamine circuitry known from independent studies to be critical for reinforcement and motivation but also descending systems from the basal forebrain. Drugs that have reinforcing effects may increase or decrease the reward value of ICSS—effects that are reflected in increases or decreases in lever pressing for the brain stimulation or changes in the threshold level of electrical current required to maintain lever pressing. One must be sure that these drug effects do indeed reflect a change in the reward value of the current rather than an inability to respond to the lever. Various ICSS paradigms have been developed to determine the minimal electrical intensity (termed the *reward threshold*) for which the animal is prepared to respond. This can be identified for each rat and is central to experimental studies of the various aspects of the addictive process. Acute administration of major drugs of abuse lowers the reward threshold, whereas withdrawal from addictive drugs after chronic administration usually elevates the reward threshold. The current intensity or frequency at which resetting occurs indicates the reward threshold. Another widely used procedure is the rate-frequency curve-shift procedure. This technique relies on the observation that if one holds either current intensity or frequency constant, increasing the value of the other parameter leads to an increased response rate. Curve shifting refers to treatment-induced changes in this relationship between frequency (or intensity) of electrical stimulation and the rat's rate of responding. Drugs that enhance the rewarding effect of the stimulation shift the curve to the left (i.e., rats press more vigorously at a given frequency), whereas drugs that reduce reward efficacy cause a rightward shift in the curve (Fig. 20–4). Both of these methods yield very similar results and control for motor effects of the drugs on lever pressing. Amphetamine and related dopamine agonists shift the curve to the left, whereas dopamine antagonists have the opposite effect. A discrete trial procedure has been developed from the classical psychophysical method of limits used so widely in sensory physiology. It also provides a reward threshold measure and control for motor effects of the drugs on lever pressing. At the start of each trial, the rat receives an experimenter-administered electrical stimulus and is allowed 7.5 seconds to turn a wheel one-fourth of a rotation to obtain a contingent stimulus identical to the previously administered noncontingent stimulus. Stimulus intensity (usually current)varies according to the psychophysical method of limits. As well as threshold measurements, the latency to turn the wheel after the delivery of the noncontingent electrical stimulus provides a measure of motor performance deficits. Rewarding drugs lower the threshold for ICSS, indicating an amplification of reward signals in the brain. In contrast, withdrawal from extended exposure to these drugs results in a gradual decrease in the sensitivity of the brain reward systems.

Behavioral Studies of Chronic Administration of Addictive Drugs

The study of addictive drugs and the addictive process has become one of the most sophisticated areas of contemporary behavioral pharmacology. Animal models of relevance to the progression from sporadic drug taking to addiction are of particular significance. They are important in trying to understand the neurobiological basis of addiction and in evaluating new treatments. Many parameters

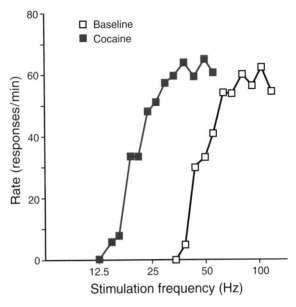

FIGURE 20–4. Intracranial self stimulation (ICSS).
In rats with intracranially implanted electrodes, the rate at which animals press a lever to obtain self-stimulation increases as the frequency of the self-stimulation current increases. Animals treated with cocaine (15 mg/kg intraperitoneally) self-stimulate at a lower current frequency than was previously rewarding. (Modified from Wise et al., 1992.)

influence this complex process, leading to a syndrome with the various criteria for *substance dependence* in the *Diagnostic and Statistical Manual of Mental Disorders*, fourth edition (*DSM-IV*), or the International Statistical Classification of Diseases and Related Health Problems (ICD-10; World Health Organization, 1992) (Table 20–5). The gradual changes in the reward value of the drug, the motivation to acquire it, and the sensations associated with its withdrawal are thought to be the most critical processes, all of which can be measured in animals using the methods described previously.

A number of hypotheses of addiction continue to be discussed and researched. Attention to psychological constructs is now playing an important part in attempts to experimentally dissect the learning processes underpinning drug-seeking behavior. Robinson and Berridge (1993) have defined an important distinction between "liking" (unconditioned response to reward) and "wanting"(conditioned salience of reward stimuli) in mediating subjective pleasure as opposed to subjective craving (Fig. 20–5).

The aim is to discover how reward drives the motivation to seek drug or to relieve withdrawal and how goal-directed behavior regresses into simple habit. The motivational factors for the development, maintenance, and persistence

TABLE 20–5. ICD-10 Diagnostic Criteria for Alcohol and Drug Dependence

Three or more of the following have been experienced or exhibited at some time during the previous year:

1. Evidence of tolerance, such that increased doses are required in order to achieve effects originally produced by lower doses
2. A physiological withdrawal state when substance use has ceased or been reduced as evidenced by the characteristic substance withdrawal syndrome, or use of substance (or closely related substance) to relieve or avoid withdrawal signs
3. Difficulties in controlling substance use in terms of onset termination or levels of use
4. Progressive neglect of alternative pleasures or interests in favor of substance use; or a great deal of time spent in activities necessary to obtain, to use, or to recover from the effects of substance use
5. Continued substance use despite clear evidence of overtly harmful physical or psychological consequences
6. A strong desire or sense of compulsion to use substance

of drug addiction can be broken down into the four sources of reinforcement discussed in Chapter 3: positive reinforcement, negative reinforcement, conditioned positive reinforcement, and conditioned negative reinforcement. The various models described previously all have a role to play in untangling the complex interacting psychological and neurobiological processes that lead from impulsive drug seeking to compulsive drug intake. Three stages have been hypothesized: binge/intoxication, measured with acute self-administration; withdrawal/negative affect, measured with ICSS and place conditioning; and preoccupation/anticipation, measured with cue induced reinstatement paradigms. One influential view proposes that at the core of addiction lies a labile interaction between a brain reward system driven by natural rewards and an antireward or "opponent process" associated with withdrawal that drives aversive states (Fig. 20–6). It is this deficit state for normal rewards that is the core motivation to seek more drug, not a hyperactive or sensitized reward state for drugs per se. Withdrawal is usually characterized by responses opposite to the acute initial action of the drug. The physical signs are readily observed, but the motivational measures of abstinence have proved to be sensitive measures of this critical phase in the transition to the compulsive addictive state.

Behavioral Models for Studying the Transition from Impulsive to Compulsive Drug Taking

It has proved challenging to develop animal models of the transition from motivated drug seeking to uncontrolled compulsion. Several groups have suggested that this involves a loss of executive control mediated by the frontal cortex over subcortical circuitries in which dopamine plays a significant, but

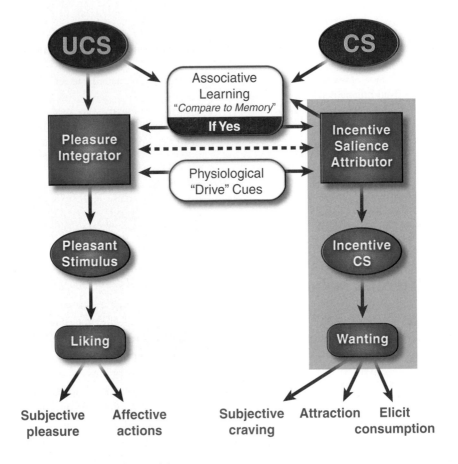

FIGURE 20–5. Addiction model.

In this model of incentive motivation, the psychological process (and neural substrate) for pleasure (*liking*) is separate from the psychological process (and neural substrate) responsible for incentive salience (*wanting*). Activation of telencephalic dopamine systems plays a direct role only in the process of wanting via the attribution of incentive salience to the perception and representation of conditioned stimuli (CS). This portion of the model (i.e., the psychological process) is sensitized by repeated drug administration. It is proposed that hyperactivation of this psychological process (incentive salience) is due to sensitization of its neural substrate by drugs, which results in the excessive attribution of incentive salience to drug-related stimuli. Whereas normal levels of incentive salience attribution result in normal wanting, hyperactivation of this system is hypothesized to result in excessive incentive salience attribution, which is experienced as *craving*. Craving is pathologically intense wanting. The major difference between this model of incentive motivation and the traditional model is that psychological processes and neural substrates responsible for pleasure (liking) are separate from those for incentive salience (wanting). Thus, natural incentives (unconditioned stimuli [UCS]) produce pleasure directly but produce incentive salience and elicit goal-directed approach behavior only indirectly (as indicated by the dashed arrow from "pleasure integrator" to the "incentive salience attributor"). (After Robinson and Berridge, 2003.)

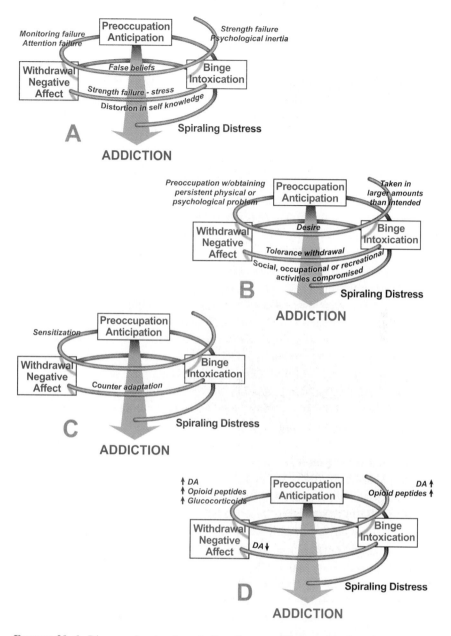

FIGURE 20–6. Diagram showing the spiraling distress–addiction cycle from four different perspectives. The addiction cycle is conceptualized as a spiral that increases in amplitude with repeated experience, ultimately resulting in the pathological state known as addiction. (A) The three major components of the addiction cycle—preoccupation/anticipation, binge/intoxication, and withdrawal/negative affect—and some sources of potential self-regulation failure in the form of underregulation and misregulation. (B) The same three components of the addiction cycle with the different criteria for substance dependence incorporated from the *DSM-IV*. (C) The places of emphasis for the theoretical constructs of sensitization and counteradaptation. (D) The hypothetical role of different neurochemical and endocrine systems in the addiction cycle. Small arrows refer to increased functional activity. CRF, corticotrophin-releasing factor; DA, dopamine. (After Koob and LeMoal, 2007.)

not exclusive, role. In humans, individual differences in the forms of impulsivity and sensation seeking have been related to the vulnerability to drug addiction. The relationship between impulsivity and compulsive drug use is uncertain but is a very important question when one considers the escalating model of addiction described in Figure 20–6. The study of individual differences in animals on measures of sensation seeking and impulsivity has opened up a new approach to this question. More than a decade ago, it was demonstrated that outbred rats with high levels of novelty-induced locomotor activity show increased sensitivity to addictive drugs and a higher propensity to self-administer psychostimulants. In the initial studies, rats were individually screened for their level of reactivity in a novel environment (a circular corridor 170 cm long and 10 cm wide, with 70-cm high walls and four photocells placed at the two perpendicular axes of the apparatus). Locomotor activity was measured every 10 minutes for 2 hours and rats were allocated to two subgroups depending on whether their activity levels were below or above the median of the entire group. Subsequently, the rats were habituated to the same apparatus for 3 hours and then injected with 1.5 mg/kg amphetamine, and locomotor activity was recorded for 3 more hours. In a second experiment, rats were screened for high or low response to novelty and then tested for acquisition of amphetamine self-administration. The locomotor response to amphetamine was greater in high responders, and self-administration of amphetamine was also greater in this group. Thus, differences in the vulnerability to addictive behavior can be predicted from the normal behavioral response to novelty and the acute response to amphetamine administration. In a more recent rat study from the laboratory of Robbins and Everitt (Belin et al., 2008), high reactivity to novelty was used as a measure of sensation seeking and premature responding in the 5-choice serial reaction time task (5-CSRTT) as a measure of one phenotype of impulsivity. They showed that with these animal models it is possible to identify within a population a "vulnerable phenotype" that predisposes to compulsive cocaine intake. Rats were screened for high impulsivity (HI) or low impulsivity (LI) on the 5-CSRTT and for high reactivity (HR) or low reactivity (LR) in the novelty-induced locomotor task. These groups were then compared on acquisition of cocaine self-administration and on three addiction criteria: increased motivation to take drug, inability to refrain from drug seeking, and maintained drug use despite aversive consequences. After 40 days of cocaine self-administration, each rat was classified as showing one, two, or three of these behaviors. It was found that HI and LI rats did not differ in their novelty-induced locomotor activity and that HR and LR rats were not impulsive. However, HR rats were more prone to acquire cocaine self-administration, as had been shown earlier with psychostimulants, but HR did not predict the transition to compulsive drug taking. By contrast, although HI and LI rats did not differ in acquisition of cocaine self-administration, HI did predict the transition to compulsive cocaine seeking even in the face of punishment. These results are in accord with the observation that in the addict population, high impulsivity is overrepresented and may predate compulsive drug use, and that comorbidity of drug addiction is seen with other disorders such as attention deficit hyperactivity disorder, also characterized by impulsive behavior (see Chapter 16). The dissociation between acquisition of cocaine self-administration and subsequent drug taking suggests that the initial exposure to the drug does not predict progression to addiction. This reinforces the view that a number of distinct behavioral and neural processes underpin the spiraling decline to compulsive drug taking.

Theories of Addiction

As a result of the advances described previously, several plausible theories of addiction are being actively investigated. Another key development has been the development of a behavioral model in rodents and nonhuman primates that predicts the potential for drug abuse in humans and provides a basis for an analysis of human addiction. A recent trend has been to model more closely in animals those aspects of human drug abuse that are based on definitions in the *DSM-IV* criteria for substance dependence (e.g., in terms of the intoxication/binge cycle and compulsivity).

The nucleus accumbens provides an interface between parts of the brain mediating motivation and reward and those producing behavioral output. One element common to most of the theories is that addiction is, in part, due to the ability of addictive drugs to "hijack" brain mechanisms involved in learning and memory. As a result, aberrant learning patterns are established. This common theme of learning explains the propensity to relapse: Behavioral conditioning triggers memories of drug-related experiences that elicit further drug-seeking and drug-taking behavior. Learning theory, based on both animal and human studies, has been invoked to understand and also to treat addiction. A central concept of this theory is that the addicted user comes impulsively to prefer small immediate rewards to potentially larger but delayed rewards. For example, an addicted user might seek the "rush" that follows the use of a substance and ignore the risk of serious ill health and possibly death. There is considerable evidence that drug addicts discount other forms of reward in an impulsive manner, suggesting hyperactivity in those neural mechanisms of impulsive choice. The recent focus on relapse and reinstatement has renewed interest in the neural systems involved and in such processes as memory consolidation and reconsolidation and extinction.

Based on a large amount of evidence, addiction is now recognized as a "chronic relapsing brain disorder." This evidence-based concept contrasts with earlier, judgmental, views concerning addiction and its treatment, which emphasized such factors as individual violation and social context rather than medical and neurobiological factors.

The Brain Circuitry and Neural Process Involved in Addiction

In recent years, there have been major developments in our understanding of the neural bases of addiction (for a review, see Koob and LeMoal, 2006). The work that led to these advances was initially performed in experimental animals (mainly rats and monkeys). However, through the use of neuroimaging techniques, many of the findings in animals have been shown to apply to humans. These advances come from studies on the main drugs of abuse, including psychomotor stimulants such as cocaine and amphetamine, opiates such as morphine and heroin, alcohol, nicotine, MDMA (Ecstasy), cannabis, and benzodiazepines such as diazepam. It now appears that although the subjective effects and primary receptors of the drugs are different, many drugs activate the same neural system in the base of the forebrain (Fig. 20–7). This common system includes a structure in the ventral striatum called the nucleus accumbens that appears to be critical for the reinforcing effects of drugs. This part of the dopamine system controls flexible goal-orientated behavior, such as the acquisition of lever pressing for cocaine reward. However, as the addictive process develops, control is lost and behavior becomes compulsive or habit-like—the form of behavior known to be controlled by the dopamine system of the dorsal, rather than the ventral, striatum. In this framework, compulsive drug taking is seen as a shift in control from the ventral to the dorsal striatum.

Brain Changes Associated with Drug Misuse

Prolonged use of drugs such as methamphetamine and alcohol can result in neurotoxic changes that occur at cellular, systems, and behavioral levels in experimental animals and in humans. These changes can be detected in humans by neuroimaging, postmortem pathology, or neuropsychological tests. However, many problems arise when interpreting these studies.

It is not easy to know whether drug-induced changes in nerve cells or neural systems lead to permanent impairments in cognitive and neurological functions. A further difficulty is encountered when attempting to determine cause-and-effect relationships. For example, the reduced binding of striatal dopamine D_2 receptors in a cocaine-dependent subject might be a result of abusing cocaine, but it might also have been present before the subject had been exposed to any psychoactive substance. Indeed, the low D_2 receptor binding might have predisposed the subject to misuse cocaine and other drugs that stimulate dopamine function.

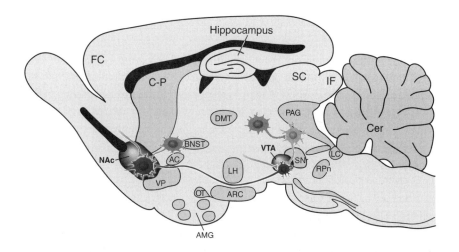

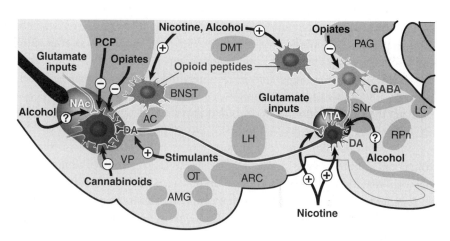

FIGURE 20–7. Sagittal section of a rat's brain illustrating the essential neural circuits underlying the reinforcing effects of addictive drugs. The critical sites are the dopaminergic (DA) neurons of the ventral tegmental area (VTA), the local and remote afferents to these neurons, and their projections to the neurons of the nucleus accumbens (NAc) and their local afferent projections. Nicotine can directly activate the dopaminergic VTA neurons, an effect that is strengthened by activation of local opioid peptide neurons that inhibit local GABA-ergic neurons, thereby disinhibiting the VTA neurons. This activation sends the rewarding DA signal to the neurons of the nucleus accumbens. Alcohol similarly indirectly activates VTA neurons and enhances their effects on nucleus accumbens neurons through opioid signaling in the VTA and in the accumbens. Likewise, opiates activate VTA dopamine neurons through disinhibition of local GABA neurons. Psychostimulants enhance the DA signals to nucleus accumbens neurons through increased local DA release in accumbens and blockade of re-uptake there. PCP and cannabinoids act on their receptors within accumbens to simulate the rewarding signals. Other brain structures shown for spatial perspective are not involved in the reinforcing effects of these addictive drugs (AC, anterior commissure; AMG, amygdala; ARC, arcuate nucleus of the hypothalamus; BNST, bed nucleus of the stria terminalis; Cer, cerebellum; C-P, caudate nucleus and putamen; FC, frontal cortex; Hippo, hippocampus; LC, locus ceruleus; PAG, periaqueductal Grey; RPn pontine raphé nucleus; SC, superior colliculus; SNr, Substantia Nigra pars reticulata). (Modified with permission from Koob, 1999.)

Animal studies have often used very high doses of drugs—far higher than those encountered in human subjects. In animals, methamphetamine causes damage to neurons containing dopamine and also to neurons containing 5-HT. Similar findings of 5-HT damage have been made for MDMA (Ecstasy). However, it is unclear if such effects are relevant to human Ecstasy users because of the high doses needed to produce these toxic effects in animals (see Chapter 21).

VULNERABILITY TO DRUG ABUSE

There is considerable evidence from the social sciences and clinical studies of predisposing factors for human addiction including social experience and context. A rich neurobiological literature, based on human and animal studies, links changes in self-administration behavior to such influences as stress and early social experience. Studies with nonhuman primates showed that low dopamine D_2 receptor number may be a vulnerability marker for cocaine abuse. Socially subordinate monkeys have lower levels of striatal dopamine D_2 receptors than their socially dominant peers and also showed a greater propensity to self-administer cocaine than did their socially dominant peers. These studies are relevant to parallel studies of normal human subjects. Drug-naive human volunteers with relatively low striatal dopamine D_2 receptors exhibited more euphoric reactions to an intravenously administered psychomotor stimulant, methylphenidate, than did normal volunteers with higher striatal dopamine D_2 receptors. The hypothesis derived from both animal and human studies is that low striatal dopamine D_2 receptors may be a risk factor for stimulant abuse. This factor may operate as a tendency to optimize the functioning of the dopamine D_2 system through self-medication.

PHARMACOLOGICAL TREATMENT OF ADDICTION

Virtually all existing medicines for the treatment of addiction are based on the principle of harm reduction—replacing the addictive drug with another that has similar effects on the brain but is less harmful (Table 20–6). For example, nicotine patches or chewing gum are used for cigarette smokers, and for heroin addicts the long-acting weaker opiates, such as methadone or buprenorphine, are used as heroin substitutes. Heroin has been provided to addicts in Germany and Switzerland as part of a harm-reduction program, and the results over the short term (several months) have been promising for heroin addicts who have been resistant to other forms of treatment.

TABLE 20–6. Medicines Approved for Treatment of Addiction

TARGET DRUG	THERAPEUTIC AGENT AND MECHANISM	INDICATIONS
Alcohol	Benzodiazepines	Withdrawal, seizures, delirium
	Antiepileptic agents (e.g., carbamazepine)	Withdrawal, seizures
	Acamprosate—glutamate antagonist	Maintenance of abstinence, relapse prevention
	Naltrexone—opiate antagonist	Maintenance of abstinence, relapse prevention
	Disulfiram—aldehyde dehydrogenase inhibitor	Maintenance of abstinence, relapse prevention
	Selective SSRIs	Maintenance of abstinence, relapse prevention, treatment of comorbid depression
Benzodiazepines	Carbamazepine	Treatment of withdrawal
Nicotine	Nicotine replacement products	Smoking cessation, maintenance therapy
	Bupropion—dopamine transporter inhibitor	Smoking cessation
	Varenicline—selective nicotinic receptor agonist	Smoking cessation
Opiates	Methadone—opiate agonist	Withdrawal symptoms, maintenance therapy
	Buprenorphine—mu-opiate receptor partial agonist	Withdrawal symptoms
	Clonidine and lofexidine— α-adrenoceptor agonists	Withdrawal symptoms
	Naltrexone—opiate antagonist	Relapse prevention

SSRIs, selective serotonin reuptake inhibitors.

Where effective, people who receive available treatments have reduced drug use and drug harms such as crime compared to those receiving minimal or no treatment. However, compliance is often poor, and relapse is common. In general, approximately two-thirds of those in treatment have had previous treatment. Substitution of heroin by methadone or buprenorphine has a success rate of 50–60% after 3 months in maintaining subjects heroin-free, but a smaller percentage achieve complete abstinence. Similarly, treatments with nicotine replacement products achieve only 10% success after 12 months, although this is still significantly better than the success rate achieved without treatment.

FUTURE ADDICTION MEDICINES

Several novel potential treatments for addiction have arisen from neuroscience research. The development of more sophisticated models of addiction is allowing the targeting of drug-induced euphoria, cue-induced craving, or drug seeking. The following are examples:

1. Naltrexone, an opiate receptor antagonist, represents a promising treatment for certain forms of alcoholism. This clinical use was based on the previous preclinical findings that naloxone blocked the anticonflict effect of alcohol in rats and that it extinguished alcohol self-administration in rhesus monkeys. Alcohol acutely increases opioid activity, and opiate mu-receptor knockout mice fail to self-administer alcohol.

2. In rats, treatment with a dopamine D_3 receptor partial agonist reduced cocaine-seeking behavior maintained by drug-associated cues. The treatment did not impair drug-taking behavior (i.e., self-administration) per se. Such studies make the D_3 receptor a viable target for research and development by pharmaceutical companies.

3. The possible efficacy of rimonabant, a cannabinoid CB1 receptor antagonist, as a potential treatment for cigarette smoking and other forms of drug abuse derives from a program of research on cannabinoid receptors. These receptors, which are located in different parts of the neural "reward" system, are implicated in nicotine, opioid, and perhaps food-related addictions (see Chapter 24).

4. Also in the realm of potential treatments are $GABA_B$ agonists, which have proved efficacious in animal models of cocaine self-administration.

Some of the other products under development are scientifically less novel but may offer important practical advances in the treatment of addictions. In particular, the development of depot-injectable formulations of the opiate antagonists nalmofene and naltrexone or the partial agonist buprenorphine should allow enhanced compliance with the treatment regime since these products can provide up to 1 month's worth of treatment in one injection. The ability to treat addicts in outpatient clinics or doctors' offices on a once-a-month basis should make treatment cheaper and more widely available, although such a regime may only be practical for the long-term maintenance of addicts who have already successfully been detoxified.

A particularly innovative approach to the treatment of addictions is the development of drug-specific vaccines. The principle behind this approach is to link a psychoactive drug to a larger protein molecule to generate a vaccine that will stimulate the immune system to make antibodies. These would recognize and neutralize the psychoactive drug. This principle could be applied to any psychoactive drug, but so far research has focused on vaccines for cocaine or for nicotine. The most advanced projects have involved the development of vaccines for nicotine to aid cessation of cigarette smoking. The vaccine triggers the patient's immune system to produce circulating antibodies that bind to nicotine and form a large molecule, the antibody–nicotine complex, which cannot cross the blood–brain barrier and thus cannot gain access to the central nervous system.

Preliminary clinical trial results have been encouraging, but whether these or other similar vaccine products will actually help to reduce long-term relapse rates in the treatment of cigarette smoking or other addictions remains to be seen.

SELECTED REFERENCES

Belin, D., A. C. Mar, J. W. Dalley, et al. (2008). High impulsivity predicts the switch to compulsive cocaine-taking. *Science* 320, 1352–1355.

Caine, S. B., R. Lintz, and G. F. Koob (1993). Intravenous drug self-adminisration techniques in animals. In *Behavioral Neuroscience: A Practical Approach* (A. Saghal, Ed.). IRL Press, Oxford, Vol. 2, pp. 117–143.

Everitt, B. J. and T. W. Robbins (2005). Neural systems of reinforcement for drug addiction: From actions to habits to compulsion. *Nature Neurosci.* 8, 1481–1489.

George, S. and E. Day (2007). Buprenorphine in the treatment of opioid dependence. *Br. J. Hosp. Med. (London)* 8, 4–7.

Goodman, A. (2008). Neurobiology of addiction. An integrative review. *Biochem. Pharmacol.* 75, 266–322.

Hejazi, N. S. (2007). Pharmacogenetic aspects of addictive behaviors. *Dialogues Clin. Neurosci.* 9, 447–454.

Kenny, P. J. (2007). Brain reward systems and compulsive drug use. *Trends Pharmacol. Sci.* 28, 135–141.

Kleber, H. D. (2007). Pharmacologic treatments for opioid dependence: Detoxification and maintenance options. *Dialogues Clin. Neurosci.* 9, 455–470.

Koob, G. F. and M. LeMoal (2005). Plasticity of reward neurocircuitry and the "dark side" of drug addiction. *Nature Neurosci.* 8, 1442–1444.

Koob, G. F. and M. LeMoal (2006). *Neurobiology of Addiction.* Academic Press, Amsterdam.

Maurer, P. and M. F. Bachmann (2007). Vaccination against nicotine: An emerging therapy for tobacco dependence. *Expert Opin. Investig. Drugs* 16, 1775–1783.

Piazza, P. V., J.-M. Deminiére, M. LeMoal, and H. Simon (1989). Factors that predict individual vulnerability to amphetamine self-administration. *Science* 245, 1511–1513.

Robinson, T. E. and K. C. Berridge (2003). Addiction. *Annu. Rev. Psychol.* 54, 25–53.

Shannon, H. E. and S. G. Holtzman (1976). Evaluation of the discriminative effects of morphine in the rat. *J. Pharmacol. Exp. Ther.* 198, 54–65.

Shippenberg, T. S. and G. F. Koob (2002). Recent advances in animal models of drug addiction. In *Neuropsychopharmacology: The Fifth Generation of Progress* (K. L. Davis, D. Charney, J. T. Coyle, and C. Nemeroff, Eds.). Lippincott Williams & Wilkins, Philadelphia.

Swerdlow, N. R., D. Gilbert, and G. F. Koob (1989).Conditioned drug effects on spatial preference: critical evaluation. In *Psychopharmacology. Neuromethods* (A. A. Boulton, G. B.
Baker, and A. J. Greenshaw, Eds.). Humana Press, Clifton, NJ, Vol. 13, pp. 399–346.

Wise, R. A., P. Bauco, W. A. Carlezon, and W. Trojniar (1992). Self stimulation and drug
reward mechanisms. *Ann. N. Y. Acad. Sci.* 652, 192–198.

Psychostimulants

This chapter focuses on the three most common illicit psychostimulants, as opposed to the legal compounds caffeine (coffee and tea) (see Chapter 16) and nicotine (Chapter 26). Cocaine, amphetamines, and Ecstasy share many common features with regard to their mode of action and psychopharmacology. All three act by stimulating monoamine mechanisms in brain indirectly by promoting the release of these neurotransmitters (amphetamines and Ecstasy) or by slowing their inactivation through reuptake mechanisms (cocaine). Amphetamines and Ecstasy also share a common molecular structure—a benzene ring with a phenylethylamine side chain.

Cocaine is a naturally occurring alkaloid from the coca plant, and it has been used for centuries in tonics and other preparations to allay fatigue, sustain performance, and treat a variety of ailments. Along with caffeine, cocaine was a key ingredient of the original Coca-Cola, but it was removed in 1903. As the dangers of cocaine were recognized, cocaine was banned in 1914 as a dangerous "narcotic" in the United States and soon thereafter elsewhere. Cocaine continues to have a legitimate medical use as a local anesthetic and vasoconstrictor. Although we now know cocaine to be a dangerous drug of addiction, its illegal use has continued to increase, partly because many users wrongly believe it to be a harmless nonaddictive stimulant.

The amphetamines, of which Ecstasy is one, are synthetic chemicals. Benzedrine (*DL*-amphetamine) was introduced in the 1930s as a cold remedy to clear stuffy noses. For a while, amphetamine and a variety of related chemicals found a huge market as appetite suppressants. This part of the amphetamine story, however, ended tragically with the introduction of an amphetamine combination treatment for obesity, the notorious "phen-fen" mixture (phentermine plus fenfluramine), which led to thousands of cases of heart valve damage and some premature deaths, triggering one of the largest civil lawsuits in history (for review, see Iversen, 2008). However, amphetamine derivatives are still used medically as appetite suppressants. Children suffering from attention deficit hyperactivity disorder (ADHD; see Chapter 16) also represent a large and growing medical use of amphetamines.

Almost as soon as benzedrine first became available as a medicine, many people found that they liked the psychostimulant effects that it produced. They felt more alert, had more energy, and could keep going at full speed for longer. It took some time to realize that amphetamines are potentially dangerous drugs of addiction. The modern versions of methamphetamine ("ice" and "crystal meth"), which can be smoked or injected, have proved particularly dangerous.

The amphetamine-like drug Ecstasy has had its own impact on the social scene, becoming intimately associated with the "rave dance" culture that flourished toward the end of the 20th century, facilitating social interactions with all-night-long "energy."

The illegal use of cocaine reached a peak in the mid-1980s, when as many as 25% of U.S. adults admitted having experimented with the drug. The misuse of cocaine has grown again recently in Europe, particularly in Britain, where cocaine use by celebrities is viewed as fashionable. In 2005, an estimated 752 tons of cocaine were seized worldwide. The first-ever United Nations global survey on Ecstasy and amphetamines in 2003 revealed a striking picture of increased production and drug trafficking. Seizures of amphetamines increased more than 10-fold in a period of 10 years to almost 40 tons in 2000–2001. Estimated worldwide production is now more than 500 tons per year, with more than 34 million users of amphetamine-like stimulants and 8 million users of Ecstasy.

CHEMISTRY

Amphetamine is a simple synthetic derivative of the naturally occurring substance phenylethylamine; it differs only in possessing a methyl group ($-CH_3$) attached to the side chain (Figure 21–1). Cocaine is a more complex substituted phenylethylamine. Phenylethylamine is consumed in many foodstuffs,

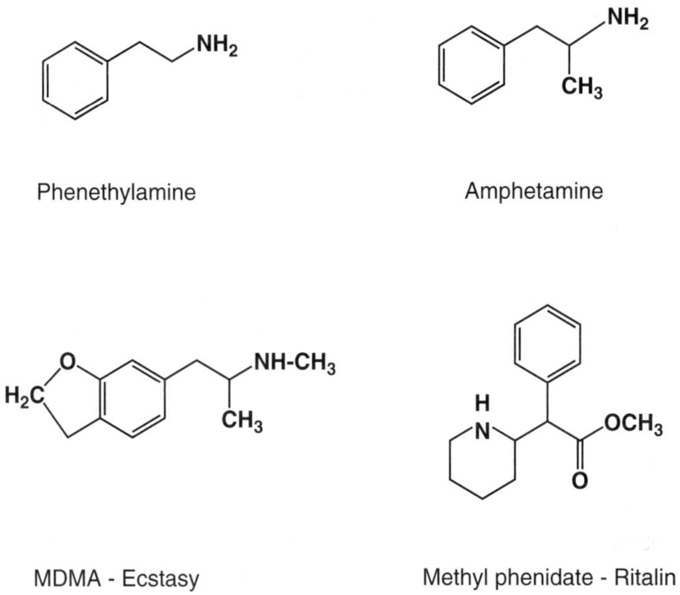

Phenethylamine

Amphetamine

MDMA - Ecstasy

Methyl phenidate - Ritalin

FIGURE 21–1. Amphetamines and their derivatives.

particularly in cheeses and wines, but has little or no effect because it is rapidly degraded in the liver by the enzyme monoamine oxidase. The addition of substituent groups on the side chain is a very significant alteration because this protects amphetamine from degradation by monoamine oxidase, and hence the drugs can enter and persist in the bloodstream and exert a variety of biological effects.

Amphetamines and cocaine exist in two different stereoisomers. *d*-Amphetamine and *d*-methamphetamine are far more biologically active than the levo-isomers. *d*-Amphetamine is also referred to as S(+)amphetamine, dexamphetamine, or dexedrine. In the case of cocaine, the L(−)isomer is the more active form. Addition of a second methyl group to the basic nitrogen of the side chain in amphetamine leads to methamphetamine, which has even more potent stimulant actions (see Fig. 21–1); again, the dextro-isomer is the more powerful. Further chemical alterations to the benzene ring lead to 3,4-methylenedioxy-methamphetamine (MDMA), commonly known as "Ecstasy" (see Fig. 21.1), and the related compound 3,4-methylenedioxy-amphetamine (MDA).

However, these are only a few examples of an almost unlimited number of chemical variations that can be made on this basic scaffold. The U.S. chemists Alexander and Ann Shulgin described 179 different synthetic phenylethylamines that they made and tested for their psychic effects—using mainly themselves as guinea pigs—in their remarkable book *PIHKAL* ("Phenylethyl-amines I Have Known and Loved"). Pharmaceutical companies also devel-oped a variety of compounds with somewhat more complex chemical structures that act by the same mechanism as the classical amphetamines, including methylphenidate (Ritalin), used in the treatment of ADHD (Fig. 21.1) (see Chapter 16), and phentermine and diethylpropion (Tenuate), used in the treat-ment of obesity.

ROUTES OF ADMINISTRATION

Cocaine hydrochloride is a white powder that is dissolved for intravenous injection or insufflated into the nasal cavity. Because of the rich vasculature, it is rapidly absorbed into the blood, producing intoxication in 2 or 3 minutes. "Crack cocaine" is a preparation of the free base in the form of large crystals. Unlike the hydrochloride, crack cocaine can be smoked, providing an even more rapid route of absorption and producing intoxicant effects within 10 seconds (Figure 21–2). The usual intoxicant doses are 20–50 mg.

In the medical use of amphetamines, oral administration provides a gradual absorption of drug and a prolonged duration of action. This avoids a rapid peak of drug level in the blood, which could cause excessive psychostimulant effects. However, it is precisely such effects that the amphetamine addict

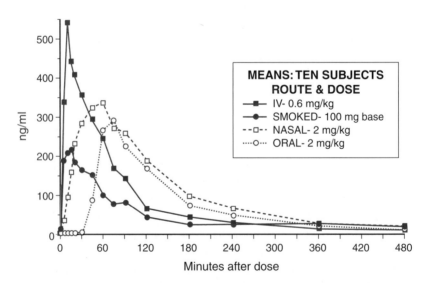

FIGURE 21–2. Absorption of cocaine following different routes of administration. Smoking (crack cocaine) or intravenous injection yields intoxicant levels of drug within seconds of administration; the oral route is considerably slower.

craves. When the drugs are abused, they are usually administered by a method that ensures rapid absorption and almost instant delivery to the brain. An obvious way of achieving this is to inject a solution containing the drug into a vein, and indeed this is how amphetamines were traditionally abused. Nowadays, with the danger of HIV or hepatitis infection associated with contaminated needles, injection is a less favored route. Users may prefer nasal insufflation with its rapid absorption and onset.

An alternative is "ice" or "crystal meth," a translucent form of pure *d*-methamphetamine hydrochloride resembling rock candy that can be smoked. The usual intoxicant dose is 5–15 mg.

The majority of Ecstasy users take the drug orally as a 100-mg tablet, although it can be insufflated or injected. Ecstasy users presumably seek a prolonged action to keep them awake for the all-night dance scene.

Cocaine and the amphetamines are readily absorbed into the bloodstream from the various routes of administration. Cocaine is fairly rapidly eliminated, with a half-life of approximately 1 hour, but the amphetamines persist for long periods of time with half-lives for elimination from the blood of 6–12 hours. *d*-Methamphetamine has a particularly long half-life of 11 or 12 hours.

MECHANISM OF ACTION

Cocaine and the amphetamines are chemically related to the naturally occurring catecholamine neurotransmitters norepinephrine and dopamine. However, neither cocaine nor amphetamines can directly activate the cellular receptors normally stimulated by the monoamines norepinephrine, dopamine, or serotonin. They act instead by making more of these naturally occurring monoamines available either by inhibiting their reuptake (cocaine) or by stimulating their release (amphetamines).

In peripheral tissues, cocaine and the amphetamines indirectly activate noradrenergic receptors, whereas in the brain the actions of norepinephrine, dopamine, and serotonin are all enhanced. Cocaine is a potent inhibitor of all three monoamine transporters (Table 21–1). *d*-Amphetamine and methamphetamine are selectively concentrated in norepinephrine and dopamine-containing nerves because they are substrates for the transporter molecules that normally recapture the catecholamine neurotransmitters after their release (see Chapter 7). Once inside the nerve cell, the amphetamines are also recognized by the separate transporter mechanisms, which help to concentrate the natural neurotransmitters inside storage vesicles in the nerve terminals. Mobilizing stored neurotransmitter from these storage vesicles causes an unusually high concentration of neurotransmitter to accumulate in the cytoplasm, and this may be amplified by the additional property of amphetamine

TABLE 21–1. Affinities of Monoamines, Cocaine, and Amphetamines at Monoamine Transporters in Rat Brain

COMPOUND	K_i, NET (nM)	K_i, 5-HTT (nM)	K_i, DAT (nM)
Dopamine	40	6,489	38
Norepinephrine	64	>50,000	357
5-HT	3013	17	2703
d-Amphetamine	39	3,830	35
d-Methamphetamine	48	2,137	114
Ecstasy (MDMA)	462	238	1572
Cocaine	779	304	478

K_i, nanomolar concentration needed to half-occupy monoamine transporter sites.
Source: With permission from Rothman and Baumann (2003).

to act as an inhibitor of the enzyme monoamine oxidase, which acts to degrade free intracellular monoamines. The increased level of free catecholamine in the cytoplasm in turn leads to a release of neurotransmitter as the transporter mechanism works in reverse to transport neurotransmitter out of the nerve terminal. The action on the cell membrane transporter (DAT) is critical. Brain slices prepared from DAT⁻/DAT⁻ knockout mice fail to show any increase in dopamine release when amphetamine is added to the incubating fluid, and administration of a high dose of amphetamine (10 mg/kg, intraperitoneally) to DAT⁻/DAT⁻ knockout mice fails to cause the normal burst of dopamine release seen in the dopamine-rich basal ganglia region of brain *in vivo*.

Cocaine acts *in vitro* with almost equal potency as an inhibitor of the two catecholamine transporters and the serotonin transporter (see Table 21–1). Its pharmacological actions may reflect a complex mixture of activation of multiple monoamine mechanisms. Amphetamine and methamphetamine, on the other hand, are recognized almost equally well by the norepinephrine and dopamine transporters but only weakly by the serotonin transporter (see Table 21–1), and they cause a release of both of the catecholamine neurotransmitters *in vitro*. In the brain, however, it seems that the ability of amphetamines to stimulate dopamine release explains most, if not all, of their psychostimulant properties.

Ecstasy (MDMA) is an unusual member of the amphetamine family because it has some ability to release dopamine and norepinephrine but has a higher affinity for the transporter in serotonin (5-HT) neurons. Thus, its main effect is to promote an increased release of serotonin in the brain (see Table 21–1). The related drug MDA promotes the release of all three monoamines.

PHARMACOLOGY OF COCAINE, d-AMPHETAMINE, AND d-METHAMPHETAMINE

Peripheral Sympathomimetic Effects

Cocaine and amphetamines interact with the norepinephrine transporter and storage in sympathetic nerve terminals to promote the availability of norepinephrine, and they may also promote central sympathetic outflow. Among other effects, cocaine and amphetamines cause an increase in blood pressure and pulse rate in both animals and humans. Other sympathomimetic effects include dry mouth, pupillary dilation, retention of urine, and sometimes increased respiratory rate. Some of the sympathomimetic effects of amphetamine can have medical benefits. In the lungs, the effect of amphetamine-induced norepinephrine release is to dilate the airways and to make breathing easier for asthma sufferers—this was one of the earliest medical uses of these drugs. Amphetamine was also used initially as a nasal decongestant based on its ability to cause norepinephrine release, which constricts the blood vessels in the nasal cavity and reduces the increased blood flow and inflammation that accompany a cold. Because of its powerful vasoconstrictor actions, a health risk associated with repeated insufflation of cocaine is damage to the palate and perforation of the nasal septum, leaving the user susceptible to infections.

The peripheral effects of cocaine and the amphetamines, especially increased pulse, are subjectively obvious to the drug user. They are also potentially life threatening and limit the dose that can safely be used. At low doses, the central nervous system (CNS) effects of methamphetamine appear to outweigh the autonomic effects, perhaps encouraging users to prefer this drug over d-amphetamine.

Psychostimulant Effects of Cocaine and Amphetamines in Animals

The psychostimulant drugs have a number of easily observed effects on animal behavior that have been extensively studied in order to understand the underlying brain mechanisms. As described in Chapter 3, the stimulant effects of amphetamine were extensively studied in pigeons operantly conditioned on different schedules of reinforcement. Amphetamine induces rate-dependent increases in responding, an effect also demonstrated with lever pressing in rats. More frequently, however, these stimulant effects have been studied in rats and mice using measures of unconditioned motor behaviors. Low doses of cocaine or d-amphetamine cause a dose-dependent stimulation of activity in these animals, and higher doses can lead to prolonged running activity. This is easily quantified in automated activity cages and provides a simple model system (see Chapter 3). The response is particularly notable since the tests are normally carried out during the day when the rodents, which are nocturnal animals, are not normally very active.

Higher doses of cocaine or *d*-amphetamine cause an entirely different pattern of behavior in animals characterized by the continuous repetition of purposeless movements, referred to as "stereotyped behavior." The pattern of movements is characteristic for different species. In rodents, stereotyped behavior normally consists of continuous head swaying, sniffing, licking, and gnawing. Instead of the purposeful running activity seen after lower doses of the drug, animals exhibiting stereotyped behavior will often stay in one part of the cage and continuously repeat these items of behavior.

An unusual feature of the behavioral responses to cocaine and amphetamine is that they show "sensitization" on repeated administration of the drug (Fig. 21–3). Thus, repeated daily administration of the drugs leads gradually to exaggerated running and stereotypy responses, and this effect persists for some days after repeat administration is stopped. The mechanisms underlying the behavioral sensitization are unclear. Some studies have reported an increased amphetamine-induced release of dopamine in various brain regions in sensitized animals, and a variety of explanations have been proposed, but others found that behavioral sensitization could occur even when the amount of dopamine released was unchanged. Although behavioral responses to cocaine and amphetamine appear to be triggered by a release of dopamine in the brain, the behavioral responses often persist long after the rate of dopamine release has decreased below its peak. Behavioral sensitization does not appear to be obvious in human amphetamine users, in whom the development of tolerance on repeated drug exposure seems more prominent.

Further insight into the importance of the dopamine neurons in the brain in mediating the various behavioral responses to *d*-amphetamine was provided by experiments in which the terminal fields of these neurons were selectively destroyed in different brain regions. The compound 6-hydroxydopamine is a neurotoxic analogue of dopamine that is selectively taken up and accumulated by the transporters in norepinephrine- and dopamine-containing neurons, leading to the permanent destruction of these neurons. By using very small doses administered at precise anatomical locations, it is possible to create selective damage to particular groups of norepinephrine- or dopamine-containing nerve terminals. Selective lesions of norepinephrine fibers were found to have little effect on the stimulant actions of *d*-amphetamine, but the stimulant actions were completely absent in animals with selective dopamine lesions. Further studies with 6-hydroxydopamine showed that different groups of dopamine neurons in brain are responsible for the various behavioral responses to cocaine and *d*-amphetamine. In rats in which the dopamine terminals in the striatum were destroyed by local microinjections of 6-hydroxydopamine, the

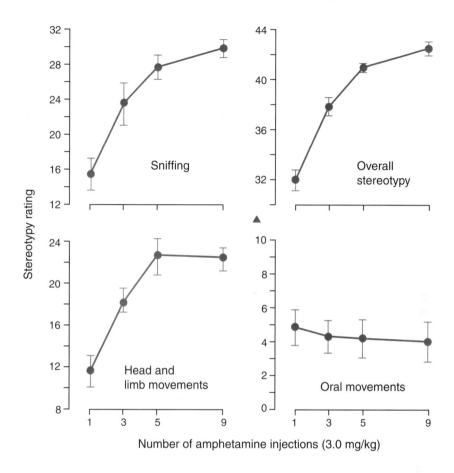

FIGURE 21–3. Sensitization of behavioral responses to amphetamine.
On repeated administration of amphetamine (3 mg/kg intraperitoneally) once every 3-4 days for a total of 9 treatments, stereotyped sniffing and head and limb movements increased significantly, whereas oral stereotyped movements did not change. Behavioral sensitization is a characteristic feature of the response to amphetamine in animals, and may be evident in chronic human amphetamine users. (Modified from Robinson and Becker, 1986.)

stereotyped behavior response to high doses of *d*-amphetamine was greatly reduced, whereas the running response remained intact. On the other hand, microinjections of 6-hydroxydopamine into the nucleus accumbens—part of a separate mesocorticolimbic dopamine-containing neural pathway—abolished the running response to *d*-amphetamine or cocaine while leaving the stereotyped behavior response to high-dose amphetamine intact.

Another experimental approach that has yielded valuable insights into the effects of amphetamine and other drugs has been the so-called drug discrimination procedure (see Chapter 3). Rats trained to recognize *d*-amphetamine show complete cross-generalization when methamphetamine, methylpheni-date, or other related amphetamine-like drugs are substituted. However, these rats do not recognize MDMA or fenfluramine, amphetamine derivatives that act predominantly via a serotoninergic rather than a dopaminergic mecha-nism. The rats do cross-generalize to cocaine, suggesting that its CNS effects are similar in important respects to those elicited by d-amphetamine. Rats trained to recognize cocaine will similarly cross-generalize to d-amphetamine and show partial cross-generalization to MDMA, reflecting the role that 5-HT release plays in the actions of cocaine. One can also ask which of the several different types of dopamine receptors in the brain is most important in mediating the amphetamine cue. Drugs that act as direct stimulants at dopamine D_2 recep-tors (e.g., quinpirole and pergolide) substitute well for cocaine or d-amphetamine in drug discrimination tests, but drugs that act on dopamine D_1 or D_3 receptors do not. As expected, antagonist drugs that block dopamine actions at D_2 recep-tors also abolish the animals' ability to discriminate cocaine or d-amphetamine from saline. Rats trained to recognize cocaine or d-amphetamine showed complete cross-generalization to direct microinjections of cocaine (for cocaine-trained rats) or dopamine (for d-amphetamine-trained rats) into areas of the frontal brain mesolimbic system, such as nucleus accumbens, whereas injec-tions into another dopamine-rich brain region, the striatum, were not recog-nized in this way.

Other neurotransmitters in brain interact with the primary dopamine mechanism triggered by d-amphetamine. Thus, for example, whereas d-amphetamine has little ability to directly stimulate serotonin (5-HT) release from brain, the 5-HT system in brain appears to act as a brake on dopamine-mediated responses. Treatment of rats with drugs that inhibit the biosynthesis of 5-HT (e.g., parachlorophenylalanine) or selective 5-HT neurotoxins (e.g., 5,6-dihyroxytryptamine) leads to exaggerated behavioral responses to d-amphetamine. This interaction with 5-HT is also apparent with cocaine, which, unlike amphetamine, leads to increased levels of extracellular 5-HT in brain because of its inhibition of the 5-HT transporter, 5-HTT. Knockout mice that lack expression of 5-HTT show increased locomotor responses to cocaine.

The use of knockout mice lacking either the dopamine transporter DAT or 5-HTT or both has provided valuable distinctions between the CNS effects of cocaine and d-amphetamine. As summarized in Table 21–2, the results for d-amphetamine are fairly simple. DAT knockout mice show no locomotor response to d-amphetamine and the place preference rewarding effects of the drug are abolished, whereas 5-HTT knockout animals continue to respond nor-mally to d-amphetamine. For cocaine, the results are more complex. DAT knock-out animals show no locomotor response to cocaine but continue to exhibit place preference (Figure 20–2). Surprisingly, 5-HTT knockout animals also show

TABLE 21–2. Effects of Monoamine Transporter Knockouts on Behavioral Effects of Cocaine

KNOCKOUT MICE	COCAINE-INDUCED INCREASED LOCOMOTOR ACTIVITY	COCAINE-INDUCED PLACE PREFERENCE BEHAVIOR
DAT⁻/DAT⁻	Abolished	Intact
5-HTT⁻/5-HTT⁻	Enhanced	Intact
5-HTT⁻/5-HTT⁻ + DAT⁻/DAT⁻	Abolished	Abolished

cocaine place preference. It is only in animals lacking both DAT and 5-HTT that the rewarding effects of cocaine are lost, as evidenced by loss of place preference. It seems that the ability of cocaine to cause increases in either dopamine or 5-HT is by itself sufficiently rewarding to induce place preference behavior.

Effects of Cocaine and Amphetamines on Human Mood and Performance

Whereas studies of cocaine and *d*-amphetamine responses in animals have provided important insights into the brain mechanisms involved, studies of the effects of these drugs on the human brain demonstrate the complexity of such effects. Low doses of insufflated cocaine or oral *d*-amphetamine produce similar psychic responses, but the effects of cocaine are of shorter duration. The most commonly reported drug effects are a euphoric sense of well-being and a feeling of exhilaration, and lessened fatigue in reaction to work. The latter effect is more pronounced with *d*-amphetamine because of its long duration of action, leading to an ability to undertake prolonged physical or mental tasks without fatigue or boredom.

These are typical of the effects of relatively low doses of cocaine or amphetamine in normal healthy people. With somewhat larger doses, all of these effects are intensified but the feeling of "relaxed alertness" is replaced by a "driven" feeling. Thoughts cascade rapidly through the mind and the capacity to concentrate is diminished. A sense of earnestness and decreased frivolity are often felt, and the user may feel compelled to bore others with increased talkativeness about serious or inappropriate subjects.

However, these relatively benign effects of the drugs are not what the addict craves. Cocaine or amphetamine abusers use high doses of the drug taken intravenously or by some other means that ensure rapid delivery to the bloodstream and brain (smoking or insufflation). The resulting "rush" is a far more intense euphoria, a much-prized event by the addict, and often compared to the pleasure of orgasm. The intensity of the rush is dose related, and this often leads addicts to increase the drug dosage and enter into a "binging" cycle.

As with most other psychoactive drugs, there is considerable variability in individual responses to cocaine or amphetamines. Not everyone finds their effects pleasant; some experience little subjective response at all, whereas others find that amphetamine provokes anxiety rather than euphoria. Some of the underlying neurobiological reasons for such individual differences are beginning to be understood, and genetic differences have been found to play an important part. For example, minor genetically determined variants in the gene coding for the dopamine transporter protein may be important. It was found that people who possessed two copies (one from each parent) of the so-called "9-repeat" version of the gene experienced virtually no subjective responses to d-amphetamine (10 or 20 mg) in terms of either euphoria or anxiety. This version of the gene is also known to result in lower levels of expression of the dopamine transporter protein, a key target to amphetamine's effects. It has also been reported that children who have the 9-repeat version of the dopamine transporter gene showed blunted responses to the amphetamine-like stimulant methylphenidate. Other studies have shown that people who found amphetamine pleasant tended to have lower levels of dopamine D_2 receptors in their brains (assessed by positron emission tomography imaging techniques), suggesting the possibility that their brain dopamine system could benefit most from a drug-induced "boost."

As in the animal drug discrimination studies described previously, human subjects can learn to discriminate the "drug cue" from placebo. After such training with d-amphetamine, other amphetamines were able to substitute fully, although higher doses were required, with potency ratios as follows: phenmetrazine, 2.5; phenylpropanolamine (norephedrine), 7.5; and methylphenidate, 2.0. These drugs are all capable of mimicking the dopamine-releasing effect of d-amphetamine. On the other hand, fenfluramine, which acts predominantly via serotonin release, substituted only partially for d-amphetamine as a drug cue.

Effects of Amphetamines on Cognitive Performance

One of the most common reasons cited by students, truck drivers, soldiers, or businessmen for taking amphetamines is that they enhance performance and stave off normal fatigue. A considerable experimental literature on animals and human subjects has sought to document this effect.

In animal models of learning and memory, it is not always easy to demonstrate an enhancement of performance with drugs. With highly trained animals, their performance is near perfect with very few errors, so drugs cannot improve it further. Low doses of amphetamine consistently speed up performance, so reaction times are shortened and latencies to respond decrease. This often occurs without any loss of accuracy, although in some tests speeded-up responses can lead to errors. The performance-enhancing effects of amphetamine are most apparent in tasks that require sustained attention.

Different doses of amphetamine have a variety of effects on rat behavior. Performance-enhancing effects are generally seen only after relatively low doses (0.1–0.4 mg/kg); higher doses (0.4–1.0 mg/kg) increase rates of responding but not necessarily accuracy. After very high doses (>3.0 mg/kg), performance is usually completely disrupted by the emergence of persistent stereotyped behavior.

Studies of amphetamine in human subjects were stimulated by the use of the drug by the military of both the Allied Powers and the Axis countries during World War II to counteract effects of fatigue and sleep deprivation during long missions. The general conclusion of these studies was that low doses of amphetamine improved performance in tasks that required long periods of sustained attention and could restore performance that had deteriorated because of fatigue or sleep deprivation. The performance-enhancing effects of the drug were most apparent in situations in which subjects were required to undertake simple, prolonged, repetitive, and often boring tasks. The performance-enhancing effects of d-amphetamine were seen most dramatically in sleep-deprived subjects. Performance on a variety of cognitive and motor performance tasks is reduced after overnight sleep deprivation, and even more marked deficits are seen after more severe sleep deprivation (up to 60 hours); d-amphetamine (20 mg) is able to completely reverse such deficits, even after severe sleep deprivation. Amphetamines dramatically decrease sleepiness, increase latency to fall asleep, and increase latency to onset of rapid eye movement (dreaming) sleep. These effects underlie the use of amphetamines by those who need to stay awake and remain vigilant for long periods of time (e.g., truck drivers and military personnel).

There are considerable individual differences in the effects of amphetamines on human cognitive performance. Some of the underlying neurobiological and genetic reasons for these differences have become apparent in recent years. It is generally thought that the effects of amphetamine on attention and cognition are mediated principally by the drug-induced release of dopamine in the prefrontal cortex. Studies on experimental animals suggest that dopamine impacts on prefrontal cortex function in accordance with an "inverted-U" dose–response curve—the response being optimum within a narrow range of released dopamine, with too little or too much having deleterious effects (Figure 16–5). It has been found that in human subjects d-amphetamine improved brain function and memory (assessed with a variety of psychological tests) only in those people who had relatively low working memory capacity at baseline, whereas in subjects with a high working memory capacity at baseline the drug worsened performance. Some of these individual differences in drug response may be genetically determined. For example, different variants of the enzyme catechol-*O*-methyltransferase (COMT) may determine the levels of responsiveness to the memory-enhancing actions of amphetamine. COMT degrades dopamine to an inactive metabolite 3-methoxytyramine. Animal studies have shown that COMT plays an important role in the inactivation of dopamine in the brain, particularly in the prefrontal cortex, where levels of the dopamine reuptake transporter are relatively low. Mice that are genetically engineered to eliminate expression of the COMT enzyme have increased levels of dopamine in prefrontal cortex but not in the striatum, where dopamine reuptake sites are abundant. In humans, COMT exists in two genetically determined variants, which differ by only one amino acid at position 158 in the protein. The Val158 form of the enzyme is fully active, but the Met158 variant (in which methionine substitutes for valine) is very much less active. People homozygous for the Met158 form of the enzyme (one copy inherited from each parent) tended to have above average prefrontal cortex function and working memory capacity and to show no positive response to *d*-amphetamine. In contrast, individuals homozygous for the Val158 form of COMT had lower initial performance levels but showed significant cognitive improvements in response to amphetamine. The results suggest that Met158 COMT homozygotes have an impaired ability to dispose of dopamine in the brain and are thus normally exposed to higher baseline levels of dopamine; further drug-induced rises in dopamine are deleterious rather than beneficial (i.e., they are already at the top of the proposed inverted-U relationship). These are important genetic differences since approximately one-fourth of the population are Met158 homozygotes and may thus be expected to react unfavorably to amphetamines.

As described above, individual differences in subjective responses to amphetamines have also been attributed in part to genetically determined differences in the dopamine transporter protein, a key mediator of the drug's actions.

Stereotyped Behavior in Human Psychostimulant Users

The Swedish psychiatrist G. Rylander suggested the term *punding* to define a form of amphetamine-induced stereotyped behavior in Swedish abusers in whom "an organized goal-directed but, nevertheless, meaningless activity" took place as "an automatic behavior with something of the compulsive factor, which is typical for obsessive–compulsive states." Cocaine may also lead to such stereotyped behavior, but more rarely. Amphetamine users place great emphasis on the pleasurable nature of punding and may continue these activities for extended periods of time. Self-injurious behaviors are also sometimes seen, such as self-biting, head banging, scratching, cutting, hair pulling, and other injurious acts. Chronic amphetamine/methamphetamine users may develop sores and skin abscesses on their bodies from repeated scratching at "crank bugs" in response to the common delusion that bugs are crawling under the skin (formication).

Effects of Cocaine and Amphetamines on Sexual Function

The effects of cocaine and amphetamines on sexual function are as variable as those of alcohol, and they depend on dosage, personality, previous sexual experience, degree of normality of predrug sexual adjustment, and the setting. Some users report a decreased interest in sexual relations or even impotence. They may find the drug to be more rewarding than sex, and many experienced users describe the cocaine or amphetamine high as resembling an intense orgasm. Similar brain mechanisms are involved in both the natural and the drug-induced pleasure.

However, it is also clear that many cocaine or amphetamine users experience a definite increase in libidinal drive that may be accompanied by delayed ejaculation or delayed female orgasm. Promiscuity, compulsive masturbation, and prolonged intercourse with few orgasms may result—perhaps a form of the drug-induced stereotyped behavior described previously. Many intravenous d-amphetamine users report that they became more sexually excited when on the drug and had prolonged intercourse and intensified orgasms.

Methamphetamine use appears to be particularly attractive to gay and bisexual men. The drug-induced release of inhibitions, delayed ejaculation, and heightened sexual pleasure are motivating factors. In the United States, methamphetamine use by gay men is reported to be associated with high rates of anal sex, low rates of condom use, multiple sex partners, sexual marathons, and anonymous sex. Use of the drug is associated with particular environments in which sexual contact among gay men is promoted, such as sex clubs and large "circuit" parties. Unfortunately, the tendency for drug-induced unprotected sex means that methamphetamine use in the gay community may exacerbate the already serious HIV/AIDS epidemic in this group.

Appetite Suppression

Both cocaine and amphetamines decrease appetite. The first positive results from clinical trials of amphetamine in the treatment of obesity were published in 1938, and amphetamines soon became widely adopted medically as appetite suppressants. d-Amphetamine and subsequently a series of other synthetic amphetamine-like drugs were very widely used as appetite suppressants during the 1950s and 1960s. At least initially the amphetamines can lead to significant weight loss. However, the appetite suppressant effect tends to wane after weeks of treatment and users may compensate by increasing the dose, thus exposing themselves to a heightened risk of becoming dependent on the drug. Furthermore, as with other antiobesity drugs, when amphetamine use is terminated body weight tends to revert back to the starting baseline.

Exactly how cocaine or amphetamines cause appetite suppression is not clear. Complex nerve circuits in the hypothalamus, a small region lying at the base of the frontal part of the brain, control the balance between hunger and satiety, which ultimately determines body weight. There has been a significant increase in scientific understanding of these mechanisms in recent years, and we now know that a series of hormones generated in the stomach, gut, and fat tissues act on appetite-stimulating and -suppressing regions of the hypothalamus to maintain normal body weight. The principal site of action of cocaine and amphetamines seems to be within the hypothalamus, and their ability to stimulate the release of dopamine, norepinephrine, and serotonin may contribute. The amphetamine derivative fenfluramine, which for a while was a highly successful antiobesity drug, appears to act principally through its ability to cause a release of serotonin.

One of the effects of cocaine and amphetamine administration in animals is to cause an increase in the synthesis of a brain chemical known as "CART peptide," which stands for "cocaine and amphetamine regulated transcript." It was discovered by researchers who were trying to determine which gene products were switched on in response to cocaine or amphetamine. CART is a particularly potent appetite suppressant (see Chapter 10), and it is present in the relevant parts of the hypothalamic circuits involved in appetite control. It is also found in regions of the brain associated with pleasure and reward mechanisms, which are dopamine-rich areas. It is likely that the increased synthesis of CART, turned on indirectly by cocaine or amphetamine via dopamine release, plays an important part in the anorectic actions of the amphetamines.

Tolerance and Dependence

For several decades after the introduction of cocaine and amphetamines as medicines, it was widely believed that they were not addictive. This was largely due to the erroneous belief that addiction must always be accompanied by physical withdrawal signs when drug use stops—as is the case for heroin and related opiates. We now use the term "substance dependence" rather than "addiction" (see Chapter 20), and under the criteria drawn up in the *Diagnostic and Statistical Manual of Mental Disorders*, fourth edition, by the American Psychiatric Association, it is clear that chronic use of cocaine or amphetamines can lead to dependence. Cocaine and/or methamphetamine have become second only to cannabis as the most common drug of abuse in many countries. Surveys by the National Institute on Drug Abuse suggest that

10–15% of those who have ever used cocaine eventually become abusers. There is also an increasing abuse of methamphetamine, particularly in the United States and Southeast Asia.

It is important to stress, however, that not all regular users of cocaine or amphetamines become dependent on the drugs. Millions of adults and children have used amphetamines medically without becoming dependent, and large numbers of people have taken low doses of amphetamines to enhance performance in the military, in sports, and in the many other ways in which these drugs have been casually employed without suffering adverse effects or dependence. Some people may insufflate powdered cocaine occasionally at fashionable dinner parties without becoming dependent. It is the persistent use of high doses of cocaine or amphetamines that distinguishes drug abuse and dependence. High-dose users become tolerant to the effects of the drug and tend to escalate the dose. The resulting high doses are incompatible with normal functioning and carry with them liabilities of toxicity, severely disturbed behavior, dysphoria, and psychosis.

There is little doubt that the route of administration is very important. The rapidity and intensity of onset of the drug effect after intravenous injection or smoking increase the rate and strength of development of psychological dependence. The rush or "flash" following such rapid routes of administration, often described as a "whole body orgasm," is highly prized. However, as the rush declines, restlessness, nervousness, and agitation replace nirvana. Irritability progresses to paranoia, fatigue, and depression as the rush comes to an end. The urge to repeat the drug experience is often irresistible. A "binge" can last for several days at a time, during which the user is unable to eat or sleep until he or she "crashes" into a deep sleep that can last for 18 hours. Repeated binging can lead to cycles of unproductive frenzied activity, stereotyped behavior, or psychosis alternating with exhaustion, extended sleep, and subsequent dysphoric lethargy. Repeated cycles of binging can lead to a severe form of dependence and a complete preoccupation with the drug and its effects.

The brain mechanisms underlying dependence are discussed in Chapter 20. All drugs capable of causing dependence are readily self-administered by experimental animals. Cocaine and amphetamines are no exception: Both monkeys and rats can readily be trained to self-administer these drugs. Usually this involves training the animals to press a lever to self-inject a small dose intravenously. Rats or monkeys given unrestricted access to cocaine or amphetamine will overdose to the exclusion of all other behavior. The compulsive nature of self-administration behavior for cocaine and amphetamines in animals accurately reflects the high abuse potential of these drugs. In rats, administration of these drugs readily leads to place preference behavior (see Chapter 20) and reduces the threshold for intracranial self-stimulation (Fig. 20–4).

The animal models of self-administration also provide further insights into the process of addiction. Rats given access to cocaine for a limited period each day (less than 3 hours) stabilize to a constant intake of the drug over long periods. However, animals given access to cocaine for periods of more than 6 hours behave quite differently, gradually escalating their drug intake while becoming less responsive to rewarding stimuli, either from the drug or from intracranial self-stimulation electrodes. The threshold current needed to elicit self-stimulation gradually rises as the cocaine intake increases. This "hedonic insensitivity" persists for several days after cocaine access is stopped. A comparable phenomenon in human drug users may help to explain why they escalate to increasingly higher doses during a binge session.

Animal experiments have shown that cocaine and amphetamines trigger dopamine release in the shell of the nucleus accumbens, in common with several other drugs with abuse/dependence liability (see Chapter 20). Brain imaging studies using functional magnetic resonance imaging have also shown that a low dose of intravenous methamphetamine (0.15 mg/kg) in drug naive volunteers causes highly selective and localized activation of brain activity in the medial orbitofrontal cortex, anterior cingulate cortex, and ventral striatum—all regions thought to represent key parts of the "reward circuitry."

A further complication in understanding the role of dopamine in drug dependence is that dopamine neurons appear to fire in two different modes, known as "tonic" and "phasic." In the tonic mode, neurons fire slowly, giving rise to low levels of dopamine both in the regions associated with synaptic contacts with other cells and in nonsynaptic regions. This is in contrast to phasic firing, which occurs in bursts of impulses and gives rise to a "spike" in dopamine release, particularly important in regulating postsynaptic neurons. The ability of intravenously administered or smoked drugs to mimic this phasic release of dopamine may help to explain why such routes of drug administration are more likely to lead to drug dependence.

Adverse Effects and Toxicity of Cocaine and Amphetamines

Overdose

Cocaine or amphetamine/methamphetamine overdose is seen in thousands of hospital emergency departments and leads to hundreds of deaths each year. The features of amphetamine/methamphetamine overdose may include chest pains, loss of speech, paralysis, coma, convulsions, shock, decreased urine output, and high fever (>40°C). The most common cause of death is due to multiple organ failure resembling that from heatstroke. This is also the case in experimental animals, in which high doses of amphetamine also cause increases in body temperature and death; mortality is greatly reduced if the animals are kept in a cold environment. Norepinephrine release in peripheral blood vessels and in the heart can also lead to cardiovascular collapse secondary to ventricular fibrillation or cerebral stroke and hemorrhage caused by a drug-induced rise in blood pressure. Overdosing is rare among experienced drug users. Repeated use of cocaine or amphetamines leads to a high degree of tolerance, particularly to the dangerous sympathomimetic effects. The dangers increase when an abuser takes a high dose after a period of withdrawal, when tolerance has been diminished.

Amphetamine psychosis

Another acute effect of high-dose amphetamines is their ability to induce psychosis. The syndrome most commonly seen by clinicians is a paranoid or paranoid hallucinatory psychosis in a setting of clear consciousness in which formal aspects of thought are relatively intact but delusion and hallucinations frequently invoke intense fear. Amphetamine psychosis is frequently associated with auditory hallucinations that resemble those experienced by patients with schizophrenia, including hearing vague noises and voices and occasionally having conversations with the voices. However, amphetamine psychosis is also commonly associated with visual hallucinations often involving faces, the tactile hallucination known as formication, and occasionally olfactory hallucinations. In contrast with the mainly auditory hallucinations of the patient with schizophrenia who may have blunted or inappropriate emotional responses, amphetamine psychosis is often associated with extreme anxiety and fear reactions. The drug taker seems to retain some insight into his or her state with a clear, if delusional, thought process. The relation between amphetamine-induced psychosis and the "dopamine hypothesis" of schizophrenia was nevertheless an important link in the development of this hypothesis.

A transient paranoid psychosis with delusions and hallucinations is also associated with chronic high-dose cocaine abuse but has been less well characterized. Both amphetamine- and cocaine-induced psychosis occur after prolonged high-dose abuse, suggesting an underlying sensitization mechanism.

Neurochemical markers

Although animal studies have shown consistent evidence for persistent changes in neurochemical markers of dopaminergic nerves in brain after exposure to high doses of amphetamine or methamphetamine, the doses used are much higher than those used in human users. Several brain imaging studies have found marked reductions in levels of the dopamine transporter (DAT) and dopamine D_2 receptors in chronic cocaine or amphetamine users, and reduced levels of DAT binding are still seen in some subjects even after several years of abstinence. It was suggested that this was evidence of irreversible neurotoxic damage to dopamine nerves. However, an alternative could be that the amphetamine abusers were drawn to the drug because they had deficits in dopaminergic function (i.e., the inverted-U relationship); the imaging studies have no baseline "predrug" measurements.

Neurocognitive impairment

The question of whether the chronic abuse of amphetamines leads to long-term impairments in cognitive function is difficult to disentangle since acute administration of these drugs can enhance some aspects of cognitive function. However, there have been several reports of impaired cognitive function in long-term amphetamine users, with significant deficits in verbal and visual memory tasks and impairments on various attention-based response measures. Methamphetamine users appear to have an impaired ability to focus attention and to manage distraction. Some of these deficits may recover gradually during a period of abstinence; the evidence for any persistent cognitive deficits in amphetamine users and ex-users is inconclusive.

Violent and criminal behavior

There is a considerable literature relating cocaine and amphetamines to violence and crime. Cocaine can be shown to increase aggressiveness under controlled laboratory conditions. Murders may be committed by psychostimulant users while intoxicated, with paranoid thinking, emotional lability, panic, and lowered impulse control induced by the drug as instrumental factors. High doses of cocaine or amphetamines cause the subject to focus on immediate, close-range stimuli. This may lead to impulsive reflex-like lashing out at innocent bystanders. The addict becomes apt to perceive anyone who seems to be interfering with his or her immediate drug-related pursuits as intolerably threatening. The result is a markedly increased risk of antisocial behavior. Apart from the random violence induced by intoxication with cocaine or amphetamines, the need for an ongoing supply of the drug can also lead to crime.

PHARMACOLOGY OF MDMA (ECSTASY)

> Ecstasy: An overwhelming feeling of joy or rapture; an emotional or religious frenzy or trance-like state
>
> —*Concise Oxford Dictionary*, ninth edition (1995)

Chemistry and History

Ecstasy is the popular name for the methamphetamine MDMA (see Fig. 21–1). Ecstasy and the related amphetamine derivative MDA are very widely used recreational drugs. Like the other amphetamines, Ecstasy and MDA are relatively easy to manufacture. It is estimated that as much as 100 tons of the precursor chemical piperonyl methylketone are smuggled into Europe every year, which is enough to make 100 million Ecstasy tablets that are sold for approximately $5 each. Because the U.S. Drug Enforcement Administration exerts strict monitoring of the chemical precursors needed for Ecstasy manufacture, there are few illegal Ecstasy labs in the United States. Supplies of the drug are imported from The Netherlands, largely via Canada; Ecstasy tablets cost approximately $15–$20 each in the United States. Tablets come in a variety of colors, shapes, and sizes and have an average MDMA content of approximately 100 mg, although the content of active drug is highly variable and contamination with other drugs—notably MDA, methamphetamine, caffeine, and aspirin—is common. The organization DanceSafe provides information on the testing of Ecstasy tablets available illegally in the United States. In 2007, it reported that only one-third of those tested contained only Ecstasy, almost one-fourth contained none at all; and the rest contained Ecstasy or MDA with a variety of other compounds.

MDA and MDMA are not new drugs. MDMA was first patented by the German pharmaceutical company Merck in 1914 as a chemical intermediate in the synthesis of other compounds. Both MDA and MDMA were assessed by the U.S. Army during the 1950s,which was interested in discovering a "truth serum" to be used in interrogating enemy captives. The psychedelic effects of these drugs have been known since the 1960s. MDA became one of the popular psychedelics in the U.S. drug scene of the late 1960s. MDA was known as the "hug drug" and was said to stand for "Mellow Drug of America." Alexander Shulgin was among the first to report the psychedelic effects of Ecstasy (MDMA) in the late 1960s, and it too became widely used among U.S. university students. During the late 1970s, MDMA was widely used by psychotherapists associated with the Esalen Institute in California who believed that it had "substantial potential as an adjunct to psychoanalysis." This pseudomedical use spread widely among psychotherapists in the United States. By the early 1980s, more than 1000 private psychotherapists in the United States were using MDMA in their clinical practice.

In July 1985, the U.S. Drug Enforcement Administration, apparently alarmed by accounts of increasing addiction to Ecstasy and by scientific reports that the related drug MDA might cause brain damage, placed an immediate ban on Ecstasy and MDA. They were placed in the most restrictive category of all, reserved for damaging and addictive drugs without medical use, and this was followed by similar moves in most other countries. Despite this ban, Ecstasy was increasingly used as a key component of the "rave dance" scene in Europe and the United States in the 1980s and 1990s.

Effects in Animals

As previously summarized (see Table 21–1), Ecstasy has a preferential affinity for the serotonin transporter, and its effects are largely due to its ability to promote serotonin release in the brain. Ecstasy-induced release of serotonin can be demonstrated in the intact animal brain using the technique of implanted microdialysis probes and by measurements of the depletion of serotonin stores in animal brain following drug administration. The involvement of the serotonin transporter was confirmed by the finding that pretreatment with the serotonin uptake inhibitor fluoxetine greatly reduced the ability of Ecstasy to cause release of serotonin in rat brain. At higher doses, Ecstasy also causes a release of dopamine in rat brain that can be measured by the microdialysis probe technique.

That Ecstasy-induced serotonin release in the brain plays a major role in the effects of the drug is supported by the observation that laboratory animals treated with the drug display the so-called "serotonin behavioral syndrome." This was first described following administration to rats of an inhibitor of monoamine oxidase together with the serotonin precursor *l*-tryptophan. The syndrome consists of hyperactivity, head weaving, forepaw treading, penile erection, salivation, and defecation. Ecstasy causes all of these acute behavioral features in rats in a dose-dependent manner. The human equivalent of the serotonin syndrome is also a real phenomenon—it can occur, for example, by the inadvertent combination of serotoninergic drugs, such as a monoamine oxidase inhibitor and a serotonin uptake inhibitor (e.g., fluoxetine). The symptoms include hyperactivity, agitation, hyperpyrexia (fever), shivering, tremor, and slowing and increased heart rate. Several of these symptoms can be seen in Ecstasy users in a milder form.

The ability of Ecstasy to cause an increase in body temperature has proved to be an important factor in the acute toxicity of the drug and is thought to have contributed to the deaths of some human users. In rats and mice kept at normal room temperature (20–22°C), Ecstasy causes an increase in body temperature of 1 or 2°C. In humans, this is the equivalent of developing the sort of fever associated with a bad bout of flu. The effect in laboratory animals is dependent on the ambient temperature. Rats kept in a cold room (10°C) show either no change or a small decrease in body temperature in response to Ecstasy. On the other hand, animals kept in a warm environment (30°C) exhibit an exaggerated increase in body temperature in response to the drug. The effect of Ecstasy on body temperature seems to be due to its ability to enhance dopamine release in the brain rather than serotonin. The increase in body temperature elicited by the drug in rats was not prevented by pretreatment with serotonin receptor antagonists or the serotonin uptake inhibitor fluoxetine (Prozac) but was blocked by pretreatment with dopamine receptor antagonists. In this respect, Ecstasy resembles methamphetamine, which also causes an increase in body temperature mediated via dopamine release.

Effects of Ecstasy on Human Consciousness and Mood

Pure MDMA salt is a white crystalline solid with a bitter taste. The optimal adult dose of racemic MDMA is approximately 120–130 mg (approximately 2 mg/kg of body weight). There are gender differences in response; proportionately to body weight, women are more sensitive than men to MDMA, so their optimal dosage may be lower. The preferentially metabolized (+)-enantiomer ("mirror image") of MDMA is more active, more stimulating, and more neurotoxic than the (−)-enantiomer.

The effects of psychedelic drugs are intensely subjective and by definition difficult to describe in words. Ecstasy causes a highly unusual series of changes in consciousness. It has been described as an "empathogen" because it can promote an extraordinary clarity of introspective self-insight, together with a deep love of self and a no less emotionally intense empathetic love of others. MDMA also acts as a euphoriant. The euphoria is usually gentle and subtle, but sometimes it is profound.

On the one hand, the experience is usually intensely pleasurable, with heightened awareness of sensory stimuli, a breakdown of normal social barriers and inhibitions, and increased empathy. In addition, there is an amphetamine-like stimulant effect, allowing the user to stay awake and indulge in energetic activities for long periods of time. The onset of action can take 20–60 minutes, with peak effects usually occurring 60–90 minutes after ingestion, and the primary effects last for 3–5 hours.

The effects of Ecstasy on sexual function are subtle. Ecstasy is sensuous in its effects without being distinctively prosexual; it is more of a hug drug than a love drug. However, the drug's capacity to dissolve a lifetime's social inhibitions, prudery, and sexual hang-ups means that sex while under its influence is not uncommon. In men, orgasm is more intense than normal but delayed.

It is easy to understand why Ecstasy has proved so popular with young people. However, not every Ecstasy experience is positive. Approximately 25% of users report having had at least one adverse reaction when unpleasant feelings and bodily sensations predominated. Minor adverse reactions are also common but generally short-lived. These include mydriasis (dilated pupils), photophobia (discomfort in bright lighting), headache, sweating, tachycardia (rapid heart beat), bruxism (grinding of teeth), trismus (uncomfortable tightening of jaw muscles), and loss of appetite.

Tolerance and Dependence

There are clear differences in the pattern of drug consumption between novice Ecstasy users and the more experienced. Whereas novices use 1 or 2 tablets per session, more experienced users take 2 or 3 tablets and heavy users (lifetime use more than 100 tablets) take more than 3 tablets per session. However, although this provides evidence for tolerance, there is little evidence to suggest that many Ecstasy users become dependent on the drug, but for some users the association of the drug with the rave dance/club scene may become a way of life.

A more worrying aspect of tolerance to Ecstasy is that the use of increasing doses may tend to exaggerate the psychostimulant effects of the drug, thought to be due largely to dopamine release in the brain. Animal studies show that the drug can cause a profound temporary impairment of serotonin function in the brain, although such changes do not occur to the same extent with dopamine-related functions. The possibility that the amphetamine-like effects of Ecstasy become more prominent in heavy users may explain why some heavy Ecstasy users indulge in binging. During a binge, users may take several tablets at once, take repeated tablets during a session, or both. The binge may last for up to 48 hours, usually without sleep or food, and can involve taking up to 20 Ecstasy tablets. Some binge users "snort" the powdered drug or inject it. These heavy users of Ecstasy show signs of becoming dependent on the drug, and many suffer harmful effects—days off with illness, loss of appetite, weight loss, and depressive experiences.

Animal studies have added little to our understanding of tolerance and dependence to Ecstasy. Whether experimental animals will readily self-administer a psychoactive drug is one widely used test of whether the drug is likely to prove addictive in humans. By this criterion, Ecstasy is not likely to be addictive since animals do not usually self-administer the drug.

Ecstasy-Related Deaths

The banning of legal Ecstasy was reinforced by the first reports of Ecstasy-related deaths in the United States in 1987 and in Europe a few years later. In the early cases, drug-induced hyperthermia (abnormally elevated body temperature) appeared to be the principal cause. All those who died had been admitted to hospitals with high temperatures (40–43°C), which led to damage to the liver, heart, and other organs. In an attempt at harm reduction, advice was given that dancers at rave events should take time out, go to a "chill out" area, and drink plenty of liquid. Unfortunately, some took this advice too literally; by 1993, deaths of Ecstasy users from water intoxication began to be reported. An analysis of the risks of fatal intoxication with Ecstasy is difficult to perform. The rare deaths attributed to Ecstasy need to be considered in relation to the very large number of users of the drug. In England and Wales during the 4-year period 1997 to 2000, a total of 81 deaths were reported to be related to Ecstasy use. However, postmortem analysis revealed that most of those who died had been taking other drugs (prescribed and nonprescribed) at the same time as Ecstasy; more than half (59%) had taken heroin or a related opiate. Indeed, most of the dead were known to the welfare or medical services as drug addicts, and typically they died at home rather than at a rave dance event. Only 6 of the dead appeared to have died after taking only Ecstasy. A case series in New York City studied 19,366 deaths between January 1997 and July 2000 for which postmortem toxicological analysis was available. Only 22 were considered to be Ecstasy related. As in Britain, the presence of other drugs was common in the Ecstasy-related cases, with heroin or other opiates in 32%, alcohol in 32%, ketamine in 27%, and cocaine in 22%. The analysis is also complicated by the fact that most illegally available Ecstasy tablets contain other potentially harmful drugs (e.g., methamphetamine and cocaine).

Is Ecstasy a Serotonin Neurotoxin?

There is a large scientific literature on the effects of Ecstasy on animal brain, focusing largely on the long-term damaging effects that the drug can have on serotonin-containing nerves. The literature is complex and often confusing, partly because there are marked differences in the effects of Ecstasy in different species (the drug has little effect on the serotonin system in mouse brain, but rats, guinea pigs, and monkeys are sensitive) but also because most animal studies used doses of Ecstasy that were far higher than those taken by human drug users. Most animal studies also administered Ecstasy by injection rather than orally, which leads to faster drug absorption and higher peak levels in blood than the slower oral route employed by most human users.

Nevertheless, it is clear that high doses of Ecstasy do cause damage to serotonin nerves in both rat and monkey brain. The drug causes a depletion of brain levels of serotonin and there is a long-lasting reduction in other neurochemical markers of serotonin nerves, including the biosynthetic enzyme tryptophan hydroxylase and the serotonin transporter mechanism, suggesting damage to the serotonin-containing nerve terminals. Both of these remain depleted for weeks or months after a single dose or course of doses of Ecstasy, although there is a slow recovery to near normal values that may take up to 1 year to complete. Anatomical studies of animal brain, using selective staining methods to visualize serotonin nerve fibers, suggest that the drug "prunes" the serotonin-containing fibers in their terminal regions.

The question of whether the animal data on the neurotoxic actions of Ecstasy are relevant to human users of the drug is a vexed one. Several studies have used brain imaging techniques to assess the integrity of the serotonin transporter in the brains of Ecstasy users and have reported consistent modest reductions in the density of serotonin transporter sites in the brains of Ecstasy users. However, no reductions in serotonin transporter densities were found in people who had stopped using Ecstasy, suggesting that the changes are reversible. Other studies have suggested that the chronic, heavy, recreational use of Ecstasy is associated with sleep disorders, depressed mood, elevated anxiety, impulsiveness and hostility, and selective impairment of episodic and working memory and attention. The cognitive deficits may persist for 6 months or more of abstinence, but all symptoms appear to remit within 6–12 months.

It seems reasonable to conclude that Ecstasy causes a temporary depletion of brain serotonin stores and some degree of downregulation of serotonin function, although there is little evidence that these changes are irreversible. The conclusion that some disruption of normal serotonin function occurs after drug use is consistent with the common observation that for several days after taking Ecstasy, users complain of depressed mood and lethargy (sometimes referred to as the "midweek blues"). However, these are transient changes, with mood reverting to normal within 7 days.

SELECTED REFERENCES

Angrist, B. and A. Sudilovsky (1978). Central nervous system stimulants: Historical aspects and clinical effects. In *Handbook of Psychopharmacology* (L. L. Iversen, S. D. Iversen, and S. H. Snyder, Eds.). Plenum Press, New York, Vol. 11, pp. 99–165.

Darke, S., S. Kaye, R. McKetin, and J. Duflou (2008). Major physical and psychological harms of methamphetamine use. *Drug Alcohol Rev.* 27, 253–262.

Di Chiara, G., V. Bassareo, S. Fenu, M. A. De Luca, L. Spina, C. Cadoni, E. Acquas, E. Carboni, V. Valentini, and D. Lecca (2004). Dopamine and drug addiction: The nucleus accumbens shell connection. *Neuropharmacology* 47, 227–241.

Green, E. R., A. O. Mechan, J. M. Elliott, E. O'Shea, and I. Colado (2003). The pharmacology and clinical pharmacology of 3,4-methylenedioxymethamphetamine (MDMA, "Ecstasy"). *Pharmacol. Rev.* 55, 463–508.

Grinspoon, L. and P. Hedblom (1975). *The Speed Culture. Amphetamine Use and Abuse in America.* Harvard University Press, Cambridge, MA.

Iversen, L. L. (2008). *Speed, Ecstasy, Ritalin: The Science of Amphetamines.* Oxford University Press, New York.

Robinson, T. E. and J. B. Becker (1986). Enduring changes in brain and behavior produced by chronic amphetamine administration: A review and evaluation of animal models of amphetamine psychosis. *Brain Res.* 396, 157–198.

Rothman, R. B. and M. H. Baumann (2003). Monoamine transporters and psychostimulant drugs. *Eur. J. Pharmacol.* 479, 23–40.

Turner, J. J. D. and A. C. Parrott (2000). "Is MDMA a human neurotoxin?": Diverse views from the discussants. *Neuropsychobiology* 42, 42–48.

United Nations (2003). Ecstasy and amphetamines—Global survey. Available at www.unodc.org.

Volkow, N. D., J. S. Fowler, G. J. Wang, J. M. Swanson, and F. Telang (2007). Dopamine in drug abuse and addiction: Results of imaging studies and treatment implications. *Arch. Neurol.* 64, 1575–1579.

Volkow, N. D., G. F. Wang, J. S. Fowler, P. P. Thanos, J. Logan, S. J. Gatley, A. Gifford, Y. S. Ding, C. Wong, and N. Pappas (2003). Brain DA D_2 receptors predict reinforcing effects of stimulants in humans: Replication study. *Synapse* 46, 79–82.

22

Heroin and Other Opiates

Opium, the resinous product of the opium poppy, has been used in human medicine for thousands of years. It was one of the key ingredients in dozens of Western proprietary medicines in the 19th century, including painkillers and "cordials" and "tonics" designed to aid sleep and to keep children quiet. When the active ingredient morphine was purified from opium and subsequently chemically modified by acetylation to form heroin, the pure chemicals also became widely used in popular medicines, including the use of heroin as a powerful cough suppressant. We find this remarkable now, but it was not until the late 19th century that the dangerous addictive properties of these drugs were recognized and their use restricted. Some believe that this may have been related to the development of the hypodermic syringe in the late nineteenth century, offering opiate users a more rapid means of delivering the drug to the brain.

The opiates, natural and synthetic, remain in widespread medical use as powerful analgesics (see Chapter 18). Meanwhile, despite the legal restrictions and criminal penalties imposed on the supply or possession of opiates for nonmedical use, such use is widespread. The United Nations' *World Drug Report 2007* estimated that there are 14.6 million heroin users worldwide. Approximately half of these are in Asia, especially in central Asia and Pakistan; 1 million in Western Europe; perhaps as many as 2 million in Russia; and 1.2 million in the United States. Heroin accounts for more than 70% of opiate abuse, and its street price has decreased in recent years to approximately $200 per gram in the United States and $75 per gram in Europe. Heroin use, however, appeared to peak in the late 1970s, when 2.3 million people in the United States admitted ever having used the drug. Heroin abusers represent a significant proportion (possibly 50%) of "problem drug users," whose powerful addiction drives them to criminal activities to fund their drug habit.

In the past decade, an epidemic of nonmedical abuse of a prescription pain killer, OxyContin, occurred in the United States. OxyContin is a sustained-release formulation of the synthetic opiate oxycodone, a powerful analgesic. This formulation helped millions of patients to manage their chronic pain with a once-a-day tablet. OxyContin was considered safe enough to be prescribed in the general physician's office rather than in a specialist pain center—as for morphine and other opiates. However, nonmedical use soon flourished. The tablets were crushed and the powder was snorted or injected. By 2002, approximately 2 million people in the United States admitted having used OxyContin nonmedically, and there were more than 10,000 emergency room visits for overdose and more than 450 deaths. Other synthetic opiates, notably methadone, which is used in the treatment of heroin addiction, also have the potential for abuse.

THE DRUGS AND HOW THEY ARE ADMINISTERED

Heroin is by far the most common opiate for nonmedical use, followed by morphine and the synthetic opiates. There are three main routes of administration. Intravenous injection is favored because it gives an opiate "high" within a few seconds. Heroin is the most popular opiate because it penetrates the blood–brain barrier more readily than morphine to give instant intoxication. However, heroin is less soluble in water than morphine, and users need to heat the drug with water (typically in a spoon) to obtain an injectable solution. All of the opiates can also be insufflated into the nasal cavity ("snorted"), or they can be smoked by careful heating and inhalation of the resulting volatile drug vapor ("chasing the dragon"). Smoking or snorting have become more popular in recent years because of the increased recognition that injection, often with dirty needles, can spread viral infections, notably HIV/AIDS.

Injected heroin reaches peak levels in plasma within 1–5 minutes and then decays rapidly as it is converted in the brain and elsewhere to the monoacetyl derivative 6-monoacetyl morphine and eventually to morphine, which in turn has a half-life of approximately 20 minutes and is metabolized in the liver. Although heroin is not active at opiate receptors, the monoacetyl metabolite is a potent agonist.

Synthetic opiates supplied as prescription medicines may be crushed and snorted or injected. Some modern formulations are less easy to use in this way.

For example, a popular medicinal formulation of the powerful opiate analgesic fentanyl is in the form of a skin patch that delivers the drug throughout the day. The patch cannot be dismantled, but abusers have found that by using multiple patches they can obtain an acceptable "high."

SUBJECTIVE EXPERIENCE OF OPIATE INTOXICATION

Following injection or other rapid administration of opiates, users describe four different components of intoxication, which can overlap in time. First, there is a profound feeling of euphoria called the *rush*, occurring within approximately 10 seconds. This wave of euphoria is frequently described in sexual terms as orgasmic. The *high* follows and is a general feeling of well-being that can last for several hours after the rush. Overlapping with the high is the *nod*, a state of escape from reality that ranges from sleepiness to virtual unconsciousness. During the high and the nod, the user remains calm, detached, and uninterested in external events. In the final stage of *being straight*, the user is no longer experiencing the rush, high, or the nod but is also not experiencing the unpleasant physical and psychic effects of withdrawal that addicts experience approximately 8 hours after taking heroin.

The dose and route of administration have a profound effect on the subjective effects of opioid administration. Patients given opiate painkillers orally or in sustained-release skin patches do not experience euphoria, and unless the medication is tampered with to allow snorting or injection, they hardly ever become addicted. Volunteers given opiates by acute intravenous injection reported that faster rates of infusion and higher doses produced greater positive subjective effects. Heroin addicts given free access to self-administered heroin over a longer period showed different phases of experience. Initially, the drug caused increased elation and reduced anxiety, but after several days tolerance to the euphoriant effects developed, and the addicts increased the frequency of drug administrations. There was a profound shift to occasional pleasurable experiences interspersed with a preponderance of dysphoria, accompanied by increased anxiety, sleep disturbances, social isolation, and increased irritability and belligerence. This is the unpleasant experience of heroin addicts—no longer capable of deriving much pleasure from the drug and using it largely to prevent the even more unpleasant experiences of withdrawal.

THE NEUROBIOLOGY OF OPIATES

Animal behavioral models have been valuable in studies of the brain mechanisms underlying the rewarding properties of opiates. Laboratory animals can readily be trained to self-administer these drugs and to recognize the opiates in place preference paradigms (see Chapter 20). Rats given limited access to opiates will maintain stable levels of daily intake over long periods without any signs of physical dependence or tolerance. However, if given access to larger quantities of drug, animals will develop tolerance and become physically dependent. Self-administration studies using cannulae implanted in various brain sites have shown that the lateral hypothalamus, nucleus accumbens, amygdala, periaqueductal gray, and ventral tegmentum all support self-administration. The possible circuits involved, including the "extended amygdala," are similar to those thought to be activated by other drugs of abuse (see Chapter 20). Although opiates stimulate dopamine release in the nucleus accumbens, dopamine antagonists or 6-hydroxydopamine-induced lesions of dopamine terminals in this area do not eliminate heroin or morphine self-administration. These procedures, however, block the acquisition of opiate place preference, and place conditioning was also blocked in dopamine D_2 receptor knockout mice, suggesting a role for dopaminergic mechanisms in the rewarding effects of opiates.

Opiates act on three different receptors in the brain—mu, delta, and kappa. Studies of genetically engineered mice with selective knockouts of one or another of these receptors have provided a surprisingly clear result: The mu opiate receptor appears to be the key target for the rewarding effects of opiates. Mu receptor knockout mice do not self-administer opiates, they do not exhibit place preference, and they do not show signs of physical dependence when dosed repeatedly with opiates. Many of the other actions of morphine, including analgesia, respiratory depression, and constipation, are also absent in such animals. Knockouts of the other opiate receptors do not show these effects. The potencies of opiate drugs at the mu receptor (Table 22–1) also predict their potencies in animal models of reward. Opiate drugs can also be ranked by how similar their effects are to morphine in animals trained to discriminate morphine from saline (see Fig. 20.3, Chapter 20). It is not clear what role the endorphin systems in brain play with regard to opiate effects, but a role for the endomorphins in the endogenous reward circuits with which heroin and morphine interact has been suggested because of the unique potency and selectivity that these neuropeptides have for mu opiate receptors, for which they exhibit subnanomolar affinities and selectivity for mu versus delta or kappa receptors in excess of 1000 (see Chapter 10).

Animals treated repeatedly with opiates or allowed to self-administer large amounts of these drugs become tolerant to both the rewarding and the physical effects of the drugs. Dependence is defined dramatically by the syndrome that appears upon rapid withdrawal of opioid administration or the administration of a mu receptor antagonist such as naloxone or naltrexone. In rats, the syndrome includes the appearance of ptosis, teeth chattering, "wet dog shakes," and diarrhea. In addition to these signs of physical withdrawal, motivational withdrawal

Table 22–1. Affinities of Opiates for Human Mu-Opioid Receptors

RECEPTOR	K_i (nM)
Etorphine	0.18
Diprenorphine	0.18
Buprenorphine	0.51
Naloxone[a]	1.4
Fentanyl	1.9
Levorphanol	1.9
Morphine	2.0
Codeine	65.0

[a]Antagonist.
Source: With permission from Raynor et al. (1995).

includes elevations in thresholds for intracranial self-stimulation (see Chapter 20), disruption of operant behavior for food reward; and the development of place aversion for the mu antagonist used to precipitate withdrawal.

The neurobiological substrates for physical and motivational withdrawal can be separated. Thus, local injection of an opiate antagonist into the nucleus accumbens or amygdala of rat brain does not elicit physical signs of withdrawal but disrupts operant food-rewarded behavior and causes place aversion. The extended amygdala seems to play a key role in precipitated withdrawal, with extensive activation of neurons in the amygdala (measured by c-Fos expression). Several pharmacological systems are involved. Dopamine release is decreased in the nucleus accumbens but increased in medial prefrontal cortex. Norepinephrine, corticotropin-releasing factor (CRF), and neuropeptide Y (NPY) (see Chapter 10) are also involved. β-Adrenergic receptor antagonists or CRF antagonists reduce the place aversion normally associated with precipitated withdrawal, and this is also attenuated by intracerebral administration of NPY.

ADDICTION AND WITHDRAWAL

A popular misconception is that any repeated opioid use, whether medical or nonmedical, inevitably leads to intractable physiological dependence and addiction. This is simply not true. The medical use of opiates rarely leads to dependence, perhaps because the drugs are administered orally rather than by injection and the amounts given are strictly controlled. Among nonmedical users, the "capture ratio" (see Chapter 20) for heroin is estimated to be 23%; that is, approximately one-fourth of those who have ever used the drug may end up becoming dependent on it. Three groups of nonmedical users can be distinguished. *Marginal* users may experiment with the drug occasionally but have no steady pattern of use. A large group of *controlled* users take the drug regularly for its pleasurable effects but not on a daily basis. They may use heroin only on weekends or a few times each week, may hold full-time jobs, and budget carefully to fund their drug use. Heroin use is planned ahead of time, and dangerous routes of administration, such as injection, are avoided. Controlled users may maintain a stable pattern of drug use over many years without becoming addicted. If challenged with naloxone, they do not show signs of withdrawal, indicating the absence of substance dependence. However, they may be classified by the *Diagnostic and Statistical Manual of Mental Disorders*, fourth edition, under the milder category of "substance abuse." Some controlled users may go on to become *compulsive* users. They use heroin on a daily basis and are physically and psychologically dependent on the drug. This is the relatively small group of "problem drug users" who cause the most damage to themselves and to society. There are at least as many controlled users as addicts. Opiate addiction is remarkably stable over time. Alan Leshner, former director of the National Institute on Drug Abuse, described addiction as a "chronic relapsing brain disorder," which describes the typical heroin addict, who tends to show repeated cycles of remission and resumption over long periods of time. For some people, heroin addiction may persist for 20 years or more, or it may become a lifelong condition. A 20-year follow-up of 100 heroin addicts in New York City found that 23% had died, 25–35% were still using drugs, and 35–42% had achieved stable abstinence.

The brain mechanisms underlying the development of opiate addiction remain obscure (see Chapter 20). However, studies of populations of heroin users have suggested that genetic factors may be associated with an increased risk of addiction. One particular polymorphism of the mu receptor gene, the A118G SNP, was found in 90% of heroin users in a European Caucasian population. Other studies have pointed to a polymorphism in the gene encoding proenkephalin that leads to increased expression of this neuropeptide precursor, found in 79% of heroin users. These findings suggest that dysfunction in the mu opioid receptor/endorphin systems may be a key factor underlying heroin addiction.

One of the reasons why compulsive users continue to take the drug is to avoid the unpleasant withdrawal syndrome that they experience if drug use is abruptly stopped. The opiate withdrawal syndrome consists of both physical and mental components. Physically, there are major disturbances largely of autonomic nervous system origin, including lacrimation, rhinorrhea, perspiration, gooseflesh, tremor, dilated pupils, anorexia, nausea, emesis, diarrhea, dehydration, elevated temperature and blood pressure, and yawning. These symptoms accompany a negative mental state of dysphoria, depression, and anxiety. Addicts in withdrawal experience intense craving and seek by every means to obtain a continuing supply of the drug. Craving occurs within a few hours of the last dose. Mild autonomic signs begin after 8–12 hours and peak in intensity in the first 24 hours. More severe physical signs reach a peak at 36–48 hours and continue up to 72 hours. Waves of gooseflesh result in the skin looking like a plucked turkey—hence the term *cold turkey*. Muscle spasms, uncontrolled muscle twitching, and kicking movements may occur. Without treatment, the withdrawal syndrome is complete in 7–10 days, although some autonomic disturbances may persist for several months.

OTHER ADVERSE EFFECTS OF OPIATES

Acute Toxicity

Heroin is dangerously toxic because the safety margin between the lethal dose and the pharmacological dose is narrow—a ratio of only 6. Death occurs because opiates depress respiration, and many thousands of opiate users die each year because of accidental overdose. This can occur because the illegal sources of heroin and other opiates are of varying quality and users cannot judge the correct dose, and inexperienced users may not have learned how to administer a safe dose. Heroin is also often taken in a lethal combination with other drugs, most commonly alcohol. Experienced users who had previously become tolerant to the respiratory depressant effects may use the drug again after a period of abstinence and misjudge the dose. Heroin users are at increased risk of a fatal overdose in the time period immediately after prison release or treatment cessation. Nonlethal overdose cases requiring admission to hospital emergency rooms also number many thousands annually.

Autonomic side effects can be distressing, especially chronic constipation, difficulty in initiating urine flow, and postural hypotension.

Chronic Toxicity

Apart from the dangers of addiction—leading to a loss of job, family relationships, and self-respect—there are other health hazards associated with opiate abuse. Injecting drug users are at high risk of infection from contaminated needles and risk transmitting or acquiring a number of diseases, including HIV, hepatitis B, hepatitis C, and various bacterial infections. The majority of cases of hepatitis C are due to the use of contaminated needles, and a substantial proportion of heroin users have this disease (as many as 40%). This is a slow-developing infection, and most of those infected do not realize they are infected until much later. Repeated injections can also lead to skin infections and, in some cases, septicemia.

PHARMACOLOGICAL TREATMENT OF OPIATE ADDICTION

The most widely used treatment for opiate addiction is to replace the heroin or other opiate with methadone, administered under controlled conditions in a treatment center. Methadone is a potent mu receptor agonist, but it is given orally and it is slowly absorbed and does not generate an intense "high." By using methadone as a substitute for heroin, the addict avoids the unpleasant withdrawal syndrome, and it is hoped that methadone use can be tapered off to reach full abstinence. However, addiction to opiates is a powerful phenomenon and difficult to break. Even with the best-regulated methadone programs, a relapse rate of more than 50% after 3 months is not unusual. An alternative to methadone is levo-alpha-acetylmethadol (LAAM), another potent mu receptor agonist. LAAM has the advantage of being long acting so that treatment needs to be given only three times a week.

A recent innovation has been the introduction of buprenorphine for the treatment of opiate addiction. Buprenorphine has a high affinity for the mu opiate receptor, but it acts as a partial agonist—that is, it cannot produce the same maximum effects produced by full agonists such as morphine or methadone. This makes it a useful drug for treating opiate addiction since it is relatively safe (i.e., death from overdose is unlikely), and although it has sufficient agonist activity to reduce the risk of withdrawal signs, as a partial agonist it does not produce a full-blown opiate "high." Furthermore, it is given orally so the absorption is slow. Buprenorphine was considered sufficiently safe to be administered in physicians' offices, which greatly expanding the availability of medical treatment outside the otherwise restricted treatment centers. However, as with OxyContin, addicts learned how to crush the buprenorphine tablets and to snort or inject the resulting powder. Another ingenious pharmacological maneuver was introduced to prevent such diversion. The drug Suboxone combines buprenorphine with the potent mu receptor antagonist naloxone. It might seem paradoxical to combine a mu agonist with a powerful antagonist, but the rationale is that naloxone is barely absorbed at all when taken by the oral route. Therefore, if the product is used correctly, it does not have any effect. However, if the addict tries to tamper with the medicine and to inject the drug, the naloxone will immediately precipitate very unpleasant withdrawal signs. Desperate to reduce crime and other social harm caused by heroin addiction, some European countries have introduced the use of heroin administered by injection in carefully controlled treatment centers. The rationale is that although this is not a treatment for the addiction, it does eliminate the need for addicts to indulge in crime to fund their habit. Also, by administering the drug under hygienic conditions, the risk of transmitting infectious disease can be avoided. However, this is a controversial and expensive program (heroin needs to be given several times a day to avoid withdrawal), and it remains to be seen how widely adopted this will become. Opiate addiction remains a major problem and none of the available treatments are completely effective.

SELECTED REFERENCES

Amato, L., M. Davoli, C. A. Perucci, M. Ferri, F. Faggiano, and R. P. Mattick (2005). An overview of systematic reviews of the effectiveness of opiate maintenance therapies: Available evidence to inform clinical practice and research. *J. Subst. Abuse Treat.* 28, 321–329.

Compton, W. M. and N. D. Volkow (2006). Major increases in opioid analgesic abuse in the United States: Concerns and strategies. *Drug Alcohol Depend.* 81, 103–107.

Ersche, K. D. and B. J. Sahakian (2007). The neuropsychology of amphetamine and opiate dependence: Implications for treatment. *Neuropsychol. Rev.* 17, 317–336.

Ikeda, K., S. Ide, W. Han, M. Hayashida, G. R. Uhl, and I. Sora (2005). How individual sensitivity to opiates can be predicted by gene analyses. *Trends Pharmacol. Sci.* 26, 311–317.

Kenna, G. A., D. M. Nielsen, P. Mello, A. Schiesl, and R. M. Swift (2007). Pharmacotherapy of dual substance abuse and dependence. *CNS Drugs* 21, 213–237.

Koob, G.F. and LeMoal, M. (2006). *Neurobiology of Addiction*, Academic Press, Amsterdam.

Lingford-Hughes, A. (2005). Human brain imaging and substance abuse. *Curr. Opin. Pharmacol.* 5, 42–46.

Martin, M., R. A. Hurley, and K. H. Taber (2007). Is opiate addiction associated with long-standing neurobiological changes? *J. Neuropsychiatry Clin. Neurosci.* 19, 242–248.

McClung, C. A. (2006). The molecular mechanisms of morphine addiction. *Rev. Neurosci.* 17, 393–402.

Shearer, J. (2008). The principles of agonist pharmacotherapy for psychostimulant dependence. *Drug Alcohol Rev.* 27, 301–308.

Vadivelu, N. and R. L. Hines (2007). Buprenorphine: A unique opioid with broad clinical applications. *J. Opioid Manag.* 3, 49–58.

Psychedelics

Of all the psychoactive drugs, the psychedelics are perhaps the strangest. These are chemicals that are capable of inducing profound changes in the state of consciousness, with altered perception and strange illusions. The drug state has been likened by some to a mystical experience but viewed by others as a form of psychosis—hence the alternative term *psychotomimetic* to describe these drugs. This is a diverse group of drugs whose effects are not all identical, but to be included in this class, the following criteria should be fulfilled:

1. The main effect is on thought, perception, and mood.
2. There is only minimal intellectual or memory impairment.
3. Stupor or psychostimulation is not an integral part of the drug action.
4. Autonomic side effects are not disabling.
5. There is little or no dependence liability.

CHEMICAL CLASSES OF PSYCHEDELICS

Space does not permit a detailed review of the chemistry of the different classes of psychedelics. More than 200 psychedelic drugs are known; some are of natural origin from plants, but many others are man-made synthetic chemicals (Fig. 23–1). The following are the main classes:

1. Lysergic acid derivatives, of which LSD is the prototype.

2. Phenylethylamine derivatives, of which the plant product mescaline is the prototype. The chemist Alexander Shulgin has described more than 100 synthetic chemicals in this class and reported their psychedelic properties (Shulgin and Shulgin, 2000). The best known synthetic phenylethylamine is 3,4-methylenedioxy and methamphetamine (MDMA or "Ecstasy"; see Chapter 21).

3. N-substituted indoleamines, of which the plant product psilocybin is the prototype. Shulgin has described more than 50 synthetic indoleamine derivatives with psychedelic properties.

4. Other indole derivatives, such as the harmine alkaloids or ibogaine.

5. Piperidyl benzilate esters, such as Ditran.

6. Glutamate NMDA receptor antagonists, such as phencyclidine and ketamine.

THE EFFECTS OF PSYCHEDELICS

By far the most famous and thoroughly studied psychedelic drug is LSD (*d*-lysergic acid diethylamide), and this will serve as a good example of the entire class. Many readers know the story of how its psychedelic properties were

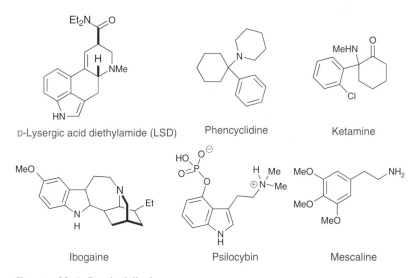

D-Lysergic acid diethylamide (LSD)   Phencyclidine   Ketamine

Ibogaine   Psilocybin   Mescaline

FIGURE 23–1. Psychedelic drugs.

discovered by the Swiss chemist Albert Hoffmann (who died in 2008, aged 102). Working for the Swiss company Sandoz, he synthesized the compound as a derivative of the fungal product ergotamine and unwittingly received a minute dose through the skin. He reported his subsequent experience to his boss Professor Stoll as follows

> Last Friday, April 16, 1943, I was forced to interrupt my work in the laboratory in the middle of the afternoon and proceed home, being affected by a remarkable restlessness, combined with a slight dizziness. At home I lay down and sank into a not unpleasant intoxicated-like condition, characterized by an extremely stimulated imagination. In a dreamlike state, with eyes closed (I found the daylight to be unpleasantly glaring), I perceived an uninterrupted stream of fantastic pictures, extraordinary shapes with intense, kaleidoscopic play of colors. After some two hours this condition faded away. This was, altogether, a remarkable experience both in its sudden onset and its extraordinary course. It seemed to have resulted from some external toxic influence; I surmised a connection with the substance I had been working with at the time, lysergic acid diethylamide tartrate.
>
> Hoffmann, *LSD: My Problem Child* (1980), NY: McGraw Hill

Subsequent studies in volunteers who usually received a typical dose of 100 µg LSD confirmed and extended Hoffmann's observations. The effects of the drug include the following:

Somatic symptoms: Dizziness, weakness, tremors, drowsiness, paresthesias, and blurred vision

Perceptual symptoms: Altered shapes and colors, difficulty in focusing on objects, a sharpened sense of hearing, and, rarely, synesthesia (seeing words or music as colors, or other mixed sensory experiences)

Psychic symptoms: Alterations in mood (happy, sad, or irritable at varying times), tension, distorted time sense, difficulty in expressing thoughts, depersonalization, dreamlike feelings, and visual hallucinations

These effects are essentially the same as those induced by another well-known psychedelic, mescaline, apart from the fact that it requires a dose that is approximately 100 times higher. The subjective experience elicited by psychedelic drugs illustrates the importance of the setting, a factor that also applies importantly to other psychoactive drugs. Literary-minded subjects who had read Huxley's book *The Doors of Perception* and expected the wonders that he described often reported some form of mystical experience. On the other hand, naive subjects, who had been warned of the possible dangers, often had a very negative experience accompanied by fear and panic.

A BRIEF HISTORY OF LSD IN THE UNITED STATES

The Swiss company Sandoz, hoping that LSD might find some medicinal use, supplied the drug free of charge to investigators in the United States for approximately 20 years beginning in 1950. This was an era before the now-familiar antidepressant, antipsychotic, and anxiolytic drugs were available, although chlorpromazine and the first antidepressants followed soon after. Psychiatrists were keen to try new remedies. Psychiatry in the 1950s was dominated by psychoanalytical theories, and LSD was perceived to be a mind-altering agent that might help the therapist reveal the patient's unconscious thoughts and fears. In the case of schizophrenia, it was thought that inducing a form of drug-induced psychosis might reveal new insights into the patient's mind. LSD was enthusiastically taken up by the medical/scientific community. Particularly important were the pioneering studies of Sidney Cohen and Betty Eisner in California, who pioneered the use of LSD in psychotherapy and in the treatment of alcoholism. Important psychiatric studies of LSD, particularly in the treatment of alcoholism, were also undertaken by Hoffer and Osmond in Canada. The CIA also sponsored a series of studies on the possible use of LSD as a "truth serum" that might be used to brainwash and interrogate enemy prisoners of war. One of the more bizarre medical applications of LSD was in the treatment of autism in children. Some remarkable benefits were claimed, both in the treatment of psychiatric patients and in treating alcoholism and autism. However, the concept of controlled clinical trials, with groups receiving active drug or placebo in a blinded manner, did not develop until much later—when the thalidomide disaster in the 1960s forced government regulatory agencies to introduce far stricter rules for the approval of new medicines. Much of the clinical work with LSD was also not published in peer-reviewed medical journals. It is thus almost impossible today to make any judgments on whether or not LSD has any genuine medical applications. On balance, this seems unlikely; the positive benefits claimed in the 1950s and 1960s were probably due to the suggestibility of patients and the preconceived expectations of clinicians.

Apart from the medical benefits claimed for LSD, other nonmedical uses increased rapidly during the 1960s. A group of Californian intellectuals, of whom Aldous Huxley was a leading figure, viewed LSD as a gateway to mystic experiences and metaphysical insights. Huxley's earlier experience with mescaline led him to write lyrically about the psychedelic experience in his books *The Doors of Perception* (1954) and *Heaven and Hell* (1956). He claimed that psychedelic drugs allowed one to transcend the mundane world and enter the elevated state of consciousness usually reserved for poets, artists, and saints. There was also a belief that LSD could be used to enhance creativity in the arts. The influence that Huxley's writing had was significant; his books on mescaline became cult classics, and the nonmedical use of LSD as a doorway to "enlightenment" increased. The claims grew increasingly more exaggerated. Some users reported a vivid sense that they were revisiting ancient Egypt, India, or Greece, and Huxley and colleagues convinced themselves that these were actual memories—proof of reincarnation. This culminated with Harvard professor Timothy Leary, who promoted the widespread use of LSD with messianic fervor. Soon after, Sandoz withdrew its sponsorship of supplies of LSD, and the drug was only available from street vendors. It was the rapid spread of the use of LSD and other psychedelics among students and other young people that eventually led the U.S. government to criminalize LSD and all the other psychedelic drugs, placing them in the category liable to the most severe criminal penalties. Governments throughout the developed world rapidly followed suit. This also effectively ended any further research on the possible medical applications of these drugs.

Despite being illegal, young people continued to use psychedelic drugs. Mescaline and LSD became firmly embedded in the "rave dance" culture that swept through Europe and the United States in the 1980s and 1990s. Recently, there appears to have been a decline in the popularity of LSD. Ecstasy has remained the drug of choice for the club dance culture, although use of another psychedelic drug, ketamine, has increased.

MECHANISM OF ACTION

For obvious reasons, it is difficult to use animal models to study the pharmacology of psychedelic drugs: We cannot assess whether or not an animal is experiencing a change of consciousness or having hallucinations. Monkeys treated with LSD behave oddly, staring into space as if seeing visions, but this is not behavior that can readily be quantified. Nevertheless, animals can be trained to recognize the subjective effects elicited by psychedelic drugs and to distinguish them from saline in drug discrimination tests. Rats or mice trained to recognize LSD will cross-generalize to a range of phenylethylamine and indoleamine psychedelic agents, suggesting a common mode of action. The important role of the 5-HT_{2A} receptor is shown by the fact that selective 5-HT_{2A} antagonists prevent animals from recognizing LSD as a discriminative cue, whereas antagonists acting selectively at 5-HT_{1A} or 5-HT_3 receptors do not have this ability. Neurophysiological studies comparing the effects of LSD with those of 5-HT at a single neuron level have shown that LSD acts as a potent partial agonist at 5-HT_{2A} sites. Drug discrimination studies have also been used to attempt to localize which brain regions mediate the subjective effects of LSD and related drugs. Animals trained to recognize systemically administered LSD will cross-generalize to LSD locally administered into certain brain regions, with the anterior cingulate cortex being a particularly effective site. Similarly, local injections of a 5-HT_{2A} antagonist into this brain region can prevent trained animals from recognizing systemically administered LSD. Activation of 5-HT_{2A} receptors in cortex may indirectly block synaptic responses to glutamate via NMDA receptors. Note that the NMDA receptor antagonists phencyclidine and ketamine are psychedelic drugs that act independently of 5-HT mechanisms. Their psychotomimetic effects have provided important clues about the importance of the glutamatergic mechanism in schizophrenia (see Chapter 15).

Is partial agonism at the 5-HT_{2A} receptor the whole story? There are some discrepancies, notably the fact that other drugs that act as agonists at this receptor (e.g., lisuride) do not possess psychedelic properties. When screened against a range of 5-HT receptor subtypes, LSD exhibits a large array of activities, showing some affinity for 5-HT_{1A}, 5-HT_{1B}, 5-HT_{1D}, 5-HT_{1E}, 5-HT_{1F}, 5-HT_{2A}, 5-HT_{2C}, 5-HT_5, 5-HT_6, and 5-HT_7 receptors. However, LSD is an extraordinarily potent drug and the human dose is 1 or 2 µg/kg, with a peak plasma level less than 10 ng/ml. To be a plausible target, LSD must show an interaction at subnanomolar concentrations, which is not the case for most of these 5-HT receptors. It has been shown that in addition to 5-HT_{2A} receptors, LSD activates 5-HT_{1A} autoreceptors on 5-HT neurons, leading to a slowing of firing of these cells in the raphe nucleus. A heteromeric dimer receptor containing 5-HT_{2A} and mGluR2 receptors may also be a key target for LSD and other psychedelic drugs. There is also evidence that LSD interacts potently with dopamine D_2 receptors, suggesting the possibility that activation of dopamine systems plays a role in its actions. There is no unequivocal evidence of the mechanism of action of these strange drugs.

ADVERSE EFFECTS OF PSYCHEDELIC DRUGS

Acute Toxicity

LSD is very safe in the sense that there have been few, if any, documented cases of death from overdose. Some of the other psychedelic agents, notably phenylethylamines, are less safe. For example, there have been a small number of highly publicized deaths from Ecstasy overdose (see Chapter 21).

LSD can induce an acute panic reaction in inexperienced users, which lasts for a few hours. More serious is the ability of these drugs to induce a toxic psychosis resembling paranoid schizophrenia, including thought disorder, auditory hallucinations, aggressive behavior, and paranoid delusions. In some cases, this psychosis can persist for several weeks and requires hospital treatment.

Users of LSD may also experience "flashbacks"—sudden recurrences of illusions and other phenomena experienced under the drug; these can occur unpredictably even weeks or months after the last dose.

Long-Term Effects

As was the case for cannabis, the use of psychedelic drugs roused storms of emotion and irrationality among those who believed that such drugs might ruin the lives of a generation of young people. Cannabis was claimed to interfere with sex hormones and lead to sterility. Similarly, LSD was alleged to accelerate breaks and gaps in human chromosomes, thus possibly damaging the germ cells on which future generations depend or causing cancer in drug users. Few poorer examples of experimental technique or scientific argument could be imagined; the methods were fraught with artifacts and the results impossible to interpret. Nevertheless, such claims raised a storm of controversy in the 1960s and 1970s until finally put to rest.

The most comprehensive survey of the long-term effects of LSD was undertaken by Sidney Cohen, who pioneered the use of the drug in psychiatry. Worried by the increasing nonmedical use of LSD, he sent a questionnaire to 62 researchers in the United States, 44 of whom replied. He asked whether any of their subjects had died, committed suicide, or experienced mental breakdown or other serious adverse effects. The responses provided valuable data on the then legal use of LSD and mescaline in medical practice. Researchers reported having administered 25,000 doses to approximately 5000 patients. Although there had been occasional panic attacks, 10 prolonged psychotic episodes, and some flashbacks, no deaths were reported. A key statistic was suicides; lurid reports were circulating of users dying by jumping out of windows in the belief that they could fly. However, Cohen concluded that of the five suicides reported, only two were directly caused by the drug. His report, published in 1960, despite its anecdotal nature, seemed to give LSD a remarkably safe profile. Those in favor of the wider nonmedical use of LSD used Cohen's report as ammunition. However, Cohen was subsequently increasingly concerned about the growing availability of street LSD, the hazards of its use by nonmedical practitioners, and the growth of LSD clinics run for profit. He issued a warning in 1962 about the hazards of suicide, prolonged psychotic episodes, and drug-induced antisocial behavior, but by then it was too late to stop the tide, which was only halted by federal government laws later in the decade.

Although both animal and human users show tolerance to repeated doses of LSD, there is no evidence of a withdrawal syndrome, and users do not appear to develop dependence.

SELECTED REFERENCES

Appel, J. B., W. B. West, and J. Buggy (2004). LSD, 5-HT (serotonin), and the evolution of a behavioral assay. *Neurosci. Biobehav. Rev*. 27, 693–701.

Baumann, M. H., J. Pablo, S. F. Ali, R. B. Rothman, and D. C. Mash (2001) Comparative neuropharmacology of ibogaine and its O-desmethyl metabolite, noribogaine. *Alkaloids Chem. Biol*. 56, 79–113.

Dyck, E. (2005). Flashback: Psychiatric experimentation with LSD in historical perspective. *Can. J. Psychiatry* 50, 381–388.

Fantegrossi, W. E., K. S. Murnane, and C. J. Reissig (2008). The behavioral pharmacology of hallucinogens. *Biochem. Pharmacol*. 75, 17–33.

González-Maeso, J., R. L. Ang, T. Yuen, et al. (2008). Identification of a serotonin/glutamate receptor complex implicated in psychosis. *Nature* 452, 93–99.

Nichols, D. E. (2004). Hallucinogens. *Pharmacol. Ther*. 101, 131–181.

Passie, T., J. Seifert, U. Schneider, and H. M. Emrich (2002). The pharmacology of psilocybin. *Addict. Biol*. 7, 357–364.

Shulgin, A., and Shulgin, A. (2000) *PIHKAL*, Transform Press, Berkeley, CA.

24

Cannabis

Marijuana (cannabis) is among the most widely used of all illicit psychoactive drugs. It is derived from the plant *Cannabis sativa*. In 1964, Gaoni and Mechoulam showed that virtually all of the pharmacological activity in cannabis extracts can be attributed to a single compound, (−)delta-9-tetrahydrocannabinol (THC), although as many as 60 different naturally occurring cannabinoids are present in plant extracts.

The cannabis plant is either male or female, and THC is most highly concentrated in the resin glands concentrated in the female flower head. The most potent preparation derived directly from the plant is "hashish," which represents the THC-rich cannabis resin obtained by scraping the resin-containing glands from the flower heads (Table 24–1).

Nowadays, culture of cannabis often takes place indoors, where nutrients, lighting, and temperature conditions can be optimized. Strains of plants bred for high THC content are grown in specially enriched soils or with hydroponics, and their growth cycle has been shortened to less than 4 months. The product has a higher THC and lower cannabidiol content than that of traditional imported cannabis. The THC content of herbal marijuana in the United States or Europe is approximately 5%, and cultivated forms of cannabis are three or four times more potent (10–20% THC) (Table 24–1).

TABLE 24–1. Cannabis Preparations

NAME	PART OF PLANT	% THC
MARIJUANA (CANNABIS, BHANG, DAGGA, KIF)	LEAVES, SMALL STEMS	4.0–6.0
SENSIMILLA (SENSEMILLA)	FEMALE FLOWER HEADS	9.0–12.0
RESIN (HASHISH, CHARAS, POLM)	CANNABIS RESIN[a]	10.0–15.0[a]
Cultivated plants ("skunk," "Nederwiet")	Indoor cultivation	15.0–20.0

[a]Street samples of cannabis resin are often of poor quality and may contain 5% THC or less; freshly prepared "polm" can contain >30% THC.

ROUTES OF ADMINISTRATION

Smoking

Smoking is an especially effective way of delivering psychoactive drugs to the brain. THC has no difficulty in penetrating into the brain by this route, and within seconds of inhaling the first puff of marijuana smoke, active drug is present on the cannabis receptors in brain. Peak blood levels are reached at approximately the time that smoking is finished.

Oral Absorption

Taking THC by mouth is less reliable as a method of delivering a consistent dose of the drug. THC is absorbed reasonably well from the gut, but the process is slow and unpredictable, and most of the absorbed drug is rapidly degraded by metabolism in the liver before it reaches the general circulation.

An officially approved medicinal formulation of synthetic THC (known pharmaceutically as dronabinol) is in the form of capsules containing the drug dissolved in sesame oil—a product called Marinol. This and other orally administered cannabis products have not proved consistently effective in their medical applications, and both patients and recreational users generally prefer smoked marijuana.

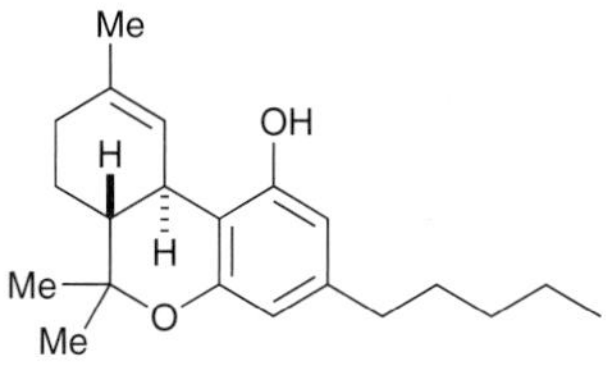

Δ^9-tetrahydrocannabinol (THC)

FIGURE 24–1. Structure of THC.

MECHANISM OF ACTION

THC is an agonist for two closely related receptors in the G protein-coupled class, CB-1 and CB-2, whose natural ligands are the endocannabinoids (see Chapter 12). The CB-1 receptor is the predominant form in brain, whereas the CB-2 receptor is mainly associated with the immune system in the periphery. These receptors can be studied in a test tube by radioligand binding, using a radiolabeled form of the potent synthetic agonist CP-55,940, or by measuring the inhibition of adenylate cyclase activity on activation of the receptors. THC and the psychoactive metabolite 11-hydroxy-THC displace radiolabeled CP-55,940 from CB-1 receptor sites at very low concentrations, but cannabidiol and other inactive cannabinoids or the less active (+)CP-55,940 have lower affinities (Table 24–2). The cannabis receptor in brain (CB-1) is not related in any obvious way to any previously known receptors for neurotransmitters or neuropeptides in brain. It is possible that additional cannabinoid receptors remain to be discovered. It is notable that cannabidiol, often present in equal amounts to THC in the plant, interacts only weakly with either the CB-1 or the CB-2 receptor. Nevertheless, cannabidiol has been reported to possess anticonvulsant activity in some animal models of epilepsy, and in some animal and human psychopharmacology experiments cannabidiol has been found to possess antianxiety properties. It has also been proposed as a possible treatment for schizophrenia.

An important development has been the discovery of a variety of synthetic chemicals that act as selective antagonists at either CB-1 or CB-2 receptors. The most widely used of these is the CB-1 antagonist rimonabant.

Neuroanatomical Distribution of CB-1 Receptors in Brain

The distribution of CB-1 receptors has been mapped in rat and human brain by autoradiographic studies using the radioligand [H^3]CP-55,940, which binds

TABLE 24–2. Cannabis Receptor (CB-1) Binding Profiles- [H^3]CP-55,940 Assay Rat Brain Membranes

DRUG	K_i CONCENTRATION FOR HALF OCCUPANCY OF RECEPTOR BINDING SITES (nM); 10^{-9} M)
(−)CP-55,940	0.068
(+)CP-55,940	3.4
THC	1.6
11-hydroxy-THC	1.6
Cannabinol	13.0
Cannabidiol	>500.0

with high affinity to CB-1 sites, and by immunohistochemistry using antibodies generated against the CB-1 receptor protein. The mapping and imaging of CB-1 receptors in the living human brain will likely be possible soon using positron emission tomography brain imaging technology. Mapping studies in rat and human brain have shown that CB-1 receptors are mainly localized to axons and nerve terminals and are largely absent from the neuronal cell bodies or dendrites, consistent with the postulated role of cannabinoids in modulating neurotransmitter release. In both animals and humans, the highest densities of CB-1 receptors are seen in the cerebral cortex, particularly the frontal regions, basal ganglia, hypothalamus, cerebellum, hippocampus, and anterior cingulate cortex. The relative absence of the cannabinoid receptors from brain stem nuclei may account for the low toxicity of cannabinoids when given in overdose.

PHARMACOLOGY OF THC

Inhibition of Neurotransmitter Release

In the brain, THC or other cannabinoids act on CB-1 receptors located presynaptically on nerve terminals to inhibit the stimulus-evoked release of various neurotransmitters, including the inhibitory amino acid GABA and the amines norepinephrine and acetylcholine. The mechanism underlying the inhibition of neurotransmitter release may be activation of N-type calcium channels by THC.

Although cannabinoids generally inhibit neurotransmitter release, this does not mean that their overall effect is always to dampen down activity in neural circuits. For example, reducing the release of the powerful inhibitory chemical GABA would have the opposite effect by reducing the level of inhibition. Studies in rodents have shown that acute THC causes an increase in the release of both acetylcholine and dopamine and an increase in dopamine turnover in PFC, whereas chronic administration caused a reduction in dopamine and acetylcholine release and dopamine turnover.

Effects on the Heart and Blood Vessels

THC acts on CB-1 receptors in blood vessels, causing a relaxation that leads to vasodilatation and a decrease in blood pressure. This in turn triggers an increase in heart rate in an attempt to compensate for the decrease in blood pressure. The vasodilatation caused by THC in human subjects is readily seen as a reddening of the eyes caused by the dilated blood vessels in the conjunctiva. The cardiac effects can be quite large, with increases in heart rate in humans equivalent to as much as a 60% increase over the resting pulse rate. Although this presents little risk to young healthy people, it could be dangerous for patients who have a history of heart disease, particularly those who have previously suffered a heart attack or heart failure. Another feature commonly seen after high doses of cannabis is "postural hypotension," which can cause dizziness or even fainting. The cardiovascular effects are absent in CB-1 receptor knockout mice, suggesting that this receptor plays a key role.

Effects on Pain Sensitivity

The ability of cannabinoids to reduce pain sensitivity represents an important potential medical application for these substances. THC and synthetic cannabinoids are effective in many animal models of both acute pain (mechanical pressure, chemical irritants, and noxious heat) and chronic pain (e.g., inflamed joint following injection of inflammatory stimulus or sensitized limb after partial nerve damage). In all these cases, the pain-relieving (analgesic) effects of cannabinoids are prevented by cotreatment with the antagonist rimonabant and absent in CB-1 receptor knockout mice, indicating that the CB-1 receptor plays a key role. In these animal models, THC is often found to be approximately equal in potency to morphine. However, the opiate and cannabinoid systems appear to be parallel but distinct, although there are links between the two systems. Cannabinoids and opiates act synergistically in producing pain relief; that is, the combination is more effective than either drug alone.

Effects on Motility and Posture

Cannabinoids cause a complex series of changes in animal motility and posture. At low doses, there is a mixture of depressant and stimulatory effects, and at higher doses there is predominantly CNS depression. In small laboratory animals, THC and other cannabinoids causes a dose-dependent reduction in spontaneous running activity. This may be accompanied by sudden bursts of activity in response to sensory stimuli, reflecting a hypersensitivity of reflex activity. Groups of mice in an apparently sedate state will jump in response to auditory or tactile stimuli; as animals fall into other animals, they resemble corn popping in a popcorn machine. At higher doses, the animals become immobile and will remain unmoving for long periods, often in unnatural postures—a phenomenon known as *catalepsy*. Human marijuana users may also sometimes withdraw from contact with other members of the group and remain unmoving for considerable periods of time.

Human Psychopharmacology

We can be reasonably confident that the psychic effects of cannabis are due to activation of the CB-1 receptor in brain. In a controlled study of healthy cannabis users who smoked either a THC-containing or placebo marijuana cigarette, the CB-1 antagonist rimonabant blocked all of the acute psychological effects of the active cigarettes.

The various stages of marijuana intoxication can be classified as the "buzz" leading to the "high" and then the "stoned" states and, finally, the "come-down." The buzz is a transient stage, which may arrive fairly quickly when smoking. It is a tingling sensation felt in the body, head, and often the arms and legs, accompanied by a feeling of dizziness or lightheadedness. The increase in heart rate caused by the drug may also be perceived as a pounding pulse. Marijuana smokers also commonly feel a dryness of the mouth and throat and may become very thirsty. The influence of the drug on the mind is far-reaching and varied; the marijuana high is a very complex experience. The drug is a powerful euphoriant, and mental and physical excitement and stimulation usually accompany the initial stages of the "high." As the level of intoxication progresses from "high" to "stoned" (if the dose is sufficiently large), users report feeling relaxed, peaceful, and calm. Their senses are heightened and often distorted. They may have apparently profound thoughts, and they experience a curious change in their subjective sense of time. As in a dream, the user believes that far more time has passed than in reality has. The distortion of the sense of time can be reproduced in animal experiments and is the exact opposite of the effect of alcohol. The disorientation of time sense may represent a key action of the drug, from which many other effects flow. Loss of the normal sense of time may be related to the rush of ideas and sensations experienced during the marijuana high. The user will become unable to maintain a continuous train of thought and no longer able to hold a conversation. An increased sensitivity to visual inputs tends to make marijuana users favor dimly lit rooms or dark sunshades because they find bright light unpleasant. The analysis of sensory inputs by the cerebral cortex also changes. For example, as intoxication becomes more intense, sensory modalities may overlap so that sounds may be seen as colors and colors contain music—a phenomenon psychologists refer to as *synesthesia*. The peak of intoxication may be associated with hallucinations (i.e., seeing and hearing things that are not there). Cannabis does not induce the powerful visual hallucinations that characterize the drug LSD, but fleeting hallucinations can occur, usually in the visual domain. At the most intense period of the intoxication, the user finds difficulty in interacting with others and tends to withdraw into an introspective state. Thoughts tend to dwell on metaphysical or philosophical topics, and the user may experience apparently transcendental insights. As the effects of the drug gradually wear off, there is the "coming down" phase. This may be preceded by a sudden feeling of hunger ("munchies"), often associated with feelings of emptiness in the stomach. There is a particular craving for sweet foods and drinks, and there is an enhanced appreciation and enjoyment of food. The cannabis high is often followed by sleep, sometimes with colorful dreams.

However, the cannabis experience is not always pleasant. Inexperienced users in particular may experience unpleasant physical reactions. Nausea is not uncommon, and it may be accompanied by vomiting, dizziness, and headache. As users become more experienced, they learn to anticipate the wave of lightheadedness and dizziness that are part of the "buzz." Even regular users will sometimes have very unpleasant experiences, particularly if they take a larger than normal dose of the drug. The reaction is one of intense fear and anxiety, with symptoms resembling those of a panic attack and sometimes accompanied by physical signs of pallor (the so-called "whitey"), sweating, and shortness of breath. The psychic distress can be intense.

ACUTE ADVERSE EFFECTS OF CANNABIS

Toxicity

Unlike other recreational psychoactive drugs, cannabis is very safe in the sense that there have been few, if any, documented cases of death from overdose. Long-term toxicity studies sponsored by the National Institutes of Health in the 1960s, in which rats received high daily doses of THC every day for 3 months or 2 years, revealed no serious organ toxicity, impairments of reproductive function, or increased incidence of cancer.

Cognitive Function

In simple mental arithmetic tasks, or repetitive visual or auditory tasks that require the subject to remain attentive and vigilant, acute intoxication with cannabis seems to have little effect on performance. By far the most consistent and clear-cut acute effect of marijuana is to disrupt short-term memory. For example, if test subjects are asked to repeat increasingly longer strings of random numbers, words, or other items both in the order in which they are presented and backwards, cannabis produces a dose-dependent impairment in most studies. People intoxicated with cannabis characteristically exhibit "intrusion errors"; that is, they tend to add items to the list that were not there originally. The drug-induced deficits in these tests become even more marked if subjects are exposed to distracting stimuli during the delay interval between presentation and recall. Marijuana makes it difficult for subjects to retain information on line in working memory in order to process it in any complex manner.

Psychosis

A more serious acute reaction is a form of toxic psychosis. The symptoms can be severe enough to lead to admission to emergency psychiatric wards. In some of the psychiatric literature, this is referred to as *cannabis psychosis*. It almost always results from taking large doses of the drug, often in food or drink, and the condition may persist for days. The initial diagnosis can be confused with schizophrenia since patients may display some of the characteristic symptoms of schizophrenic illness, including delusions of control, grandiose identity, persecution, thought insertion, auditory hallucinations (hearing sounds, usually nonverbal in nature), changed perception, and blunting of the emotions. Cannabis is not unique in sometimes causing acute psychotic reactions. Similar effects are commonly seen with amphetamines, cocaine, ketamine, phencyclidine, and alcohol.

LONG-TERM ADVERSE EFFECTS

Tolerance and Dependence

The casual user, taking the drug infrequently, or those using small amounts for medical purposes seem to develop little, if any, tolerance. Tolerance seems only likely to become important for heavy users who are taking gram quantities of resin on a daily basis.

The question of whether regular users become "dependent" on the drug has proved to be one of the most contentious in the field of cannabis research. According to modern definitions, neither tolerance nor physical dependence need necessarily be present to make the diagnosis of "substance dependence." This has particularly changed the way in which cannabis is viewed nowadays. It has often been argued that since neither tolerance nor physical dependence are prominent features of regular marijuana users, the drug cannot be addictive. However, in the *Diagnostic and Statistical Manual of Mental Disorders, fourth edition (DSM-IV)*, or *International Statistical Classification of diseases and Related Health Problems, tenth edition* (ICD-10), the diagnosis of "substance dependence" is made as the result of a carefully structured interview, and the diagnosis rests on the presence or absence of various items from a checklist of symptoms (see Table 20–5, Chapter 20). When such assessments are made on groups of regular marijuana users, a surprisingly high proportion are diagnosed as dependent—perhaps as many as 10% of regular users. Both major classifications of mental disorders—the *DSM-IV Text Revision* and the *ICD-10*—include a diagnosis of cannabis dependence.

There have also been developments in basic animal research that point to similarities between cannabis and other drugs of addiction. A behavioral withdrawal syndrome can be seen in animals that have been treated repeatedly with THC or other cannabinoid when they are challenged with the antagonist drug rimonabant. The withdrawal signs in rats include "wet dog shakes," scratching and rubbing of the face, compulsive grooming, arched back, head shakes, spasms, and backwards walking. Carefully controlled studies have also shown that a reliable and clinically significant withdrawal syndrome does occur in human users. The symptoms include craving for cannabis, decreased appetite, sleep difficulty, and weight loss. The syndrome may sometimes be accompanied by anger, aggression, increased irritability, restlessness, and strange dreams.

Another series of experiments in animals revealed that in common with other drugs of addiction, THC is able to selectively activate nerve cells in the ventral tegmentum region of rat brain, and this is accompanied by an increased dopamine release from the nucleus accumbens and prefrontal cortex of the rat brain (see Chapter 20). The THC-induced release of dopamine from the nucleus accumbens seems to involve an opioid mechanism because the effect of THC could be prevented by treatment of the animals with naloxonazine, a drug that potently and selectively blocks opioid receptor sites in brain. Additional support for the concept of a link between the cannabinoid and opioid systems in brain has come from studies of CB-1 receptor knockout mice. These animals survived quite normally without the CB-1 receptor, but as expected, they were unable to show any of the normal central nervous system responses to THC (analgesia, sedation, and hypothermia). Interestingly, the mice were also less responsive to morphine. Although morphine was still analgesic, it was less likely to be self-administered, and the mice displayed a milder opiate withdrawal syndrome.

Cognitive Function

Considerable attention has focused on the possibility that there might be more persistent effects of marijuana on intellectual function. However, there are many methodological difficulties inherent in such studies. In addition to other confounding factors, comparisons have to be made between groups of drug users versus nonusers whose baseline performance is impossible to match. Most studies have been done within a period of 12–48 hours after last drug use, but the results may simply reflect a residual effect of the drug, or the withdrawal symptoms that heavy users suffer when they stop taking marijuana could also impair their cognitive performance during the immediate period after drug cessation. Although persistent impairments in various cognitive tests have been reported, these are generally modest and not consistent from one study to another.

Cannabis and Mental Illness

A number of studies have addressed the controversial question of whether cannabis use can precipitate long-term psychiatric illness. The strongest evidence came from a study in Sweden that involved taking detailed medical records and information about the social background and drug-taking habits of more than 50,000 conscripts on entry to the Swedish army at age 18 to 20 years (1969–1970) and following up their subsequent medical history over a 15-year period. A disproportionate number of the 246 cases of schizophrenic illness diagnosed in the overall group on follow-up were attributed to former cannabis users; the relative risk of schizophrenia was 2.4 times greater in users than in nonusers. Also, for the small number of heavy users who had taken the drug on more than 50 occasions, the relative risk of schizophrenia increased to 6.0. The authors concluded that cannabis was an independent risk factor for schizophrenia. Since then, a number of other similar reports involving smaller numbers of subjects have all reached the same conclusion. A meta-analysis of pooled data from all of these studies, discounting as many confounding factors as possible, concluded that the overall odds ratio linking cannabis use to subsequent psychosis was 1.4; that is, cannabis use is associated with a 40% increased risk of developing a schizophrenia-like psychosis in later life. At first glance, these findings seem convincing, but they do not necessarily prove that a cause-and-effect relationship exists between cannabis use and psychosis. If cannabis use were an important cause of schizophrenia, one might expect to have seen an increase in the incidence of schizophrenia as cannabis use became more common during the past 30 years, but there is no evidence that this has occurred. Indeed, an analysis of the incidence of schizophrenia and psychotic illness in Britain showed a decline during the past decade rather than an increase (http://drugs.homeoffice.gov.uk/publication-search/acmd/acmd-cannabis-report-2008).

Special Hazards of Smoked Marijuana

Although THC appears to be a relatively safe drug, the same cannot be said about cannabis smoke, which is very similar in chemical composition to tobacco smoke. In addition to the large number of chemical components present in the dried plant material, hundreds of additional chemicals are created during the process of combustion (carcinogens). Some reports have indicated that two of the most potent known carcinogens in tobacco smoke, benzanthracene and benzpyrene, are present in similar amounts in cannabis smoke. Because of differences in smoking behavior and the absence of filters in cannabis joints, compared with smoking tobacco, smoking cannabis results in a fivefold greater absorption of carbon monoxide and four or five times more tar is retained in the lungs. Various studies have been undertaken in human cannabis smokers, but they have been confounded by the fact that many consume the drug with tobacco, making it difficult to disentangle the effects of the two agents. However, follow-up studies of tobacco versus cannabis smokers show that although both tobacco and cannabis smoke cause irritation of the airways, bronchitis and cough, unlike tobacco smokers, cannabis smokers did not develop obstructive pulmonary disease or emphysema. A meta-analysis also found no indication of an increased incidence of cancer of the lungs or upper airways in cannabis smokers, despite the fact that some subjects had smoked cannabis daily for more than 30 years.

CANNABIS-BASED MEDICINES

Cannabis was widely used in ancient Chinese and Indian medicine, and it was popular in Western medicine for approximately 100 years beginning in the mid-19th century. At the time cannabis was banned in the United States by the Marijuana Tax Act of 1937, approximately 28 different medicines contained it as an ingredient, many with no indication of its presence. Despite a paucity of scientific evidence for its efficacy, large numbers of patients with multiple sclerosis, HIV/AIDS, and other painful conditions smoke marijuana in the belief that it helps their symptoms. In the United States, 12 states have sanctioned such medical uses, despite opposition by the federal government.

Interest in the potential medical uses of cannabis has been reawakened in recent years. Influential reviews by the British Medical Association, the U.S. Institute of Medicine, and the Royal College of Physicians, London, have concluded that there are genuine medical indications. The synthetic cannabinoids THC (Marinol) and nabilone (Cesamet) have been available as prescription medicines for years for the treatment of nausea and vomiting associated with cancer chemotherapy or AIDS wasting syndrome, but these products have not been widely used because of the unpredictable absorption from the oral route of administration and the availability of new and more powerful medicines. However, the first properly controlled randomized clinical trials of herbal cannabis for various indications have been performed in recent years.

Multiple Sclerosis

The British Medical Research Council sponsored a large clinical trial involving more than 600 patients that compared a herbal cannabis extract to pure THC or placebo, all administered orally. After 15 weeks of treatment, patients' subjective ratings showed significant benefit for THC or herbal cannabis over placebo for pain, spasticity, sleep disorders, and activities of daily life.

However, the objective measure of limb spasticity on the Ashworth scale failed to show significant benefit, although after 1 year of treatment there were significant improvements in the patients receiving pure THC. A number of other smaller scale clinical trials have tested the medicinal product Sativex, a liquid extract of herbal cannabis containing equal amounts of THC and cannabidiol, delivered sublingually by metered spray. Significant improvements in spasticity and pain scores have been reported, and the product has been approved for use in the treatment of pain associated with multiple sclerosis in Canada. It will likely be approved in Europe in the near future for treatment of pain and spasticity in multiple sclerosis.

Pain

Although there are many different pharmacological approaches to the management of pain (see Chapter 18), many patients fail to respond to any of the currently available medicines. Historically, pain was one of the main indications for the medical use of cannabis. Controlled clinical trials of Sativex have reported significant benefits over placebo in the treatment of neuropathic pain and cancer-associated pain, and the product is approved in Canada for the latter indication. It is likely that approval will be granted in Europe, and large-scale phase III clinical trials of Sativex are under way in the United States for cancer-associated pain.

Other Indications

There are various other medical conditions for which cannabis-based medicines may possibly be used. These include nausea and vomiting associated with cancer chemotherapy, AIDS wasting syndrome, glaucoma, epilepsy, bronchial asthma, and depression. However, none of these conditions have the same priority given to pain or multiple sclerosis because other effective and safe medicines exist to treat these conditions.

SELECTED REFERENCES

Barnes, M. P. (2006). Sativex: Clinical efficacy and tolerability in the treatment of symptoms of multiple sclerosis and neuropathic pain. *Expert Opin. Pharmacother.* 7, 607–615.

Bellochio, L., G. Mancini, V. Vicennati, et al. (2006). Cannabinoid receptors as therapeutic targets for obesity and metabolic diseases. *Curr. Opin. Pharmacol.* 6, 586–591.

Iversen, L. L. (2008). *The Science of Marijuana*, 2nd ed. Oxford University Press, Oxford.

Joy, J. E., J. Watson Jr., and J. A. Benson, Jr. (Eds.) (1999). *Marijuana and Medicine: Assessing the Science Base*. National Academy Press, Washington, DC.

Macleod, J., R. Oakes, A. Copello, et al. (2004). Psychological and social sequelae of cannabis and other illicit drug use by young people: A systematic review of longitudinal, general population studies. *Lancet* 363, 1579–1588.

Moore, T. H. M., S. Zammit, A. Lingford-Hughes, et al. (2007). Cannabis use and risk of psychotic or affective mental health outcomes: A systematic review. *Lancet* 370, 319–328.

Pertwee, R. G. (2005). Pharmacological actions of cannabinoids. *Handb. Exp. Pharmacol.* 168, 1–52.

25

Alcohol

W hen textbooks of chemistry describe alcohol, they refer to any organic compound consisting of carbon and hydrogen in which the hydroxyl group -OH is attached to the carbon atom. When textbooks of pharmacology refer to alcohol, the substance cited is ethyl alcohol, or ethanol, the main alcohol present in alcoholic beverages such as beer, wine, or hard liquors such as whiskey, gin, vodka, and brandy. The acute and chronic effects of beverage alcohol, ethanol, are widely held to be socially acceptable when consumed in moderation but are physically and criminally dangerous when consumed in excess consistently. Finding the scientifically validated boundary between acceptable moderate use and excessive consumption is a matter of individual metabolism, history of consumption, cultural environment, and, often, family history.

Compared to the other recreational drugs discussed in this book, alcohol produces subjective cognitive and other physiological effects on human performance at blood levels between 25 and 100 mM, whereas drugs such as nicotine, cannabinoids, opiates, and psychedelics produce effects in the low micromolar range. In most U.S. states, the legal limit for drivers is a blood alcohol concentration of 80 mg/100 cc of blood, or 0.08 g% as conventionally expressed (equal to a molar concentration of slightly less than 20 mM), whereas blood levels greater than 400 mg% can be lethal depending on the consumer's history of drinking (Fig. 25–1).

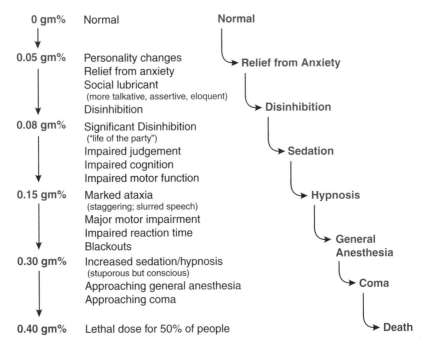

FIGURE 25–1. The relationship of blood alcohol levels to physiological and cognitive performance (Modified from Koob and LeMoal, 2005).

Given the long human experience with alcoholic beverages, it is clear that the population differs substantially in their willingness to imbibe. In a national survey in the United States, more than half the population had had an alcoholic drink in the past month; more than 20% had indulged in binges of drinking, taking up to five drinks on an occasion; and nearly 7% admitted to heavy drinking, consuming more than five drinks per occasion in the past month. More than one out of seven of those polled admitted to driving under the influence at least once in the past year.

The high dose requirements, the chemically simple nature of the chemical being imbibed, and the lack of pharmacological tools to affect the response to alcohol have made it extremely difficult to study. The social consequences of chronic excessive use of alcohol are enormous—more than 100,000 deaths per year, a third of all deaths, of which approximately 15,000 are attributable to driving while intoxicated. Legal attempts after World War I to ban the use of beverage alcohol were recognized as socially unacceptable. Beginning in the late 1970s, the high social costs of alcohol use led to increased research by the National Institutes of Health to determine the basis of alcohol's actions and the then almost unthinkable possibilities of therapeutic medications to suppress its consumption.

It is a testimony to this research that at least three medications have now been approved for the treatment of alcoholism and alcohol abuse.

PHARMACOKINETICS OF ALCOHOL

Beverage alcohol, as the name implies, is taken by ingestion, although in many of the studies described later in this chapter, comparable effects with different time parameters could be observed after systemic or inhaled ethanol administration. The common dose equivalency is the extracellular levels reached at the site of the observed effects. Therefore, one 16-ounce glass of beer (with an alcohol content of 3.5%), one 4-ounce glass of wine (with an alcohol content of 14%), or one 1½-ounce jigger of 50% (100 proof) whiskey will produce legally intoxicating blood alcohol levels close to 0.10% in a 150-pound (70-kg) male. As the so-called universal solvent, ethanol taken by mouth is readily absorbed in the stomach and small intestine at rates that are dependent on whatever other foodstuffs are present. Alcoholic beverages are absorbed much better on an empty stomach than when the stomach contains ingredients with high lipid content that can transiently absorb the ethanol. Females who drink the same amount as males will derive slightly higher blood alcohol levels initially because their stomachs contain lower amounts of the ethanol-catabolizing enzyme, alcohol dehydrogenase.

Once absorbed, alcohol is further catabolized largely by passage through the liver's alcohol dehydrogenase, yielding acetaldehyde, which in turn is almost immediately degraded by acetaldehyde dehydrogenase to acetic acid, carbon dioxide, and water. The acetic acid component enters the 2-carboxylic acid pathway contributing to the synthesis of lipids. The first treatment for alcoholism (Antabuse; disulfiram) was based on the inhibition of acetaldehyde dehydrogenase yielding aversively high blood levels of acetaldehyde causing severe flushing, sweating, and nausea. A naturally occurring mutation in this enzyme is seen in Asian populations that almost exactly, and inversely, parallels the incidence of serious alcoholism in those populations: The higher the mutation rate, the lower the incidence. However, in no population is the incidence zero, suggesting that with sufficient motivation for self-intoxication, the genetic adversity can be overcome.

Alcoholic beverage consumption varies widely across cultural and national boundaries, being highest in Western Europe and lowest in the Middle East and India. Historians have noted that every population has found some natural vegetative source to undergo fermentation, except for the Alaskan Indians because no suitable agricultural substrate could be found. This deficit was later overcome by commercial beverage alcohol.

Another important distinction between the neuropsychopharmacology of ethanol and other drugs of abuse, aside from the doses required to evoke behavioral changes, is the lag between ingestion and the onset of the behavioral results. Typically, on an empty stomach, ingestion of an intoxicating dose of alcohol does not reach even suboptimal intoxicating levels for at least 20–30 minutes, but absorption from that single dose will continue for 3 or 4 hours. As a result, the inexperienced imbiber may perceive that the dose just consumed has had no effect and will re-dose expecting negligible consequences. As subsequent doses lead to more seriously intoxicating blood levels, the consumer will be intoxicated until liver metabolism (operating at the rate of approximately half a drink dose per hour) or gastric distress (and emesis) deal with the alcohol. However, when blood alcohol levels are monitored against self-perception of intoxication or actual coordinated motoric performance, it is clear that a central nervous system (CNS) acute tolerance develops, with the result being that an ascending blood alcohol level in the early stages of consumption is much more incapacitating than the same blood level on the descending side of the dose–response curve. These metabolic facts will not, however, dissuade the legal justice system that an elevated blood alcohol level is acceptable.

ALCOHOL TOLERANCE

Repeated use of alcoholic beverages leads to both metabolic and central nervous system tolerance, well beyond the acute tolerance that develops during a given drinking session. In the liver, a second ethanol-catabolizing pathway is induced by repeated alcohol exposure that augments alcohol dehydrogenase. This second pathway, the microsomal ethanol oxidizing system, is catalyzed by one of the cytochrome P450 oxidizing enzymes, CYP. With repeated exposure to alcohol, this system's capacity can more than double within 2 weeks, and it may remain elevated even with abstention from drinking for several more weeks.

Aside from the metabolic tolerance, repeated drinking episodes also lead to more rapid tolerance to the intoxicating effects of alcohol. Rats that are selectively bred for alcohol preference also show much more rapid development of CNS tolerance whether gauged by motor tasks or by maze performance. Humans with family histories of alcoholism and alcohol abuse, who often exhibit excessive consumption in late adolescence or early adulthood, also show tolerance in the self-perceived effects of their consumed alcohol, suggesting a basis for their motivation to continue drinking. The heritability of the susceptibility to alcohol dependence in both humans and animal models is explored in greater detail later in this chapter.

In an interesting experiment, rats were trained to walk on as automated treadmill to avoid a foot shock they would receive if they failed to maintain their walking pace. After training, the animals were divided into two groups that received the same doses of ethanol by intraperitoneal (i.p.) injection, with one group of rats being injected 1 hour before their treadmill walk and the other group walking the treadmill for the same hour and then receiving their i.p. injections of alcohol on return to their home cages. Since these two groups received the same daily doses of alcohol for 3 weeks, their metabolic tolerance development should have been equivalent. However, on day 24 of the experiment, both groups received the same i.p. doses of ethanol before being placed on the treadmill. Those that had practiced walking the treadmill while intoxicated showed very few errors in maintaining their pace on the treadmill. The rats that had previously only been given alcohol after walking the treadmill showed as many errors in maintaining their pace as did rats of the same size who had been trained for the treadmill walk but never previously been exposed to alcohol (Fig. 25–2). This learned task tolerance may partially explain why adult humans can sometimes appear to drive their vehicles perfectly well while intoxicated even though it is illegal to do so.

Animals allowed alcohol exposures for prolonged periods and humans who are allowed ad libitum consumption can "learn" to tolerate increasingly high blood alcohol levels—levels that in fact would be lethal to naive drinkers. When inexperienced college students enter the liberating environments of

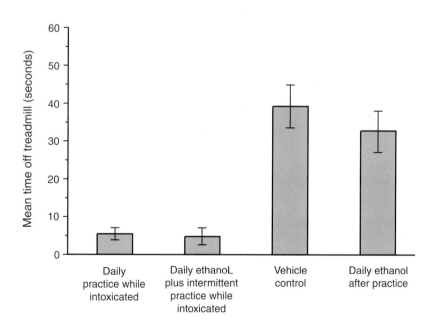

FIGURE 25–2. Mean performance (± standard error) of the various groups of rats on day 24 (2.2 g of ethanol per kilogram was injected i.p. 1 hour before testing). The group sizes were adjusted to include only those rats that absorbed ethanol adequately. (Modified from Wenger et al., 1981.)

their upper classmates, the mismatch in prior alcohol tolerance can lead to fatal alcohol intoxication.

The brains of the chronically inebriated appear to be somewhat sober due to the adaptive mechanisms that are subtly activated in an attempt to stay abreast of events in their environments. When they are finally overwhelmed by intoxication, and blood levels begin to fall, these ongoing adaptive mechanisms are revealed by the *alcohol withdrawal reaction*, which includes sweating, anxiety, tremulousness, frank withdrawal seizures, and hallucinatory behaviors (delirium tremens), with activation of the hypothalamic–pituitary stress axis. Experimental animals also show elevation of the threshold for activating intracranial self-stimulation.

HOW DOES ALCOHOL REWARD CONSUMPTION?

Alcohol research increased in the late 1970s contemporaneously with the discovery of several relevant neuropeptides, namely the neuropeptides of the proopiomelanocortin, proenkephalin, and prodynorphin families, as well as several other novel neuropeptide systems (see Chapter 9). Early studies revealed two behavioral consequences of modest doses of ethanol:

1. An anxiolytic effect observed when experimental animals were trained in "conflict" tests. Typically, food- or water-deprived animals were allowed to lever press to receive the missing nutrient, but each lever press elevated a foot shock applied to the floor of their cage. When administered known anxiolytics such as the benzodiazepines (see Chapter 14), rats continued to take punishment well beyond that tolerated by untreated animals, and ethanol had the same results, albeit less potently and with doses similar to those that impair motor performance. In an era in which there was an obsession with the opioid peptides, it was remarkable, but unexplainable, that the opiate antagonist naloxone reduced the anticonflict effects of both alcohol and a benzodiazepine.

2. A rewarding effect of alcohol seen in both nonhuman primates and rats, especially in those inbred substrains selectively bred for their preference for voluntary consumption of ethanol. Again, the surprising result was obtained that in those animals that did engage in alcohol self-administration, opiate antagonists would reduce the amounts of alcohol that animals would self-administer.

In the rat models with alcohol-preferring subjects, and in some cases with standard rat strains, using the behavioral model of lever pressing for consumption of alcohol versus neutral or artificially sweetened fluids as the dependent variable, it was possible to challenge animals so trained with intracerebral injections of neurotransmitter agonists and antagonists to define sites and transmitter systems that would enhance or diminish alcohol self-administration. These studies established that dopamine-containing neurons of the ventral tegmental area projecting to the nucleus accumbens are important for the rewarding effects. In animals bred for alcohol preference, merely placing them in environments in which they had previously lever pressed for alcohol solutions to drink was sufficient to cause the release of dopamine in the nucleus accumbens, as detected by microdialysis. Antagonists of the 5-HT$_3$ receptor will suppress voluntary ethanol self-administration, as will antagonists of the CRF-1 receptor and the endocannabinoid CB1 receptor (see Chapter 12). Ongoing clinical trials of the lead CB-1 antagonist, SR141716 (Rimonabant), are evaluating the short-term appetite for alcohol in subjects whose blood alcohol has been raised to subintoxicating levels; a more potent analogue, SR147778, is in the pipeline.

HOW DOES ALCOHOL CHANGE NEURONAL FUNCTION AND ALTER BEHAVIOR?

Attempts to explain the effects of ethanol and other alcohols on the CNS have historically emphasized similarities between this class of drug and general anesthetics. As recently as 1980, a classic textbook of pharmacology stated, "Despite popular belief in its stimulant properties, ethanol is entirely depressant in its actions on neurons of the central nervous system. In fact, its actions are qualitatively similar to those of a general anesthetic" (Bowman and Rand, 1980). When considered under the Meyer–Overton rule, the pharmacological potency of an alcohol, like some general anesthetics, was held to be proportional to its lipophilicity, and lipophilicity is in turn directly related to the chain length and other physicochemical properties of the alcohol. Although no consensus mechanisms ever emerged for how these physicochemical properties of alcohols and anesthetics actually "explained" their effects on cellular and organismic function, the inference was that the primary sites of action of these substances took place within the lipid matrix of the plasma membranes.

However, in the mid-1980s, new research methods indicated that actions based exclusively on drug–lipid permeation were inadequate to explain the experimental observations and that the composition of neurons offers selective sites for presumptive protein–lipid interactions that were not detectable in nonneuronal membranes. Analysis of the molecular mechanisms that have been shown to be modified by doses of acutely administered alcohols that are pharmacologically relevant to the time course and dose–response course of alcohol intoxication indicates that the sensitivity of specific mammalian neurons to ethanol varies over a wide dose range. Those neurons most sensitive to ethanol (whose threshold doses fall within the minimum human intoxicating dose range) show specific changes in selected intracellular mechanisms mediating responses to neurotransmitters. Several transmitter-selective effects of ethanol on neuronal function, as well as selected alterations in transmitter biochemistry in animals bred for preference for alcohol consumption, were then reported. These observations became a starting point from which to assemble the molecular and cellular events leading to intoxication and alcohol dependence (or, more commonly and generally, alcohol addiction).

ACTIONS ON GABA TRANSMISSION

For the past two decades, the intoxicating and behaviorally rewarding effects of ethanol have been linked most closely to the actions of the major CNS excitatory transmitter, GLU, and to the major inhibitory transmitter, GABA, although in ways that were not initially obvious. The GABA-mimetic actions of ethanol were inferred from the pharmacological synergism between alcohol and barbiturates and benzodiazepines, in which the latter two drug classes had been shown to be linked to specific subunits of the GABA receptor. This line of thinking was further strengthened by reports that in brain homogenates enriched for "synaptoneurosomes" composed of a synaptic terminal with some dendritic membrane component still attached, GABA would stimulate uptake of Cl−, and this effect was further enhanced by ethanol and antagonized by a benzodiazepine inverse agonist.

Nevertheless, in cellular studies of the effects of GABA *in vivo*, little or no potentiation by ethanol within the range of intoxicating blood levels could be seen in cerebellum, hippocampus, or the lateral septal nucleus, whereas it was seen occasionally in neurons of the medial septal nucleus. However, despite the view that there were perhaps select $GABA_A$ receptors with differing sensitivity to ethanol, *in vitro* data began to accumulate that ethanol was not directly influencing $GABA_A$ receptors on neurons from brain regions in which ethanol influenced GABA function *in vivo*. For example, the GABA-gated currents from neurons isolated from medial septum responded to ethanol *in vivo* but not *in vitro*. Other neurons respond to ethanol *in vitro* only if $GABA_B$ receptors in those brain regions were previously antagonized, or only at lethal concentrations.

In studies on neurons of the central nucleus of the amygdala (CeA), which is a part of the extended amygdala studied for its role in addictive drug reinforcement effects, combined electrophysiological and biochemical methods with microdialysis revealed an unexpected avenue for GABA potentiation by low-dose ethanol, namely enhanced synaptic release from presynaptic GABA terminals. Although ethanol had no effects on the release of glutamate, glycine, or taurine in alcohol naive rats, in animals studied after 10–14 days of continuous exposure to intoxicating blood alcohol levels, glutamate release was initially enhanced and later decreased as GABA release again increased during stages of acute withdrawal.

As summarized in Figure 25–3, the presynaptic effect of ethanol on GABA release in mouse CeA neurons appears to be further regulated by the neuropeptide corticotrophin-releasing factor (CRF), which is known to coexist in approximately half of the GABA neurons of the CeA. At 10–100 nM of CRF, there is electrophysiological and biochemical evidence of enhanced GABA release like that produced by ethanol, and the effects of both CRF and ethanol are blocked

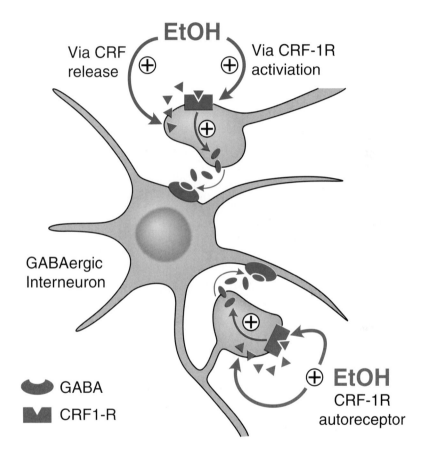

FIGURE 25–3. Schematic of hypothetical ethanol action on GABAergic synapses in the central amygdala. (Top synapse) Ethanol could enhance the release of GABA (blue/light gray) from another GABAergic interneuron either via (1) the release from the same terminal of CRF (red/dark gray) that then acts on CRF-1R on the terminal to elicit the release of more GABA (small arrow) or via (2) the direct activation of CRF-1R to elicit the release of more GABA. (Bottom synapse) A terminal (or dendrite) could feed back onto the same neuron to act on GABAergic autoreceptors. Ethanol may then enhance GABA release onto these GABA receptors via CRF release or via direct CRF-1R receptor activation, as in the top synapse. Thus, ethanol may augment the autoinhibition of this inhibitory interneuron, leading to the excitation of downstream neurons by disinhibition. (From Siggins and Roberto, 2005.)

in mice in which the expression of the CRF-1 receptor gene has been geneti-cally eradicated or by CRF-1 antagonists. Of further functional interest, mice lacking a CRF-1 receptor show enhanced stress-induced ethanol consumption that is progressive throughout their adult life span; these mice also show evi-dence for upregulation of the NR2B subunit of the NMDA receptor, leading us back to the second major transmitter system affected by ethanol. A rela-tively new member of the superfamily of opioid peptides, nociceptin/orphanin FQ, has been shown to act presynaptically to decrease GABA transmission in the central nucleus of the amygdala and also to block the ability of alcohol to increase GABA release from this site.

ACTIONS ON GLU TRANSMISSION

Many early electrophysiological studies of the effects of ethanol *in vivo* or on slice preparations *in vitro* pointed to generally inhibitory effects on GLU-mediated events in spinal motoneurons responding to dorsal root stimulation, in hippocampal neurons responding to K^+-induced or synaptically released GLU, or to NMDA-R initiated long-term potentiation. Low concentrations of ethanol, well within the range of human intoxicating doses, reduce evoked non-NMDA-mediated excitatory postsynaptic potentials. Studies of the direct effects of ethanol on NMDA responses on cultured hippocampal neurons have re-tested the Meyer–Overton rule using a series of aliphatic alcohols to show that although potency of the NMDA blockade increases exponentially for alcohols with one to five carbons, this potency peaks at six to eight carbons and then disappears with still longer alcohols. These effects have been interpreted to indicate that the site of alcohol action on the NMDA receptor is within the hydrophobic pockets on the receptor protein at sites of its interaction with the membrane phospholipids.

Ethanol also inhibits NMDA responses on neurons within the core of the rat nucleus accumbens, another critical element in the drug reinforcement circuitry, whereas much higher levels of ethanol are required to affect responses to direct applications of AMPA or quisqualate. This disparity has been suggested to reveal a presynaptic effect of the ethanol action, more sensitive to ethanol than the postsynaptic actions. In CeA neurons from alcohol naive rats, superfusion of 5–66 mM of ethanol decreases GLU-mediated excitatory postsynaptic poten-tials, and based on both biochemical and electrophysiological evidence, this effect was interpreted as likely to be postsynaptic. However, in animals chroni-cally exposed to ethanol for 2–4 weeks, an additional acute local superfusion of ethanol produced both biochemical and electrophysiological evidence for increased GLU release and perhaps provided a basis for the increased expres-sion of NMDA receptors seen in mice lacking CRF1 receptors.

ETHANOL EFFECTS ON OTHER TRANSMITTER SYSTEMS

Although diminished cerebellar function in the intoxicated individual forms the basis for the hand-to-nose and heel-to-toe roadside performance tasks, actions of alcohol on cerebellar neurons have been found to be surprisingly subtle. After single injections of ethanol (1–4 g/kg i.p. yielding blood alcohol levels of approximately 100–400 mg%), single-unit extracellular recordings of rat cerebellar Purkinje cells showed dramatically increased frequency of climbing fiber bursts but only occasional increases in simple spike firing rate. These effects of ethanol are not observed in rats chronically treated with the alcohol by vapor chamber administration for 11–14 days. Here, firing patterns for the first 3 hours after the last ethanol administration did not differ significantly from those of controls. However, rats chronically treated and then withdrawn from ethanol show significant, progressive decreases in climbing fiber activity and overall firing rates from 3 to 32 hour after the last ethanol administration. These effects on cerebellar Purkinje cell firing appear to be physiological correlates of the phenomena of ethanol intoxication, tolerance, and dependence, but the effects are primarily elicited from neurons such as the inferior olivary nucleus or the locus ceruleus that project onto cerebellar cortical neurons and not due to effects of ethanol on the cerebellar cortical neurons. Both cerebellar afferent nuclear effects of ethanol have been directly observed: Inferior olivary neurons accelerate after systemic intoxicating doses of alcohol, whereas neurons of the locus ceruleus progressively lose their high-fidelity responsiveness to random sensory stimuli as blood alcohol levels increase.

A LOST HYPOTHESIS OF ETHANOL MEDIATION

At first glance, there seem to be two alternative concepts of how alcohols, and ethanol the drug, affect neurons to produce the biologic effects that eventuate in the forms of altered behavior recognized as intoxication, dependence, and tolerance: Either ethanol interacts with selected proteins, such as enzymes, transmitter receptors, or structural proteins, in or on the membrane of neurons or ethanol interacts with the lipids of the membrane. However, a third alternative does exist theoretically, which in overview creates many alternatives and will therefore be presented as a brief digression from the main theme: Rather than viewing ethanol per se as the agent causing the effects that emerge upon consumption of ethanol, an "active catabolite" could be formed in the body in the presence of ethanol, and this active catabolite could then interact with a host of receptive target systems. In the most notorious version of this hypothesis, the "tetrahydroisquinoline hypothesis," either a condensation product of a brain amine with acetaldehyde or other hypothetical condensation products of monoamine catabolism resulting from ethanol effects on brain redox systems was proposed to generate an active intermediate agent that was then responsible for the pharmacology of ethanol and was thus unconstrained by the physical properties of ethanol. To the degree that such an intermediate could be documented, the greater specificity of its receptor interactions would tend to support a protein site of action. For its supporters, increasingly more sensitive detection methods that failed to find any such intermediate attested to how potent the invisible intermediates must be.

A variant of this general concept is the class of steroidal substances formed in the brain that varies in concentration with behavioral manipulations but not peripheral sources of gonadal or adrenal steroids (see Chapter 12). The original end product of the brain neurosteroid pathway, dehydroepiandrosterone (DHA; see Chapter 12), is rapidly depleted by intoxicating doses of parenteral ethanol but not by other CNS depressants. Since the concentrations of δ5-pregnenolone, the precursor neurosteroid to DHA, are not affected by ethanol, it is conjectured that an alternative metabolic neurosteroid pathway has been utilized in the presence of ethanol. Indeed, some synthetic steroids are known to be useful anesthetics.

Similarly, we have already noted that acute intoxication acts to speed the firing of neurons of the inferior olive, and a similar effect has been observed to follow the effects of the 5-HT-selective monoamine oxidase inhibitor harmaline. Since the rodent inferior olivary complex is heavily innervated with 5-HT-containing fibers, an indirect mediation of the ethanol effect on inferior olive could thus be attributed to a hypothetical metabolite of ethanol, such as a harmaline-like β-carboline (formed by condensation of acetaldehyde and serotonin), whose effects would be presumed to derive from more typical transmitter receptor actions. However, this hypothesis is not correct.

THE GENETIC BASES OF ALCOHOLISM

National surveys in the United States have established alcohol dependence, or alcoholism, as one of the most prevalent adult psychiatric disorders. Although anecdotal evidence for alcoholism running in families or in particular ethnic lines is abundant, replicated studies of family, twin, and adoption studies have provided compelling evidence that genes play an important role in the development of alcohol dependence. Heritability estimates of 50–60% for both men and women have been reported.

Research clinicians define the phenotypic characteristics of alcoholism and alcohol dependence as a maladaptive pattern of substance use leading to clinically significant impairment or distress as manifested by three or more of the following occurring at any time in the same 12-month period:

1. Need for markedly increased amounts to achieve intoxication or desired effect; or markedly diminished effect with continued use of the same amount
2. The characteristic withdrawal syndrome to relieve or avoid withdrawal symptoms
3. Persistent desire or one or more unsuccessful efforts to cut down or control substance use
4. Substance use in larger amounts or over a longer period than the person intended
5. Important social, occupational, or recreational activities given up or reduced because of substance use
6. A great deal of time spent in activities necessary to obtain, to use, or to recover from the effects of substance use

Using these diagnostic criteria, a multiuniversity consortium on the genetics of alcoholism reported on a systematic single nucleotide polymorphism screen for alcohol dependence genes in 262 densely affected Caucasian families. Four of the eight most significant genes were located in or very close to the gene *ACN9*, located near the centromere of human chromosome 7. Although discovered in yeast unable to employ the acetate moiety as a carbon source, little is known of its functions in humans, and other unknown genes within the targeted region of chromosome 7 may be responsible for the vulnerability phenotype.

Studies of experimental rodents have yielded useful experimental models of selective inbreeding based on initial preference for drinking high ethanol-containing solutions (>10%) generally eschewed by control rats. At least four sets of such inbred lines have been reported: the P versus NP, preferring and nonpreferring rats; the HAD and LAD rats (high acceptance drinking versus low acceptance drinking), both raised at the University of Indiana Alcohol Research Center; the AA (alcohol accepting) and ANA (alcohol nonaccepting) rats developed in Finnish laboratories; and the Sardinian alcohol-preferring rat raised at the University of Sardinia. All of these lines have proven useful as experimental models of dependence and withdrawal but have yielded no common genetic or other molecular commonalities. Three genes seem to account for the phenotypic differences between the P and NP lines, of which two have been identified—α-synuclein and glutathione *S*-transferase 8-8.

Substantial effort has also gone into the study of ethanol consumption, tolerance, and withdrawal in mice, where the availability of multiple strains and recombinant inbred substrains can potentially provide even greater molecular understanding of the behavioral responses to drugs. Prior literature indicated that mice of the C57BL strains are unique in their willingness to self-administer ethanol to blood levels that yield behavioral intoxication as evidenced by balance beam walking and rotorod motor dysfunction. These mice exhibit low chronic withdrawal severity and low ethanol taste aversion. Determining the genetic basis for these strain differences offers a great opportunity for further insight.

THE EMERGENCE OF PHARMACOLOGICAL THERAPIES

We conclude with some promising developments in alcohol neuropsychopharmacology that have emerged in part from the scientific studies of its intoxicating and rewarding cellular and molecular mechanisms and in part from the essential element of drug discovery—fortuitous observations.

Antabuse

We have already mentioned that blocking the catabolism of alcohol with Antabuse (disulfiram) will suppress consumption by causing a highly adverse reaction to the accumulation of acetaldehyde. This effect was an unexpected side effect of a drug that had been developed as an antiparasitic drug but for which the volunteers had not been warned to avoid alcoholic beverages. Similar adverse side effects to alcohol have been reported with certain sulfonylurea compounds in the treatment of diabetes mellitus and with cephalosporin antibiotics. The respiratory distress and severe nausea that result in the unwarned can be extremely aversive and may be life threatening. Daily doses of 100–500 mg are prescribed to be taken in the mornings when the resolve not to drink may be stronger. However, nothing about the actions deals with the underlying craving of the alcohol-addicted person, and compliance is difficult to enforce.

Acamprosate

Given the long suggestive history of a mediator relationship between alcohol and GABA systems, the developers of acamprosate (Ca-N-acetylhomotaurine) set out to screen for amino acid analogues that might diminish the consumption of alcohol in spontaneously drinking rats. Having observed such an effect for this taurine analogue and whose effects in that regard could be blocked by the GABA antagonist bicucculine, clinical trials were implemented on alcoholic subjects who had been detoxified after hospitalization for acute alcohol abuse. Of 37 subjects in the treatment arm, 20 had not relapsed after 3 months, whereas only 12 in the 30 control group remained similarly abstinent. After many clinical trials, primarily from Western Europe, had been published, meta-analysis showed that after 6 months, daily treatment with acamprosate produced more abstinent patients than placebo (36% versus 24%). Soon thereafter, in 2004, based primarily on the European data, the U.S. Food and Drug Administration (FDA) approved the drug for the treatment of alcohol dependence under the name Campral. Clinical trials in the United States have not shown comparable effectiveness, and the 1.3- to 2.0-g daily dose requirement is another barrier to strict compliance. Further basic research on animals made dependent on alcohol suggests that rather than being GABA related, acamprosate works by being both an NMDA and mGLUR5 antagonist.

Naltrexone

We have already noted that in the early days of post-1970s alcohol research, two observations in 1980 indicated the pharmacological link between endogenous opioid systems and alcohol: suppression of alcohol-induced effects on the conflict test and suppression of alcohol self-administration in nonhuman primates. These results led to several clinical trials seeking effective doses in humans and to controlled clinical trials in which naltrexone, an orally active form of naloxone and an equally good mu receptor antagonist, was reported to reduce alcohol craving and relapsed heavy alcohol consumption. After a replication of this clinical result, the FDA approved naltrexone for the treatment of alcoholism in 1992.

Subsequently, nearly 30 additional clinical studies were reported, with the drug showing reduced craving for alcohol in virtually all but with only modest and highly variable effects overall. In 1996, a study of family history-positive but nonalcoholic adults found that those with a family history of alcoholism showed a greater release of anterior pituitary β-endorphin in response to systemic alcohol than did those with no family history. This greater response has been attributed to allelic variation in the mu receptor, with the Asp40/Asp40 homozygous allele showing greater sensitivity to alcohol. In a retrospectively analyzed clinical trial of patients responding to naltrexone for alcoholism treatment, those with the greater therapeutic response were found to have this receptor allele. A genomically stratified clinical trial based on this allele has been reported in which the results confirm and extend the prior observations that the Asp40 allele can predict naltrexone responding in alcoholic subjects. A long-lasting (once per month) injectable form of naltrexone was approved by the FDA in 2005. Thus, a long and winding road from basic research observations has eventuated into three potentially valid treatment options for a chronic, relapsing addictive disorder once, and not so long ago, regarded as an untreatable matter of willpower.

SELECTED REFERENCES

Anton, R. F., G. Oroszi, S. O'Malley, D. Couper, R. Swift, H. Pettinati, and D. Goldman (2008). An evaluation of mu-opioid receptor (OPRM1) as a predictor of naltrexone in the treatment of alcohol dependence. *Arch. Gen. Psych.* 65, 135–144.

Bloom, F. E. (1991). Alcohol and anesthetic actions: Are they mediated by lipid or protein? In *Neuropharmacology of Ethanol—New Approaches* (R. E. Myers, G. F. Koob, M. J. Lewis, and S. M. Paul, Eds.). Birkhäuser, Boston, pp. 1–19.

Bowman, W. C. and M. J. Rand (1980). *Textbook of Pharmacology.* Blackwell Scientific Publications, Oxford, pp. 8.12–8.16.

Breese, G. R., H. E. Criswell, M. Carta, P. D. Dodson, H. J. Hanchar, R. T. Khisti, M. Mameli, Z. Wing, A. L. Morrow, R. W. Olsen, T. S. Otis, L. Parsons, S. N. Penland, M. Roberto, G. R. Siggins, C. F. Valenzuela, and M. Walner (2006). Basis of the GABAmimetic profile of ethanol. *Alcohol Clin. Exp. Res.* 30, 731–744.

Fleming, M., S. J. Mihic, and P. A. Harris (2006). Ethanol. In *Goodman and Gilman's The Pharmacological Basis of Therapeutics* (L. Brunton, J. S. Lazo, and K. L Parker, Eds.). McGraw-Hill, New York, 11th ed., pp. 591–206.

Johnson, B. A. (2008). Update on neuropharmacological treatments for alcoholism: Scientific basis and clinical findings. *Biochem. Pharmacol.* 75, 34–56.

Koob, G. F. and M. Le Moal (2006). Alcohol. In *Neurobiology of Addiction.* Elsevier, New York, pp. 173–241.

Koob, G. F., R. E. Strecker, and F. E. Bloom (1980). Effects of naloxone on the anticonflict properties of alcohol and chlordiazepoxide. *Substance Alcohol Actions/Misuse* 1, 447–457.

Peoples, R. W. and F. F. Weight (1995). Cutoff in potency implicates alcohol inhibition of *N*-methyl-D-aspartate receptors in alcohol intoxication. *Proc. Natl. Acad. Sci. USA* 92, 2825–2829.

Roberto, M. and G. R. Siggins (2006). Nociceptin/orphanin FQ presynaptically decreases GABAergic transmission and blocks the ethanol-induced increase of GABA release in central amygdala. *Proc. Natl. Acad. Sci. USA* 103, 9715–9720.

Rogers, J., G. R. Siggins, J. A. Schulman, and F. E. Bloom (1980). Physiological correlates of ethanol intoxication, tolerance and dependence in rat cerebellar Purkinje cell. *Brain Res.* 196, 183–198.

Siggins, G. R., M. Roberto, and Z. Nie (2005). The tipsy terminal: Presynaptic effects of ethanol. *Pharmacol. Ther.* 107, 80–98.

Wenger, J. R., T. M. Tiffany, C. Bombardier, K. Nicholls, and S. C. Wood (1981). Ethanol tolerance is learned. *Science* 213, 575–577.

26

Nicotine

The long, odious history of nicotine abuse is intimately connected with the Spanish, Portuguese, and English explorations of the New World, whose inhabitants were already deeply committed to the cultivation and enjoyment of tobacco on first encounters with the Europeans. A Mayan pottery vessel dating to the 11th century depicts a man smoking a roll of tobacco plants tied with a string known as a *sik-ar*. Among the gifts received by Christopher Columbus on the island of San Salvador were "certain dried leaves that gave off a distinct fragrance"; Columbus threw the leaves away. However, a few days later his men observed the natives smoking the leaves and also chewing them. On Columbus' second trip to the Americas, one of his companions, Ramon Pane, wrote the first descriptions published in Europe of the smoking habits of the Indians. It may be of more than passing interest that the nicotine alkaloid is produced in the roots of the tobacco plant to be concentrated in the leaves, where it acts as a potent antiherbivore to which insects rarely exhibit tolerance.

Following Columbus' beachhead in the Caribbean, Portuguese sailors began to plant tobacco seeds at every trading post, transplanting hardier varieties from the Central American mainland to the islands of the Caribbean and to their posts in Brazil. In the mid-16th century, the French ambassador to Portugal, Jean Nicot de Villemain—for whom the active ingredient was eventually named—returned home with tobacco plants and products.

English sailors soon brought the habit home as well. Tobacco use became so widespread that early in the 17th century, King James I wrote the first treatise to try to restrict its use: "A custom loathsome to the eye, hateful to the nose, harmful to the brain, dangerous to the lungs, and in the black stinking fumes thereof, nearest resembling the horrible Stygian Smoke of the Pit that is bottomless." Parliament constrained him from his attempted ban on tobacco use but could not ban the tax he imposed. When the Virginia colony became established in Jamestown, Brazilian tobacco seeds were available for planting, an effort aided by the importation of African slaves to clear the land and tend the crops. Exportation began with 9 tons in 1617, increasing to 10,000 tons per year by 1700. During the American Revolutionary War, not only was the tobacco tax one of the instigations of the revolt but also 5 million pounds of Virginia tobacco constituted the collateral employed by Benjamin Franklin to procure a loan from France.

During the American Civil War, a mutant form of the *Nicotiana tabacum* plant, which was the prevalent form in cultivation at that time, was recognized and termed "white Burley" because it was low in chlorophyll and proved to be exceptionally flavorful in chewing tobacco. Congressionally imposed taxes on tobacco were in part used to support the Civil War effort. Unfortunately, after three or four planting seasons, the soil becomes exhausted, and the barren soil is subject to erosion, requiring 20 years to become revitalized. As tobacco farmers moved west in search of fresh planting land, they encountered light sandy soil that produced a thin, lightly flavored and yellow tobacco leaf that soon became the mainstay of the U.S. tobacco industry, named "Bright leaf" for the bright yellow color that characterizes this tobacco after curing. Flue curing of Bright leaf tobacco is done in tobacco ovens (originally wooden shacks) at temperatures of approximately 100–130°F over 5–10 days, depending on ambient conditions. (In contrast, other tobacco types, such as Burley, are air cured over a longer period of time without the addition of heat.) Legend has it that the flue-curing process was initially discovered by accident on a North Carolina tobacco plantation in 1839 by a slave who fell asleep while fire curing tobacco (yet another curing technique) and hastily added charcoal to a dying fire. The increased heat and absence of smoke from the charcoal burning turned the leaf a bright yellow. The mild flavor of the resulting product fetched a high price at the local tobacco auction, and Bright leaf or Bright Yellow tobacco was born.

TOBACCO PRODUCTS: PREPARATION AND USES

Until the discovery of flue curing of American tobacco, most tobacco was consumed by smoking cigars or pipes or by chewing, in which the nicotine is absorbed slowly through the mucous membranes of the mouth or nose. Snus is a form of steam-cured tobacco that results in a moist powder; it is used largely in Scandinavian countries by placing a small sachet under the upper lip, and the nicotine is absorbed through the mucosa without causing hypersalivation or a need for spittoons. Although these forms of tobacco use were widely popular, especially among males, and especially during wars, the use of tobacco vastly increased after the discovery of the effects of the curing method and the mass manufacturing of the cigarettes that resulted (Figure 26–1).

Flue curing, especially of tobaccos such as Bright Yellow, changes the acid–base chemistry of nicotine. In tobacco smoke, nicotine can be found in both the smoke particulate matter and the gas phase of the smoke in three pH-dependent forms: diprotonated, monoprotonated, and unprotonated ("freebase"). The fraction of freebase nicotine in particulate matter increases with the alkalinity. In the gas phase, nicotine is found only as freebase nicotine, whereas it is the particulate matter that serves as a carrier transporting protonated nicotine into the lower respiratory tract, where the majority of deeply inhaled smoke nicotine is retained. The more nicotine delivered to the lungs, the greater the initial dose strength and the greater the addiction potential. The amounts of tobacco-specific nitrosamines, believed to be one of the major oncogenic substances in tobacco smoke, also depend on the level of heat and the relative humidity of the curing oven.

Approximately 50 years after the development of flue curing, most tobacco use remained pipes and cigars. When Spanish troops returned from the Crimean War (1853–1856), they brought with them the habit of smoking small sticks of tobacco wrapped in paper, and the use of cigarettes with their deeply inhaled quick jolts of nicotine soon became the rage limited only by the speed at which "tobacco girls" could hand roll the smokes (approximately five per minute). As cigarettes grew in popularity, tobacco companies began the search for a mechanical method of manufacturing them rapidly. In 1880, 18-year-old James Bonsack, a schoolboy in Virginia, developed a machine to make cigarettes at the rate of 70,000 per hour. Initially, his machine was unreliable, but the Duke family of Durham, North Carolina, refined the device and revolutionized the cigarette industry.

Addiction to tobacco products is a worldwide health hazard, both to the smoker and to those in the smoker's household environment. Although anti-smoking campaigns persuade many middle-aged smokers to attempt to quit, their numbers are replaced by adolescents who try their hand at the legal adult recreational drug. Moreover, many countries lack the active preventive campaigns seen in the United States, Canada, and the United Kingdom, and the number of smokers is rapidly increasing in China, India, and other Asian countries (Figures 26–2 and 26–3).

The Centers for Disease Control and Prevention (CDC) estimates that 371 billion cigarettes were consumed in the United States in 2006. Total U.S.

US Tobacco Product Output and Consumption (1950 - 2005)

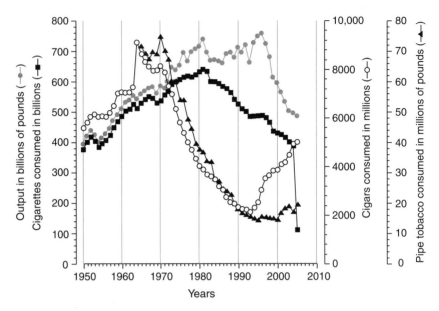

FIGURE 26–1. Historical trends in per capita consumption of various tobacco products used in the United States. (From U.S. Department of Agriculture, *Tobacco Situation and Outlook Report 1950–2005.*)

expenditures on tobacco were estimated to be $88.8 billion in 2005, of which $82 billion was spent on cigarettes. Also in 2005, the advertising budget of cigarette companies was more than $36 million per day—nearly $300 for every U.S. smoker. Finally, cigarette smoking results in 5.5 million years of potential life lost annually in the United States.

PHARMACOKINETICS OF SMOKING

Given the variety of forms in which nicotine-containing tobacco products are taken, it is obvious that the absorption, distribution, and metabolism will vary with the route of administration.

Cigarettes

Depending on the brand and properties of the cigarette (tobacco, length of cigarette, and filter), each puff inhalation can deliver 20 mg to more than 300 mg of nicotine to the lungs, and experienced smokers will feel the CNS

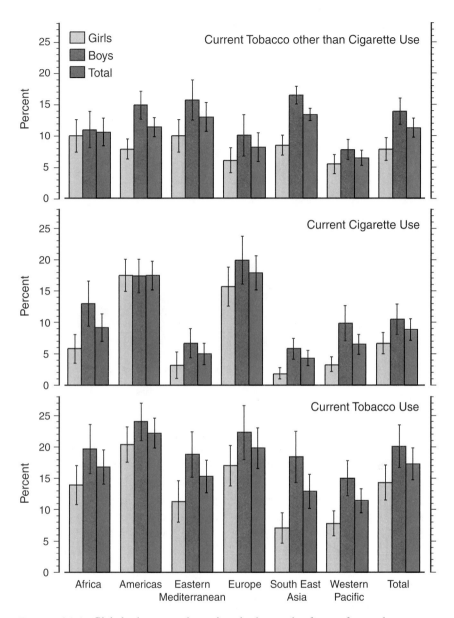

FIGURE 26–2. Global tobacco use by nations in thousands of tons of raw tobacco averaged for 1998–2000. (From the report *Raw Tobacco* from the Commission of the European Communities, Brussels, 2008.)

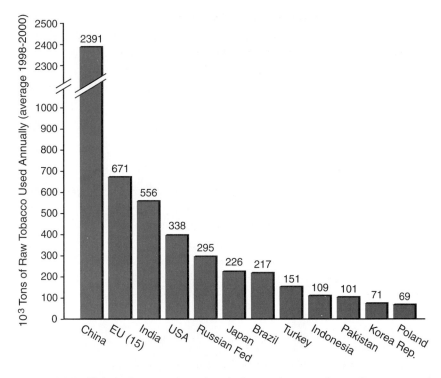

FIGURE 26–3. Global tobacco use by nations in thousands o tons of raw tobacco averaged for 1998–2000. (From the report Raw Tobacco from the Commission of the European Communities, Brussels, 2008.)

stimulant effects of that puff in 7–10 seconds as the arterial flow delivers the dose directly from the lungs to the brain. The concentrations of nicotine, or its main catabolite cotinine, in venous blood will reach a peak approximately 5–10 minutes into the cigarette, depending on how many puffs the smoker takes, and then begin to fall quite rapidly, with a half-life of approximately 15 minutes. This rapid decline represents the redistribution of nicotine from blood to liver, kidney, and salivary glands as well as nicotine binding to peripheral tissues with nicotinic cholinergic receptors, principally the adrenal medullary chromaffin cells and sympathetic ganglion neurons. The rate of disappearance from venous blood gradually slows, with an elimination rate of approximately 5 ng/ml/hour, but depending on the smoker's frequency of use, it can accumulate in plasma. Cotinine levels in plasma or urine, as well as a complex of carbon monoxide with hemoglobin (carboxyhemoglobin), persist for hours after a smoking episode and represent biomarkers for an active smoker. The elevated carboxyhemoglobin may be the cause of the increased cardiovascular disease found in smokers.

For the novice smoker, aversive side effects accompany initial nicotine usage, including dizziness, tachycardia, palpitations, nausea, progressing to emesis, sweating, and piloerection. Many of these adverse effects can be attributed to the stimulation of the adrenal medulla releasing epinephrine into the general circulation, as well as the direct stimulation of sympathetic ganglia. However, repeated use leads to rapid tolerance to these effects due to peripheral and central receptor desensitization.

Cigars and Pipes

Both of these forms of tobacco deliver the unprotonated nicotine more slowly by dissolution into the saliva and absorption of the higher levels into the buccal mucosa and then the general circulation of nicotine in cigar and pipe tobacco. If the tobacco stays lit, a full pipe load or high-density cigar can produce a venous blood level close to that produced by cigarettes but peaking 20–30 minutes after commencing to smoke and declining somewhat more slowly since tissue distribution is already ongoing as the smoking continues.

Snuff, Snus, and Chewing Tobacco

The tobaccos used for these forms of nicotine use are all much higher in nicotine content than that used for cigarettes, whereas the absorption rate is approximately the same as that for cigars and pipes. However, the swallowing of saliva containing nicotine may delay gastric emptying time and thus represents another source for absorption. Although users of so-called smokeless tobacco avoid the carcinogenic effects of inhaled tobacco particulate matter on the lungs, the prolonged exposure of the oral cavity to tobacco in snuff and chewing tobaccos leads to a much increased prevalence for cancers of the tongue and esophagus and gingivitis. The National Cancer Institute asserts that smokeless tobacco contains hundreds of carcinogenic substances, many derived from the reaction of tobacco and saliva. On the other hand, the formulation of nicotine in snus has thus far shown no such increase in oral cancers, and in Sweden, where it is mainly used, the prevalence of cigarette smoking is relatively low.

EXPERIMENTAL NICOTINE SELF-ADMINISTRATION

For each of the other psychoactive recreational drugs discussed in this text, demonstration that experimental animals will work to access self-administration of the drug represents an important avenue in determining the sites and mechanisms of the drug's reinforcing capacity. In fact, until 1981, there was no reliable evidence that nicotine could function as a reinforcer of any animal drug self-administration, but the manner of the initial successful self-administration paradigm revealed an explanation for the prior failures.

Reasoning that the reinforcing properties of nicotine may be amplified by the smell, taste, and environmental associations that the smoker experiences, Goldberg and colleagues placed permanent intravenous catheters in chaired squirrel monkeys and trained them to press a lever 10 times within 1 minute to force a green light to change to amber on a panel for 1 second, during which they received an intravenous injection of 30 mg of nicotine/kg body weight. A 3-minute time-out followed each injection. The monkeys readily learned to perform the task at high rates of responding. Their responses would extinguish if saline was injected instead of nicotine, and the effects of the nicotine reinforcement were blocked if the centrally active nicotine antagonist, mecamylamine, was injected 30 minutes before starting the behavioral task. The secondary signal of the visual stimulus played an important role, driving the monkeys to lever press twice as often during the signal that accompanied the drug injection.

In subsequent similar experiments in rats, animals were placed in cages with two levers to press, one of which delivered intravenous doses of nicotine at 30 mg of nicotine/kg body weight and the other did nothing. Rats learned to press both levers at comparable rates. However, when the dose injected per lever press was reduced to 3 or 10 mg/kg, they quickly learned to press only the active (drug delivery) lever.

These experiments established two principles of experimental self-administration of nicotine: (1) The drug must be injected somewhat infrequently, and (2) it must be administered at low doses per injection. Subsequent experiments established that too high an initial dose may in fact be so aversive that lever pressing is reduced from the negative reward.

With reproducible models of self-administration in hand, it became possible to investigate the sites and transmitter systems involved in maintaining the self-administration behavior. Corrigal and colleagues, following paradigms employed with other abused drugs, found that injections of the dopamine denervation toxin, 6-hydroxydopamine, into the nucleus accumbens of rats would promptly and permanently block nicotine self-administration. Furthermore, when a cholinergic nicotinic receptor antagonist, dihydro-β-erythroidine, was microinjected into the ventral tegmental area where the dopamine neurons whose axons innervate the nucleus accumbens are located, the nicotine self-administration was blocked, as it was with prior administration of dopamine antagonists.

As described in Chapter 6, the nicotinic acetylcholine receptor is one of the most thoroughly studied molecular mechanisms in neurophysiology and neuropharmacology. These receptors belong to the ligand-gated, multisubunit ion channel category of receptors composed of a pentameric structure, with each of the five subunits exhibiting four transmembrane domains, an extracellular ligand recognition site, and a cytoplasmic domain subject to phosphorylation that enhances desensitization. Central nervous system nicotinic receptors are made up of variable numbers of the α and β receptor subunits. The $\alpha_4\beta_2$ receptor, although relatively rare, is intensely expressed on the dopamine neurons of the ventral tegmental area (VTA). Transgenic mice in which the expression of the α_4 or β_2 subunit cannot occur will not self-administer nicotine. When the β_2 subunit is reexpressed in β_2 receptor knockout mice by stereotaxically injecting them in the VTA with a lentiviral vector of the β_2 subunit gene, nicotine-induced dopamine release and electrophysiologically responsive nicotinoceptive neurons are restored. When expression of the immediate early gene, c-*fos*, is mapped by immunocytochemistry in animals that self-administer nicotine, sites in the cingulate and piriform cortex and the superior colliculus are activated along with the ventral shell of the nucleus accumbens.

Thus, the basis for the molecular, cellular, and neuronal circuitry aspects of nicotine action appears to be solved. The important question that remains is why otherwise reasonable, sentient individuals would continue to abuse their bodies by acquiring and persisting in the use of tobacco products for their nicotine addiction. In rats, but not in humans, a rest period of 3 weeks is sufficient to extinguish nicotine-seeking behaviors. Furthermore, in rats, intracerebral injection in VTA or accumbens of antagonists to the mGLUR2/3 receptor will also reduce nicotine self-administration. This pharmacology represents a possible link to the excess smoking seen in patients diagnosed with schizophrenia, for whom the same receptor agonists have been proposed as novel antipsychotic agents.

CENTRAL AND PERIPHERAL ACTIONS OF NICOTINE

As noted in Chapter 6, acetylcholine acting at postsynaptic nicotinic receptors is the neurotransmitter for the preganglionic innervation of neurons of the sympathetic and parasympathetic autonomic nervous systems and the adrenal medulla. These autonomic nicotinic receptors, as at the neuromuscular junction, are the peripheral nervous system's equivalent of fast synaptic transmission. Nicotinic receptors are also found in the central nervous system but in a much more restricted distribution than the cholinergic muscarinic receptors and a somewhat different physiology than those in the periphery. Except for a modest excitatory input to GABAergic interneurons of the hippocampal formation, most central nicotinic receptors appear to function presynaptically to regulate the release of almost all other synaptic transmitters, including the monoamines GLU and GABA (see Chapter 6).

NICOTINE DEPENDENCE AND TREATMENT

Given the repeated observation that more than three-fourths of adults who are smokers began their habit before the age of 20 years, and the epidemiological evidence that significant decreases in adult smokers derive from delaying the onset of smoking, much effort has been expended to try to determine what humans find reinforcing about tobacco use. Tobacco products are legal for adults, and like alcoholic beverages, taxes on them provide a great deal of support to state and federal governments in the United States and elsewhere. Given their general availability, it is not difficult for children to access tobacco, and the prevalence of teenagers who smoke increases with age, approaching 30% by age 18 years (Fig. 26–2). No matter how averse are the early exposures to tobacco, tolerance to the autonomic side effects develops quickly—even more quickly with greater use.

Two theories have emerged to explain what maintains the smoking habit after regular smoking patterns have been established. Cigarette smokers who are heavily dependent will seek to maintain a given blood level of nicotine to which they have become accustomed, although both stress and boredom can elevate consumption. The theory of positive reward posits that due to either biological or behavioral consequences, the nicotine in tobacco is reinforcing or, in human terms, "pleasurable." Smokers also report a relaxation effect that approaches that produced by anxiolytics but without loss of attention or frank sedation, as well as an anorectic effect.

A second approach posits that although these pleasurable effects—following completion of the development of tolerance to the autonomic side effects—are the motivators to persist usage initially, most smokers, including youthful smokers, acknowledge that when they try to stop smoking or cut back, they experience extreme restlessness, irritability, increased appetite, insomnia, and an inability to concentrate, all of which are relieved by resumption of smoking. For other dependency-causing drugs, this state is withdrawal; however, this realization was very slow to come to the nicotine field.

Switching to low-nicotine cigarettes increases the number of cigarettes smoked and increases the exposure of the lungs and family members to more tars and particulate matter. The avoidance of these withdrawal states comes to represent a more beneficial state to smokers than the cognitive recognition that the act of smoking is unhealthful, and they develop the misbelief that if they really wanted to stop, at a later time, they could "always" do so. On the biological level, Koob and colleagues found that regardless of the drug to which a given animal has been made dependent and then withdrawn, there is a common elevation of corticotropin-releasing factor (CRF) and that CRF antagonists may act to diminish these withdrawal states. Because the somatic signs of nicotine withdrawal can be precipitated experimentally by opiate antagonists and reversed by injection of opiates, there is a presumption that endogenous opioids may be involved in nicotine dependence.

Clearly, the human condition is often a complex one that may, in a given individual, have differing origins. Some hold that there is a complex trait of vulnerability to addiction that has genetic influences that transcend specific licit or illicit drug usage, and the specific drug to which a given addict commits depends to a great degree on what drugs are currently fashionable to the person's social or peer group.

Treatments for nicotine dependence are relatively weak and recidivism is quite high, with verified abstinence rates 6 months after quitting of 20% or less. According to O'Brien, when ex-smokers "slip" and begin smoking a little, they usually relapse quickly to their prior level of dependence. Treatment consists of nontobacco nicotine replacement by chewing gum, nasal spray, or transdermal patches. The antidepressant bupropion, a norepinephrine/serotonin transporter inhibitor, has in lower doses been reported to be more effective than nicotine replacement therapies, especially when combined with behavioral group therapy. In 2006, the FDA approved the $\alpha_4\beta_2$ nicotine receptor partial agonist varenicline (sold as Champix in Western Europe and as Chantix in the United States) for the treatment of nicotine addiction based on several successful clinical trials. In animal studies, varenicline reduces the nicotine-induced release of dopamine (see Chapter 6). However, in 2008, the manufacturer stated that although it successfully helps treat nicotine addiction, some patients have experienced serious neuropsychiatric symptoms, including changes in behavior, agitation, depressed mood, suicidal ideation, and suicidal behavior. As with alcohol and appetite control, there are ongoing clinical trials of the cannabinoid receptor 1 antagonist rimonabant, the results of which are not yet known.

SMOKING, LUNG CANCER, AND SMOKING PREVENTION

Given the long history of nicotine's social acceptability and pervasive presence in cultures throughout the world, not to mention the free distribution and encouragement of cigarette use by the military in World War II, it is important to recognize the extreme skepticism with which society in general, and physicians in particular, regarded the initial reports that virtually all men dying with bronchial carcinoma in the late 1940s were chronic smokers. Although there had been prior suggestions of such a cause-and-effect relationship, when Wynder and Graham reported on a series of 684 cases in 1950, they concluded that "excessive and prolonged use of tobacco, especially cigarettes, seems to be an important factor in the induction of bronchiogenic carcinoma" but were themselves hesitant to claim a causal role.

According to the CDC, the incidence of men dying with lung cancer in 1930 was less than 5/100,000 deaths, but by 1990 it had increased to 75.6/100,000 deaths. In 1964, after more than 7000 reports had appeared linking smoking and disease, an advisory committee to the U.S. Surgeon General concluded that smoking is a cause of lung and laryngeal cancer in men, a probable cause of lung cancer in women, and the leading cause of chronic bronchitis in both sexes. A 50-year follow-up of 40,000 British doctors showed that cigarette smoking not only increased the risk of death from lung cancer but also increased the risk of dying from 23 other causes. Annual cigarette consumption in the United States, which had increased from 54 cigarettes per person in 1900 to more than 4300 per person in 1963, decreased by half between 1964 and 1998 following the Surgeon General's report (Fig. 26–1), aided no doubt by increased taxes on tobacco products and increased prices across the industry.

The Surgeon General's report also led to changes in the manufacture and marketing of cigarettes, with filters to reduce the inhaled tars of the particulate matter and reduced nicotine content. The latter proved to increase the frequency and depth of inhaling as chronic smokers sought to maintain their preferred nicotine blood levels. The 1998 Master Agreement between the tobacco industry and the Attorneys General of 46 of the U.S. states represented a general acknowledgment by the industry of the prior harm caused by their products. Although the settlements were to compensate states for the increased health care costs for their addicted patients, very few states have used the funds in that manner.

Tobacco use is still responsible for one out of four adult deaths annually, and it remains highest among those who are at the lower levels of the socioeconomic scale and is growing worldwide (Fig. 26–3). Federal subsidies to tobacco farmers in the United States ended in 2003 but still continue in the European Union for farmers in Greece and Italy, despite the World Health Organization's 2008 *Report on the Global Tobacco Epidemic* proclaiming that this "entirely preventable epidemic must rank as a top priority for public health and for political leaders in every country of the world." Clearly, tobacco/nicotine addiction remains a fertile field for future drug development.

SELECTED REFERENCES

Borio, G. (2007). *The Tobacco Timeline*. Available at www.tobacco.org/resources/history/tobacco_history.html; accessed March 2, 2008.

Centers for Disease Control and Prevention (1999). Tobacco Use—United States, 1900–1999. *JAMA* 282, 2202–2207.

Cox, B. M., A. Goldstein, and W. T. Nelson (1984). Nicotine self-administration in rats. *Br. J. Pharmacol.* 83, 49–55.

Dani, J. A. and D. Bertrand (2007). Nicotinic acetylcholine receptors and nicotinic cholin-ergic mechanisms of the central nervous system. *Annu. Rev. Pharmacol. Toxicol.* 47, 699–729.

Doll, R., R. Peto, J. Boreham, and I. Sutherland (2005). Mortality from cancer in relation to smoking: 50 years observations on British doctors. *Br. J. Cancer* 92, 426–429.

Goldberg, S. R., R. D. Spealman, and D. M. Goldberg (1981). Persistent behavior at high rates maintained by intravenous self-administration of nicotine. *Science* 214, 573–575.

Hayford, K. E., C. A. Patten, T. A. Rummans, D. R. Schroeder, K. P. Offord, E. D. Glover, D. P. Sachs, and R. D. Hurt (1999). Efficacy of bupropion for smoking cessation in smokers with a former history of major depression or alcoholism. *Br. J. Psychiatry* 174, 173–178.

Koob, G. F. and M. Le Moal (2005). Nicotine. In *The Neurobiology of Addiction*. Elsevier, New York, pp. 243–287.

Liechti, M. E., L. Lhuillier, K. Kaupmann, and A. Markou (2007). Metabotropic glutamate 2/3 receptors in the ventral tegmental area and the nucleus accumbens shell are involved in behaviors relating to nicotine dependence. *J. Neurosci.* 27, 9077–9085.

O'Brien, C. P. (2004). Drug addiction and drug abuse. In *Goodman and Gilman's The Pharmacological Basis of Therapeutics* (L. L. Brunton, J. S. Lazo, and K. L. Parker, Eds.). McGraw-Hill, New York, 11th ed., pp. 607–627.

Tiffany, S., C. A. Conklin, S. Shiffman, and R. R. Clayton (2004). What can dependence theories tell us about assessing the emergence of tobacco dependence? *Addiction* 99(Suppl. 1), 78–86.

Uhl, G. R., T. Drgon, C. Johnson, O. O. Fatusin, Q.-R. Liu, C. Contoreggi, C.-Y. Li, K. Buck, and J. Crabbe (2008). "Higher order" addiction molecular genetics: Convergent data from genome-wide association in humans and mice. *Biochem. Pharmacol.* 75, 98–111.

World Health Organization (2008). *WHO Report on the Global Tobacco Epidemic, 2008— The MPOWER package.* World Health Organization, Geneva. (Available online at www. who.int/tobacco/mpower/en)

Wynder, E. L. (1997). Tobacco as a cause of lung cancer: Some reflections. *Am. J. Epide-miol.* 146, 687–694.

Index

Note: Page numbers followed by *f* indicate a figure; by *t* a table.